Biomaterials: Interfacial Phenomena and Applications

Biomaterials: Interfacial Phenomena and Applications

Stuart L. Cooper, EDITOR
University of Wisconsin

Nicholas A. Peppas, EDITOR
Purdue University

Allan S. Hoffman, ASSOCIATE EDITOR
University of Washington

Buddy D. Ratner, ASSOCIATE EDITOR
University of Washington

Based on a symposium sponsored by the Materials Engineering and Sciences Division and the Committee on Fundamentals of Life Sciences of the American Institute of Chemical Engineers at Their 73rd Annual Meeting in Chicago, Illinois, November 1980.

ADVANCES IN CHEMISTRY SERIES **199**

AMERICAN CHEMICAL SOCIETY
WASHINGTON, D. C. 1982

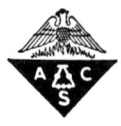

Library of Congress Cataloging in Publication Data
American Institute of Chemical Engineers. Meeting
  (73rd: 1980: Chicago, Ill.)
Biomaterials, interfacial phenomena and applications.
  (Advances in chemistry, ISSN 0065-2393; 199)

  "Based on a symposium sponsored by the Materials Engineering and Sciences Division and the Committee on Fundamentals of Life Sciences of the American Institute of Chemical Engineers at their 73rd Annual Meeting in Chicago, Illinois, November 1980."
  Includes bibliographies and index.

  1. Biomedical materials—Congresses. 2. Biomedical materials—Physiological effect—Congresses.
  I. Cooper, Stuart L., 1941-   . II. Peppas, Nicholas A., 1948-   . III. American Institute of Chemical Engineers. Materials Engineering and Sciences Division. IV. American Institute of Chemical Engineers. Committee on Fundamentals of Life Sciences. V. Title. VI. Series: Advances in chemistry series; 199. [DNLM: 1. Biocompatible materials—Congresses. 2. Blood—Congresses. 3. Proteins—Congresses. 4. Surface properties—Congresses. QT 34 B61155 1980]

QD1.A355 no. 199   [R857.M3]   540s   [610'.28]
                                          82-6763
ISBN 0-8412-0631-7 AACR2 ADCSAJ 199 1-540
                                          1982

Copyright © 1982

American Chemical Society

All Rights Reserved. The appearance of the code at the bottom of the first page of each article in this volume indicates the copyright owner's consent that reprographic copies of the article may be made for personal or internal use or for the personal or internal use of specific clients. This consent is given on the condition, however, that the copier pay the stated per copy fee through the Copyright Clearance Center, Inc. for copying beyond that permitted by Sections 107 or 108 of the U.S. Copyright Law. This consent does not extend to copying or transmission by any means—graphic or electronic—for any other purpose, such as for general distribution, for advertising or promotional purposes, for creating new collective work, for resale, or for information storage and retrieval systems.

The citation of trade names and/or names of manufacturers in this publication is not to be construed as an endorsement or as approval by ACS of the commercial products or services referenced herein; nor should the mere reference herein to any drawing, specification, chemical process, or other data be regarded as a license or as a conveyance of any right or permission, to the holder, reader, or any other person or corporation, to manufacture, reproduce, use, or sell any patented invention or copyrighted work that may in any way be related thereto.

PRINTED IN THE UNITED STATES OF AMERICA

Advances in Chemistry Series

M. Joan Comstock, *Series Editor*

Advisory Board

David L. Allara

Robert Baker

Donald D. Dollberg

Robert E. Feeney

Brian M. Harney

W. Jeffrey Howe

James D. Idol, Jr.

Herbert D. Kaesz

Marvin Margoshes

Robert Ory

Leon Petrakis

Theodore Provder

Charles N. Satterfield

Dennis Schuetzle

Davis L. Temple, Jr.

Gunter Zweig

FOREWORD

ADVANCES IN CHEMISTRY SERIES was founded in 1949 by the American Chemical Society as an outlet for symposia and collections of data in special areas of topical interest that could not be accommodated in the Society's journals. It provides a medium for symposia that would otherwise be fragmented, their papers distributed among several journals or not published at all. Papers are reviewed critically according to ACS editorial standards and receive the careful attention and processing characteristic of ACS publications. Volumes in the ADVANCES IN CHEMISTRY SERIES maintain the integrity of the symposia on which they are based; however, verbatim reproductions of previously published papers are not accepted. Papers may include reports of research as well as reviews since symposia may embrace both types of presentation.

ABOUT THE EDITORS

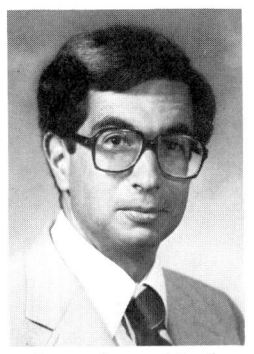

STUART L. COOPER received his B.S. at Massachusetts Institute of Technology and his Ph.D. in chemical engineering at Princeton University. While at Princeton, his research was directed by Arthur V. Tobolsky in the area of polymer physical chemistry. He is currently professor of chemical engineering at the University of Wisconsin where, since 1967, he has been active in polymer research. He has published more than 80 papers on topics covering polyurethane block polymers, inomers, polymer yield mechanisms, composites, and fiber physics. His current research includes studies of protein and thrombus deposition on polymers used in biomedical applications. Professor Cooper is a Fellow of the American Physical Society and has served on the Board of Trustees of Argonne Universities Association.

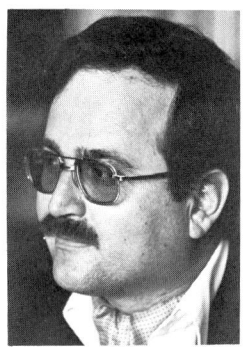

NICHOLAS A. PEPPAS, a native of Greece, studied chemical engineering at N.T.U., Athens (Dipl. Eng., 1971) and at Massachusetts Institute of Technology, from which he received his Sc.D. in 1973. He joined Purdue University in 1976 where he is currently Professor of Chemical Engineering. He is a member of the editorial boards of *Biomaterials* and the *Journal of Applied Polymer Science*. He has co-authored more than 90 publications in his areas of research interest, which include diffusion in polymers, polymer network structures, membrane science, and biointerfacial phenomena. In 1982–83 he will be Zyma Foundation Visiting Professor at the University of Geneva, Switzerland.

CONTENTS

Preface xiii

BLOOD–MATERIALS INTERACTIONS

1. Blood–Biomaterial Interactions: An Overview 3
   A. S. Hoffman

2. Surface Characterization of Materials for Blood Contact Applications .. 9
   B. D. Ratner

3. A New Model for In Vivo Platelet and Thrombus Kinetics 25
   R. Rodvien, J. Robinson, R. R. Mitchell, P. Litwak, and D. C. Price

4. Platelet Retention on Polymer Surfaces: Some In Vitro Experiments ... 35
   E. W. Merrill, E. W. Salzman, V. Sa Da Costa, D. Brier–Russell, A. Dincer, P. Pape, and J. N. Lindon

5. Thrombus Formation on Surfaces in Contact with Blood 43
   J. S. Schultz, S. M. Lindenauer, and J. A. Penner

6. Thrombotic Events on Grafted Polyacrylamide–Silastic Surfaces as Studied in a Baboon 59
   A. S. Hoffman, T. A. Horbett, B. D. Ratner, S. R. Hanson, L. A. Harker, and L. O. Reynolds

7. Plasma Interaction on Block Copolymers as Determined by Platelet Adhesion 81
   M. N. Helmus, O. P. Malhotra, and D. F. Gibbons

8. A Critical Study of Segmented Polyurethanes 95
   E. W. Merrill, V. Sa Da Costa, E. W. Salzman, D. Brier–Russell, L. Kuchner, D. F. Waugh, G. Trudel, III, S. Stopper, and V. Vitale

9. The Effect of Polyether Segment Molecular Weight on the Bulk and Surface Morphologies of Copolyether-Urethane–Ureas 109
   K. Knutson and D. J. Lyman

10. Hydrogel Formation from Copolyether-Urethane–Ureas Salt Complex: Morphology Effects of Lithium Bromide 133
    R. Benson, S. Yoshikawa, K. Knutson, and D. J. Lyman

11. The Fate of Surface Bound Heparin 147
    M. F. A. Goosen and M. V. Sefton

12. The Anticoagulant Activity of Derivatized and Immobilized Heparins .. 161
    C. D. Ebert, E. S. Lee, J. Deneris, and S. W. Kim

13. Hemocompatibility Effect of Molecular Motions of the Polymer Interface 177
    W. M. Reichert, F. E. Filisko, and S. A. Barenberg

14. Thrombogenesis: An Ionic Steric Phenomenon 195
   S. A. Barenberg and K. A. Mauritz

15. Alteration of Polymorphonuclear Neutrophil Leukocyte Response to Shear Stress Exposure In Vitro: Effects of Prostaglandin E_1 and Dipyridamole Derivative RA-233.................................. 209
   D. J. Stockwell, L. V. McIntire, and R. R. Martin

16. A Method to "Count" Flow-Resistant Blood Microemboli 221
   K. A. Solen and B. L. Betteridge

PROTEIN ADSORPTION ON BIOMATERIALS

17. Protein Adsorption on Biomaterials............................... 233
   T. A. Horbett

18. Protein Structure and the Kinetics of Interaction with Surfaces 245
   A. G. Walton and B. Koltisko

19. Proteins, Plasma, and Blood in Narrow Spaces of Clot-Promoting Surfaces 265
   L. Vroman, A. L. Adams, G. C. Fischer, P. C. Munoz, and M. Stanford

20. Influence of Red Blood Cells and Their Components on Protein Adsorption 277
   S. Uniyal, J. L. Brash, and I. A. Degterev

21. Protein Adsorption on Polymers: Visualization, Study of Fluid Shear and Roughness Effects, and Methods to Enhance Albumin Binding.... 293
   R. C. Eberhart, M. E. Lynch, F. H. Bilge, J. F. Wissinger, M. S. Munro, S. R. Ellsworth, and A. J. Quattrone

22. Plasma Proteins: Their Role in Initiating Platelet and Fibrin Deposition on Biomaterials....................................... 317
   B. R. Young, L. K. Lambrecht, S. L. Cooper, and D. F. Mosher

23. Probing Protein Adsorption: Total Internal Reflection Intrinsic Fluorescence 351
   R. A. Van Wagenen, S. Rockhold, and J. D. Andrade

24. Fourier Transform Infrared Spectroscopy for Protein–Surface Studies... 371
   R. M. Gendreau, R. I. Leininger, S. Winters, and R. J. Jakobsen

25. Analytical Methods for the Determination of Biologically Derived Absorbed Species in Biomedical Elastomers 395
   D. R. Owen, R. Zone, T. Armer, and C. Kilpatrick

26. Effect of Electrical Signals on the Adsorption of Plasma Proteins to a High Copper Alloy... 413
   H. J. Mueller

27. Adsorption of Proteins from Artificial Tear Solutions to Poly(methyl methacrylate–2-hydroxyethyl methacrylate) Copolymers............... 453
   F. H. Royce, Jr., B. D. Ratner, and T. A. Horbett

28. Structure, Testing, and Applications of Biomaterials 465
    N. A. Peppas

29. Design Principles and Preliminary Clinical Performance of an
    Artificial Skin.. 475
    I. V. Yannas, J. F. Burke, M. Warpehoski, P. Stasikelis,
    E. M. Skrabut, D. P. Orgill, and D. Giard

30. Collagenase Immobilized on Cellulose Acetate Membranes 483
    Y. Chen, N. S. Mason, R. E. Sparks, D. W. Scharp, and
    W. F. Ballinger

31. A System for Heparin Removal 493
    R. Langer, R. J. Linhardt, P. M. Galliher, M. M. Flanagan,
    C. L. Cooney, and M. D. Klein

32. Implantable Micropump for Insulin Delivery: Effect of a
    Rate-Controlling Membrane....................................... 511
    M. V. Sefton

Index... 523

PREFACE

The field of biomaterials presents unique and challenging problems to investigators. Because the field is interdisciplinary, researchers with diverse backgrounds must be brought together. This has been done to the extent that one can now identify many clinical applications of biomaterials and a growing high technology biomaterials industry. The success of new biomaterials systems is highly dependent on the correct selection, design, and fabrication of the biomaterials components. However, the fundamental principles that govern the biocompatibility of devices have not been fully developed. This situation is particularly true for those systems designed to contact blood. In order to understand blood-material interactions, it was thus desirable to focus attention on the biomaterials interface, and review advances in this area in a special symposium.

Because a significant portion of the fundamental biomaterials research in the United States is occurring in chemical engineering departments, it was timely that the topic of biomaterials was selected as the subject of a 3-day symposium at the 73rd annual meeting of the American Institute of Chemical Engineers (AIChE) in November 1980. Participating in this symposium were researchers in engineering, medicine, pharmacy, and chemistry. Thus a wide spectrum of research and viewpoints was presented at this meeting.

This volume contains manuscripts based on 28 of the 32 contributions presented at the Chicago AIChE Biomaterials Symposium. These manuscripts are organized into three major sections: Blood–Materials Interactions, Protein Adsorption on Biomaterials, and New Biomaterials Systems and Applications. Introductory chapters are placed at the beginning of each section of the book to provide nonspecialists with background material and a perspective into these evolving research areas.

The blood-materials interactions section contains a review article dealing with surface characterization. Consideration of the surface structure of biomaterials is critical to every study in this volume. This section contains 16 chapters dealing with the choice of in vivo and in vitro methods of biomaterials evaluation, biomaterials selection and modification, and cellular interactions with candidate surfaces. Individual papers dealing with the use of dogs, baboons, and goats for in vivo blood-materials evaluation can be found together with in vitro methods. There are also several contributions on polyurethanes, which are prime candidates for use in blood contacting devices.

The second section on protein adsorption is introduced by a review on protein adsorption. The 11 chapters under this heading are an excellent collection of current research in this area. Chapters on protein conformation, cellular interactions, and the interaction of some less common but very important proteins with surfaces can be found. In addition, several chapters on the latest spectroscopic methods for studying protein adsorption and conformation are included.

The section on new biomaterials systems and applications includes a discussion of material advances in new applications such as wound closure and drug delivery systems.

We have thus attempted through the symposium and this volume to bring together current research and ideas in the design and interactions of biomaterials. This volume will benefit nonspecialists with an interest in this area and will provide an extensive source of information for specialists in the field.

The editors wish to thank the individual contributors and reviewers for their cooperation. We wish also to acknowledge the superb editorial assistance provided by the American Chemical Society Books Department.

STUART L. COOPER
University of Wisconsin
Madison, Wisconsin

NICHOLAS A. PEPPAS
Purdue University
West Lafayette, Indiana

November 1981

BLOOD–MATERIALS INTERACTIONS

Blood–Biomaterial Interactions: An Overview

ALLAN S. HOFFMAN

University of Washington, Center for Bioengineering and Department of Chemical Engineering, Seattle, WA 98195

A wide number and great variety of clinically important cardiovascular implants and devises exist. Some (e.g., catheters) may only contact the blood once, and for a relatively short time; others (e.g., kidney dialyzers and blood oxygenators) may be exposed to blood for hours, while tissue implants (e.g., heart valves and vascular grafts) will hopefully last for years, or the lifetime of the patient. All of these implants and devices contain materials that are recognized by blood as foreign; the result is a process of thrombosis often followed by formation of thromboemboli. This process generally involves a sequence of protein adsorption steps followed by blood cell interactions (especially involving platelets).

Three possible routes to the formation of blood thrombi may be delineated: (1) the "intrinsic" blood coagulation system involving a series or "cascade" of enzymatic activation steps presumed to begin with the surface activation of a glycoprotein, Factor XII (Hageman Factor), and ending with the formation of fibrin on this surface; (2) the "extrinsic" blood coagulation system, initiated by the release of a tissue factor (thromboplastin) that can trigger a cascade of enzyme reactions (in a sequence similar to part of the intrinsic system), again leading to fibrin deposition; and (3) the adhesion and aggregation of platelets at the foreign interface, leading to the formation of a platelet thrombus on that surface.

High shear rate (arterial) flow conditions promote thrombi composed largely of platelets; such deposits are called "white thrombi." Low shear rate (venous) flow conditions promote thrombi composed of red cells and platelets entrapped in a fibrin mesh, referred to as "red thrombi." Sometimes, a smooth layer of fibrin also may be deposited. Embolization of the white or red thrombi may produce ischemia and infarction in distal circulatory beds.

The causative mechanisms and prevention of thrombosis and embolization at foreign surfaces continue to be elusive goals of a significant number of researchers worldwide. Most researchers in this field will agree that there are three key system components that can interact in varying ways and to varying degrees, leading to the process of thrombosis and embolization at foreign interfaces. They are (1) the biomaterial, (2) the nature of the blood flow (or hemodynamics), and (3) the biological environment. These factors are detailed in Table I.

Table I. Factors Influencing Blood Interactions at Foreign Interfaces

The Biomaterial
- Surface composition
  - —(polar vs. apolar groups)
  - —(acidic vs. basic groups)
  - —(H-bonding groups)
  - —(immobilized biomolecules, drugs)
  - —(double layer effects)
  - —(γ_c; $\gamma^d + \gamma^p + \gamma^H$)
  - —(presence of impurities, particles)
- Water sorption
  - —(surface water structure)
- Surface crystalline/amorphous structure
- Surface smoothness, roughness, and porosity
- Mechanical compliance of surface, bulk
- Regular or irregular distribution of surface "domains" of the above
- Bulk leachables (including biomolecules, drugs), degradation products

Blood Flow Effects (Hemodynamics)
- Shear rate
- Pulsed or irregular flow
- Flow separation, turbulence, and stasis
- Augmented diffusion of blood components
- Biomaterial wall motion

The Biologic Environment
- In vitro vs. ex vivo vs. in vivo
- Species and history
- Whole blood, plasma, serum, proteins, and cells
- Anticoagulants, drugs
- Radiolabeled species (^{3}H, ^{14}C, ^{51}Cr, ^{111}In, ^{125}I, etc.) and techniques
- Air interface, dissolved gas

Various researchers, at various times, have described the mechanism of blood coagulation at foreign interfaces in terms of each of the material factors listed under the first heading in Table I. Others have claimed that hemodynamic factors may dominate over any one or all of the material factors. In addition to these contrasting viewpoints, a relative few have attempted to compare different animal species, with material and flow conditions presumably remaining the same. These studies continue to indicate that each of the biological environment factors can have a significant influence on (if not effect entirely) any conclusions reached from studies testing hypotheses based on biomaterial or hemodynamic factors. In fact, there may be a number of valid but distinctly different mechanisms leading to thrombosis and embolization on foreign surfaces, depending on the material and system involved. (One case in point is the contrast between in vivo canine vena cava ring tests and ex vivo baboon shunt tests for Silastic or acrylamide-grafted Silastic materials. The Silastic rings are plugged rapidly with deposited thrombus, while Silastic shunts exhibit very low platelet consumption in the baboon; the opposite is true for the acrylamide-grafted Silastic—*see* Chapter 6 in this book.)

A number of general hypotheses have emerged from the many studies over the past twenty years. Some of these have actually become a part of the generally accepted "conventional wisdom" in this complex field. Table II lists some of the more common ones that have been proposed. Hopefully this volume will help clarify or modify, and maybe even shorten this list.

Table II. Blood–Foreign Material Interactions: Some "Conventional Wisdom" and Some Unresolved Hypotheses

General
- The overall processes of in vivo thrombogenesis, thromboembolization, and subsequent endothelialization on a foreign surface are dominated by surface properties rather than by hemodynamics (or by hemodynamics rather than by surface properties).
- No foreign material can ever be truly "blood compatible." (Corollary: Drugs will always be needed.)

Materials
- A material with a critical surface tension around 25 dyn/cm will have a low thrombogenic potential.
- A small negative surface charge lowers material thrombogenicity.
- High water content materials have a low thrombogenic potential due to the lowered free energy of the hydrated interface.
- High water content materials may continually expose a fresh, foreign interface, leading to a high thrombogenic potential; however, they also tend to exhibit low thromboadherence due to their low interfacial free energy.
- H-bonding groups in a surface lead to strong interactions with biological species and therefore endow a surface with a high thrombogenic potential.
- A surface with a high apolar/polar ratio is desirable for low thrombogenic potential.
- Thrombus is nucleated in regions of the surface where a specific spatial distribution of specific chemical (electrostatic) groups is present.
- Flexible (as opposed to stiff) polymer chain ends and loops in the material interface lower the thrombogenic potential of the foreign surface.

Materials and Hemodynamics
- Thrombi will always be generated at surface imperfections due to flow disturbances, surface compositional differences, and/or trapped gas bubbles.
- Smooth surfaces in arterial flow conditions may release thromboemboli before they grow too large to be dangerous. (Corollary: High shear rates can detach thromboemboli before they have grown too large.)
- Certain rough or textured surfaces may form and retain fibrin thrombus, leading to a "passivated" surface.

Table II *(continued)*

Hemodynamics
- Thrombi will always be generated in regions of low flow or flow separation.
- Low shear rates can lead to regional accumulation of activated protein coagulation factors and subsequent thrombogenesis on a nearby surface.
- High shear rates can be destructive to blood cells (e.g., shear rates can initiate platelet activation and lead to thrombogenesis).
- In a tubular flow field, the platelets tend to accumulate preferentially near the wall and the red cells near the central core. (Corollary: The red cells enhance the rate of collision of platelets with the wall.)

Protein Adsorption
- Protein adsorption comprises the initial interaction of a foreign material with blood.
- The composition and organization of the initial protein layer is determined by the surface properties of the material.
- The composition and organization of the initial protein layer mediates subsequent platelet interactions in vivo, and may also determine long-term effects.
- In vitro protein adsorption studies are relevant to in vivo behavior in humans.
- The heat evolved on adsorption of proteins can lead to their denaturation on the surface; the magnitude of the heat evolved may be determined by the surface composition.
- Hydrophobic surfaces will tend to adsorb proteins more "strongly" than hydrophilic surfaces, leading to greater denaturation of proteins on the hydrophobic surfaces.
- Fibrinogen dominates the initial protein layer on most foreign materials, and fibrinogen adsorption leads to high thrombogenic potential for that surface.
- A layer of adsorbed albumin reduces in vitro platelet adhesion; materials that preferentially adsorb albumin will be antithrombogenic in vivo.
- Certain other specific proteins may also adsorb and have a significant influence on subsequent events (e.g., CIG, or fibronectin, VWF, complement factors, high molecular weight kininogen, lipoproteins, etc.).
- The various carbohydrate components of adsorbed glycoproteins may play an important role in the recognition of the biomaterial as foreign and in the subsequent events leading to thrombus deposition.

Platelets
- Platelet adhesion on a foreign surface is a necessary precursor to platelet aggregation on that surface.
- High platelet adhesion on a foreign surface is bad.
- In vitro platelet adhesion is related directly to in vivo thrombus formation and embolization on foreign surfaces.
- Platelets adhere with different strengths on different sites.

Table II *(continued)*

- Platelet adhesion and release reactions at foreign interfaces occur when specific platelet membrane receptor sites "recognize" specific groups on the foreign surface. (Corollary: Platelet adhesion is not a random process.)
- Some platelet release factors (e.g., serotonin and ADP from dense granules) enhance platelet aggregation on foreign surfaces, while the roles of others (platelet factor 4 with its heparin neutralizing activity (HNA) and β thromboglobulin from α granules) remain to be clarified.

Erythrocytes and Leukocytes
- The role of leukocytes in thrombogenesis may be related to their ability to recognize a particular biomaterial surface as "foreign" after certain proteins and/or platelets have adhered to that surface.
- Red blood cells may play only a minor role in the thrombogenic process.

Heparinized Surfaces and Drugs
- Heparinized surfaces must leach heparin to be nonthrombogenic. (General corollary: "Immobilized" antithrombogenic drugs are ineffective unless they leach into the flowing blood.)
- Heparinized surfaces that bind antithrombin III do not need to leach heparin to be nonthrombogenic.
- There may be a synergistic interaction between specific drug therapies and specific biomaterials such that reduced drug regimens may be indicated in combination with the use of specific biomaterials in devices or implants.
- The natural endothelium is nonthrombogenic because endothelial cells produce the powerful antiplatelet aggregation agent prostacyclin (PGI_2).

Calcification
- Calcification may be initiated at points of high mechanical strain in a foreign material (such as a blood pump diaphragm).
- Calcification in foreign materials is a biological process; γ-carboxy glutamic acid is a necessary amino acid in one key protein involved in this process.

Species Differences
- The dog model is relatively inexpensive and convenient, but may lack relevance to humans.
- The baboon model is relatively expensive and unavailable, but is relevant to humans.
- Similarity of platelet function, the concentration and activity of clotting factors, and the hematocrit should be the primary determinants for deciding which species are most relevant to humans.

Note: Part or all of any of these statements may be accepted or disputed.

Acknowledgment

The author would like to thank Steven R. Hanson for his helpful comments on the manuscript.

Literature Cited

1. Vroman, L.; Leonard, E. F. Eds.; *Ann. N. Y. Acad. Sci.* **1977** *283*.
2. "Proceedings of the Devices and Technology Branch, Contractor's Meeting 1979," U. S. Department of Health and Human Services, N.H.L.B.I., N.I.H., **1980**, No. 81-2022/November.
3. "Guidelines for Blood-Material Interactions," U.S. Department of Health and Human Services, Devices and Technology Branch, N.H.L.B.I., N.I.H., **1980**, No. 80-2185/September.
4. "Guidelines for Physicochemical Characterization of Biomaterials," U.S. Department of Health and Human Services, Devices and Technology Branch, N.H.L.B.I., N.I.H., **1980**, No. 80-2186/September.

RECEIVED for review April 4, 1981. ACCEPTED May 4, 1981.

2
Surface Characterization of Materials for Blood Contact Applications

BUDDY D. RATNER

University of Washington, Department of Chemical Engineering, Seattle, WA 98195

In recent years the surface characterization of biomaterials has been forcefully emphasized (1–3). Unfortunately, a clear understanding of how surface characterization can be of value to biomaterials research, development, and production has, in many cases, not been realized. This chapter addresses the subject of surface characterization of biomaterials by considering three aspects of the problem: first how surfaces differ from the bulk of materials; second, how the important parameters of surfaces can be measured and what new techniques might be developed; and finally, how surface characterization can help in understanding and predicting the biocompatibility (and in particular, the blood compatibility) of synthetic materials.

Unique Properties of Surfaces

The surfaces of materials are almost always different in structure and chemistry from the bulk or interior of the materials. These differences result from surface contamination (a consequence of surface chemistry), molecular orientation, and surface reaction. The driving force for this surface/bulk differentiation can be explained (at least for the first two factors) by considering surface energetics from a thermodynamic standpoint—the interfacial energy of any system tends to be reduced. Examples will be presented to show how each of these three factors can alter the nature of a surface.

Surface contamination is ubiquitous and almost unavoidable. Even in ultrahigh vacuum environments, the question is not if a surface will become contaminated, but when. For high-energy surfaces, such as metals and inorganics, the driving force for reducing the interfacial energy is extremely high. A "clean" metal surface will recontaminate with a monolayer of organic material in a vacuum environment at 10^{-6} Torr in approximately 1 s. Contamination at the monolayer or multilayer level will occur essentially instantaneously in a laboratory environment at atmospheric pressure.

Surface contamination can take a number of forms. We are surrounded by a complex mixture of hydrocarbon molecules as a consequence of both our industrial and natural environments. Low surface energy silicones (e.g., vacuum greases and pump oils) are commonly present in the laboratory environment. Silicone contamination is particularly troublesome and is found on many surfaces because few materials have surface energies lower than silicone compounds.

Polymers have significantly lower surface free energies than metals or inorganics. Therefore, the driving force to reduce interfacial energy is lower and, consequently, contamination in a laboratory environment is slower. However, such contamination still exists for most systems. For materials such as Teflon, the surface free energy is very low. A substance with a surface energy lower than that of Teflon would have to adsorb to the surface to reduce the interfacial energy. Since few such substances are present in the atmosphere, contamination for such fluoropolymers can be negligible.

Two important points might be made about environmentally propagated surface contamination which we must, in most cases, live with. First, some level of contamination is unavoidable, but contamination beyond this background level is unnecessary. For example, in a study of the effectiveness of various techniques for cleaning glass, relatively stable glass surfaces could be prepared in an ordinary laboratory environment with surface carbon/silicon ratios ranging from 0.19 to 2.2 (4). Glass with a carbon/silicon ratio of 2 would be unnecessarily contaminated while glass with a carbon/silicon ratio of 0.2 would be as clean as can be readily achieved under reasonable working conditions. Obviously, the lower the ratio, the more desirable the glass surface for studying biological interactions with glass. The biomaterials scientist is responsible for reducing contamination to the lowest possible levels and for insuring that all specimens in an experiment (and in later experiments) have reproducible (low) levels of contamination. Second, even though glass, platinum, and poly(ethylene terephthalate) might all be contaminated with an apparently similar layer of hydrocarbon-like material from the atmosphere, the essential properties indicative of these three substances still manifest themselves at their surfaces. Thus "clean" glass which has at least one monolayer of organic carbon compounds at its surface is "glass-like" and not "hydrocarbon-like" (e.g., "polyethylene-like") in its interactions with proteins and cells (4). The mechanisms by which the properties of a specific substance are propagated to the surface through contaminant films are not completely clear. Still, the intrinsic properties are visible at the surface and can, for moderately clean materials, be exploited to study or influence biological systems.

Molecular orientation at the surface of biomaterials has received increased attention in recent years. Again, as for surface contamination, the driving force for the surface reorientation observed often can be explained in thermodynamic terms as a mechanism for reducing the interfacial energy.

For polymeric systems, chain segments or pendant functional groups migrate to or from the surface in many instances. Thus, for block copolymers containing siloxane chain segments, the tendency is for these low-energy blocks to migrate to the surface (5). For other block copolymer systems in which the surface energies of the two blocks differ by smaller amounts, preferred surface localization of the lower surface energy block can be influenced by the casting solvent used or by the nature of the substrate against which they are cast (6, 7). For some polymeric systems in which a degree of chain flexibility exists, rapid chain configurational alterations might occur as polar side groups or the nonpolar chain backbones respond to the nature of the environment. For example, for poly(hydroxyethyl methacrylate), hydroxyl groups are apparently exposed at the surface in an aqueous medium (liquid–solid interface) while the chain backbone orients itself towards the surface in the dehydrated (gas–solid interface) situation *(8–10)*.

Other levels of induced molecular surface organization for polymeric systems have been observed. For example, casting a polymer system onto a given surface permits that surface to act as a molecular template which can orient the polymer chains (7, 11). Such "template-induced" surface structures may relax slowly when the template is removed. The casting solvent may significantly affect the outermost surface of even simple polar polymers such as poly(methyl methacrylate) (PMMA), as experiments that utilized inverse gas chromatography suggest (12). In these studies, PMMA cast from five solvents onto gas chromatographic supports shows vastly different specific retention volumes. Finally, anisotropies in the molecular chain orientation may be induced by casting (13).

These and other related observations lead to a number of conclusions and considerations concerning polymer chain surface orientation. First, the nature of the surface differs, in most cases, from that of the bulk. Second, the surface can change in response to the environment such that a probe of surface structure (e.g., a drop of liquid used for measuring contact angles) may alter that which it was intended to measure. Third (and related to the second item), the environment in which a biomaterial is studied may direct the surface structure—an appropriate environment for biomaterials study is an aqueous medium. Fourth, surface structures may relax (and change) in response to the environment; depending on the kinetics of this process, irreproducible surface measurements could occur. Finally, the level of surface characterization (depth of penetration) suitable for biomaterial characterization must be considered. Examples given in this section have described surface/bulk differentiations ranging from microns to angstroms. Considering the ability of bulk material properties to propagate themselves through thin surface layers, to what depth must we analyze a surface? This question may be answerable when we learn more about the sensitivity of proteins and cells to small chemical perturbations.

Surface chemical reactions are also important considerations in trying to understand how the surface of materials differs from the bulk. Certainly the most common surface reaction is oxidation. An oxidized layer exists at the surface of many polymers and metals. Polyethylene, which might be viewed as the simplest polymer from a chemical standpoint, has a rather complex surface structure due to such oxidation. The carbon/oxygen ratios at the surfaces of a number of nominally pure polyethylene specimens stored in air range from 300 to 9 (*14*). These surfaces contain several different types of carbon–oxygen bonds. The simple $(CH_2-CH_2)_n$ structure that is often assigned to polyethylene seems meaningless, considering the variety of rather polar structures with which cells and proteins might interact at the polyethylene surface. Similar surface complexity as a result of oxidation will be expected for many other polymers. This oxidation has been explored in a systematic way on only a few systems.

Other surface reactions also can be anticipated. Surface acidic or basic structures can exist in an ionized and/or neutral form. The ratio of the ionized to neutral form will depend strongly on a material's environment and previous history. Also, any compound with ionic charges can complex or couple with many ions and some neutral molecules; even neutral polymers can have strong, rather specific interactions with ions (*15*). Finally, molecules such as SO_2 and NH_3 commonly are found in the urban and/or laboratory environment. Such reactive molecules can, again, completely alter the nature of a surface. Of course, some reactions are purposely performed on surfaces to alter their properties. A large number of grafting and chemical reactions come under this category. Such reactions are described elsewhere (*3*).

Three major mechanisms were described in this section by which surfaces alter their chemical properties compared to the bulk: contamination, molecular orientation, and reaction. Since, a priori, the nature of a surface cannot be predicted because of these factors, tools are needed to study surfaces. Such techniques for analyzing surface structure are discussed in the next section.

Techniques for Surface Characterization

The development of new methods for studying surfaces is progressing rapidly, precipitated by the phenomenal growth and interest in surface physics and chemistry which was stimulated, in part, by the need for clean, well-characterized surfaces for microelectronic and other high-technology applications. The biomaterials field should be able to capitalize upon this plethora of new methods which have appeared primarily in the past 15 years. In particular, many of the new techniques measure surface chemistry directly, in contrast to older methods which often required indirect or thermodynamic data. At the present stage of development in the field of surface analysis, a "picture" of a surface must be built up by using a variety of methods. Combinations of the "classic" surface analysis methods (e.g., contact angle determination) and the newer methods have the potential to describe the nature of a surface adequately for biomaterials investigation (1, 16).

Surface analysis techniques are categorized in Table I. Figure 1, often called a Propst diagram, illustrates the "probes" and emitted species that can be measured in many of the new techniques for surface analysis. More than 40 of the possible combinations have been explored; many others have not yet been tried. Figure 2 presents an approximate comparison of the various techniques with respect to their depth of analysis. Only the techniques that have shown success or show promise for use in biomaterials characterization will be considered in more detail in this review.

Table I. Surface Analysis Methods

- *Thermodynamic Analysis*
— Contact angle—surface energetics (17, 18)
— BET—surface area

- *Surface Electrical Properties (1)*
— Zeta potential (streaming potential)
— Faraday cup
— Surface potential difference
— Rest potential
— Vibrating electrode
— Cascade device for measuring triboelectric charging (19)

- *Surface Chemistry Analysis*
— ESCA (electron spectroscopy for chemical analysis)
— AES (Auger electron spectroscopy)
— SIMS (secondary ion mass spectroscopy)
— ISS (ion scattering spectroscopy)
— ELS (electron loss spectroscopy)
— ATR-IR (attenuated total reflectance infrared analysis)

- *Spatially (Laterally) Resolved Surface Chemistry Analysis*
— SAM (scanning Auger microprobe)
— SIMS (also called ion microprobe)
— EDXA (energy dispersive x-ray analysis)

- *Surface Topography*
— Light microscopy
— SEM (scanning electron microscope)
— Optical heterodyne profilometry (20)
— Profilometry (stylus technique)

- *Surface Crystallinity and Atomic Organization*
— LEED (low energy electron diffraction)
— SEXAFS (surface extended x-ray absorption fine structure)
— FEM (field ion microscopy)

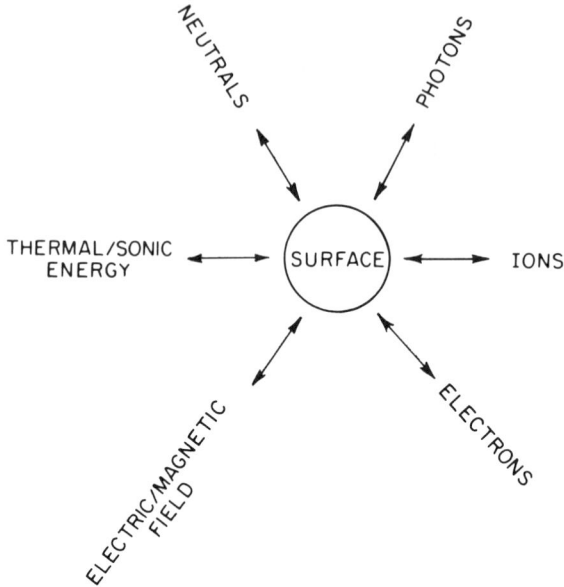

Figure 1. Propst diagram as a representation of the possible spectroscopies that might be used to study surfaces. Each spectroscopy is represented by an arrow in and an arrow out.

Electron Spectroscopy for Chemical Analysis (ESCA). ESCA is the most valuable technique presently available for the study of biomaterial surfaces, and particularly for materials intended for blood contact applications, for the following reasons:

1. The sampling depth for ESCA covers a relevant surface region for biomaterials (~ 10–100 Å depending on the mean free path of the emitted photoelectrons and the angle of the sample with respect to the analyzer).
2. Many levels of information can be obtained from a single ESCA experiment (*see* Table II).
3. Samples can be studied in a hydrated (frozen) condition (8).
4. Sample preparation is simple.
5. The technique, if used with some care, is nondestructive.
6. High sensitivity can be obtained.
7. The theoretical basis for ESCA, particularly as it applies to the use of ESCA as an analytical technique, is well established.
8. ESCA is the only technique that (to date) allows a direct correlation to be made between surface chemistry and in vivo blood interaction (21–23).

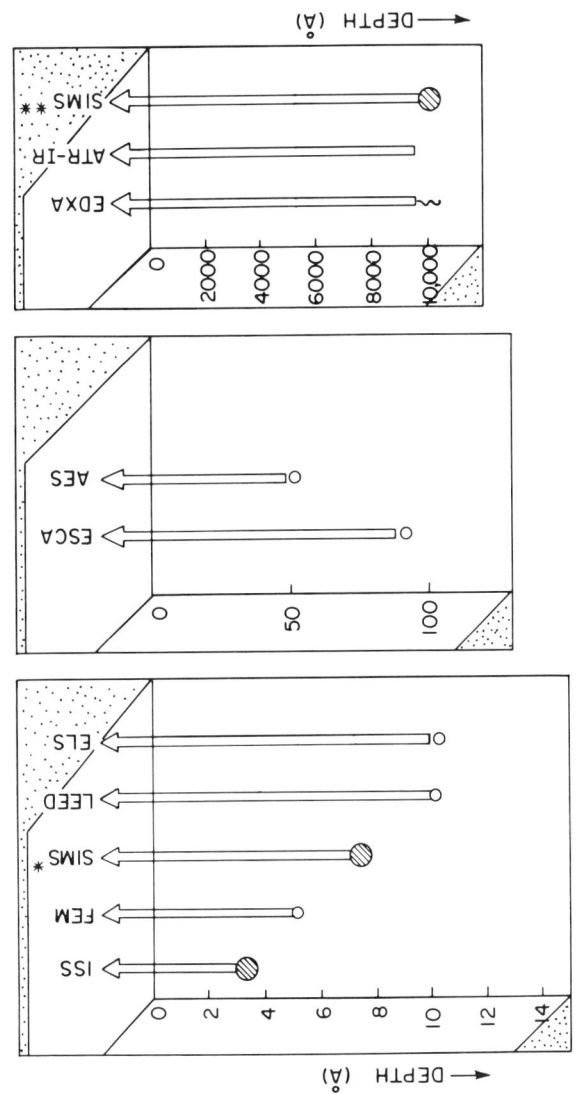

Figure 2. Comparison of some surface analytical methods with respect to depth of analysis. Key: *, static SIMS; **, dynamic SIMS (destructive); ●, ion; ○, electron; and ⚡, x-ray.

The ESCA experiment has its basis in the photoelectron effect—matter bombarded with x-rays (electromagnetic radiation) will emit photoelectrons with an energy:

$$E_{\text{photoelectron}} = h\nu - \text{binding energy} - \phi$$

where $h\nu$ is the energy of the bombarding x-ray, ϕ is a work function that is established for each spectrometer, and $E_{\text{photoelectron}}$ is the kinetic energy of the photoelectron which is measured by the ESCA instrument. Thus, the binding energy of the ejected electron can be determined. This binding energy is a sensitive function of the atomic environment, where the environment is defined by the nature of atom with which the ejected electron was associated and by the atoms bound to the atom that has suffered the photoemission. By measuring the intensity and energy distribution of the photoemission, the information listed in Table II can be obtained. A diagram illustrating the components of an ESCA spectrometer is presented in Figure 3. A number of good reviews describing the ESCA technique exist (24, 25). In addition, reviews directed particularly toward the unique aspects of ESCA for studying polymeric systems also have been written (26). The significance of ESCA for biomaterials investigations is discussed in the next section.

The ability to work with hydrated (frozen) samples is an important advantage of the ESCA technique for biological studies. The importance of experiments on hydrated biomaterials is supported by studies indicating that certain surfaces radically change their character (probably due to alterations in side group and backbone orientation) upon dehydration (8,–10). At liquid nitrogen temperatures all significant chain backbone and side group motion in polymers (and proteins) is inhibited. Therefore, by rapid freezing, a chain conformation similar to that at the liquid–solid interface should be frozen in place. Distortions in this hydrated interface configuration may, in fact, be

Table II. Information Derived from an ESCA Experiment

- All elements present (except hydrogen and helium)
- Approximate surface concentrations of elements ($\pm 10\%$)
- Bonding state (molecular environment) and/or oxidation level of most atoms
- Information on aromatic or unsaturated structures from shake-up ($\pi \rightarrow \pi^*$) transitions
- Information on surface electrical properties from charging studies
- Nondestructive depth profiling and surface heterogeneity assessment using (1) photoelectrons with differing escape depths and (2) angular-dependent ESCA studies
- Destructive depth profile using argon etching (for inorganics)
- Positive identification of functional groups using derivatization reactions
- "Fingerprinting" materials using valence band spectra

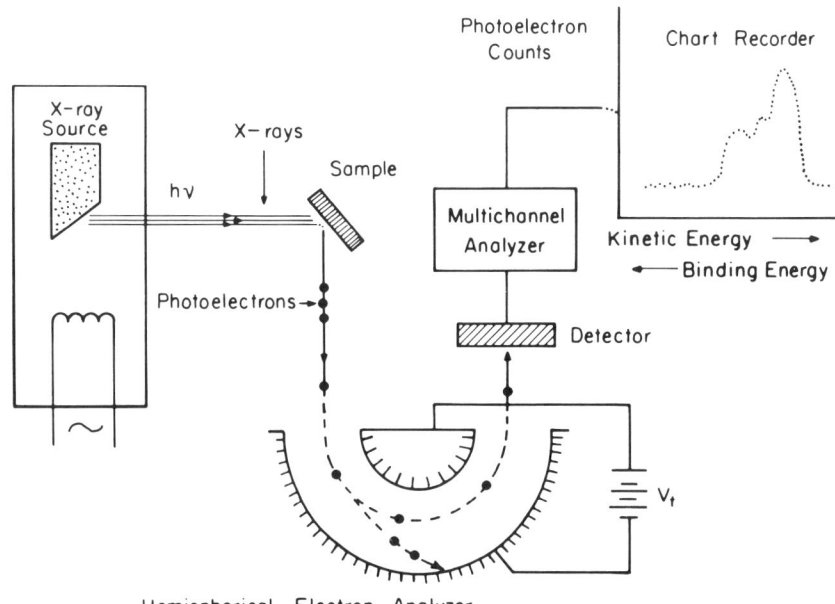

Figure 3. Representation of an ESCA instrument using a hemispherical electron analyzer ($E_{\text{photoelectron}} = h\nu -$ binding energy).

introduced by a restructuring of the water during freezing or by ice-crystal formation. However, if the freezing is rapid, such distortions would be expected to be minimal because the mobility of the side group and backbone segments of the polymer chains quickly goes to zero. Ideally, studies on frozen hydrated biomaterials should be performed in the following fashion (8). The sample is rapidly frozen in the ESCA instrument with a visible layer of water at its surface. At this stage, by ESCA, only oxygen can be observed. The temperature is then gradually raised (to $\sim -100°C$) until water begins to sublime from the sample. When the carbon signal from the polymer can be detected, the temperature is reduced again to $-160°C$. At this point a thin, frozen-water film (~ 50 Å) showing little tendency to sublime further should be covering the sample, and the desired interface (water/polymer) is exposed for analysis. By allowing the specimen to warm to room temperature in situ, molecular rearrangements at the interface due to dehydration can be studied.

Auger Electron Spectroscopy (AES). If a material is bombarded by electrons, an electron can be removed from a core level of an atom. A higher-energy electron can then drop down to fill the orbital vacancy. The energy reduction that occurs in this process can be balanced by the ejection of an electron. This ejected electron is referred to as an Auger electron and has an energy characteristic of the atom from which it emerged. By measuring the energy of and counting ejected Auger electrons, one can obtain a spectrum that characterizes the elemental composition of a surface. Because the impinging electron beam can be finely focused, high spatial resolution can be achieved permitting compositional analysis of small particles or inclusions on surfaces. In the high spatial resolution mode this technique is often referred to as scanning Auger microprobe (SAM). Many reviews of the AES and SAM techniques exist (27, 28).

AES and SAM studies probably are seen in the scientific literature more frequently than any other technique for applied surface analysis. However, SAM is, in almost all cases, so destructive to polymeric systems that meaningful analyses are particularly difficult to make. In addition, the information content is low compared to ESCA. With some exceptions, one can only determine which elements are present. SAM can be valuable for nonpolymeric biomaterials, and has been used successfully in many studies, particularly where its high spatial resolution could be exploited.

Secondary Ion Mass Spectrometry (SIMS). In the SIMS experiment a surface is bombarded by accelerated ions (frequently argon or neon). These ions, by transference of their energy to the surface atoms or molecules, can induce bond breakage and/or sputtering at the surface of a material. By detecting the number and mass of the surface-ejected (sputtered) ions, the nature of the surface species can be inferred (29, 30).

The SIMS technique has great potential for the analysis of polymeric biomaterials surfaces, but the complete interpretation of SIMS data for polymeric materials is not yet possible. Ideally, sputtered fragments of polymers that might correspond to expected higher stability ionic fragments from the polymer would occur. For example, from poly(ethyl methacrylate), the fragments $CH_3CH_2O^-$, $CH_3CH_2^+$, and CH_3^+ would all be expected. With increasing ester side chain lengths, increasing fragment size should be observed.

In actuality, the situation is more complex (31). The high-energy argon beam may be generating a plasma-like state at the surface of materials, leading to a process more akin to pyrolysis than fragmentation. Still, the SIMS spectra generated in polymer experiments could be used for fingerprinting many polymers (31). Recent experiments have suggested that the ability to detect expected fragments may indeed be developed by using appropriate ion bombardment conditions (32). If the fundamental aspects of polymer SIMS could be clarified, the result would be a desirable surface analytical method because of its high detection sensitivity, extreme surface orientation (surface sensitivity), high chemical information content, excellent spatial resolution (including imaging capabilities), and depth profiling capabilities.

A related technique, ion scattering spectroscopy (ISS), is frequently coupled with SIMS because both the excitation source and vacuum system are shared in common (33). Extreme surface sensitivity is the primary advantage of ISS for studies of interest to biomaterials scientists. The surface orientation of polar and nonpolar groups on a polymer chain may possibly be detected using ISS.

Attenuated Total Reflectance Infrared (ATR-IR) Spectroscopy. A vibrational spectrum of a surface can be obtained by placing it in intimate contact with an optical element of high refractive index through which internally reflected infrared radiation is traveling. The absorption of the infrared radiation by the material under study at reflectance points on the crystal surface can be measured and used to construct a spectrum that is rich in chemical information. This technique has a relatively long history of application for biomaterials research and characterization. Monographs and articles exist describing ATR-IR in detail and demonstrating its value for particular types of investigations (34, 35).

The ATR-IR method has not been particularly successful as a technique for characterizing materials with regard to surface contamination or biocompatibility (see, for example, Ref. 36). However, new developments may alter this picture. In particular, Fourier transform infrared instruments (FTIR) offer much higher signal-to-noise (S/N) ratios than older dispersive instruments. The ATR method is generally inefficient in its use of the infrared source output. Increased signal-to-noise ratios allow investigators to work at higher internal reflection angles and with crystal materials of high refractive index such as germanium. Both of these conditions reduce the depth of sampling. Since earlier infrared studies generally were performed at sampling depths in the range of 1–5 mμ, the designation "surface analysis" was questionable. A cylindrical ATR element geometry may reduce sampling depths to 500 Å (34, 37). Thus, ATR-IR will begin to approach sampling depths observed in ESCA under some conditions (e.g., using a titanium x-ray anode). The high information content of ATR-IR coupled with reduced depths of penetration, high resolution, computer subtractive capabilities, and relatively modest cost may increase the application of this technique for biomaterials characterization. For examples of recent studies effectively exploiting the capabilities of FTIR, see Refs. 11 and 38.

Contact Angle Measurement. Contact angle measurement is one of the oldest techniques used to characterize surfaces. Its value lies in its simplicity, low cost, and extreme surface orientation. It is remarkably sensitive in detecting surface contamination (39, 40). Also, high degrees of correlation between contact angle measurements and various biological interactions have been made (41–48). The value of contact angle measurement is expanded upon in the next section.

A review that puts contact angle measurement techniques in a contemporary context has been published by Good (18). With respect to biomaterials studies, the following limitations of contact angle measurements should be kept in mind during data analysis and interpretation:

1. Contact angle measurements are artifact-prone. Inaccuracies in the measurements can be induced by contamination of the measurement liquids (by the surface under study or from the environment), by surface roughness, by penetration of the measurement liquid or swelling induced by it, and by the relative humidity during the measurement.
2. The liquids used in contact angle measurement can actually alter the surface under study. For polar polymers that have (at ambient temperatures) a reasonable degree of chain mobility, or have chain mobility due to plasticization by the measurement liquid, the polymer chains will undergo configurational transitions to minimize interfacial energy. Thus, the orientation of the polymer groups with respect to the surface (the precise factor that produces a surface of given character) will be altered in a different way by each measurement liquid.
3. Contact angle measurements require extensive operator training to obtain reproducible, accurate results.
4. Contact angle measurements are tedious.
5. The relationship between contact angle data and surface structure is always inferential and is, therefore, subject to interpretational difficulties and biases.

The Significance of Surface Characterization in Biomaterials Science

Three primary reasons why surface characterization is important to biomaterials science are: (1) surface identification (chemistry, structure, and reproducibility assurance), (2) contamination detection (reproducibility assurance), and (3) correlation between surface structure and biocompatibility.

As documented in the previous sections, tools now exist to detect contamination to very low levels and to characterize many of the parameters that define surface chemistry and structure. Both of these aspects of characterization are essential to insure surface reproducibility in biomaterials investigations and for commercial medical devices. The most work remains to be done in the area of correlation between surface structure and biocompatibility.

Many interesting correlations have been established between the critical surface tension of materials (or other approximations of surface free energy) and protein adsorption, cell adhesion, and thrombus formation (41–48). Unfortunately, very few studies in which a biological response has been related to a specific surface chemistry exist. One study in which such a relationship was established, demonstrated the power of the contact angle method in analyzing surface structure related to blood compatibility (40). The blood compatibility of Stellite alloy heart valves was not due to the alloy itself, but to the closely packed methyl group structure associated with a tallow polishing compound used to finish the valve. Very recently, the power of the ESCA technique for understanding and predicting the blood compatibility of materials was demonstrated. A series of polyurethanes was analyzed by ESCA, and their surface chemistry was considered in terms of the concentrations of each of the expected chemical bond types at the surface (21, 22, 49). A linear correlation was found between the concentration of ether-type linkages at the surface and the platelet consumption of these materials as assessed in a chronic, in vivo baboon arteriovenous shunt model (21). In addition, a correlation between ESCA data on polyurethane surfaces and in vitro platelet adhesion in a glass bead column was found also (23). These studies using ESCA represent the first indications that surface chemistry (as opposed to surface energetics, a manifestation of surface chemistry) can be related to complex blood-interaction responses. They also further support the contention that surface characterization is a significant part of biomaterials development and evaluation. Surface characterization should give us the knowledge to design materials rationally for optimized biocompatibility in different implantation sites.

Conclusions

A knowledge of the surface chemistry and structure of materials should enable us to understand and predict blood compatibility, and give us the information needed to design improved materials rationally. To date, this has been demonstrated clearly, only for a limited class of materials, polyurethanes. Generalized relationships must be worked out to encompass all materials. This endeavor will require accurate identification and quantitation of all chemical groups and atomic structures at the surface of materials and an understanding of their interactions with biological systems. Synergistic interactions between different surface structures also must be considered. The sampling depth that must be observed is another area in need of research. This knowledge will help to answer questions concerning permissible levels of contamination, and propagation of the interactive effects of "buried" structures to the surface.

Acknowledgment

The author thanks T. A. Horbett for helpful discussions relating to this manuscript. NHLBI grants HL22163 and HL19419 supported some of the studies described.

Literature Cited

1. Keller, K. H.; Andrade, J. D.; Baier, R. E.; Dillingham, E. O.; Ely, J.; Klein, E.; Morrisey, B. W.; Altieri, F. D. "Guidelines for Physico-chemical Characterization of Biomaterials," NIH Publication No. 80-2186. National Heart, Lung, and Blood Institute, NIH, Bethesda, MD **1980**.

2. Hench, L. L.; *J. Biomed. Mater. Res.* **1981**, *15*, iii.
3. Ratner, B. D. *J. Biomed. Mater. Res.* **1980**, *14*, 665–687.
4. Ratner, B. D.; Rosen, J. J.; Hoffman, A. S.; Scharpen, L. H. In "Surface Contamination," Mittal, K. L., Ed.; Plenum: New York, 1980; Vol. 2, p. 669.
5. McGrath, J. E.; Dwight, D. W.; Riffle, J. S.; Davidson, T. F.; Webster, D. C.; Viswanathan, R. *Am. Chem. Soc., Polym. Prepr.* (Washington, D.C., September 1979).
6. Thomas, H. R.; O'Malley, J. J. *Macromolecules* **1979**, *12*, 323.
7. Stupp, S. I.; Kauffman, J. W.; Carr, S. H. *J. Biomed. Mater. Res.* **1977**, *11*, 237–250.
8. Ratner, B. D.; Weathersby, P. K.; Hoffman, A. S.; Kelly, M. A.; Scharpen, L. H. *J. Appl. Polym. Sci.* **1978**, *22*, 643–664.
9. King, R. N.; Andrade, J. D.; Ma, S. M.; Gregonis, D. E.; Brostrom, L. R. In *Proceedings of the Workshop on Interfacial Phenomena: Research Needs and Priorities*, University of Washington, 15–16 February 1979, National Science Foundation, Washington, DC, 1979, pp. 458–502.
10. Holly, F. J.; Refojo, M. F. In "Hydrogels for Medical and Related Applications," Andrade, J. D., Ed.; ACS Symposium Series No. 31, ACS: Washington DC, 1976, pp. 252–266.
11. Paik Sung, C. S.; Hu, C. B. In "Multiphase Structures," Cooper, S. L.; Estes, G. M.; Eds.; ACS Advances in Chemistry Series No. 176, ACS: Washington DC, 1979; p. 83.
12. Croucher, M. D.; Schreiber, A. P. *J. Polym. Sci., Polym. Phys. Ed.* **1979**, *17*, 1269–1273.
13. Prest, W. M.; Luca, D. J. *J. Appl. Phys.* **1979**, *50*, 6067.
14. Ratner, B. D. unpublished data.
15. von Hippel, P. H.; Peticolas, V.; Schack, L.; Karlson, L. *Biochem.* **1973**, *12*, 1256.
16. Dwight, D. W.; Riggs, W. M. *J. Coll. Interface Sci.* **1974**, *47*, 650.
17. Zisman, W. In "Contact Angle, Wettability, and Adhesion," Fowkes, F. M., Ed.; ACS Advances in Chemistry Series No. 43, ACS: Washington, DC, 1964; pp. 1–51.
18. Good, R. J. In "Surface and Colloid Science," Vol. II, Good, R. J.; Stromberg, R. R. Eds.; Plenum: New York; 1979 Vol. 2, p. 1.
19. Gibson, H. W.; Pochan, J. M.; Bailey, F. G., *Anal. Chem.* **1979**, *51*, 483.
20. Sommargren, G. E. *Appl. Opt.*, in press.
21. Hanson, S. R.; Harker, L. A.; Ratner, B. D.; Hoffman, A. S. *J. Lab. Clin. Med.* **1980**, *95*, 289–304.
22. Ratner, B. D. In "Photon, Electron, and Ion Probes of Polymer Structure and Properties," Dwight, D. W.; Fabish, T. J.; Thomas, H. R., Eds.; ACS Symposium Series No. 162, ACS: Washington, DC, 1981; p. 371.
23. Merrill, E. W.; DaCosta, V. S.; Salzman, E. W.; Brier-Russell, D.; Waugh, D. F.; Trudel, G., III, Chap. 8 in this book.
24. Swingle, R. S., II; Riggs, W. M. *Crit. Rev. in Anal. Chem.* **1975**, *5*, 267–321.
25. Siegbahn, K. In "Molecular Spectroscopy," West, A. R., Ed.; Heyden: London, 1977; p. 227.
26. Clark, D. T. In "Chemistry and Physics of Solid Surfaces," Vanselow, R., Ed.; CRC: Boca Raton, FL, 1979, Vol. 2, p. 11.
27. Grant, J. T. In "Characterization of Metal and Polymer Surfaces," Lee, L. H., Ed.; Academic: New York 1977; Vol. 1, p. 133.
28. Janssen, A. P.; Venables, J. A. *Scanning Electron Microsc. II* **1979**, 259.
29. Benninghoven, A. *Surf. Sci.* **1973**, *35*, 427–457.
30. Day, R. J.; Unger, S. E.; Cooks, R. G. *Anal. Chem.* **1980**, *52*, 557A.
31. Gardella, J. A., Jr.; Hercules, D. M. *Anal. Chem.* **1980**, *52*, 226–232.
32. Briggs, D., personal communication.
33. Czanderna, A. W.; Miller, A. C.; Helbig, H. F. *Scanning Electron Microsc. I* **1978**, 259.

34. Harrick, N. J. "Internal Reflection Spectroscopy," Interscience: New York, 1967.
35. Jakobsen, R. J. In "Fourier Transform Infrared Spectroscopy," Ferrarro, A., Ed.; Academic: New York, 1979; Vol. 2, p. 165.
36. Kennedy, J. H.; Ishida, H.; Staikoff, L. S.; Lewis, C. W. *Biomater. Med. Devices, Artif. Organs.* **1978**, *6*, 215–224.
37. Gendreau, M., personal communication.
38. Knutson, K.; Lyman, D. J. *Am. Chem. Soc., Div. Org. Coat. Plas. Chem. Prepr.*, (Houston, March 1980).
39. Lelah, M. D.; Marmur, A. *Am. Ceram. Soc. Bull.* **1979**, *58*, 1121.
40. Baier, R. E.; Gott, V. L.; Dutton, R. C. *J. Biomed. Mater. Res.*, **1972**, *6*, 465.
41. Chang, S. K.; Hum, O. S.; Moscarello, M. A.; Neumann, A. W.; Zingg, W.; Leutheusser, M. J.; Ruegsegger, B. *Med. Prog. Technol.* **1977**, *5*, 57–66.
42. Lyman, D. J.; Muir, W. M.; Lee, I. J. *Trans. Am. Soc. Artif. Intern. Organs.* **1965**, *11*, 301.
43. Grinnell, F.; Milan, M.; Srere, P. A. *Arch. Biochem. Biophys.* **1972**, *153*, 193–198.
44. Mohandas, N.; Hochmuth, R. M.; Spaeth, E. E.; *J. Biomed. Mater. Res.* **1974**, *8*, 119–136.
45. Carter, S. B. *Nature* **1965**, *208*, 1183–1187.
46. Yasuda, H.; Yamanashi, B. S.; Devito, D. P. *J. Biomed. Mater. Res.* **1978**, *12*, 701–706.
47. Loeb, G. I.; Wajsgras, S. *Am. Chem. Soc., Div. Org. Coat. Plast. Chem. Prepr.*, (New Orleans, March 1977).
48. Dexter, S. C.; Sullivan, J. D., Jr.; Williams, J., III; Watson, S. W. *Appl. Microbiol.* **1975**, *30*, 298–308.
49. Ratner, B. D.; Hanson, S. R.; Harker, L. A.; Hoffman, A. S.; unpublished data.

RECEIVED for review April 14, 1981. ACCEPTED July 13, 1981.

A New Model for In Vivo Platelet and Thrombus Kinetics

R. RODVIEN, J. ROBINSON, and R. R. MITCHELL—The Institutes of Medical Sciences, San Francisco, CA 94115

P. LITWAK—Thoratic Laboratories Corp., Emeryville, CA

D. C. PRICE—University of California at San Francisco School of Medicine, San Francisco, CA

> *A rapid, minimally invasive in vivo animal model was developed to evaluate continuously the process of thrombosis on biomaterials. Goats subjected acutely to bilateral polyethylene catheters are monitored for net retention of ^{111}In-oxine platelets on the separate catheters. Comparisons between continuous scintigraphic monitoring of platelet retention and thrombus recovered at catheter retrieval show that platelet retention and thrombus growth are dynamic processes for at least the first few hours of implantation, and that platelet retention is predictive for thrombus size. Mean recovered thrombus weight is 23 mg/cm, which corresponds to a 44% increase in effective radius of the catheter–thrombus combination.*

Members of the biomaterials community continue to search for experimental animal models that assess the thromboresistance of polymers. We developed a new animal model involving rapid, simple retrograde cannulation of the goat's carotid arteries. The method promises to assess potential biomaterials, evaluate drugs that may decrease thrombus growth, and measure real-time thrombus growth and dissolution. A critical aspect of this new experimental model is that the continuously monitored net platelet retention data can be modeled mathematically.

Experimental

Animals. Male neutered outbred goats weighing between 40 and 60 kg were boarded for 2–3 weeks prior to use in acute 3-h experiments. Before use, goats with anemia, leukocytosis, thrombocytopenia, and infection were excluded.

Routine Blood Tests. Complete blood counts (CBCs) (1), platelet counts (2), plasma hemoglobin (3), and fibrinogen concentration (4) were all done by standard methods modified by us for goat blood.

Radionuclide Labeling of Blood Components. Autologous platelets were isolated, labeled with ^{111}In, and reinjected 24 to 48 h prior to the experiment. Because of the fragility of goat red blood cells and the difficulty in separating platelets from these cells, the following procedures were developed to prevent hemolysis and to allow isolation of platelets:

A 50-mL aliquot of blood collected into 10 mL of anticoagulant (3.8% sodium citrate +2.45% dextrose) was centrifuged at 250 × g for 15 min at room temperature. The platelet-rich plasma was removed and recentrifuged at 1000 × g for 15 min at room temperature. After removing the platelet-poor plasma, the platelet button was suspended in 5 mL of anticoagulant isotonic saline (1:6) to produce a final platelet concentration of at least 500,000/mm^3. After exposing the suspension to ^{111}In-oxine (10–15 μg oxine/mL) for 30 min at room temperature, the suspension was centrifuged at 1000 × g for 15 min. The platelet button was washed twice with 1 mL of platelet-poor plasma and finally resuspended in 5 mL of platelet-poor plasma for injection into the animal.

Using this technique, approximately 285 μCi of ^{111}In has been injected. The labeling efficiency, defined as the counts per minute (CPM) platelet suspension/total CPM ^{111}In used, was 48 ± 14%; in vivo recoveries (1 h after injection) were 72 ± 15%. Mean platelet survival time in five goats was 118 h (5).

Goat fibrinogen isolated by repeated β-alanine precipitation at room temperature and 93% clottable was kept frozen at −70°C, and aliquots were thawed and iodinated for each study. Iodination (0.025 μg ^{125}I/mg fibrinogen) was done at room temperature by a solid-phase technique using Iodogen followed by the addition of potassium iodide and Sephadex G-15 chromatography after 5 min (6). After labeling, the clottability of the fibrinogen was 82–88%, and no change in the fibrinogen using sodium dodecyl sulfate (SDS) electrophoresis was observed. The fibrinogen half-life in eight goats was 91 ± 15 h.

Surgical Procedure. After anaesthesia (Thiamylal sodium 10 mg/kg) was induced, the goat was intubated and ventilated in the supine position with the neck fully extended. Anaesthesia was maintained using 2% halothane in nitrous oxide and oxygen (20%/80%). The lingual arteries were exposed, and then the femoral vein was exposed and catheterized to allow repeated blood sampling. Background counts of the neck were obtained and rapid catheter placement via the lingual artery of the carotid artery using a clinically used polyethylene angiographic catheter (Type P5, Lot No. 4490, Cook, Inc., Bloomingdale, Indiana) was performed bilaterally. The entire surgical procedure for bilateral catheterizations took less than 5 min. After continuous scanning of the catheters for 150–200 min, the two catheters were retrieved immediately with the thrombus intact. Technetium-99m was used on occasion just prior to catheter retrieval to demonstrate good carotid artery blood flow and to exclude vessel occlusion.

Thrombus Evaluation. The thrombus was readily stripped from the catheter, weighed, digested with 10% sodium hydroxide, and counted in a Beckman 4000 gamma counter for ^{111}In and ^{125}I. Portions of the thrombus were prepared for histologic evaluation (7).

Scintillation Camera Data Processing. Data were recorded continuously on 9-track 800-bytes per inch tape, temporarily stored on disk, and analyzed to determine individual catheter count rates as a function of time.

Results

The continuous noninvasive monitoring of net platelet retention during an acute 3-h experiment was performed successfully in 34 of 36 consecutive goats. Sequential antero–posterior scintiphotos of the neck of a supine goat are shown in Figure 1. Increasing platelet retention is shown in the sequence "A" through "E", whereas the beginning of thrombus dissolution is shown in "F". Prior to catheterization but after ^{111}In injection, this animal had a jugular venepuncture which accounts for the radionuclide localization in the right lateral neck seen in all scintiphotos.

Figure 2 shows net platelet retention measured over each of the two carotid artery catheters using "region-of-interest" computer analysis. The derived count for each 2-min frame was normalized (including background correction) to account for the difference in the size of the areas studied. A linear fit for the initial data is shown, but in three out of ten goats, a quadratic representation of the concave upward behavior for both carotid arteries provided the best fit to the data by an F test. After the peak occurred, a rapid reversal indicated a net loss in retained platelets. The data following the peak were best fit by a constant plus mono-exponential curve. The left catheter was surgically inserted 3 min after the right. Platelet retention apparently never returned to the baseline.

Figure 3 demonstrates the repeatable as well as nonrepeatable aspects of the model in different goats. In this graph, the ordinate was changed by using the ^{111}In counts/cm of thrombus recovered from the catheter and the specific radioactivity of the platelets in the blood to convert the count rate to absolute numbers of retained platelets by:

$$\text{platelets/cm} = [(\text{platelets/mL WB})/(\text{CPM/mL WB})] \times [\text{CPM/cm thrombus}]$$

where WB is whole blood. The initial slopes were highly repeatable despite differences in the initial platelet counts of the four animals. However, the maximum platelets retained on the catheter, and the time to reach that maximum varied. Generally, a monotonic continuous loss of radionuclide from the catheters was observed. Between 0.5 and 5% (mean, 2%) of the total platelet pool was found per gram of recovered thrombus. These data pertain to different goats, all of whom received polyethylene catheters.

The amount and quality of thrombus recovered varied from goat to goat. For 47 catheters, the average thrombus weight recovered was 23 mg/cm (range: 7–85 mg/cm). Grossly, the thrombus was fibrous and red even though it was essentially a "platelet thrombus" (*see* Figure 4). The whole catheter was involved evenly, and no dangling thrombotic material was seen. Fibrin was a small percentage of the thrombus weight; in an evaluation of 34 catheters, the mean was 2.5% (range: 1–7%). When two catheters were placed in one animal, the repeatability of thrombus weight/centimeter, platelets retained on the catheter/milligram of thrombus, and milligrams of fibrinogen/

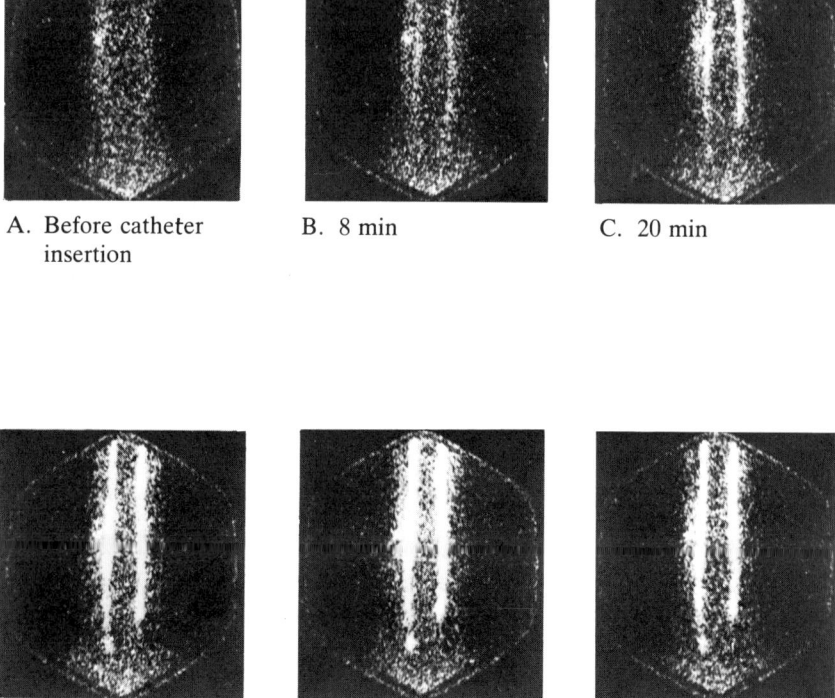

Figure 1. Sequential anterior–posterior scintiphotos of the neck of a supine goat.

Circulating radiolabeled platelets adhered and aggregated on two polyethylene catheters inserted retrograde into the carotid arteries. Increasing platelet retention is shown in the sequence "A" through "E". The beginning of thrombus dissolution is seen in "F". The small platelet collection is best shown in the precatheter sample (A). Blood was drawn from the jugular vein.

milligram of thrombus were much better than for the grouped data for all goats (*see* Table I) (8).

Catheters were assigned randomly to Group one or two. The standard deviations for the grouped data were large when compared to the means for each group, and the average pooled variance was very high when compared to the means as two independent samples. However, paired analysis is associated with a small variance. If only one catheter is placed in each animal, the number of animals to be studied to achieve similar "p" values would increase from 6- to 35-fold for the parameters listed in Table I.

Attempts were made to predict thrombus size using data obtained non-invasively. One correlation between absolute numbers of platelets retained on the catheter and thrombus weight is shown in Figure 5. Although a linear correlation appears excellent, the data near the origin suggest an overall nonlinear behavior.

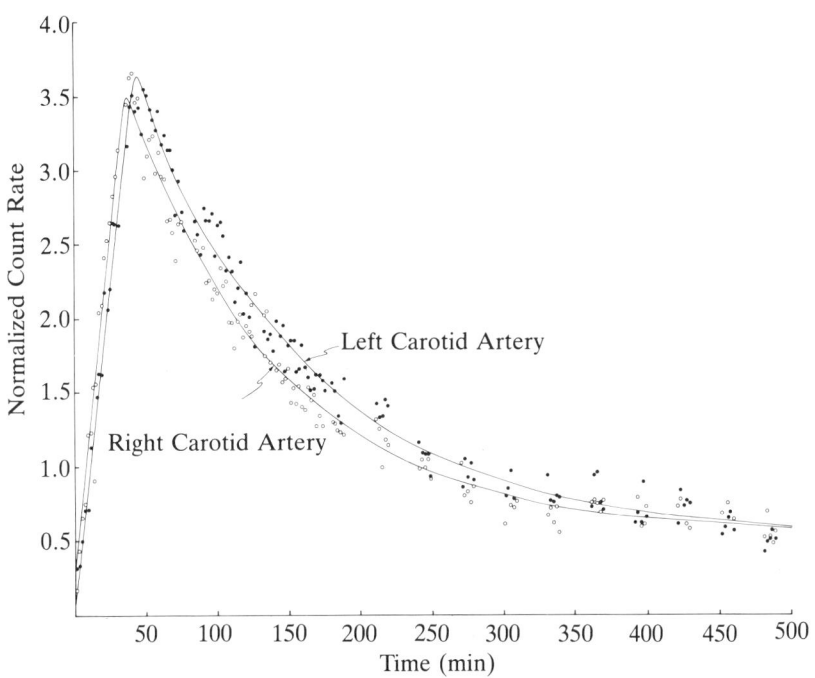

Figure 2. Thrombus growth and dissolution measured by carotid artery catheter region-of-interest scintillation counting.

The total count for each 2 min frame was normalized by the number of pixels per region. A linear fit for the initial data and a constant-plus-exponential fit thereafter are shown for each data set. The left carotid catheter was inserted surgically 3 min after the right. The repeatability, the linear initial behavior, the very narrow peak, and the monoexponential decay are shown.

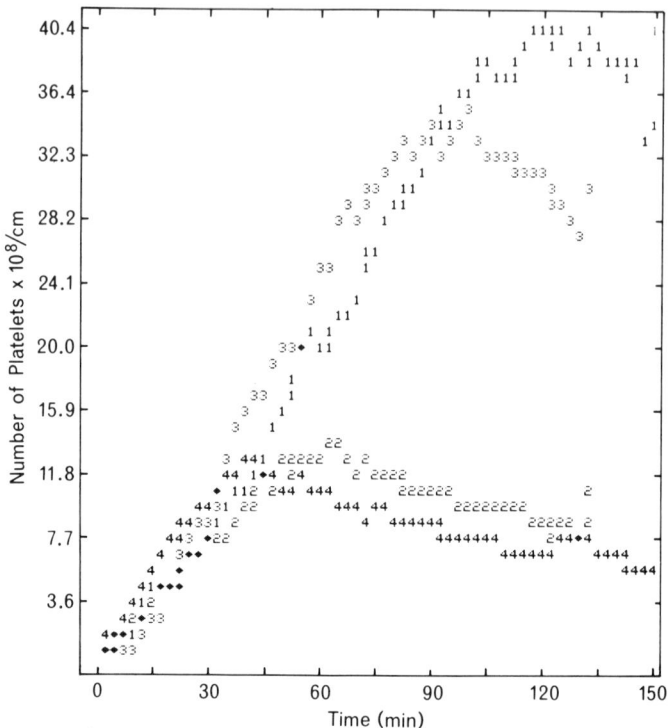

Figure 3. Net platelet retention behavior on polyethylene catheters in four goats. Thrombus platelet concentration/catheter length was used to calibrate externally detected platelet retention curves. The repeatability of the initial slope and the variable times to peak are shown. Key: 1, Goat 32; 2, Goat 36; 3, Goat 37, and 4, Goat 45.

Discussion

A model that predicts accurately thromboembolic risk associated with the use of biomaterials is still needed. Utilizing minimal surgical techniques, catheters were placed in goat carotid arteries, and subsequent analysis in real time was performed noninvasively of net platelet retention of autologously labeled ^{111}In platelets. We concentrated on acute animal studies using polyethylene catheters. Price et al. used a very similar model in dogs, obtaining similar results (9).

The large number of platelets and size of the thrombus retained by the polyethylene catheters are impressive. We calculated that in goats, 1.33% (range: 0.3–10%) of the circulating platelet pool is accumulated by the catheter. In dogs, from 4 to 7% of the pool is accumulated by a similar, but longer catheter as calculated at peak value (9). A direct comparison can be made between our model and the ex vivo model of Ihlenfeld et al. (10). In their dog

Table I. Paired Catheter Studies in 18 Goats

Grouped Data	Thrombus (mg/cm)	Platelets $\times 10^9$/g	Platelets $\times 10^8$/g	I/g
n	18	18	18	14
Catheter 1	19.76 ± 9.78[a]	41.59 ± 19.50	8.81 ± 7.53	23.05 ± 9.88
Catheter 2	18.58 ± 10.9	42.43 ± 17.97	8.82 ± 8.72	23.39 ± 10.97
Average pooled variances	107.27	351.54	66.43	107.99
Paired Data				
Mean difference	1.17	0.84	0.02	0.35
Variance	31.67	19.80	9.63	12.83
t	0.885	0.181	0.097	0.3619

[a]Mean ± 1 s.d.
Note: Two catheters were placed into the carotid arteries of one animal within 5 min of each other. The results are similar for the two catheters. Note the large average pooled variance obtained by analyzing the results as independent groups, compared with the small variance of difference obtained by analyzing as paired groups.

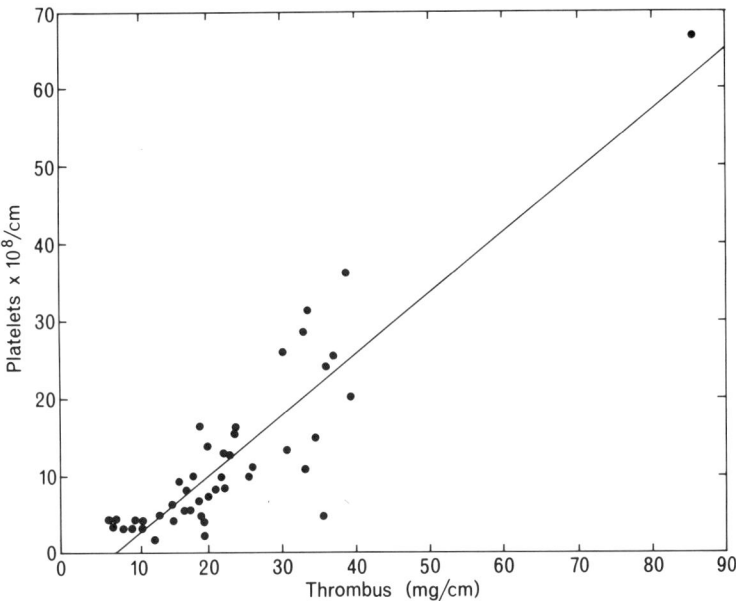

Figure 4. Correlation of thrombus platelet concentration and thrombus weight. The positive correlation suggests that thrombus weight can be predicted from the number of platelets retained. These thrombi were retrieved 2–3 h after catheter placement. Conditions: $m = 0.80$ and $r = 0.90$.

model, the largest amount of platelet mass retained by any material or substrate (polyvinyl chloride pretreated with fibrinogen) was 3×10^8 platelets/cm^2 at 15 min. In contrast, peak platelet deposition on polyethylene in our in vivo goat model was 30×10^8 platelets/cm^2, an order of magnitude greater. Concerning thrombus size, assuming even distribution of thrombus along the catheter and a mean recovered thrombus weight of 23 mg/cm, the effective radius and therefore the surface area of the polyethylene catheter increased about 44% by this amount of thrombus (from $r = 0.0825$ to 0.119 cm). This extent of thrombosis is even more impressive because the thrombus size at recovery has probably diminished from its peak size. Work by others is consistent with our data: Zimmerman et al. (11), using a chemical method to induce thrombosis in rabbits, found a 50-fold increase in the platelet content of the thrombus compared to blood; we found a 100-fold increase. Olson's group found similar numbers of platelets/mg of thrombus (12). However, Niewiarowski and Stewart, using steel tube insertion in the arteries of dogs, found far fewer number of platelets/mg of fibrin than we did: 2.7×10^6 vs. 1.77×10^9 (13). The thrombotic material we recovered was nearly pure platelets histologically (see Figure 4). The average peak platelet density was 30×10^8 platelets/cm^2 of catheter, an order of magnitude larger than observed in an ex vivo model.

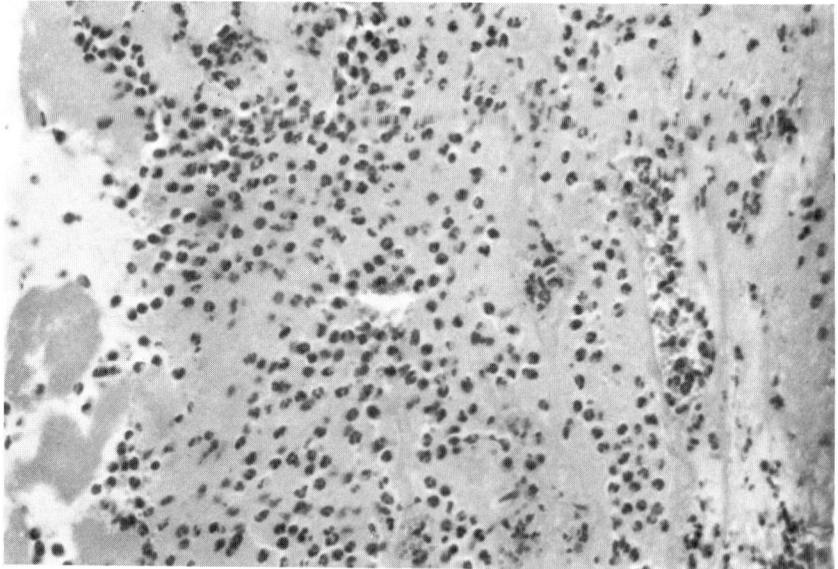

Figure 5. Histopathology of recovered thrombus. The granular acellular material (platelets) predominated, although a latticework of fibrin trapping leukocytes, red cells, and platelets did occur in discrete areas.

Our experimental model continuously evaluates net platelet accumulation, not necessarily thrombus growth and dissolution. These platelet kinetics are very unusual (*see* Figure 2):

1. The initial slope of the curve is usually linear but may be concave upward.
2. The time to the peak and the height of the peak are quite variable from animal to animal, although they are quite repeatable when identical catheters are placed in the same animal.
3. The reversal in net platelet retention is very rapid, is never complete, and is exponential in quality.
4. Net loss of platelets from the catheter may continue for hours.
5. Normalization of the platelet data from a count rate (Figure 2) to the absolute number of platelets retained/centimeter (Figure 3) reveals significant repeatability in the early upward slope.

These very unusual, yet repeatable kinetics are now being modeled mathematically to learn more about fundamental blood-materials interaction reactions (*14, 15*). Two different methods of modeling are being used, one accepting and one ignoring the conventional sequence of reactions that includes protein adhesion, platelet adhesion and aggregation, fibrin formation, and red-cell entrapment. We are using an empirical application of a stepwise regression technique called model structure determination to develop a mathematical model that characterizes the observed data. A nonlinear, second-order differential equation, similar to an enzyme reaction equation, has been derived.

Despite the fact that we are measuring net platelet retention, we can probably predict thrombus weight from platelets retained ($r = 0.9$). A similar correlation ($r = 0.88$) exists for dogs, comparing clot weight to platelet activity (%/centimeter) (*9*).

Our goat model is not only a minimally invasive procedure; the use of both a control and test catheter in the same animal produces greater sensitivity in determining differences between the catheters because animal variation is omitted. The comparable results in dogs and goats suggest species consistency. The model also has extraordinary potential flexibility—catheters can be made of different biomaterials, treated with different proteins or drugs, or implanted acutely or chronically, and multiple blood components can be evaluated. Mathematical modeling also can provide more fundamental biological knowledge concerning blood-materials interactions, and thrombus growth and dissolution in general.

Acknowledgments

The authors thank G. Bosak, H. Phillips, C. Sullivan, J. Hartmeyer, and C. Spatz for their invaluable technical support.

Literature Cited

1. Coulter, Counter ZBI-6.
2. Brecher, G.; Schneiderman, M.; Cronkite, E. P. *Am. J. Clin. Pathol.* **1953**, *23*, 15–26.
3. Harboe, M. *Scand. J. Clin. Lab. Invest.* **1959**, *11*, 66–70.
4. Lerner, R. G.; Rapaport, S. I.; Siemsen, J. K.; Spitzer, J. M. *Am. J. Physiol.* **1968**, *214*, 532–537.
5. Murphy, E. A.; Francis, M. E. *Thromb. Diath. Haemorrh.* **1971**, *25*, 53–80.
6. Fraker, P. J.; Speck, J. C. *Biochem. Biophys. Res. Commun.* **1978**, *80*, 849–857.
7. Lendrum, A. C.; Fraser, D. C.; Slidders, W.; Henderson, R. *J. Clin. Pathol.* **1962**, *15*, 401–413.
8. Snedecor, G. W.; Cochran, W. G. "Statistical Methods", 6th ed.; Iowa State Univ.: Ames, IA, 1968.
9. Price, D.; Hartmeyer, J. A.; Prager, R. J.; Lipton, M. J. presented at *Proc. Yale Symp. Radiolabelled Blood Cellular Elements, New York, 1980.*
10. Ihlenfeld, O. V.; Cooper, S. L. *J. Biomed. Mater. Res.*, **1979**, *13*, 577–591.
11. Zimmermann, R.; Zeltach, C.; Lange, D. *Thromb. Res.* **1979**, *16*, 147–158.
12. Olson, P. S.; Ljungquist, U.; Bergent; S. E. *Thromb. Res.* **1974**, *5*, 1–19.
13. Niewiarowski, S.; Stewart, G. J. In "Platelets: A Multidisciplinary Approach"; de Maetano, G; Baratteni, S., Eds.; Raven: New York, 1978; pp. 131–147.
14. Gupta, N. K.; Hall, W. E.; Treakle, T. E. *J. Guidance Control* **1978**, *1*, 197–204.
15. Hall, W. E.; Gupta, N. K.; Tyler, J. S. *AGARD Specialist Meet. Methods Aircraft State Parameter Identif., NASA, Nov. 1974.*

RECEIVED for review January 16, 1981. ACCEPTED March 24, 1981.

4

Platelet Retention on Polymer Surfaces

Some In Vitro Experiments

E. W. MERRILL, E. W. SALZMAN, V. SA DA COSTA, D. BRIER–RUSSELL, A. DINCER, P. PAPE, and J. N. LINDON

Massachusetts Institute of Technology, Department of Chemical Engineering, Cambridge, MA 02139 and Harvard Medical School and Beth Israel Hospital, Department of Surgery, Boston, MA 00215

Several polymers were evaluated in the form of a surface coating on glass beads packed in columns to determine their ability to retain platelets when whole human blood passes over the surface. This ability was measured as the platelet retention index $\bar{\rho}$, the fraction of platelets retained on the column. Lowest values of $\bar{\rho}$ were found for poly(ethylene oxide), poly(propylene oxide), poly(tetramethylene oxide) (in the form of polyurethanes), and polydimethylsiloxane. Highest values (around 0.8) were found for cross-linked poly(vinyl alcohol) and the copolymers of ethylenediamine with diisocyanates. Intermediate values were found for polystyrene and its copolymers with methyl acrylate, for polyacrylate, and for poly(methyl methacrylate). The results are interpreted in terms of possible hydrophobic and hydrogen bonding interactions with plasma proteins.

Unlike metallic and ceramic surfaces, polymer surfaces are mobile (unless very highly cross-linked), and their molecular segments can rearrange side groups or main chain groups in response to the environment (e.g., air, water) to minimize free energy (1).

Polymer surfaces, exposed to blood and blood plasma, can function like the stationary phase in partition liquid chromatography, that is, the molecular blood elements (lipids, proteins) cannot only adsorb on, but may "dissolve into" the surface layer of the polymer.

The arrangement of molecular elements of a polymeric material at a blood–polymer interface generally is not known in detail; x-ray photoelectron spectroscopy (XPS, also called ESCA) indicates that for block copolymers, polymers having large side groups of differing polarity and polyelectrolytes, the surface composition may be quite different from the bulk, stoichiometric composition (2).

This chapter deals with a specific test of blood–surface interaction: in vitro platelet retention in a column of beads (due to platelet adhesion and aggregation). Protein adsorption precedes platelet adsorption, and thus the in vitro platelet retention test involves competitive and sequential adsorption of proteins, the outcome of which produces surfaces having widely varying degrees of platelet retention. Except in the case of thrombin (3), plasma protein absorption on these surfaces has not been studied.

We hypothesize that the plasma protein molecules contain specific clusters of hydrophobic groups, cationic groups, anionic groups, hydrogen bonding groups, etc., over their surfaces that enable them to recognize and adhere to the "foreign" surfaces, thereby recruiting platelets to adhere and aggregate upon contact. According to this hypothesis, high surface concentration of certain proteins, for example, fibrinogen or fibronectin, or conformational change of the adsorbed protein could invoke platelet activity. The details of these reactions and their relation to the in vivo behavior of polymers remain to be established.

Experimental

Platelet Retention Test. The in vitro platelet retention assay device is shown in Figure 1 (4). Whole human blood, freshly drawn, citrated, and thermostatted to 37°C, was passed from the holding syringe by aliquots of 1 mL through columns packed with 0.2-mm diameter beads. The beads had been coated previously with the polymer to be tested. Each column offered a surface area of about 400 cm^2, with a void volume of about 0.5 mL. The platelet count was determined for the blood samples emerging, aliquot by aliquot, and was averaged for five aliquots and six different donors. This average, divided by the platelet count in the blood in the holding syringe, is the recovery index r, and from this the platelet retention index $p = 1 - r$, that is, the fraction of entering platelets retained on the column, was determined.

Synthesis of Polymers. All polymers used in the study were synthesized in our laboratories, except for poly(vinyl alcohol)(du Pont Elvanol 99.5% hydrolyzed). The acrylates and methacrylates were synthesized by batch polymerization in methyl ethyl ketone initiated by azobisisobutyronitrile. Molecular weights ranged between 60,000 and 150,000 (weight average). The copolymers of methyl acrylate and styrene and homopolymer polystyrene were synthesized at 60°C in solvent-free systems using benzoyl peroxide as initiator. Conversions were limited to 10% to maintain nearly constant composition of the polymer, and molecular weight averaged around 100,000 (weight average). Polymer composition (mole fraction of styrene) was determined by infrared spectroscopy and by material balance on residual monomer. Segmented polyurethanes containing polyethers were prepared by procedures given elsewhere (5). Aromatic polymers were prepared as alternating copolymers of 2,4-tolylene diisocyanate with ethylenediamine, and alternating copolymers of 4,4-diphenyl methyl diisocyanate with ethylenediamine (5, 6). Polymers synthesized in our laboratory were precipitated from the reaction medium and redissolved in appropriate solvent to remove initiator residues and oligomers.

Polydimethylsiloxane (PDMS) was synthesized from the cyclic trimer hexamethyltrisiloxane "D3" in hexane using anionic ring-opening polymerization and dilithium stilbene as initiator (7). This material was terminated by chlorovinyldimethylsilane at a molecular weight $\bar{M}_w$ of 60,000. It was then precipitated from

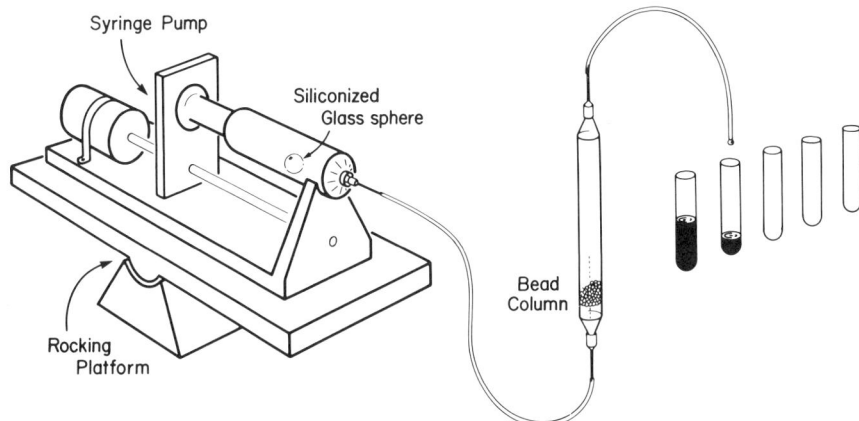

Figure 1. In vitro test for platelet retention, using plastic columns, packed with fine glass beads whose surfaces are thereafter coated with test polymer (ambient temperature = 37°C).

hexane solution by alcohol, washed with alcohol–water to remove lithium chloride, and dried.

Deposition of Polymer as a Test Surface. The test columns, packed with glass beads of 0.2-mm diameter to maximum density, were filled from below with a solution of the polymer, the concentration of which was adjusted (1 to 5 wt %) to insure that gravitational drainage in the subsequent step would be conveniently rapid. Drainage is the descent of the liquid–air meniscus through the packed column; it is "complete" when the meniscus leaves the lower end of the column. Obviously, the fluid film continued to flow down over the beads at a rate dependent on the solution viscosity, which in turn was a function of polymer concentration and molecular weight. For all polymers except poly(vinyl alcohol), the column was then attached to a source of argon gas that provided a dust-free, nonoxidizing carrier into which the solvent could evaporate. As soon as the solvent started to evaporate, the viscosity of the film of polymer solution began to rise without limit, as polymer concentration increased, and thus drainage ceased. Upon completion of solvent evaporation, (hours to several days depending on volatility), the polymer was left as a continuous coating on the bead surfaces, joining them at their junctions. For each polymer the solvent was chosen to insure that the polymer film remained homogeneous as the solvent evaporated. In general, solvents of chromatographic grade purity were used to avoid adventitious contaminants in the polymer surface. For most polymers chloroform was used, but for the segmented polyurethanes, dimethylformamide was used. The final thickness of polymer coating on the bead was between about 0.1 and a few micrometers. Hydraulic resistance of the bed of beads *after* coating was substantially unchanged. (At most, a 10% increase in pressure drop for a fixed flow rate occurred.)

Continuous coating of the glass surfaces, theoretically expected from the high critical surface tensions of acid-washed glass and the much lower surface tensions of the organic solution used, was confirmed by scanning electron microscopy combined with specific dye tests that would have revealed glass had it been exposed.

Poly(vinyl alcohol) as a 5 wt % solution in water with 1% $MgCl_2$ and 5% glutaraldehyde was coated onto the bead surfaces. After draining, the columns were heated to 60°C for 1 h, during which time the poly(vinyl alcohol) was partially cross-linked via acetal bond formation. The columns were then washed exhaustively with water to remove the $MgCl_2$ (the catalyst) and unreacted aldehyde. As a consequence, poly(vinyl alcohol) was rendered insoluble and its crystallinity was reduced significantly. Upon conditioning in isotonic saline, prior to contact with blood, the poly(vinyl alcohol) coatings swelled but remained integral and adherent to the bead surfaces.

Results

Ten polymers were studied in respect to platelet retention, as summarized in Figure 2.

The first three, polyethers in the form of the "soft segment" of segmented polyurethanes, are described in detail in another chapter in this volume (6), as is the ninth of the list, identified as aromatic polyurea, an

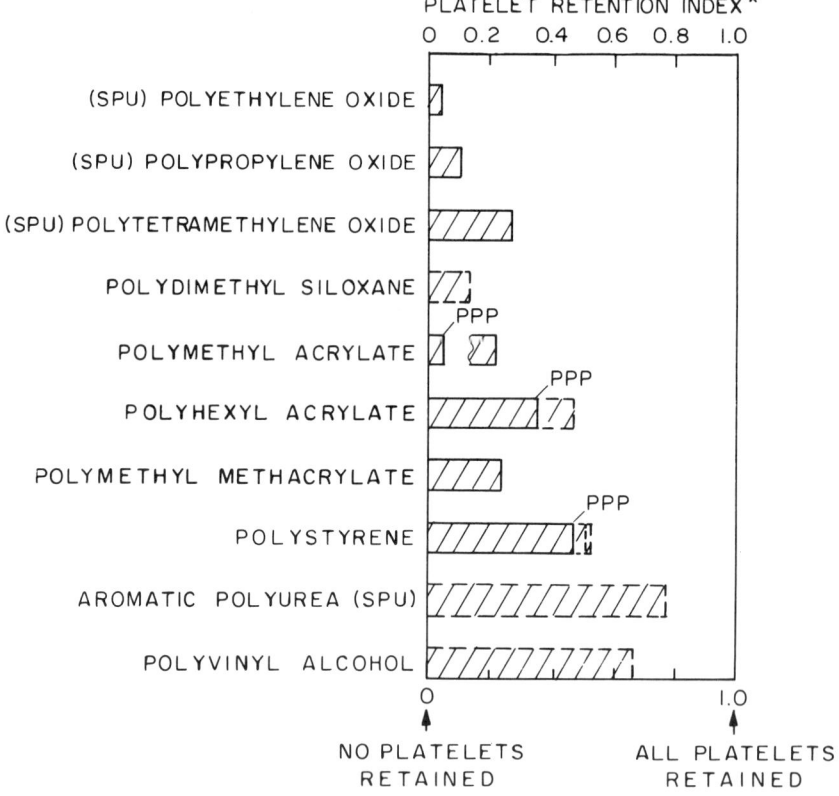

Figure 2. Composite display of average platelet retention index $\bar{p}$ for selected polymer types. The acrylates, but not polystyrenes, are significantly passivated by pretreatment with plasma (n = ≥6). Key: *, lowest value observed in each case; and PPP, preincubated in platelet-poor plasma.

analogue of the "hard segment" of the polyurethanes that contain the polyethers.

The acrylates (fifth and sixth in the list of Figure 2) are part of a series in which the alkane side chain length was varied over a range of 1 (methyl) to 16 (hexadecyl). The experiments are described completely elsewhere (8), and include a similar series on the methacrylates one of which poly(methyl methacrylate) (PMMA), is shown as seventh in the list of Figure 2.

Not reported elsewhere are results on pure PDMS (fourth in Figure 2), pure polystyrene (eighth in Figure 2), cross-linked poly(vinyl alcohol) (tenth in Figure 2), and copolymers of styrene with methyl acrylate (Figure 3).

We tested the hypothesis that the platelet retention index should increase as polymer composition varied from 100 mol % methyl acrylate to 100 mol % styrene, the respective platelet retention indices $\bar{\rho}$ being about 0.25 and 0.55 for the homopolymers. The results are shown in Figure 3, wherein $\bar{\rho}$ increases to a maximum near 40% styrene. When the surfaces were incubated in platelet-poor plasma before contact with whole blood, the values of $\bar{\rho}$ were much reduced (from 0.25 to 0.05 for methyl acrylate) for copolymers containing up to 60 mol % styrene. Copolymers of higher styrene content were not rendered significantly less retentive by plasma pretreatment.

XPS was used to evaluate the surface composition of these copolymers in relation to the bulk composition (fractions of methyl acrylate and styrene). Surface composition was essentially identical to the bulk composition. Thus, for example, when the bulk composition is 40 mol % styrene, the surface percentage of styrene is about 40. Such a surface appears to be as active as polystyrene homopolymer.

Of the polymers listed in Figure 2, cross-linked poly(vinyl alcohol) was the least well characterized. It swells to nearly twice its dry volume when in equilibrium in isotonic saline. An undetermined fraction of its secondary hydroxyl groups is converted to acetal linkages by the dialdehyde.

Discussion

The mobility of groups attached to polymer segments in response to interfacial conditions probably has much to do with the response of plasma proteins, and then platelets, to these surfaces. For example, Hoffman and Ratner described XPS spectra showing that (9, 10) acrylamide grafted to silicone rubber by radiation will predominate at the surface after equilibration in water, but that dimethylsiloxane will predominate in the surface if it has been equilibrated in air. Gregonis et al. (11) showed that even glassy PMMA, after long exposure to water, will change its contact angle (receding) from 80° to 20°, indicating significant motion of side groups.

Thus, time of water exposure prior to challenging platelets is probably important, but the matter needs further study. Our tests suggest that increasing the hydrophobic side group length increases platelet retention; in these experiments surfaces were exposed to isotonic saline solution for less

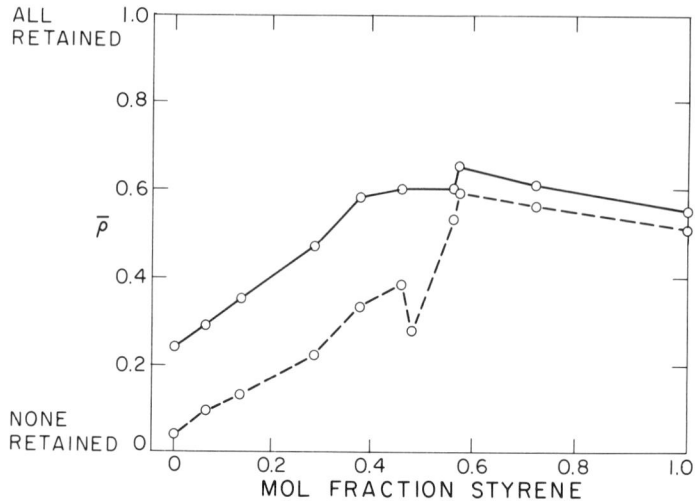

Figure 3. Average platelet retention index $\bar{p}$ as a function of mole fraction of styrene in a series of copolymers of methyl acrylate and styrene. Key: —, control and - - -, pretreated in platelet-poor plasma.

than 30 min prior to testing. Very long exposures to isotonic saline could result in a significant rearrangement of the ester linkage and alkane chain.

Preincubation of surfaces with platelet-poor plasma substantially reduced the platelet retention index of polyacrylates and polymethacrylates, but hardly altered the retention index of polystyrene or copolymers with methyl acrylate that are rich in styrene. Even without plasma pretreatment, the surface, when exposed to whole blood, was probably first contacted by molecular elements (including the proteins) before the cellular elements arrived. What then is the mode of action of plasma pretreatment? Several hypotheses, none conclusive, can be advanced, such as:

(1) Lipid adsorption during incubation alters the adsorptive capacity for certain proteins effective in binding platelets.
(2) Platelet-binding proteins desorb from the surface during incubation in favor of proteins that when adsorbed do not bind platelets.
(3) The polymer surface itself, in response to the lipids and/or proteins to which it is exposed during incubation, undergoes time-dependent conformational changes (hydrophobic side groups moved to or from the surface, for example) in such a way that a layer of proteins having more or less affinity for platelets is achieved.

The exchange of proteins (albumin, globulin, and fibrinogen) and the time course of adsorption–desorption from polymers have been studied by various researchers (*12–14*). Continual transition of, or evolution of, the surface upon prolonged contact with plasma, separate protein solutions, or blood appears to occur often.

The evidence summarized in Figure 2 shows lowest platelet retention indices for poly(ethylene oxide) (PEO), poly(propylene oxide) (PPO), and PDMS. This result implies low degrees of adsorption of specific critical plasma proteins and/or adsorption without conformation alteration of the protein. The molecular attributes these three polymers have in common appear to be:

(1) Absence of ionic groups
(2) Absence of hydrogen atoms that can form hydrogen bonds
(3) Relatively small nonpolar groups (e.g., methyl, -CH$_2$-)
(4) Regular alternation of the nonpolar groups with a polar group (the siloxane and ether oxygens)
(5) Segmental mobility (at 37°C), that is, "liquid-like" motion of units and side groups
(6) Surface activity: (PDMS can be spread as a monolayer on water; PEO will concentrate at an oil–water interface).

These observations indicate a need to refine the meaning of hydrophobicity in connection with protein interaction and platelet retention.

Reports from recent conferences sponsored by the Devices and Technologies Branch of the National Heart, Lung, and Blood Institute (*15, 16*) indicate that silicone rubber and segmented polyurethanes are among the most inert materials studied by ex vivo or in vivo methods, whereas polyethylene and polytetrafluroethylene are more active. In these latter two polymers, no conformational change of the surface can result that will expose less hydrophobic groups, whereas with PEO, PPO, and PDMS, such a result is inevitable, since high chain and segment mobility occur in the polymers, permitting response to the thermodynamic requirement of minimum free energy easily achieved by changing oxygen for -CH$_3$ or -CH$_2$- at the surface.

Polystyrene beads are known for their capacity to bind immunoglobin G globulins nonspecifically, by hydrophobic interaction, so that the immunospecificity of the F_{ab} region is preserved. Because of the dipolar nature of the phenyl ring, polystyrene probably represents a surface capable of extraordinary interaction with hydrophobic regions of proteins.

The unusual properties of PEO [including poly(ethylene glycol) (PEG)] in minimizing adsorption were described by Hiatt et al. (*17*) with respect to rabies virus, and by George (*18*) with respect to platelets. Whicher and Brash (*13, 14*) noted the low degree of adsorption by segmented polyurethanes containing PEG of albumin or fibrinogen, and the low degree of platelet retention on these surfaces. Wasiewski et al. (*19*) reported that adsorption of thrombin to glass can be prevented by adding PEG of 6000 molecular weight.

Before long-term hemocompatibility can be expected for any material, the nature of polymer surface–protein interaction must be established in more detail: the way in which the polymer surface alters itself (rotation of segments, side groups, chain refolding, etc.) in response to the protein species; the way the protein is altered in conformation (if at all) upon adsorption by the surface; and how this conformational change provokes platelet retention. Of course, longer-term ex vivo or in vivo studies also will be necessary.

Acknowledgments

The support of United States Public Health Service under Grant HL 20079 is gratefully acknowledged. J. J. Wu synthesized the PMMA and the polyacrylates. The cross-linked poly(vinyl alcohol) was prepared by John Frenz as part of his M.S. thesis (MIT, Department of Chemical Engineering, January 1980).

Literature Cited

1. Andrade, J. D.; Coleman, D. L.; Didisheim, P.; Hanson, S. R.; Mason, R.; Merrill, E. W. *Trans. Am. Soc. Artif. Intern. Organs*, in press.
2. Thomas, H. R.; O'Malley, J. *Macromolecules* **1979**, *12*, 323.
3. Sa da Costa, V.; Brier-Russell, D.; Trudell, G., III; Waugh, D. F.; Salzman, E. W.; Merrill, E. W. *J. Colloid Interface Sci.* **1980**, *76*, 594.
4. Lindon, J. N.; Rodvien, R.; Brier-Russell, D.; Greenberg, R.; Merrill, E. W.; Salzman, E. W. *J. Lab. Clin. Med.* **1978**, *92*, 904.
5. Sa da Costa, V.; Brier-Russell, D.; Salzman, E. W.; Merrill, E. W. *J. Colloid Interface Sci.* **1981**, *80*, 445.
6. Chapter 8 in this book.
7. Meyers, K. O.; Bye, M. C.; Merrill, E. W. *Macromolecules* **1980**, *13*, 1045.
8. Brier-Russell, D.; Salzman, E. W.; Lindon, J. N.; Handin, R.; Merrill, E. W.; Dincer, A. K.; Wu, J. S. *J. Colloid Interface Sci.* **1981**, *81*, 311.
9. Hoffman, A. S.; Ratner, B. D. In "Synthetic Biomedical Polymers," Szycher, M.; Robinson, W. J., Eds.; Technomic: Westport, CT, 1980; pp. 133–150.
10. Ratner, B. D. *J. Biomed. Mater. Res.* **1980**, *14*, 665.
11. Gregonis, D. E.; Smith, L. M.; Andrade, J. D. *ACS, Div. Org. Coat. Plast. Chem., Prepr.* (New York, August, 1981).
12. Cooper, S. L.; Ihlenfeld, J. V.; Mathis, T. R.; Barber, T. A.; Mosher, D. F.; Riddle, L. M.; Hart, A. P.; Updike, S. J. *Trans. Am. Soc. Artif. Intern. Organs* **1978**, *24*, 727.
13. Whicher, S. J.; Brash, J. L. *J. Biomed. Mater. Res.* **1978**, *12*, 181.
14. Brash, J. L.; Uniyal, S. *J. Polym. Sci., Polym. Symp.* **1979**, *66*, 377.
15. Contractors Meeting Proceedings, Devices and Technologies Branch, National Heart, Lung, and Blood Institute, (December 1979).
16. Ibid. (December 1980).
17. Hiatt, C. W.; Shelvkov, A.; Rosenthal, E. J.; Galimore, J. N. *J. Chromatogr.* **1971**, *56*, 362.
18. George, J. N. *Blood* **1972**, *40*, 862.
19. Wasiewski, W.; Fasco, M. J.; Martin, B. M.; Detwiler, J. C.; Fenton, J. W. *Thromb. Res.* **1976**, *8*, 881.

RECEIVED for review January 16, 1981. ACCEPTED August 10, 1981.

5

Thrombus Formation on Surfaces in Contact with Blood

J. S. SCHULTZ, S. M. LINDENAUER, and J. A. PENNER

University of Michigan, Ann Arbor, MI 48109

> *An ex vivo test method consisting of a flow-through couette cylinder placed in an arteriovenous shunt of a dog was used to evaluate the effects of shear, surface properties, spatial relationships, and drugs on thrombus formation. In whole blood, thrombus formation does not appear to be a diffusion-limited process. Increasing shear rates from 150 to 260 s^{-1} resulted in a reduction in the rate of thrombus formation. When two surfaces were placed in tandem on the central rod of the chamber, thrombus formation was independent of blood flow direction. A reduction in thrombus formation by aspirin was found only for mildly (not strongly) thrombogenic surfaces.*

Methodologies to evaluate the interaction of biomaterials with blood and blood components vary from in vitro systems, where anticoagulated blood or blood fractions are contacted with surfaces in a variety of configurations, to in vivo procedures, where tubes, sheets, etc. are inserted into the vascular system. A compendium of these techniques that seek to understand the complex interactions of blood with surfaces recently was assembled *(1)*.

An Ex Vivo Flow-Through Couette Test System

In this laboratory, an ex vivo test system was developed and utilized to delineate some of the factors affecting thrombus formation on surfaces. The system consisted of a flow-through couette device (Figure 1) placed in an arteriovenous shunt in a dog. The device was designed to allow independent control of blood flow and shear by separate control of the flow rate through the chamber, and of the rotation speed of a central rod, which is coated with the material to be studied. The validation of the method with respect to flow conditions, hematological considerations, and reproducibility has been reported previously *(2–4)*.

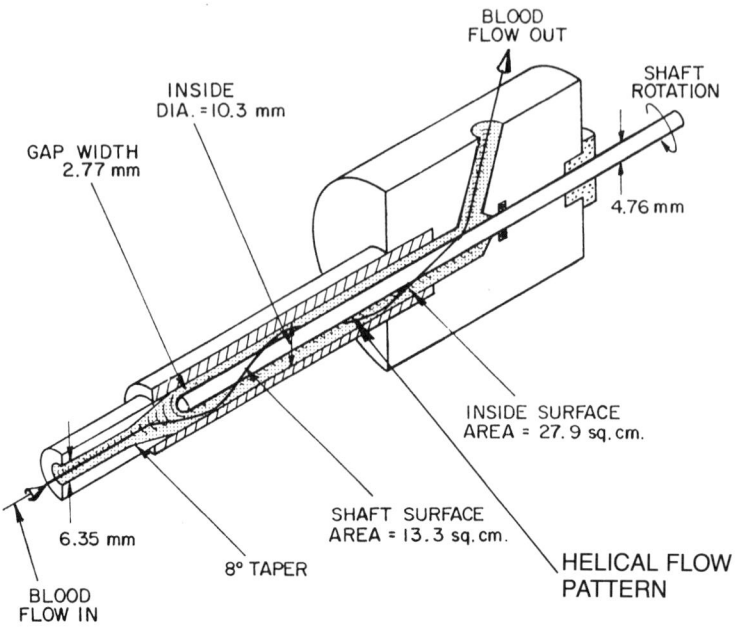

Figure 1. Ex vivo flow-through couette for evaluating thrombus formation on biomaterials.

Thrombus formed on central rod is removed and the composition measured. In experiments to evaluate the effect of shear, the rod was made of polypropylene. In other experiments, segments of rod surface were coated with different materials or vein segments placed on the rod (7).

Briefly, the important characteristics are (1) flow through the chamber was laminar over a range of rod rotation speeds from 0 to 800 rpm at a blood flow rate of 200 mL/min; (2) flow streamlines followed a helical pattern because of the additivity of the axial and rotational components of flow; and (3) shear was uniform over the entire surface of the rod and could be varied from 150 to 260 s^{-1} under these operational conditions.

Three chambers were placed in parallel in the arteriovenous shunt, by means of a manifold, so that three tests could be conducted simultaneously. The manifold feeding the chambers was designed to maintain a laminar flow condition in the blood stream from the animal to the test system. Flow visualization studies utilizing dyes placed at the entrance of the apparatus showed that fluid elements in the center of the tubing never contacted the tubing wall as the dye progressed through the tubing and the manifold into the test chambers. Thus the blood elements that bathed the surface of the rod coated with the biomaterial had minimal contact with other foreign surfaces.

Conditioned male dogs, weighing about 30 kg, were injected with human ^{125}I-labeled fibrinogen (Abbott Laboratories) 1 day before the test. This allowed for the metabolic removal of inactive fibrinogen. The next morning an aliquot of blood was removed from the animal, processed to label platelets with In-111, and reinjected. The animal was anesthestized, and direct access to a carotid artery and jugular vein was achieved by standard vascular surgical techniques. The saline-filled ex vivo test system was connected to the exposed blood vessels, clamps were removed and blood flow through each chamber was adjusted to 200 mL/min. Usually the test period was 1 h, after which the apparatus was disconnected from the animal and dismantled. The rods were removed from the chambers, rinsed, and stored for analyses. New rod test specimens were placed in the chambers and another run was initiated. Afterwards, the blood vessels were repaired and the animal was returned to the animal care facility to allow the wounds to heal. Animals could be used three to four times for these tests.

A typical hematological profile of the animals during the course of this test protocol is shown in Figure 2. The changes in hematocrit, platelets, fibrinogen, and PTT were rather minor, indicating that the integrity of the coagulation system was not compromised during this period.

Thrombus Formation Characteristics

In the inflow section of this test system, gross thrombus formation was usually limited to the surface of the rod placed in the center of the flow chamber. The tubing, manifold, and shell of the chamber do not accumu-

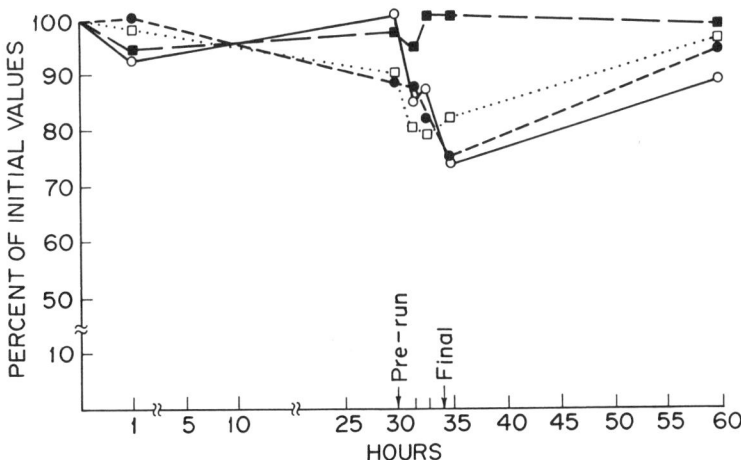

Figure 2. Hematological profile during a typical test procedure. Key: ■*, PTT;* □*, hematocrit;* ●*, platelet count; and* ○*, fibrinogen.*

late gross thrombus. This result is attributed to the low thrombogenicity of silicone rubber, which was used for the tubing and to coat the interior surfaces of the manifold and the shell of the chamber.

The thrombus that formed on the rotating rod was usually quite uniform in thickness over the apical portion, as seen in Figure 3. Measurements of the platelet and fibrinogen content per unit surface area of the rod confirmed this pattern (Figure 4) (5). The increase in deposit on the last fourth of the rod is attributed to recirculation patterns in flow around the exit port of the chamber. Because of this effect, only data from the apical three-fourths of the rods are reported and discussed.

This uniformity in deposition has important implications with respect to understanding the relative contribution of hydrodynamic factors that may be involved in thrombus formation. If diffusion of clotting factors or platelets to a surface limited the rate of thrombus formation, then the profile of thrombus probably would be maximum at the forward end of the rod and diminish toward the distal end, proprotional to $L - ⅓$ (where L is the distance from the tip of the rod) (5). The absence of this pattern indicated that factors other than diffusion dominated the process of thrombus formation in this system.

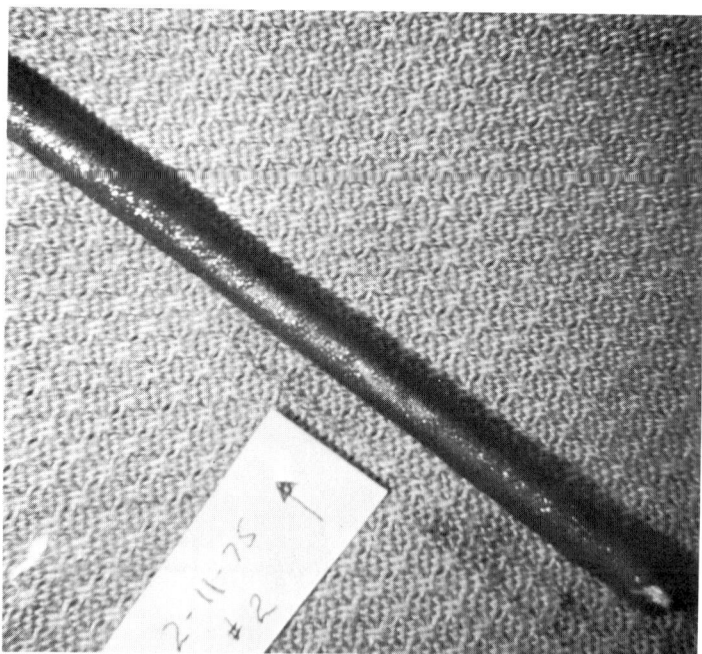

Transactions of the American Society of Artificial Internal Organs

Figure 3. *Typical pattern of uniform thrombus formation over entire surface of biomaterial coated rod* (4).

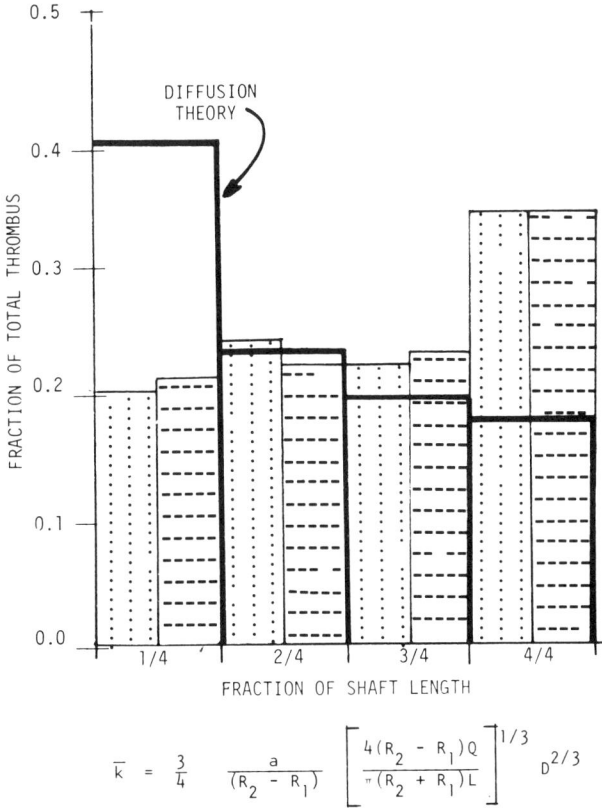

$$\bar{k} = \frac{3}{4} \frac{a}{(R_2 - R_1)} \left[\frac{4(R_2 - R_1)Q}{\pi(R_2 + R_1)L} \right]^{1/3} D^{2/3}$$

Transactions of the American Society of Artificial Internal Organs

Figure 4. Thrombus distributed over length of shaft in biomaterial test chamber as measured by relative (= = =) platelet content; (:::) wet weight (4).

The literature on this point is somewhat contradictory. Freidman and Leonard (6) found that platelet deposition did decrease in relation to position from the inlet in a tube flow configuration. However, they only considered initial rates, and eventually, after the surface becomes saturated, the thrombolic process might become kinetically controlled. Adams and Feuerstein (7) observed a marked decrease in platelet attachment along a collagen-coated tube, but observed no variation with position for a glass tube. In both studies blood was anticoagulated.

In contrast, no anticoagulants were used in our experiments. Diffusional phenomena probably did not play a controlling role when the entire coagulation system was active, and biochemical and kinetic factors most likely dominated the long-term interaction between biomaterial and blood. In ex vivo experiments using a baboon model, Harker et al. (8) also found that platelet consumption was proportional to the area of shunt surface exposed to blood, indicating that surface kinetics dominated the process.

Effects of Shear on Thrombus Formation

In most studies in which attempts have been made to investigate the relationship between hydrodynamics and thrombus formation, the flow rate of blood through the test device was changed to alter the hydrodynamics. Unfortunately, for many configurations [for example, a tube *(9)*] a change in flow rate also changed the residence time of blood in the device, the mass transfer coefficients, as well as shear rates at the biomaterial–blood interface. This simultaneous variation in hemodynamic parameters makes it difficult to assign specific cause and effect relationships to the results obtained with these methods.

In our test system, shear could be altered independently of flow rate by varying the rotation speed of the rod. In the couette device, neither the residence time of blood nor the mass transfer coefficients were changed by this maneuver *(2)*. Experiments to evaluate the effect of surface shear on thrombogenesis were performed with polypropylene rods. Polypropylene is a relatively thrombogenic material (Figure 5); the amounts of platelets, fibrinogen, and erythrocytes deposited on this material were among the highest of the many materials tested. Blood flow through all chambers was maintained at 200 mL/min, but the rod rotational speeds in the three parallel chambers were 200, 500, and 800 rpm, corresponding to shear rates at the rod surface of 150, 200, and 260 s^{-1}, respectively *(10)*.

The results of this study are shown in Figure 6, where the deposition rates of fibrinogen, platelets, and red blood cells are given relative to their respective rates at the lowest shear condition, that is, 150 s^{-1}. A similar result for each of these components of the clotting system is that all deposition rates were reduced with increasing shear. Platelets were least affected by shear; their deposition rate was reduced about 50% over this range of shear rates. Fibrinogen deposition was inhibited by about 80%, which probably accounts for the almost complete lack of red blood cells in the thrombus formed at the high shear rates. These results are consistent with the common pathological finding that thrombi in arteries (high shear) are white (mostly platelets) while thrombi in veins (low shear) are red (mostly red blood cells). A mechanism for the inhibition of thrombus formation by shear may involve the formation of fibrin fibrils from fibrinogen. Increased embolization at higher shear probably is not involved, because a SEM examination of the samples exposed to the highest shear rate did not show any large thrombi, but rather only some scattered platelets and strands of fibrin (Figure 7).

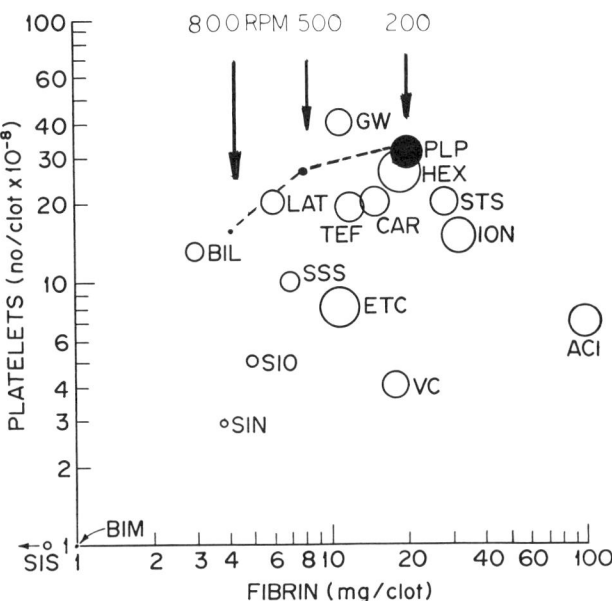

Figure 5. Composition of thrombus formed on rods coated with different materials.

Values given for the clots are for the apical 3 in. of the rod, equivalent to about 12 cm^2 of surface area. Key: SIS, siloxane on Silastic; BIM, Biomer; SIN, Silastic (1979); VC, vapor-deposited carbon GW; SIO, Silastic (1977–78); ACI, acrylamide gel; ETC, ethocellulose; SSS, siloxane on stainless steel; BIL, Biolized latex; ION, Ionomer; TEF, Teflon; STS, stainless steel; CAR, vapor-deposited carbon GA; LAT, Latex; HEX, Hexsyn; PLP, polypropylene; and GW, Gulf and Western (7).

Statistics of Thrombus Formation

Apparently because of the autocatalytic nature of thrombus formation on surfaces, the variation in amounts of thrombus found in repeated tests is fairly wide, and statistical methods are required to evaluate the reliability of the results. A common assumption is that the data are normally distributed when tests of significance or correlation are applied. However, as Downie et al. (5) suggested, the data are better fit to a log normal distribution. This behavior has been confirmed for measures of thrombogeneity; for example, in Figure 8, data on thrombus weight are plotted on probability paper along with the logarithm of the weight values (11). The log-transformed data fall more nearly on a straight line, suggesting some sort of exponential re-

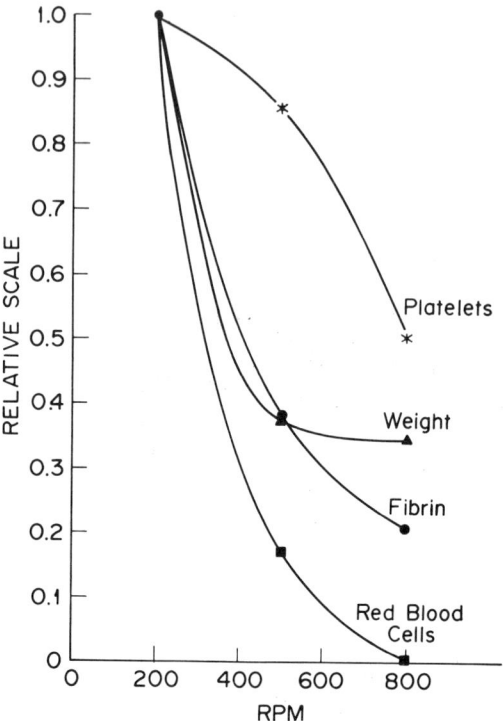

Figure 6. Effect of shear on thrombus formation. Conditions: blood flow, 200 mL/min; and material, polypropylene (7).

lationship between the rate of thrombus formation and some other key parameter of the form

$$w = a \cdot k \exp(mx) \tag{1}$$

where w is the rate of thrombus formation; x is a controlling parameter; and a, k, and m are constants. Taking logs on both sides

$$\log w = \log a + mx \cdot \log k \tag{2}$$

If x is normally distributed, then $\log w$ will be normally distributed as well. Further investigation of the kinetics of the coagulation process will be required to see if kinetic expressions of the form of Equation 1 are reasonable.

Spatial Relations in Thrombus Formation

Apparently, if a thrombus starts to form on one section of a surface, it will spread to other areas, particularly downstream of the affected re-

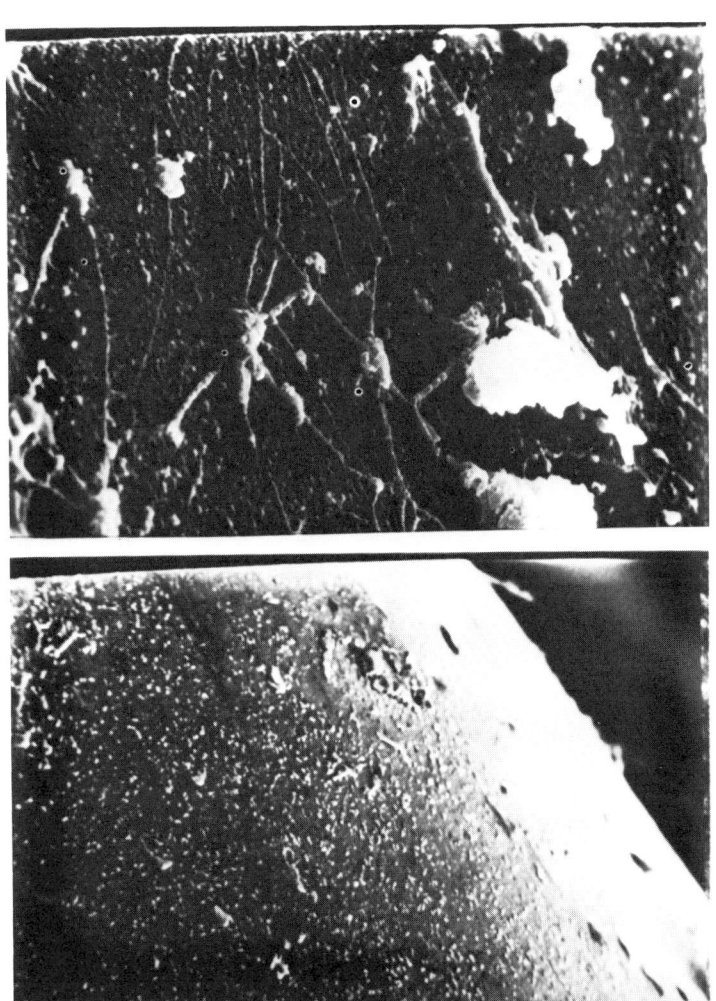

Figure 7. Scanning electron microscope photograph of polypropylene surface after 1-h exposure to flowing blood at 200 mL/min and rod rotation speed of 800 rpm.

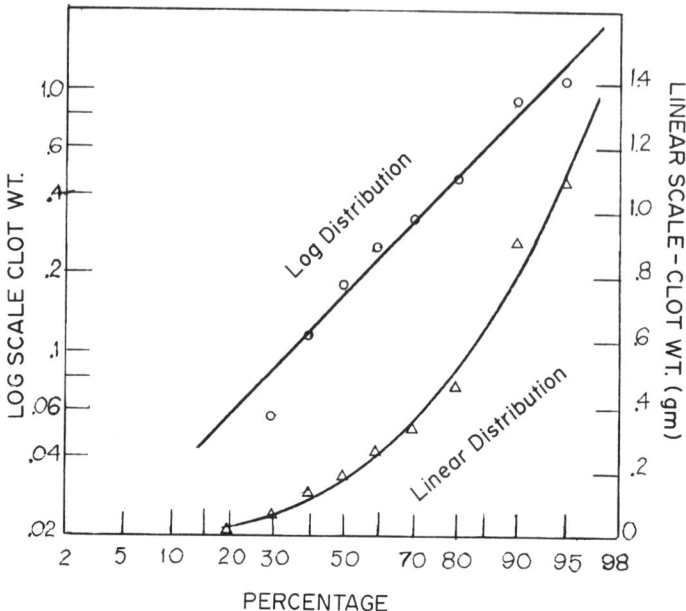

Figure 8. Clot weight distribution data for Silastic.

gion. However, the mechanism and dynamics of the propagation rate currently are unknown. In this context a distinction between two types of growth should be made.

One type of growth is primarily the result of the profileration of fibrin fibrils to the extent that hydrodynamic forces carry the macroscopic meshwork downstream of the thromoblic area. This type of proliferating thrombus usually does not adhere to downstream surfaces, and may embolize depending on the strength of the gel compared to the hydrodynamic forces acting on it. Factors that affect the strength of fibrin gels have been studied *(11)*, but little work has been done on the growth of fibrin networks into free-flowing blood.

The other type of propagation is presumably due to the sensitization of clotting factors and/or cellular elements as blood passes over a developing thrombus, and to the initiation clots in other areas due to the localized hypercoagulability of blood. To understand the magnitude of this effect, we arranged a highly thrombogenic area (polypropylene) contiguous to a relatively nonthrombogenic surface (Silastic) on the rod in our ex vivo test chamber. This arrangement was accomplished by coating either the apical or distal end of a polypropylene rod with a Silastic dispersion. The distinct difference in the thrombogenicity of these two polymers is apparent in Figure 5. The results of this study are shown in Figure 9 *(9)*.

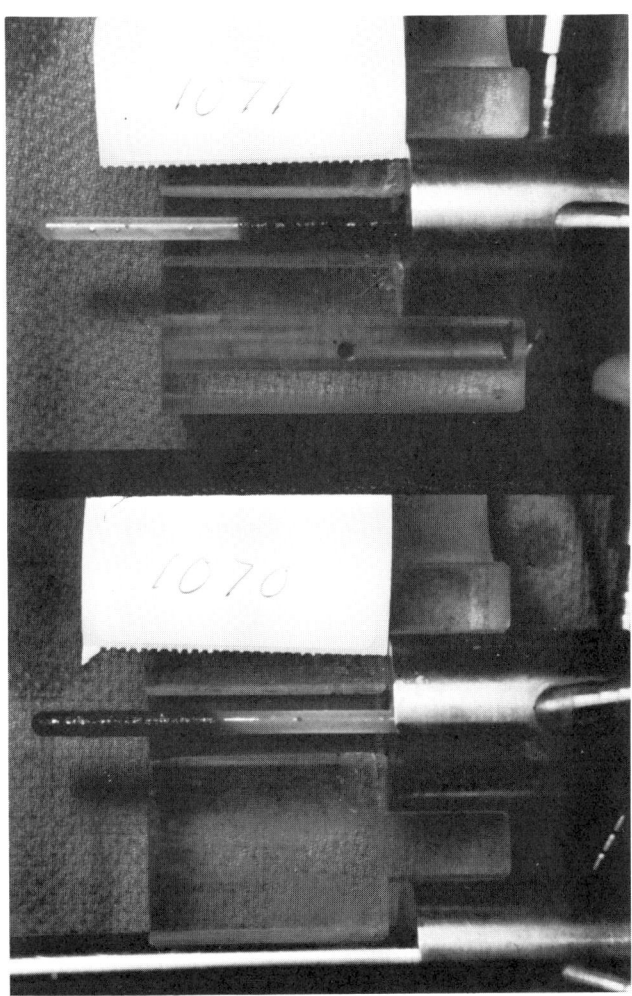

Figure 9. Segmental surface experiments to test sensitization of blood due to contact with a thrombogenic surface (7). A, the apical section of the rod is coated with Silastic and the distal end is polypropylene; and B, the apical section of the rod is polypropylene and the distal end is coated with Silastic.

When Silastic is on the front portion of the rod and blood contacts it first, little thrombus forms on the Silastic, while a distinct thrombus forms on the back polypropylene section (Figure 9a). Thus the thrombus did not propagate upstream, against the flow of blood. When the order of materials was reversed, a frank thrombus developed on the polypropylene, as expected, but the thrombus did not propagate downstream onto the surface of the Silastic. (There is a slight zone of overlap of a few millimeters.) Thus, blood sensitization was not significant.

This phenomenon is worthy of further study because it provides an opportunity to test two or more materials in the same device, and it may be important for understanding thrombus propagation in vascular prostheses.

As an extension of the first concept, autologous vein segments were placed on the rod to serve as a control comparison for biomaterial evaluations.

Some preliminary data obtained with this arrangement are given in Table I. With respect to platelet and fibrinogen deposition, Silastic is about equivalent to the endothelial surface of veins. Segments of vein with the adventitial surface exposed were included as a negative control, and developed substantial deposits of platelets and fibrinogen. When vein segments were placed on polybenzylglutamate-coated rods, the endothelial surface again was virtually free of thrombus even though it was downstream in relation to this particular polymer. Polybenyzlglutamate is more thrombogenic in the endothelium but less thrombogenic than the adventitial surface of a vein.

Effects of Drugs on Thrombus Formation

The ex vivo flow-through couette method provides a very convenient model for assessing the effect of drugs on the thrombogenic process. By directly monitoring the accumulation of radioisotope in the couette device, a direct measure of the kinetics of thrombus accumulation can be obtained. An example of the deposition of platelets on the rod surface after the administration of systemic heparin is shown in Figure 10 (4). In this experiment

Table I. Relative Thrombogenicity of Vein Segments Placed on Polymer-Coated Rods

Front section of rod			Middle section of rod		
Material	Platelets[a]	Fibrinogen[a]	Material	Platelets	Fibrinogen
Silastic	1.74	0.17	endothelium	1.15	0.15
Silastic	0.91	0.18	adventitia	2.64	1.36
PBLG[b]	1.6		endothelium	0.14	
PBLG	0.67		adventitia	3.8	

[a]Amounts relative to blood, calculated as (radioactivity CPM/cm^2 surface)/(radioactivity CPM/mL whole blood).
[b]PBLG is poly(benzyl-L-glutamate).

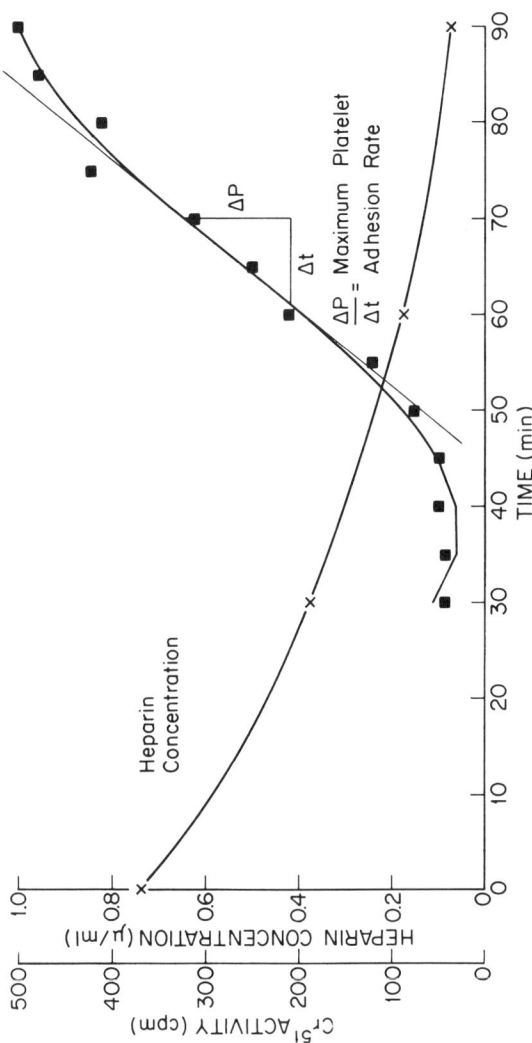

Figure 10. Heparin and ^{51}Cr levels vs. time.

heparin was injected into the animal 30 min before the test apparatus was connected to the arteriovenous shunt. The platelet deposition was delayed for about 15 min, until the heparin concentration dropped to about 0.3 units/mL. A series of dose–response experiments were conducted to evaluate the effect of heparin on thrombus development more directly, wherein the steady-state heparin level was adjusted by perfusing heparin into the animal at different rates. The results for three different materials are shown in Figure 11, leading to the conclusions that (a) the systemic heparin requirement to "neutralize" a thrombogenic material increases with the thrombogenicity of the surface and (b) the dose–response curve is semilogarithmic.

In other experiments, the animals were given 10 grains of aspirin 1 h before the biomaterial tests were initiated. The results summarized in Table II also show that the effect of this drug is different for different materials. For Silastic and polybenzylglutamate (cast from chloroform), aspirin pretreatment reduced the thrombogenicity significantly, whereas for poly-

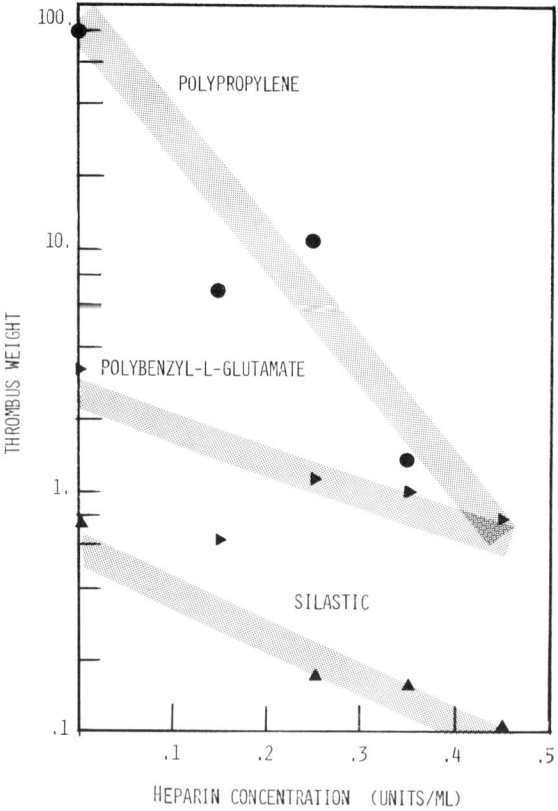

Figure 11. Effects of heparin concentration on thrombus formation.

Table II. Effect of Aspirin on Thrombogenesis

Material	Pre-Aspirin			Post-Aspirin		
	Platelets	Fibrin	Weight	Platelets	Fibrin	Weight
Silastic	2.09	6.38	0.212	0.8	2.3	0.09
PBLG[a] (cast from chloroform)	3.96	19.8	1.59	0.567[b]	(1.6)	0.052[b]
PBLG[a] (cast from dioxane)	33.5	117	8.6	37.8	59.8	2.03

[a]PBLG is poly(benzyl-L-glutamate).
[b]Differences between pre- and post-aspirin values are significant at the $P < 0.05$ level.

benzylglutamate cast from dioxane (a much more aggresive material), aspirin treatment was relatively ineffective. The solvent used to dissolve the polybenzylglutamate to prepare a coating solution had a major effect on the response of the clotting system.

Summary

At this time, an adequate understanding of the physical chemical processes involved in thrombus formation is not available. The type of effect some factors will have can be indicated, but not the magnitude of the response. For example, shear inhibits thrombus formation, and thrombus propagation on surfaces is limited for modest differences in thrombogenicity. Drugs can inhibit thrombus formation, but the magnitude of the effect is related in some fashion to the surface characteristics.

Animal models using an ex vivo shunt preparation, such as described here, will yield useful information in regard to the thombolic process. In the next few years integration of biochemical knowledge of the clotting system along with a better understanding of the physical chemical phenomena involved will result in robust models that can be used in a predictive way in the design of biocompatible devices.

Acknowledgments

This work was supported in part by NHLBI Contract No. NO1-HV-42962, Grant R01-HL 24039, and Grant R01-HL 23551. The assistance of W. Armstrong, A. Ciarkowski, and S. Barenberg is greatly appreciated.

Literature Cited

1. Report of the National Heart, Lung, and Blood Institute Working Group "Guidelines for Blood-Material Interactions," NIH Publ. No. 80–2185, Bethesda, MD., 1980.

2. Schultz, J. S.; Goddard, J. D.; Ciarkowski, A. A.; Penner, J. A.; Lindenauer, S. M. *Ann. N. Y. Acad. Sci.* **1977**, *283*, 494.
3. Schultz, J. S.; Ciarkowski, A. A.; Goddard, J. D.; Lindenauer, S. M.; Penner, J. A. "NHLBI Annual Report NO1–HB–4–2962," 1976.
4. Schultz, J. S.; Ciarkowski, A. A.; Lindenauer, S. M.; Penner, J. A.; *Trans. Am. Soc. Artif. Organs* **1976**, *21*, 269.
5. Downie, H. G.; Murphy, E. A.; Rowsell, H. C.; Mustard, J. F. *Circ. Res.* **1963**, *12*, 441.
6. Friedman, L. I.; Leonard, E. F. *Fed. Proc., Fed. Am. Soc. Exp.* **1971**, *30*, 1641.
7. Adams, G. A.; Feuerstein, I. A. *Trans. Am. Soc. Artif. Intern. Organs* **1980**, *26*, 17.
8. Harker, L. A.; Hanson, S. R.; Hoffman, A. S. *Ann. N. Y. Acad. Sci.* **1977**, *283*, 317.
9. Benis, A. M.; Anthony, M.; Nossel, M. L.; Aledort, L. M.; Koffsky, R. M.; Stevenson, J. F.; Leonard, E. F.; Shiang, M.; Litwak, R. S., *Thromb. Diath. Haemorr.* **1975**, *34*, 27.
10. Schultz, J. S.; Lindenauer, S. M.; Penner, J. A.; Barenberg, S. B. *Trans. Am. Soc. Artif. Intern. Organs* **1980**, *26*, 279.
11. Schultz, J. S.; Ciarkowski, A. A.; Lindenauer, S. M.; Penner, J. A.; Barenberg, S. B. "NHLBI Annual Report NO 1–HV–4–2962–5," 1979.
12. Ferry, J. D. *Physiol. Rev.* **1970**, *34*, 753.

RECEIVED for review February 9, 1981. ACCEPTED May 18, 1981.

6

Thrombotic Events on Grafted Polyacrylamide–Silastic Surfaces as Studied in a Baboon

ALLAN S. HOFFMAN, THOMAS A. HORBETT, and BUDDY D. RATNER—University of Washington, Departments of Chemical Engineering and Bioengineering, Seattle, WA 98195

STEPHEN R. HANSON and LAURENCE A. HARKER—University of Washington, Department of Medicine, Seattle, WA 98195

LARRY O. REYNOLDS—University of Washington, Department of Nuclear Engineering, Seattle, WA 98195

The interaction of well-characterized grafted polyacrylamide–Silastic and Silastic surfaces with blood was studied using an ex vivo, arteriovenous baboon shunt model. The consumption of autologous ^{51}Cr-labeled blood platelets was measured in the animals with test shunts. A new laser light scattering technique was developed to detect flowing platelet microemboli in real time. This technique was applied to the measurement of the size and number of microemboli generated by biomaterial cannulae in the ex vivo baboon shunt. In vitro protein adsorption studies also were carried out using a new, highly sensitive silver staining technique to visualize proteins separated by sodium dodecyl sulfate gel electrophoresis. The results suggest that the polyacrylamide–Silastic hydrogel surface is more platelet-consumptive than the Silastic surface due to a greater rate of platelet aggregation on and subsequent embolization from the hydrogel surface.

A hydrogel can be defined as a polymeric material that has the ability to swell in water and retain a significant fraction (e.g., 10–20%) of water within its structure, but that will not dissolve in water. Hydrogel materials resemble, in their physical properties, living tissue more than any other class of synthetic biomaterial. In particular, their relatively high water contents and their soft, rubbery consistency give them a resemblance to living soft tissue. On the basis of these properties, hydrogels have been investigated extensively in a variety of biomaterial applications (1–3).

Polyacrylamide hydrogels are among the most highly hydrated gels, and often exhibit water contents ranging from 60 to 95%. They have been tested for blood compatibility by a number of researchers, including our own group, using a wide variety of in vitro and in vivo test techniques and animal models (4–11). Despite these numerous studies, no general consensus concerning the blood compatibility of polyacrylamide surfaces exists. This chapter brings together our previous and most recent studies of grafted polyacrylamide surfaces in contact with blood and its components, and attempts to reach a general conclusion concerning the blood compatibility of this interesting biomaterial.

The studies described in this chapter were conducted as four separate projects to describe the sequence and mechanistic aspects of the short- and long-term thrombotic events that occur when synthetic materials contact blood. The first project was responsible for the development, synthesis, and surface characterization of all materials used for subsequent studies. This assured that all investigators were examining identical materials and that a careful record was kept of the surface structure of each specimen tested. Short-term interactive events after exposure to blood were considered in the second project. These events included protein deposition, initial cell adhesion, and thrombus buildup. Purified baboon proteins (in vitro) and baboon blood (both in vitro and in vivo) were used for all experiments. The baboon was chosen as the sole animal model for this project because of its hematological similarity to humans (12). The third project examined chronic events occurring when materials in tubular form were connected to an arteriovenous (AV) shunt in the baboon. In particular, platelet consumption by the implanted materials received the most attention. The fourth project explored the mechanism by which the platelets were consumed by materials. A laser light scattering system was developed and used to measure the number, density, and size distributions of emboli generated by the AV shunt during both the acute and chronic phases of embolization. Using the same materials and a relevant, reproducible animal model allowed a systematic picture of the complete thrombotic process to be assembled.

Experimental

Preparation of Polymers and Materials Characterization. Techniques have been developed previously for the grafting of acrylamide to polymer substrates (13). These techniques were adapted so that the luminal surfaces of long tubes could be grafted. Silastic tubing (medical-grade Silastic, Dow Corning Inc., 0.125 in. i.d.) was cleaned by sonicating with Ivory soap solution (0.1%) flowing at 100 mL/min through the tube lumen. Three water rinses with flow and sonication followed. A portion of this tubing was radiation grafted to produce a polyacrylamide hydrogel luminal surface using a flow grafting apparatus described previously (14). (Electrophoresis-grade acrylamide monomer was obtained from Eastman Kodak.) A cupric nitrate solvent solution was used to inhibit homopolymerization during the grafting (15). A radiation dose of 0.25 Mrad was used, and the grafting temperature averaged 48°C over the course of the reaction.

Graft levels and graft water controls were measured using methods described previously (16). Scanning electron micrographs (SEMs) were taken using a JEOL JSM25 instrument with gold–palladium control specimens. Electron spectroscopy for chemical analysis (ESCA) spectra were taken on a Hewlett–Packard Model 5950B ESCA system. An 0.8-kW monochromatized x-ray beam from an aluminum anode was used for all spectra. An emission from an electron flood gun was used to neutralize static charge buildup on nonconducting polymeric surfaces. All aliphatic carbon 1s peaks were assigned a binding energy of 285.0 eV to correct for the energy shift resulting from the electron flood gun. Other element peak positions were shifted an amount corresponding to 285.0 eV (observed carbon 1s peak position).

Protein Adsorption Studies. Grafted or ungrafted Silastic materials in tubular form, each approximately 100 cm long × 0.3 cm i.d. were used. Baboon plasma was prepared from fresh baboon blood (anticoagulated by drawing it into 0.1 volume of acid citrate dextrose or ACD) by centrifugation, and was stored at −70°C. The buffer used for prefilling and rinsing was 0.01M citrate, 0.01M phosphate, 0.12M sodium chloride, and 0.02% sodium azide (CPBSz). Adsorbed proteins were eluted with 1% sodium dodecyl sulfate, 0.01M trisphosphate, pH 7 (SDS sample buffer). Immersible molecular sieves (Millipore, Immersible CX) were used to concentrate the eluates. SDS–polyacrylamide slab gel electrophoresis was done with the same buffers and chemicals described previously (17, 18), and with an apparatus obtained from Biorad (Model 220). The gels were 1.5 mm thick and contained 7.5% acrylamide. Staining the proteins with silver was based on a published procedure (19).

Adsorption of plasma proteins was studied by pumping 37°C plasma through the tubes (prefilled with degassed buffer at 37°C) for 2 h at 100 mL/min. Rinsing was done by pumping 37°C buffer through the tubes for 1 min. The tube was drained of the buffer, filled with SDS sample buffer, immersed in an ultrasonic bath kept at 50°C, and sonicated for 1 h. The eluate from each tube was then concentrated approximately tenfold and frozen at −70°C until electrophoresis was done.

Measurements of Platelet Consumption. A baboon AV shunt model was used to assess quantitatively the effects of physicochemical properties associated with polyacrylamide grafted substrates. In this model, measurements of platelet consumption using ^{51}Cr-labeled platelets were steady state, reproducible between test animals, and unaffected by the surgical procedure (8, 10). The methodology involved in the use of AV baboon shunts has been described previously (8, 10). We concluded that this primate model simulates arterial thrombotic processes in humans and is suitable for the in vivo evaluation of biomaterial thrombogenesis (10).

Laser Light Scattering Detection of Microemboli. To elucidate the mechanism of platelet destruction by grafted polyacrylamide–Silastic surfaces, an optical scattering technique was developed (20) to observe and quantitate the sizes and size distributions of microaggregates in blood produced within the AV baboon shunt. Presumably, any such flowing microaggregates represent platelet microemboli.

The optical scattering cuvette with which these measurements were made was placed at the distal tip of the biomaterial test shunt (Figure 1). The cuvette was constructed of a 1.0-mm diameter medical-grade Silastic tube, 5 mm long (Figure 2). Two 3-mm diameter Teflon tubes were used to connect the cuvette to the baboon shunt. The cuvette was encased in an aluminum housing that held three optical fibers in contact with and orthogonal to the Silastic flow tube. Light from a helium–neon laser was focused on one of the optical fibers, and the scattered intensity detected by the orthogonal arrangement of the other fibers was analyzed to determine the size and number density of thromboemboli produced in the shunt.

The formation of microaggregates by any particular shunt was determined by a series of optical sizing measurements consisting of 50 data acquisitions (25 60-s measurements were taken during the first hour, beginning immediately after the

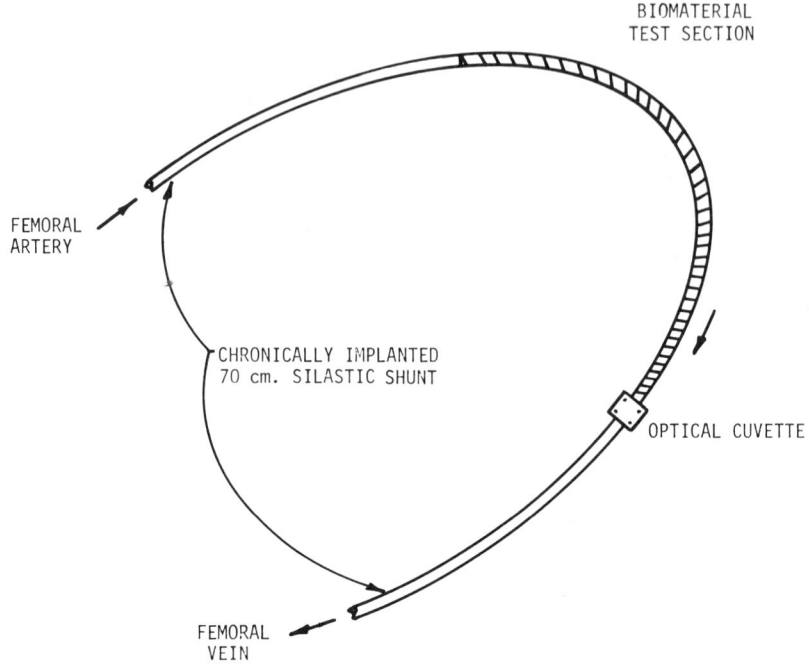

Figure 1. Schematic of optical scattering cuvette at distal end of shunt.

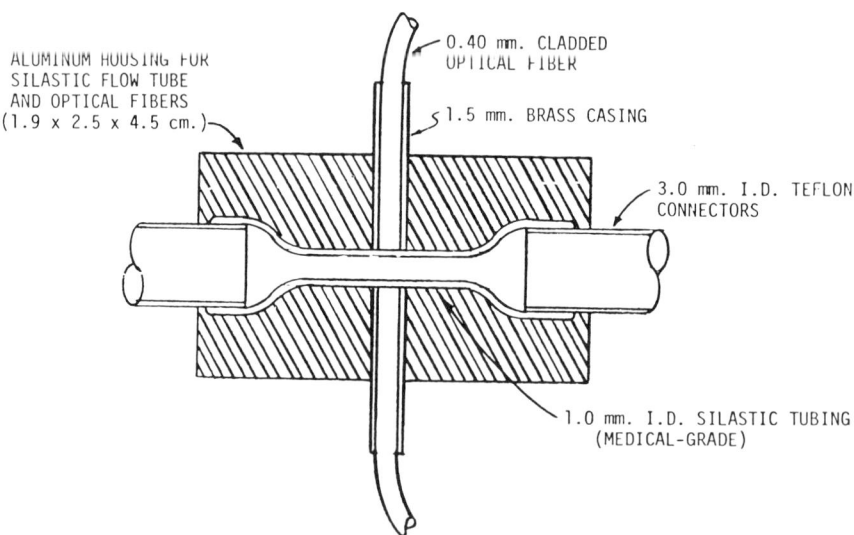

Figure 2. Detail of optical scattering cuvette.

initial blood–biomaterial interaction, and 25 data acquisitions, each 120 s long, were taken in the following 2 h). The size distribution of microaggregates from 20–800 μm in diameter and the number of emboli were measured during each datum acquisition. The system was calibrated using polystyrene microspheres before each experiment. (For details on this technique, see Ref. 20.) From the size distribution measurements, an equivalent rate of platelet thromboembolization (platelets/day) was calculated assuming that the thromboemboli were spheres composed of close-packed spherical platelets.

Results

Material Preparation and Characterization. The effect of cupric ion on acrylamide graft level, as determined in an experiment separate from the tubing preparation, is shown in Figure 3. Based on this result, a cupric nitrate concentration of $0.01M$ in the solvent was chosen.

Graft level (measured gravimetrically) as a function of distance from the pump is shown in Figure 4. The first 200 cm of tubing was discarded, resulting in a length of tubing with a graft level of 2.90 ± 0.34 mg/cm^2.

SEMs were used to compare, in a qualitative sense, the surface texture of the acrylamide-grafted Silastic and the ungrafted Silastic. Similar surface textures were noted in both cases (Figure 5). Because the acrylamide graft was dehydrated for SEM analysis, the graft also was observed in a hydrated

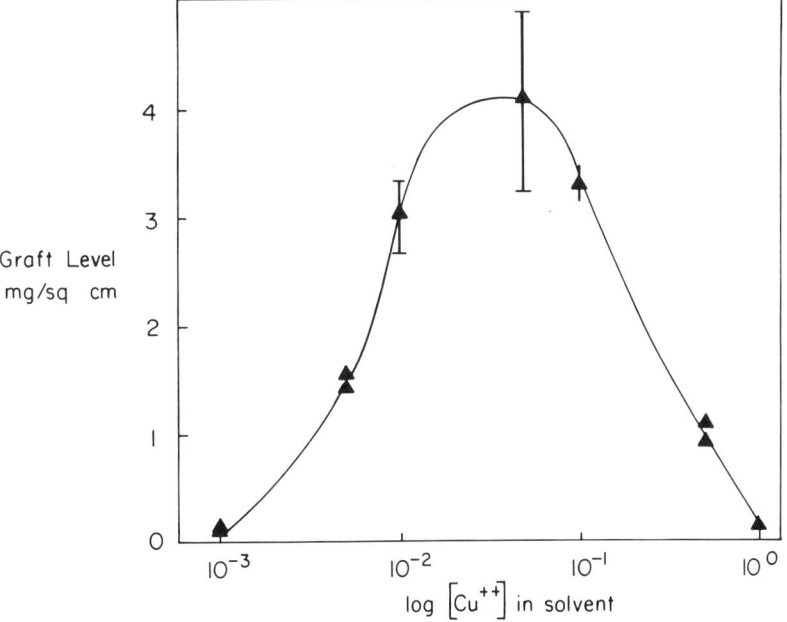

Figure 3. Effect of Cu^2 concentration on acrylamide grafting to 10-mil Silastic (0.375 Mrad).

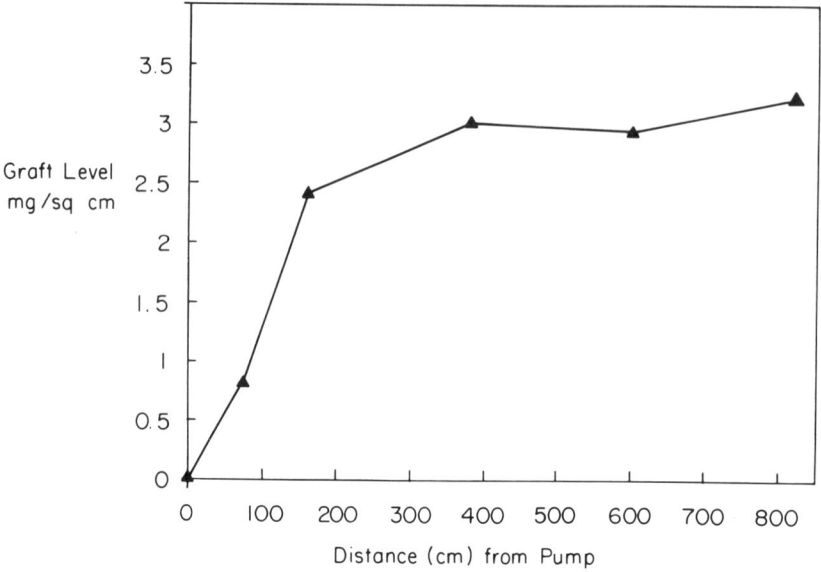

Figure 4. Graft level as a function of length along the shunt for polyacrylamide–Silastic shunts prepared using the flow-grafting apparatus described in Ref. 14.

state with a light stereomicroscope. Taking into account the resolution limits of such an instrument, the general surface texture of both surfaces still appeared to be similar.

Graft and substrate polymer surface chemistries were examined by the ESCA technique. ESCA spectra are shown in Figures 6 and 7. Surface elemental ratios determined by ESCA are compared with those expected, based on the stoichiometry in Table I. Close agreement exists between experimentally determined values and theory for untreated Silastic. However, the acrylamide graft surface is a mixture of polyacrylamide and polydimethylsiloxane. Earlier experiments using frozen, hydrated grafts have shown that, in the hydrated state, a much larger fraction of the graft surface will be attributable to polyacrylamide than in the dehydrated state (*21*) (Table I, Figure 8). However, silicon can be detected even in the hydrated state.

Further information on the surface chemistry of these materials can be obtained by examining the carbon 1s spectra in Figures 6 and 7. For Silastic, only one symmetrical peak with a full width at half maximum (fwhm) of 1.2 eV is expected in the carbon 1s spectrum; this peak is observed. For polyacrylamide, the comparison between a curve-resolved carbon 1s spectrum of a pure polymer sample (Figure 9a) and the dehydrated graft used in this study (Figure 7a) is instructive. The higher binding energy peak due to the carbon atom π-bonded to oxygen in the amide functionality is almost un-

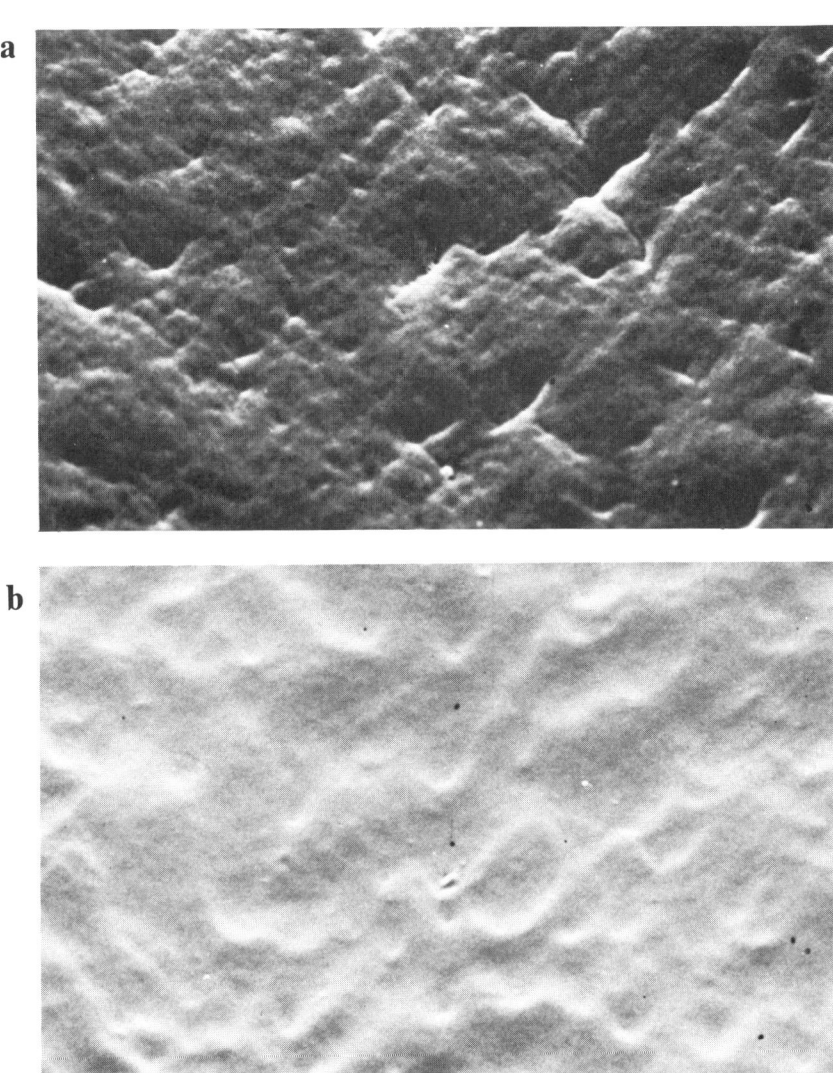

Figure 5. SEMs of (a) Silastic tubing, luminal surface, 100 ×, and (b) polyacrylamide–Silastic, luminal surface, 100 × (white bar = 100 μm).

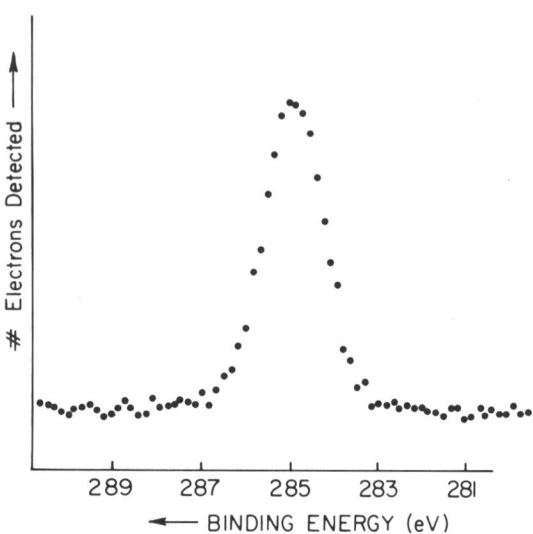

Figure 6a. ESCA C 1s spectrum of the luminal surface of Silastic tubing.

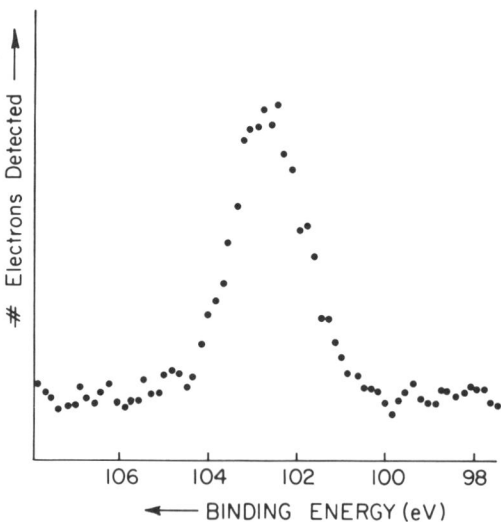

Figure 6b. ESCA Si 2p spectrum of the luminal surface of Silastic tubing.

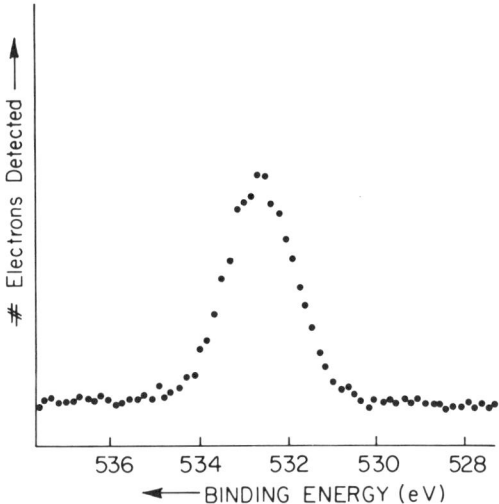

Figure 6c. ESCA O 1s spectrum of the luminal surface of Silastic tubing.

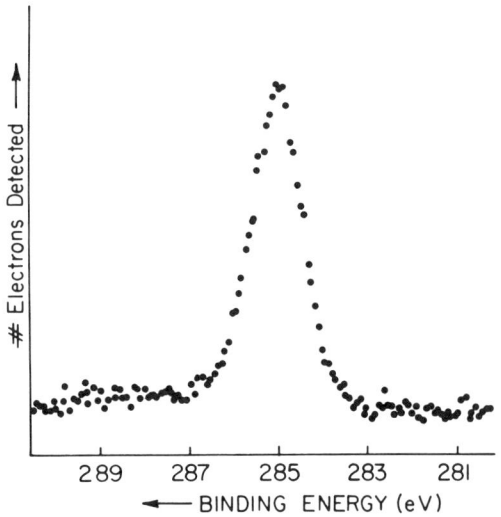

Figure 7a. ESCA C 1s spectrum of the luminal surface of polyacrylamide–Silastic tubing in the dehydrated state.

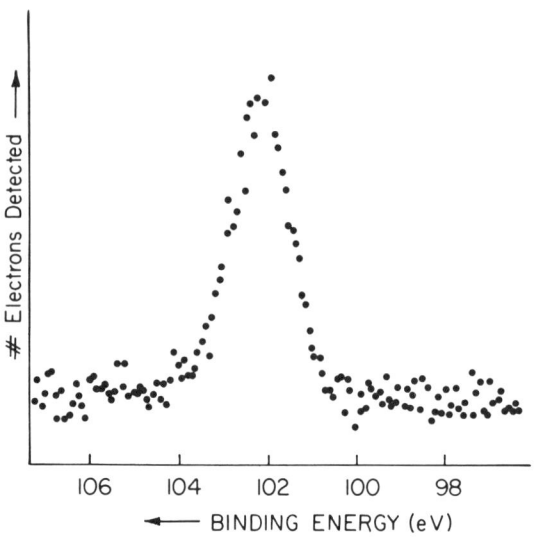

Figure 7b. ESCA Si 2p spectrum of the luminal surface of polyacrylamide–Silastic tubing in the dehydrated state.

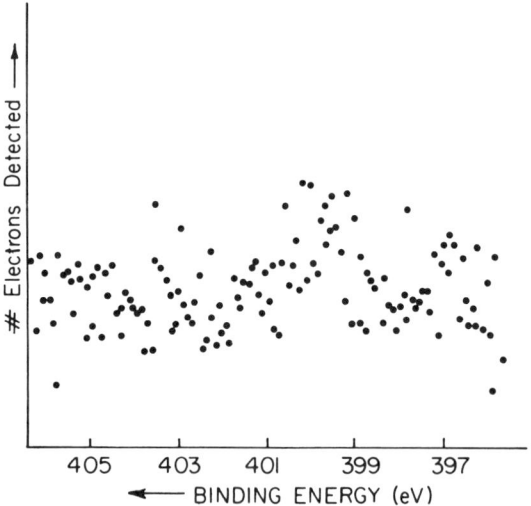

Figure 7c. ESCA N 1s spectrum of the luminal surface of polyacrylamide–Silastic tubing in the dehydrated state.

Table I. ESCA Elemental Ratios for Silastic and Acrylamide-Grafted Silastic

	Silastic		Acrylamide-Grafted Silastic (Dry)		Acrylamide-Grafted Silastic (Hydrated, 160K)	
	Theory	Experimental	Theory[a]	Experimental[b]	Theory[a]	Experimental[c]
C/O	2.0	2.1	3.0	—	—	0.41[d]
C/Si	2.0	1.7	∞	2.3	∞	2.5
C/N	—	—	3.0	54.9	3.0	3.41

[a] Complete coverage of the Silastic by a polyacrylamide film is assumed.
[b] Data from Figure 7.
[c] Data from Ref. 21, see Figure 8.
[d] The high levels of oxygen in this film indicate that the polymer is hydrated.

detectable at the graft surface. Again, in the hydrated state, an increased ratio of this peak to that at 285.0 eV occurred (Figure 8). A comparison of the nitrogen 1s signal for the dehydrated graft on Silastic (Figure 7c) and the pure polymer (Figure 9b) is also interesting in this regard. (This hydration–dehydration effect was discussed in the previous paragraph.)

Protein Adsorption. Since protein adsorption is the earliest event in the thrombotic response of the blood to polymers, the types of proteins adsorbed from plasma to polyacrylamide–Silastic and Silastic tubes were examined. As described in the Experimental section, plasma was recirculated through the tubes for 2 h at 37°C and rinsed away with buffer. The proteins adsorbed to the polymers were eluted with SDS, separated by SDS–polyacrylamide slab gel electrophoresis, and silver-stained using a new extremely sensitive method (19). Figure 10 shows the results of these assays.

A mixture of proteins of known molecular weights was separated on the polyacrylamide gel (#3 in Figure 10). The calibration plot obtained with this mixture was used to assign molecular weights to the unknown proteins in the eluates from the test surfaces. Approximately 0.08 μg of each calibration protein were needed to give a very clearly stained protein band, which is only 1% of the amount needed with other stains, such as Coomassie blue. In addition, in other experiments, fibrinogen, immunoglobulin G (IgG), albumin, and hemoglobin mixtures were separated on similar gels (not shown). Fibrinogen remained at the top of the gel, IgG occurred as a band between 102,000 and 132,000 Daltons, albumin occurred at 58,000 Daltons, and hemoglobin displayed a diffuse band centered at 15,000 Daltons. These molecular weights deviated from those usually observed for these proteins in SDS gel electrophoresis because the disulfide bonds were not reduced in the experiments reported here.

The eluate from polyacrylamide–Silastic had six distinct proteins in it (Gel 2 in Figure 10). The most prominent bands had molecular weights of

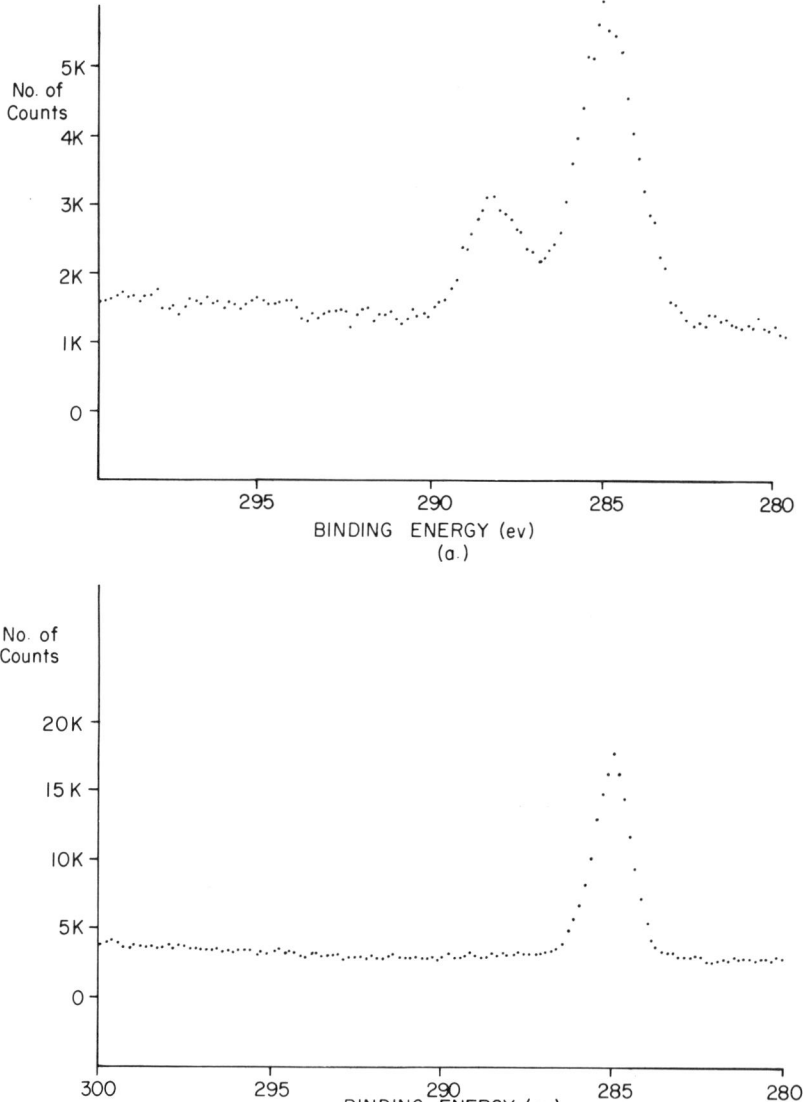

Figure 8. ESCA C 1s spectra for polyacrylamide–Silastic (21). Key: a, 160 K (hydrated) and b, 303 K (dehydrated).

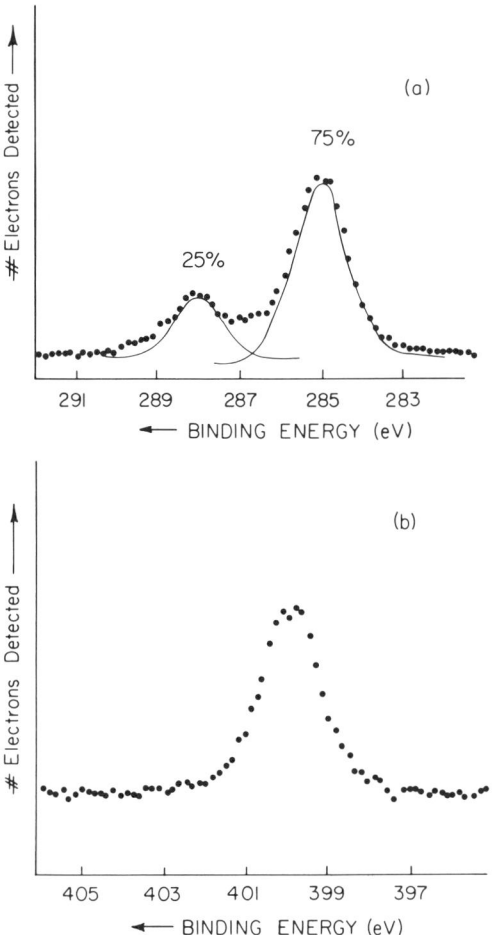

Figure 9. ESCA spectra of pure polyacrylamide film cast on glass. Key: a, C 1s spectrum resolved (using a DuPont 310 analog curve resolver) into its component peaks; and b, N 1s spectrum.

132,000, 58,000, and 21,000. Bands of lower intensity also occurred at 93,000, 70,000, and 16,000 Daltons.

The eluate from Silastic (Gel 1 in Figure 10) had only three visible bands, each of which was much less intense than the corresponding bands in the eluate from polyacrylamide–Silastic. Two of the bands from Silastic occurred at 131,000 and 58,000 Daltons, and had approximately the same stain intensity. A third band of even lower intensity occurred at 95,000 Daltons.

Measurements of Platelet Consumption. When the extent of grafting of acrylamide on Silastic was varied, cannular platelet consumption increased

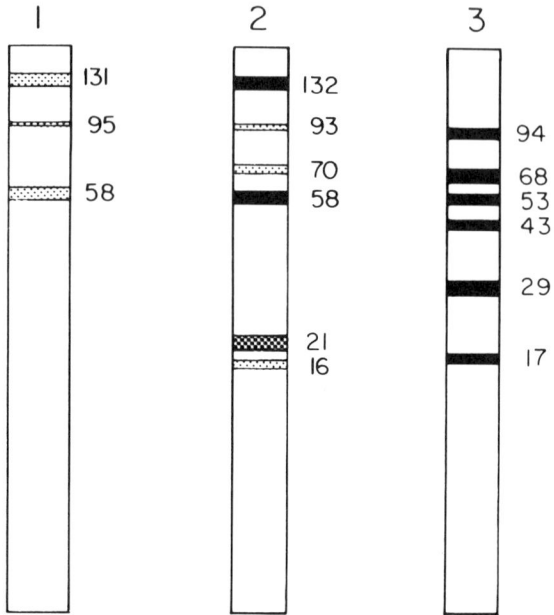

Figure 10. Analysis of adsorbed proteins with SDS-polyacrylamide gel electrophoresis.

Proteins eluted from Silastic (Gel 1) or polyacrylamide–Silastic (Gel 2) after exposure to plasma, and a mixture of known proteins (Gel 3), were separated and stained. The approximate positions, stain intensities, and molecular weights ($\times 10^{-3}$) are indicated in the diagram.

sharply as graft level increased from 0 to 1 mg/cm², and remained level thereafter (Figure 11). Thus, all grafted tubes in this study were grafted to levels well above 1 mg/cm².

Table II shows the effect on platelet consumption of increasing lengths of the polyacrylamide–Silastic tubing. The acrylamide surface is much more destructive to platelets than is the Silastic surface. Table II also shows that platelet consumption increases linearly with shunt area for both the polyacrylamide–Silastic shunts.

A series of shunts with radiation and ceric ion–initiated grafts of polyacrylamide on the luminal Silastic surface, and having water contents varying between 51–83% were also studied. Table III shows these data. The platelet consumption increases linearly with the gel water, such that the ratio of platelet consumption to graft water content remains relatively constant.

Laser Light Scattering Detection of Microemboli. The optical scattering technique was used to assess in vivo the thromboembolic propensity of polyacrylamide–Silastic and Silastic shunts of varying lengths. In four baboons, control measurements of the number and size distribution of thromboemboli produced by the 35-cm proximal section of the chronically

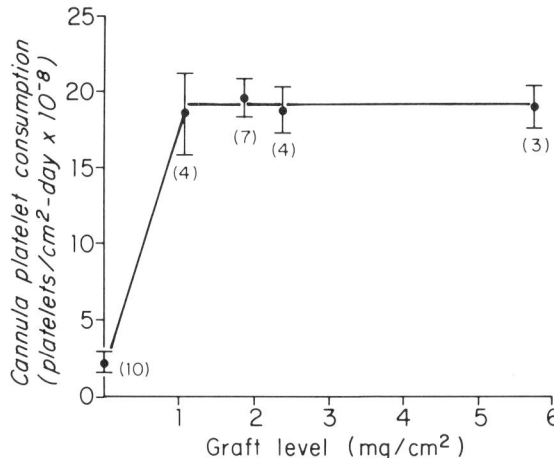

Figure 11. Platelet consumption vs. graft level of polyacrylamide–Silastic shunts (9). (Numbers in parentheses refer to the number of shunts tested for each value reported.)

implanted Silastic shunt were made during the acute phase of thromboembolization. This measurement also included endogenous circulating platelet aggregates. The baseline value of $(1.75 \pm 0.77) \times 10^9$ platelets/day, estimated from these measurements, subsequently was subtracted when calculating the total rate of production of embolus mass of a given test material. Good agreement existed between this baseline value and the rate of thromboembolus mass produced by a short 35-cm Silastic biomaterial test section placed proximal to the optical cuvette ($(2.14 \pm 0.07) \times 10^9$ platelets/day). Therefore, thromboemboli are generated on the basis of biomaterial surface area and are not effected significantly by the surgical procedure, the connectors, or any flow disturbance caused by the optical cuvette.

Table II. Effect of Cannula Composition and Area on Platelet Consumption (8)

Exposed Area (cm^2)	Mean Platelet Survival Time (days)	Cannula Platelet Consumption (platelets/day $\times 10^{-10}$)	Cannula Platelet Consumption/ Unit Area (platelets/cm^2 day $\times 10^{-8}$)
		Polyacrylamide-grafted Silastic	
16.6	4.2 ± 0.6	2.7 ± 1.5	16.3 ± 8.8
41.5	2.6 ± 0.2	7.5 ± 0.7	18.0 ± 1.6
83.0	1.5 ± 0.1	15.5 ± 1.7	18.6 ± 2.1
99.7	1.8 ± 0.4	18.2 ± 2.3	18.2 ± 2.3
		Silastic	
65.8	4.7 ± 0.1	0.8 ± 0.3	1.3 ± 0.3
131.7	4.0 ± 0.2	2.5 ± 0.4	1.9 ± 0.4

Note: Values are mean ± standard error.

Table III. Platelet Consumption by Polyacrylamide-Grafted Substrates (9)

Substrate	Method of Initiation	Water Content (W) (wt %)	Platelet Consumption[a] (PC) (platelets/cm^2-day × 10^{-8})	Ratio $\frac{(PC)}{(W)}$
Silastic/HEMA[b]	Ce^{4+}	50.8	16.4 ± 3.4 (3)	0.32
Silastic	^{60}Co rad'n.	60.8	19.0 ± 0.8 (18)	0.31
Silastic	^{60}Co rad'n.	83.0	27.2 ± 2.7 (5)	0.33

[a] Mean values are ± 1.0 standard error. The number of studies is in parentheses.
[b] Silastic pregrafted with 1.74 mg/cm^2 poly(2-hydroxyethyl methacrylate).

The analysis of the size and number of thromboemboli generated by grafts of polyacrylamide–Silastic and Silastic cannulae shows a consistent peak period of thromboembolization occurring in the first hour that is at least 3–5 times greater than the steady-state value occurring in the second and third hours. In addition, as shunt surface area increases, the average rate of platelet consumption due to embolization during the steady-state period increases linearly, for both shunt materials studied (Figure 12). Furthermore, the polyacrylamide–Silastic shunt produces significantly more thromboembolus mass than the Silastic shunt.

Discussion

Previous studies of the response of blood to polyacrylamide surfaces have demonstrated clear differences relative to other materials, especially silicone rubber. Early reports of "improved blood compatibility" of polyacrylamide were based on in vitro tests, such as Lee–White clotting times (5) and spinning-disc platelet adhesion results (7). This impression was reinforced when canine vena cava rings with grafted polyacrylamide–Silastic surfaces remained patent for 2 weeks, while untreated Silastic rings were occluded within 2 h (22, 23). However, when similar polyacrylamide–Silastic rings were implanted just above the canine renal arteries, numerous kidney infarcts were noted (23). Luminally grafted polyacrylamide–Silastic tubes were implanted subsequently as ex vivo AV shunts in sheep, and these tubes induced significantly greater platelet destruction than did the ungrafted Silastic (24). Taken together, these earlier studies suggested that contrary to the "conventional wisdom," polyacrylamide surfaces are in fact thrombogenic, but are not strongly thromboadherent. Such important differences in blood responses to polyacrylamide and Silastic surfaces have lead us to examine in greater detail the differences in their surface properties before, during, and after exposure to plasma proteins and blood, using a wide range of experimental protocols including the ex vivo baboon AV shunt model.

The radiation grafting technique used to prepare the polyacrylamide–Silastic grafts is a practical method for immobilizing the mechanically weak

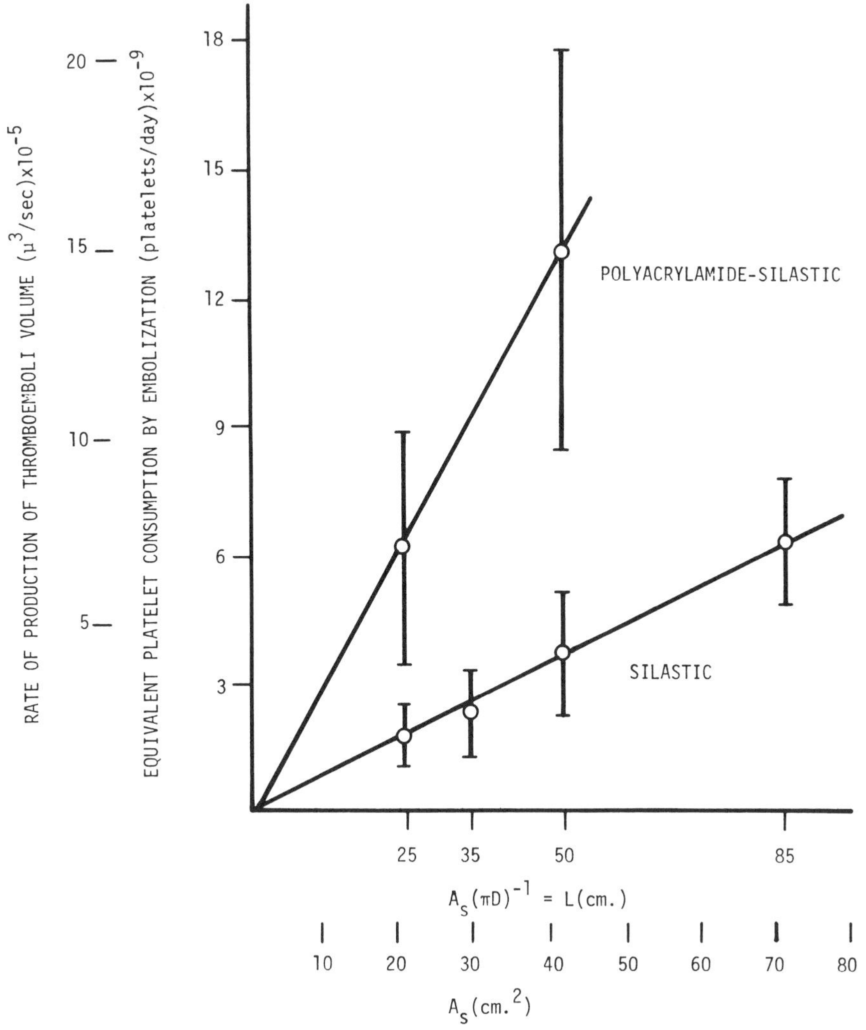

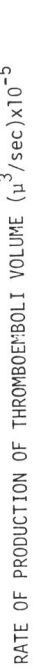

Figure 12. Rates of production of thromboemboli volume (μ^3/s) and equivalent platelet consumption by embolization (platelets/day) vs. surface area for two biomaterials: Silastic (bottom) and polyacrylamide–Silastic (top). The equivalent steady-state platelet consumption is $(3.0 \pm 0.2) \times 10^8$ (platelets/day-cm^2) for polyacrylamide–Silastic and $(0.8 \pm 0.1) \times 10^8$ (platelets/day-cm^2) for Silastic.

polyacrylamide hydrogel on the strong Silastic support. The use of cupric ion to inhibit acrylamide homopolymerization is essential to achieve significant grafting levels of polyacrylamide. Elemental analyses of the grafts show that no significant level of copper ion is retained in these grafts.

The surface chemistry of this acrylamide graft cannot be examined in the dehydrated state by ESCA in a biologically meaningful way (Table I, Figure 8) (*see* Ref. *21*). In the hydrated state, the graft surface is composed of polyacrylamide intermixed with polydimethylsiloxane. This complex surface raises some questions as to whether these graft surfaces are a good model for polyacrylamide. Two observations support our contention that these surfaces are, indeed, valid models for polyacrylamide. First, silicone rubber is among the most passive of materials we have seen with respect to platelet consumption. Therefore, silicone rubber chains in the graft surface probably would not influence the platelet consumption of a more consumptive material such as polyacrylamide. Second, baboon platelet consumptivities of a wide variety of hydrogels (not just polyacrylamide) grafted lumenally in Silastic and polyurethane shunts increase linearly with hydrogel water content (*9*). If the silicone chains were affecting the platelet consumption process, hydrogels grafted onto two different substrates probably would not have platelet consumptions governed only by graft water content.

The adsorption of plasma proteins to polymers precedes the interaction of blood cells with the surfaces, and therefore, is likely to be an important initial event in the response of blood to polymers (*25, 29*). At present, however, little is known about the adsorbed protein layer, even though it has been studied in some detail in recent years (*30–36*). Because protein adsorption from blood plasma is a competitive process, differences in the adsorbed layer on different polymer substrates could be a primary cause of differences in thrombogenicity. Previous studies of the composition of the adsorbed protein layer have employed ^{125}I-labeled protein added to plasma (*37–39*), antibody binding (*34*) to detect individual proteins, or electrophoretic analysis of detergent-elutable proteins (*17, 33, 35*). The procedure used in this study does not require the large surface areas used in previous work (*35*), nor does it rely on incorporation of radiolabels (*36*) into adsorbed protein. Instead, a staining method at least 100-fold more sensitive than these other techniques has been used.

The eluates from both polyacrylamide–Silastic and Silastic contained a protein occurring at the same molecular weight as albumin (58,000). Relatively large amounts of this protein in plasma give this protein a considerable competitive advantage over other plasma proteins, making its presence on biomaterial surfaces quite predictable (*37–39*). Albumin adsorption is generally thought to make surfaces less adhesive to platelets. The more intense staining observed for albumin in the eluate from polyacrylamide–Silastic compared to Silastic presumably indicates that the total amount of albumin is greater on polyacrylamide–Silastic than on Silastic. In previous studies, fluorescein-labeled protein uptake by polyacrylamide–Silastic films was used to distinguish absorption into the polyacrylamide gel from adsorption onto the gel surface (*40*). Albumin did not enter the gel, while chymotrypinogen (MW = 26,000) did. Therefore, the results presented here for proteins above this molecular weight most likely reflect surface adsorption. The greater absolute adsorption of albumin on polyacrylamide–Silastic may explain why these surfaces were not as thromboadherent as Silastic in the canine vena cava ring and renal embolus experiments.

The eluates from both polyacrylamide–Silastic and Silastic also contained a major protein at molecular weight 132,000, within the range observed for the IgG group. Because this group of glycoproteins is the next most common plasma after albumin, the presence of these molecules on surfaces is also not surprising (*34–36, 38, 39*). Recent experiments in a number of laboratories have suggested an important role for leukocytes in the process of thrombogenesis on artificial surfaces (*41–43*), and have indicated a role for IgG in mediating the white cell response at foreign interfaces (*44, 45*).

Because fibrinogen remains at the gel top in the electrophoresis system used here, we cannot assess its importance because staining artifacts frequently occur at the gel top. However, adsorption of ^{125}I-fibrinogen to polyacrylamide–Silastic shunt surfaces from baboon blood in vivo is much greater than adsorption to Silastic shunt surfaces (*46*).

When the greater adsorption of albumin to polyacrylamide–Silastic (as observed by the electrophoresis technique) is taken together with the higher fibrinogen adsorption on these surfaces (as observed in the baboon shunt), the following explanation of the greater thromboembolic potential of polyacrylamide–Silastic surfaces may be proposed: Platelets encountering this surface may become activated by the high local concentration of fibrinogen at its surface, leading to aggregation on or near the sites of platelet aggregation. However, these platelet aggregates do not adhere very long or very strongly because of the high level of adsorbed albumin in the vicinity. Alternatively, the role of other proteins observed in the eluate from polyacrylamide–Silastic, such as IgG and other minor proteins at molecular weights 93,000, 70,000 (prothrombin?), 21,000, and 16,000 (hemoglobin?), may be more important than previously thought. More extensive study of the protein adsorption process clearly is needed.

The laser scattering technique is newly developed, and probably will be extremely valuable in quantitating the differences in embolic events during blood–material interactions, and thus potentially useful in elucidating the mechanisms responsible for these differences.

For example, the volume of microaggregates flowing through the cuvette at any time can be estimated from the size distribution, assuming that the microaggregates are composed of close-packed spherical platelets and that the emboli are nearly spherical. Although these assumptions, at present, are somewhat restrictive, the total volumes of embolus mass estimated from these distributions compare well with measurements of embolus volume made with the Coulter counter and with embolus mass estimated by screen filtration pressure (20). The cannula platelet consumption values are shown in Figure 11. In comparing Figures 11 and 12, the (optically) estimated platelet consumption of the polyacrylamide–Silastic cannulae is greater than the Silastic cannula only by a factor of about 3.0–4.0, while the ^{51}Cr-labeled platelet technique showed that the surfaces differed in platelet consumption by a factor of about 10.0. The difference between these two measurement techniques may be due to very small or very large platelet aggregates that are not included in the optical scattering measurements; to errors in the calculations due to the assumption of spherical platelets and microemboli; to discrepencies between the time at which the steady-state measurements were made in the two techniques (3 h in the optical technique vs. several days in the ^{51}Cr survival measurements); and/or to additional mechanisms of platelet consumption such as platelet lysis or the destruction of single cells. Additional factors include the possibility of both reversibly and irreversibly aggregated microemboli, and may represent another source of discrepancy between the ^{51}Cr data and the optical sizing measurements. Although a difference exists between the platelet consumption for polyacrylamide–Silastic estimated optically and that calculated from ^{51}Cr-labeled platelets, good agreement exists between the Silastic platelet consumptions calculated by both techniques. Both techniques predict a linear increase in platelet consumption (embolization) with an increase in cannula surface area.

Conclusions

Polyacrylamide–Silastic hydrogel surfaces are more polar, more water-swollen, and more porous to smaller molecules and proteins than the control Silastic surfaces, and they are more platelet consumptive than Silastic surfaces in the AV baboon shunt. This increased destruction of platelets is manifested by greater formation and shedding of microemboli (platelet aggregates) from the hydrogel surfaces. The polyacrylamide–Silastic surfaces adsorb more proteins overall than Silastic, and in particular, adsorb more of both albumin and fibrinogen. Thus, when compared to Silastic surfaces, the polyacrylamide–Silastic hydrogel surface probably has a combination of lower adherence to platelets (higher albumin) but higher activity toward platelet aggregation (higher fibrinogen). This situation could lead to low platelet residence times on the hydrogel surface combined with a high probability of activation and aggregation on or near the surface. On the other hand, other minor proteins observed on the polyacrylamide–Silastic surface, but not on the Silastic surface, may possibly play a significant role in thrombogenesis and embolization on the polyacrylamide hydrogel surfaces.

Acknowledgment

The authors acknowledge the support of the Devices and Technology Branch of the National Heart, Lung, and Blood Institute of the National Institutes of Health (Contract NO1–HB–2970 and Grant HL–22163).

Literature Cited

1. Hoffman, A. S. In "Polymers in Medicine and Surgery"; Kronenthal, R. L.; Oser, Z.; Martin, E., Eds.; Plenum: New York, 1975; p. 33.
2. Ratner, B. D.; Hoffman, A.S. In "Hydrogels for Medical and Related Applications"; Andrade, J. D., Ed.; ACS Symposium Series No. 31, ACS: Washington, DC, 1976, p. 1.
3. Ratner, B. D. In "Biocompatibility of Clinical Implant Materials"; Williams, D. F., Ed.; CRC: Boca Raton, FL, to be published.
4. Halpern, B. D.; Cheng, H.; Kuo, S.; Greenberg, H. In "Proc. Artif. Heart. Prog. Conf.," Hegyeli, R. J., Ed.; Washington, DC, 1969; p. 87.
5. Bruck, S. D. *Biomater. Med. Devices Artif. Organs* **1973**, *1*, 79.
6. Kearny, J. J.; Amara, I.; McDevitt, N. B. In "Biomedical Applications of Polymers"; Gregor, H. P., Ed.; Plenum: New York, 1975; p. 75.
7. Leonard, E. et al. "Coordinated Studies of Platelet and Protein Reactions in the Artificial Heart," Annual Report, NO1–HB–3–2910; available as PB–241–333/ AS N.T.I.S., Springfield, VA, Nov. 1975.
8. Hanson, S. R.; Harker, L. A.; Ratner, B. D.; Hoffman, A. S. *J. Lab. Clin. Med.* **1980**, *95*, 289.
9. Hanson, S. R.; Harker, L. A.; Ratner, B. D.; Hoffman, A. S. *Ann. Biomed. Eng.* **1979**, *7*, 357.
10. Harker, L. A.; Hanson, S. R. *J. Clin. Invest.* **1979**, *64*, 559.
11. Ihlenfeld, J. V.; Mathis, T. R.; Barker, T. A.; Mosher, D. F.; Riddle, L. M.; Hart, A. P.; Updike, S. J.; Cooper, S. L. *Trans. Am. Soc. Artif. Intern. Organs* **1978**, *24*, 727.
12. Todd, M. E.; McDevitt, E.; Goldsmith, E. J. *J. Med. Primatol.* **1972**, *1*, 132.
13. Hoffman, A. S.; Ratner, B. D. *J. Rad. Phys. Chem.* **1980**, *14*, 831–840.
14. Ratner, B. D.; Balisky, T.; Hoffman, A. S. *J. Bioengineering* **1977**, *1*, 115.
15. Ratner, B. D.; Hoffman, A. S. *J. Appl. Polym. Sci.* **1974**, *18*, 3183–3204.
16. Sasaki, T.; Ratner, B. D.; Hoffman, A. S. In "Hydrogels for Medical and Related Applications"; Andrade, J. D., Ed.; ACS Symposium Series No. 31, ACS: Washington, DC, 1976, p. 283.
17. Weathersby, P. K.; Horbett, T. A.; Hoffman, A. S. *Trans. Am. Soc. Artif. Intern. Organs* **1976**, *22*, 242.
18. Weber, K.; Osborn, M. *J. Biol. Chem.* **1969**, *244*, 4406.
19. Switzer, R. C.; Merrill, C. R.; Shifrin, S. *Anal. Biochem.* **1979**, *98*, 231–237.
20. Reynolds, L. O.; Simon, T. L. *Transfusion* **1980**, *20*(6), 669–678.
21. Ratner, B. D.; Weathersby, P. K.; Hoffman, A. S.; Kelly, M. A.; Scharpen, L. H. *J. Appl. Polym. Sci.* **1978**, *122*, 643–664.
22. Ratner, B. D.; Hoffman, A. S.; Whiffen, J. D. *J. Bioeng.* **1978**, *2*, 313–323.
23. Ratner, B. D.; Hoffman, A. S.; Hanson, S. R.; Harker, L. A.; Whiffen, J. D. *J. Polym. Sci., Polymer Symp.* **1979**, *66*, 363.
24. Hoffman, A. S. "Interaction of Natural and Chemically Modified Aortic Tissue Proteins with Blood," NHLBI Annual Report Contract NO1–HV–42970, July, 1975–June, 1976.
25. Salzman, E. W. *Bull. N.Y. Acad. Med.* **1972**, *48*, 225.
26. Bruck, S. D. *Biomed. Mater. Symp.* **1977**, *8*, 1.
27. Baier, R. E. *Ann. N.Y. Acad. Sci.* **1977**, *283*, 17.
28. Baier, R. E.; Dutton, R. C.; *J. Biomed. Mater. Res.* **1969**, *3*, 191.

29. Vroman, L.; Adams, A. L. *J. Biomed. Mater. Res.* **1969**, *3*, 43.
30. Morrissey, B. W.; Stromberg, R. R. *J. Colloid Interface Sci.* **1974**, *46*, 152.
31. Nyilas, E.; Chiu, T.-H.; Herzberger, G. A. *Trans. Am. Soc. Artif. Intern. Organs* **1974**, *20*, 480.
32. McMillan, C. R.; Sarto, H.; Ratnoff, O. D.; Walton, A. G. *J. Clin. Invest.* **1974**, *54*, 1312.
33. Lyman, D. J.; Metcalf, L. C.; Albo, D.; Richards, K. F.; Lamb, J. *Trans. Am. Soc. Artif. Intern. Organs* **1974**, *20*, 474.
34. Vroman, L.; Adams, A. L.; Klings, M.; Fischer, G. In ACS Advances in Chemistry Series No. 145, ACS: Washington, DC, 1975, p. 255.
35. Limber, G. K.; Mason, R. G. *Thromb. Res.* **1975**, *6*, 421.
36. Lee, R. G.; Adamson, C.; Kim, S. W. *Thromb. Res.* **1974**, *4*, 485.
37. Kim, S. W.; Wisniewski, S.; Lee, E. S.; Winn, M. L. *Biomed. Mater. Symp.* **1977**, *8*, 23.
38. Horbett, T. A.; Weathersby, P. K.; Hoffman, A. S. *J. Bioeng.* **1977**, *1*, 61.
39. Horbett, T. A.; Weathersby, P. K.; Hoffman, A. S. *Thromb. Res.* **1978**, *12*, 319–329.
40. Hoffman, A. S.; Horbett, T. A.; Ratner, B. D. "Interaction of Natural and Chemically Modified Aortic Tissue Proteins with Blood," Annual Report, N.T.I.S. Springfield, VA, Aug., 1977.
41. Van Kanpen, C. L.; Gibbons, D. F. *J. Biomed. Mater. Res.* **1979**, *13*, 517–541.
42. White, D. C.; Trepmon, E.; Kolobow, T.; Sheffer, D. K.; Reddick, R. L.; Bowman, R. L. *Artif. Organs* **1979**, *3*, 86–91.
43. Lederman, D. M.; Cumming, R. D.; Petschek, H. E.; Levine, P. H.; Kunsky, N. I. *Trans. Am. Soc. Artif. Intern. Organs* **1978**, *25*, 557–560.
44. Barber, T. A.; Mathis, T.; Cooper, S. L.; Ihlenfeld, J. V.; Mosher, D. F. *Scanning Electron Microsc. II* **1978**, 431–440.
45. Barber, T. A.; Lambrecht, L. K.; Mosher, D. F.; Cooper, S. L. *Scanning Electron Microsc. III*, **1979**, 881–890.
46. Cheng, C.-M., unpublished data, Master's Thesis research, University of Washington, Seattle, 1980.

RECEIVED for review January 16, 1981. ACCEPTED April 13, 1981.

Plasma Interaction on Block Copolymers as Determined by Platelet Adhesion

MICHAEL N. HELMUS[1], OM P. MALHOTRA, and DONALD F. GIBBONS

Case Western Reserve University, Departments of Biomedical Engineering and Pathology, Cleveland, OH 44106

A series of block copolymers, with controllable domain morphology, were tested to determine the effect of surface wettability, morphology, and chemistry on the attachment of platelets. The surfaces were first exposed to a plasma for 3 s or 3 min, and then to platelets suspended in Tyrode's buffer in 0.35% albumin (pH 7.4). The most hydrophobic surface, styrene–butadiene–styrene (SBS) attached the most platelets, followed by the less hydrophobic polyurethane, and lastly the hydrophilic polystyrene–poly(ethylene oxide) (PS–PEO), which attached essentially none. Phase separation in polyurethane and in SBS significantly ($P < 0.025$) increased the adherence of platelets after exposure to platelet-poor plasma, for 3 s and 3 min, respectively. No such difference was observed in PS–PEO. The SBS, with and without long-range order, attached significantly ($P < 0.025$) more platelets at 3 s than at 3 min. The SBS block copolymer, as compared with hydrophobic glass, appears to adsorb fibrinogen loosely, but more tightly than hydrophilic glass. Phase separation causes the protein to attach more strongly.

The initial event that occurs when blood contacts a foreign surface is the adsorption of plasma proteins, followed by a complex series of reactions that include the activation of blood-clotting enzymes, and adhesion and activation of blood platelets and leukocytes; desorption and/or further adsorption of proteins may occur also (1, 2). Generally, when intact plasma comes in contact with artificial surfaces, fibrinogen is the most commonly deposited protein. On hydrophilic, glass-like surfaces, but not on hydro-

[1] Current address: C. R. Bard, Inc., Bard Implants Division, Billerica, MA 01821.

phobic materials, the adsorbed fibrinogen molecules appeared to be altered by the plasma, as the molecules lost their ability to react immunologically with antifibrinogen sera. This change in response, called "conversion", was at first thought to be due to some conformational change in the fibrinogen molecules (3). Now, however, conversion is related to desorption followed by deposition of other plasma protein(s), primarily high molecular weight kininogen (4).

The change in biological response of the adsorbed fibrinogen molecule (conversion), is also noticeable with platelet adhesion studies. In confirmation of earlier studies of Zucker and Vroman (5), we found that, usually, less platelets adhered to areas of glass slides exposed to platelet-poor plasma for 3 min than areas exposed for 3 s. When, however, a gel-filtered platelet suspension was used in place of platelet-rich plasma, a dramatic difference in the number of platelets attached to the surface previously exposed to platelet-poor plasma for 3 s or 3 min occurred. Therefore, this more reproducible protocol was used to study not only the adhesion of platelets onto artificial surfaces but also as a probe of conversion. For this purpose we chose a series of block copolymers with controllable domain morphology (phase separation on a molecular scale) and different surface energies (wettability). Previous studies have shown that the degree of phase separation influences the interactions with blood components (6, 7).

Experimental

The hydrophobic polyurethane block copolymer was chosen because phase-separated samples had been shown by an in vitro assay to exhibit a greater platelet adhesion from human blood than samples having a mixed, nonphase-separated structure (7). The hydrophobic styrene–butadiene–styrene (SBS) block copolymer was chosen because of the ease with which the morphology could be controlled (8). The block copolymer having hydrophilic blocks of poly(ethylene oxide) and hydrophobic polystyrene blocks (PS–PEO) was chosen to examine the effect of the more hydrophilic blocks on the protein interaction.

The platelet assays were carried out on polymer films cast onto microscope slides precleaned in a hot sulfuric–chromic acid solution (Chromerge). The domain structures of the polymer films were characterized with transmission electron microscopy (TEM). The surface morphology of the cast films was visualized using reflected light, differential interference constrast (Nomarski) microscopy, with a Zeiss Ultraphot II microscope. The surface energy (9) and critical surface tension (10) were calculated from advancing contact angle measurements. The contact angles were measured with a goniometer telescope for a series of diagnostic liquids: water, glycerol, ethylene glycol, benzyl alcohol, and methylnaphthalene.

Polyurethane. [This polymer was supplied by R. A. Auerbach, Lord Corporation.] The polyurethane was composed of a soft segment of poly(tetramethylene glycol) with a molecular weight of 1000 and a hard segment of p-diphenylmethane 4,4'-diisocyanate (MDI), and was chain extended with ethylenediamine (7). A solution of 7 wt % polyurethane in N,N-dimethylacetamide was used to cast the films. The phase-separated samples (ANN) were prepared by annealing the film at 135°C for 90 min in a helium atmosphere, and the mixed, nonphase-separated samples (NEQ) were prepared by casting a 0.005-in. film with a Gardner casting knife and rapidly evaporating the solvent under vacuum. The MDI domains in the phase-separated state previously had been shown to be 60 Å with an interdomain distance of 120 Å (7). Normarski microscopy demonstrated that both morphologies exhibited a smooth, defect-free surface at a magnification of 770×. The surface energy and critical surface tension are given in Table I. No effect of morphology on contact angle was observed.

Styrene–Butadiene–Styrene (SBS). This polymer was provided by J. St. Clair, Shell Development Company. Kraton 1101 is a triblock copolymer composed of 30 wt % styrene, molecular weight 14,000, and butadiene, molecular weight 67,000 (8). The morphology was controlled by the evaporation rate of the solvent. A solution of 5 wt % SBS, in analytical-grade toluene, was used to cast the films. The mixed state (M) was prepared by casting a 0.005-in. film with a Gardner casting knife on slides preheated to 50°C. The phase-separated state (S) was prepared by slow evaporation of the solvent, by casting in an enclosure connected to toluene at 0°C; this process produced a constant, but low toluene vapor pressure in the enclosure, and thus a constant, slow-driving force for solvent removal. The films were heated at 55°C in vacuum for 2 days to ensure solvent removal. Thin films for TEM were prepared under similar conditions, but were cast from a 0.01 wt % solution in toluene. These films were stained with OsO_4, which preferentially stains the butadiene phase. Figure 1 is a TEM micrograph of the mixed state showing irregular and interconnected styrene-rich domains. Thus the "ideal" mixed state was not achieved and some initial segregation of the styrene was present. Figure 2 shows the phase-separated state with irregular spherical or ellipsoidal styrene domains, with approximately 200 Å dimen-

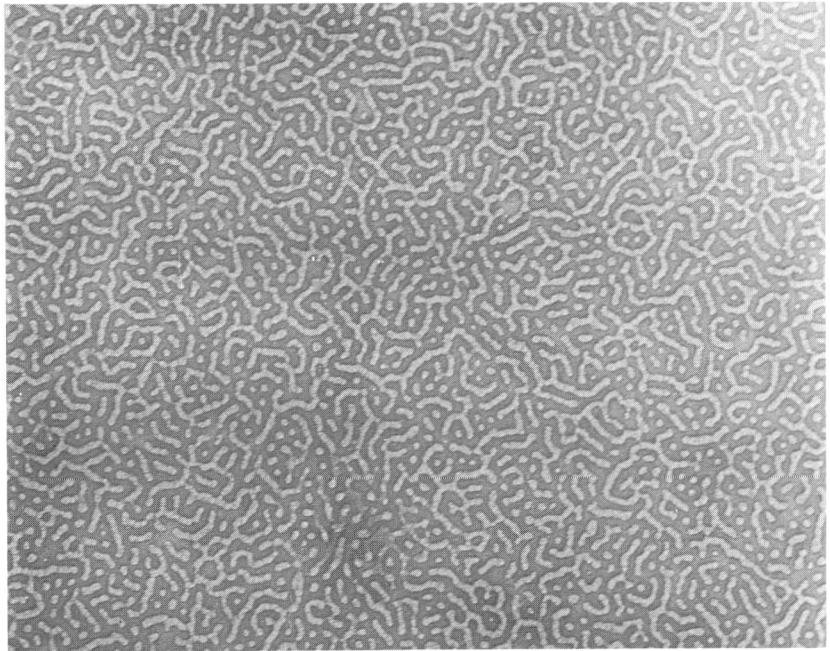

Figure 1. SBS (M) TEM micrograph of irregular styrene domains (white phase) in butadiene matrix (48,000×).

sions. The domains have a hexagonal packing in the butadiene matrix and are oriented in grains of approximately 1 μm. A small number of grains containing rods parallel to the surface were also observed (Figure 2). Nomarski microscopy showed the surface of the mixed-stated (M) film to be featureless at a magnification of 770×. However, the phase-separated state (S) showed polygonal valleys surrounded by ridges (Figure 3). Utilizing interferometry with the Nomarski optics, the height of the ridges was less than 0.15 μm, the limit of resolution for the optics used. The surface energy and critical surface tension are given in Table I. No effect of morphology on contact angle was observed.

Polystyrene–Poly(ethylene oxide) (PS–PEO). This polymer was provided by J. J. O'Malley, Xerox Corporation. The PS–PEO contained 66.7 wt % PS, and had a number-average molecular weight of 46,800 for PS and 23,400 for PEO (11). A 5 wt % solution in chloroform was used to cast the films. A 0.005-in. film was cast with a Gardner casting knife, and the solvent was evaporated under vacuum to produce the mixed state (Mx). Phase-separated films (Sty) were prepared by casting in an enclosure containing chloroform, and were maintained at low humidity with a desiccant. Before use, the films were maintained in a vacuum at 40°C for 16 h to ensure solvent removal. Thin films for TEM were prepared by casting directly onto copper grids with a 0.01 wt % PS–PEO solution in chloroform. The films were stained with OsO_4 for 4 h; the PS phase stained preferentially (11). The mixed-state samples (Mx) exhibited a uniform granular structure, all features being less than 60 Å (Figure 4). The phase-separated state (Sty) consisted of spherical polystyrene domains, 30–500 Å in di-

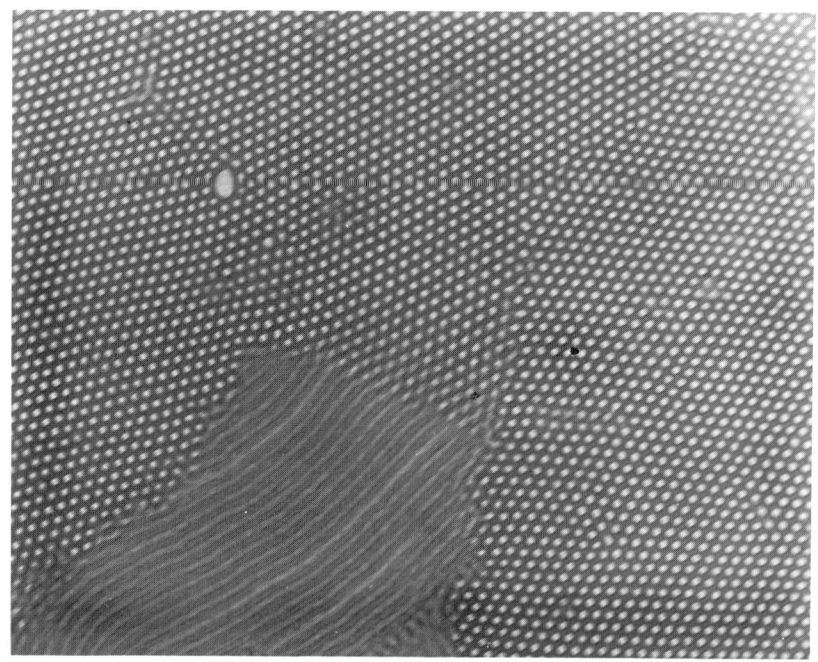

Figure 2. SBS (S) TEM micrograph of spherical styrene domains (white phase) hexagonally packed in grains of about 1.5 × 0.5 μm (48,000×).

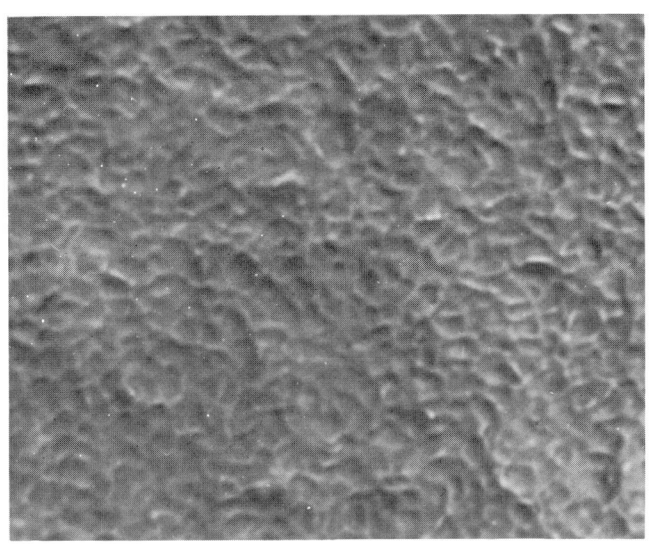

Figure 3. SBS (S) Nomarski micrograph of surface texture of polygonal valleys of 3 μm in diameter (1188×).

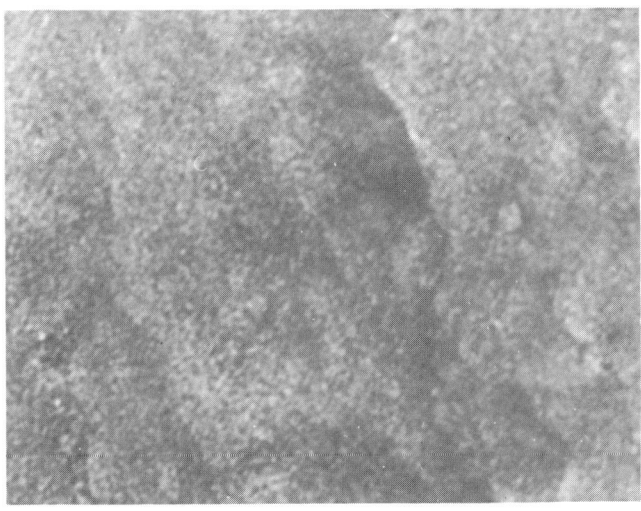

Figure 4. PS–PEO (Mx) TEM micrograph of uniform granular appearance of PS (dark phase) and PEO domains of equal size (145,000×).

Table I. Contact Angle Analysis[a]

Material	Contact Angle of Water		Surface Tension $\gamma_S \pm SE$	% Polarity (γ_p)	Critical Surface Tension (γ_C)
	Advancing	Receeding			
Styrene—butadiene—styrene—mixed spheres	94°	92°	26 ± 5 dyn/cm	12 (2)[b]	34 (3)[c] dyn/cm
	92°	38°	25 ± 5	15 (2)	33 (3)
Polystyrene—poly(ethylene oxide)—mixed spheres	73°–45°	0°	39 ± 4	1 (5)	38 (4)
	54°–45°	0°	39 ± 4	2 (5)	38 (4)
Polyurethane—nonequilibrium	70°	—[d]	39 ± 1	18 (9)	37 (5)
annealed	70°	—[d]	39 ± 1	18 (9)	37 (5)
Control glass—hydrophobic	76°	74°	—	—	—
hydrophilic	5°	0°	—	—	—

[a] A minimum of two samples of material were used for the analysis. Only liquids that did not swell or spread were used in the calculation.
[b] Number of pairs of liquids used in the analysis.
[c] Number of liquids used in the analysis.
[d] Not measured.

ameter, in a matrix of PEO (Figure 5). Nomarski microscopy showed the mixed state (Mx) to have a surface texture of approximately 1.0 μm in diameter (Figure 6). The phase-separated films (Sty) showed a rough surface texture with dimensions of 1–7 μm (Figure 7). Both morphologies exhibited smooth surfaces when equilibrated with water; however, surface patterns reminiscent of the dehydrated surface textures could still be discerned. The surface energy is given in Table I. However, because the polymer absorbed water up to 50% of its initial dry weight, the contact angle decreased with time (both morphologies approaching the same value of 45°). The other diagnostic liquids showed no observable differences in contact angles between the two morphologies.

Glass Control Surfaces. The hydrophilic control glasses were prepared by cleaning glass microscope slides with detergent (Sparkleen), and the hydrophobic control glasses were prepared by siliconizing (Siliclad) the microscope slides.

Human platelet-rich and platelet-poor plasmas were obtained from blood drawn by venipuncture into a 10-mL, siliconized Vacutainer (Becton Dickinson) anticoagulated with 0.11M sodium citrate in a 9:1 ratio. All donors had fasted overnight and had not taken medication for at least 2 weeks. Platelet-rich plasma was prepared by placing the anticoagulated blood in polypropylene tubes and centrifuging at 77 g for 10 min at room temperature. Platelet-poor plasma was prepared by centrifuging the blood at 23,000 g for 10 min. Platelet counts were performed using a Coulter counter; the platelet-rich plasma had a concentration of 270,000–320,000 platelets/mm^3.

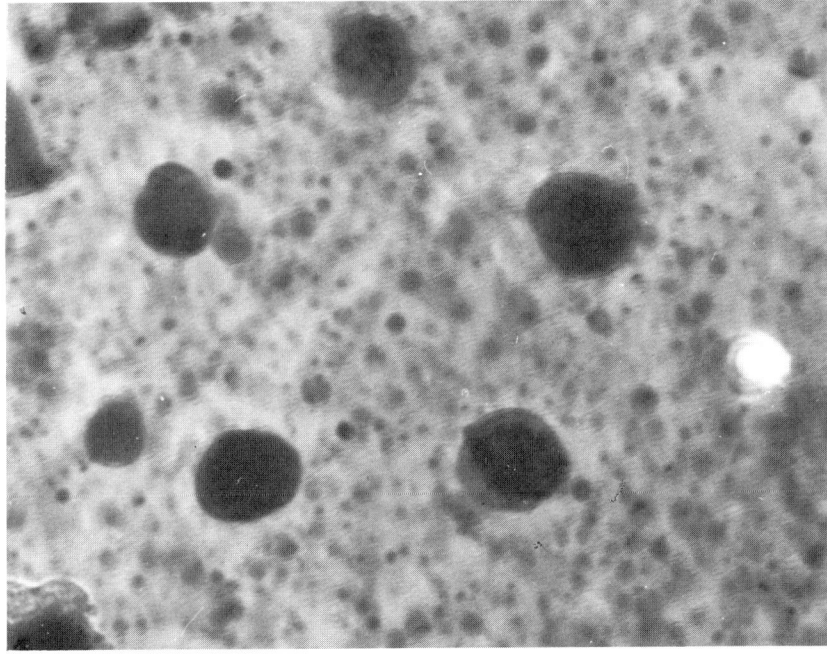

Figure 5. PS–PEO (Sty) TEM micrograph of PS domains (dark phase) of 30–500 Å (246,000×).

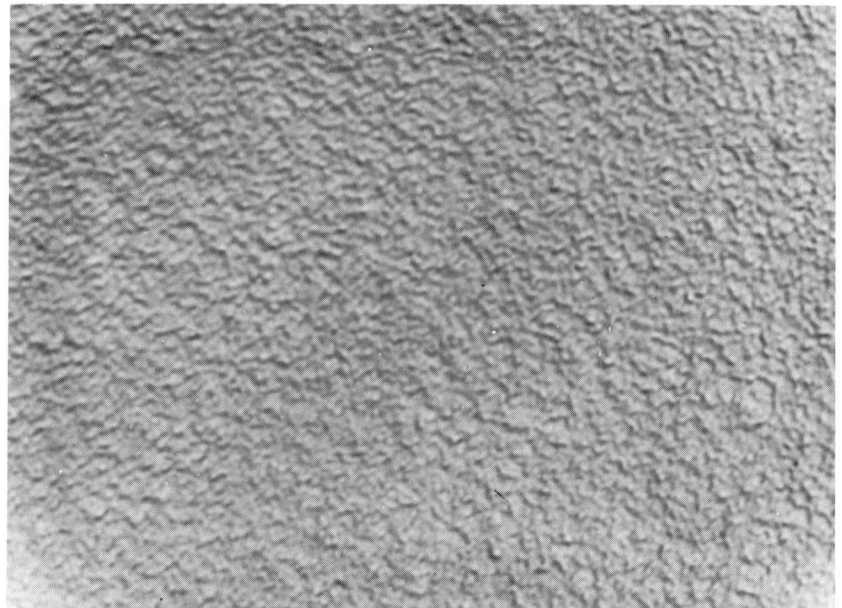

Figure 6. PS–PEO (Mx) Nomarski micrograph of surface texture of about 1-μm diameter valleys (1188×).

Platelet suspension was obtained by passing platelet-rich plasma through a sepharose 2B (Pharmacia) column (1.6 × 20 cm) equilibriated in calcium-free Tyrode buffer [0.137M NaCl, 2.7 mM KCl, 12 mM NaHCO$_3$, 0.36mM NaH$_2$PO$_4$ H$_2$O, and 5.6mM glucose (pH 7.4)] containing 0.35% bovine albumin (3 × crystallized, Sigma). Then, 1.6-mL fractions of platelets suspended in Tyrode buffer with albumin were collected at a flow rate of 0.8 mL/min. The platelet count of the platelet suspension (pooled fractions) was 186,500 ± 26,500 platelets/mm^3.

Platelet adhesion experiments, carried out at room temperature, were completed in approximately 3 h. To avoid the air interface, a drop of 0.02M sodium barbital buffer in 0.01M NaCl (pH 7.4) was placed on the material before adding a drop of platelet-poor plasma (3, 4, 12). After 3 s or 3 min of plasma exposure, the surface was rinsed with 20 mL of the buffer. After removing the buffer left around the exposed surface with filter paper (Whatman #1, qualitative), a drop of platelet suspension was placed on the surface previously occupied by platelet-poor plasma. The slides were kept in the moist chamber to prevent drying, and after 10 min, were rinsed with 20 mL of the sodium barbital buffer. The attached platelets were fixed with 0.1% gluteraldehyde, 0.12M sucrose, and 0.0625M sodium cocodylate in Ringers adjusted to pH 7.45 for 10–30 min, followed by 3% gluteraldehyde and 0.1M sodium cacodylate adjusted to pH 7.45 for 10–30 min (13). Slides were rinsed in distilled water and dehydraded by immersing them in increasing concentrations of ethanol (65%, 80%, 90%, 100%, and 100%) for about 10 min at each concentration. Some SBS samples were dehydrated in Freon 13/ethanol solutions (50%, 80%, 90%, 100%, and 100% Freon) to minimize the pitting that occasionally occurred with ethanol.

The platelets, at four random fields, were counted visually on a Zeiss Ultraphot II microscope using reflected light and Nomarski optics at a magnification of 1280× and a field of view of 7542 μm². At least four samples of each polymer were tested for each experiment, and each experiment was repeated at least once with a different donor. For the glasses, at least 1–2 samples were tested per experiment. Conversion was expressed as the percentage difference between platelet adhesion at 3 s and 3 min of platelet-poor plasma exposure with respect to the 3-s platelet-poor plasma exposure.

Statistical Analysis. All data for a particular donor were normalized with respect to the hydrophobic glass at 3 min of platelet-poor plasma exposure for that donor, that is, platelet adhesion at 3 min of platelet-poor plasma exposure to hydrophobic glass was 100%. A one-way analysis of variance was performed, using each material and time of platelet-poor plasma exposure as a variable. For each material and time, the normalized platelet counts for all the donors were summed, and Scheffe's multiple comparisons were performed. For the difference between the two SBS morphologies, a student's t test was used. Data are presented as the mean of the normalized average from each donor and the pooled standard deviation.

Results and Discussion

The surface energy data, Table I, show that polyurethane has the largest percent contribution from polar forces, and that it and PS–PEO have the

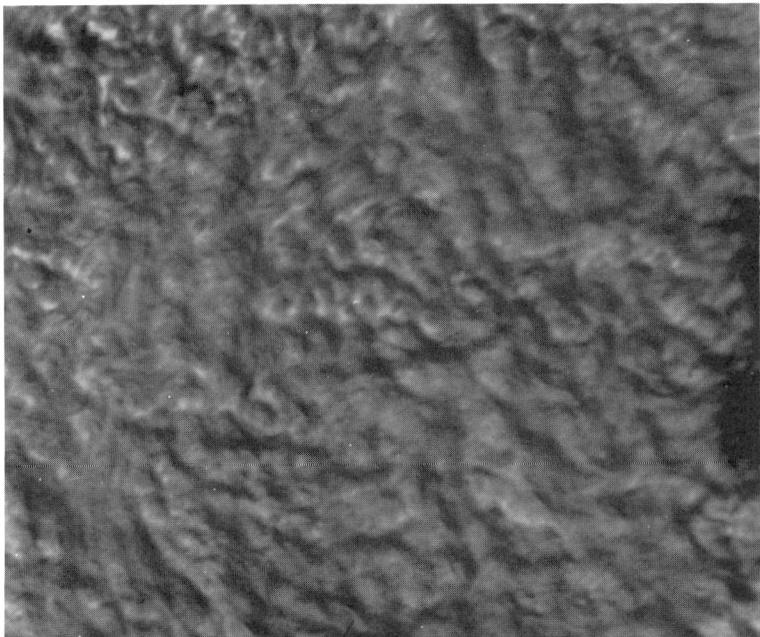

Figure 7. PS–PEO (Sty) Nomarski micrograph of surface texture, peaks spaced 1–7 μm apart (1188×).

largest total surface energy. The critical surface tensions were similar to the total surface energy, except for SBS (the critical surface tension being greater than the total surface energy). The platelet adhesion data are summarized in Table II.

At 3 s of platelet-poor plasma exposure, the most hydrophobic block copolymer, SBS, attached an average of 100 platelets, significantly ($P < 0.025$) greater than the 45 platelets (average of the numbers adhered to the NEQ and ANN morphologies) that adhered onto the relatively less hydrophobic polyurethane (Table II). The relatively hydrophilic PS–PEO block copolymer, on the other hand, did not exhibit any platelet adhesion even when the platelet-poor plasma exposure time was extended to 3 min. This observation is apparently due to the dominant role of the PEO, and not to the polystyrene phase, which is also present in the SBS. The PS–PEO polymer adsorbed up to 50% of its initial weight in water as a result of the PEO component, and for this reason the polymer behaved like a hydrogel [since hydrogels do not attach platelets (14) even though they do adsorb fibrinogen (15)]. The influence of the PEO phase was so strong that the change in the morphology of the block copolymer from mixed to phase-separated did not affect platelet adhesion.

Table II. Platelet Adhesion

Material	Number of Donors	% Platelet Adhesion 3 s	% Platelet Adhesion 3 min	% Conversion
Styrene–butadiene styrene,				
mixed (M)	3	102 ± 30	45 ± 26	56
phase-separated (S)	3	97 ± 24	64 ± 18	34
Polyurethane				
mixed (NEQ)	2	29 ± 19	37 ± 19	−28
phase-separated (ANN)	2	61 ± 26	53 ± 28	13
Polystyrene–poly(ethylene oxide)				
mixed (Mx)	2	0.4 ± 1	1 ± 2	—
phase-separated (Sty)	2	1 ± 5	6 ± 16	—
Control glass				
hydrophobic	3	104 ± 25	100 ± 31	4
hydrophilic	2	79 ± 5	1 ± 1	99

The change in morphology in SBS did not affect the platelet adhesion at 3 s, as the phase-separated and mixed morphologies both attached approximately 100 platelets. On the polyurethane surface, however, phase separation significantly ($P < 0.05$) created a twofold increase in the number of platelets attached, from 29 for the mixed state (NEQ) to 61 for the phase-separated state (ANN), as shown in Table II. However, the mixed-state morphology (NEQ) for polyurethane tended to have slightly more platelets attached at 3 min, as compared with the 3-s plasma exposure. A particular protein, presumably fibrinogen, might have been adsorbed at a slower rate on the NEQ surface, and consequently, the number of platelets at 3 min of platelet-poor plasma exposure tended to increase. The slow rate of fibrinogen adsorption could be explained if initially globulins played a significant role in competition for the surface sites on the mixed state (NEQ), and if γ-globulin were less effective in promoting platelet attachment. A much smaller degree of platelet adhesion was observed on surfaces preadsorbed with γ-globulin compared to those preadsorbed with fibrinogen (16). The role of fibrinogen in these interactions was demonstrated further by the negligible platelet adhesion onto test surfaces preadsorbed to heat-defibrinogenated plasma (56°C for 10 min)—for 3 s and 3 min (unpublished results). When purified fibrinogen (IMCO) was added to the defibrinogenated plasma, and the mixture was preadsorbed onto the test surfaces, platelet adhesion was the same as that observed on surfaces exposed to platelet-poor plasma.

The polyurethane in the phase-separated state (ANN), however, behaved in a manner similar to certain other hydrophobic surfaces (3), including siliconized glass, in that platelet adhesion was independent of the time of exposure to plasma, that is, no difference between 3 s and 3 min existed. The hydrophobic SBS block copolymer, on the other hand, attached significantly ($P < 0.025$) less platelets at 3 min of plasma exposure. The effect was relatively more predominant in the mixed state as the percent decrease in platelets attached at 3 min (conversion) was 56 compared with 34 for the phase-separated state (Table II). The conversion, however, was far less than the 99% observed on the hydrophilic glass.

On hydrophilic, but not on hydrophobic glass, fibrinogen was adsorbed loosely, and with time underwent desorption. The fibrinogen film that attracted platelets was replaced primarily by high molecular weight kininogen, and to a lesser extent with the blood coagulation factor XII. This model is consistent with the observation by Ratnoff and Saito (17) that adsorption of high molecular weight kininogen to a surface is a necessary step in the surface activation of factor XII. The factor XII could be considered as behaving as a cross-linking agent for high molecular weight kininogen, and thus stabilizing its adsorbed layer.

The physiochemical behavior of a surface, therefore, controls both the rate of the initial fibrinogen absorption and its rate of desorption. This latter process may be formalized by the desorption rate relationship,

$$\frac{dc\phi}{dt} = K[1 - E^*(\phi)_{ad}] \tag{1}$$

where ϕ is the fibrinogen molecule, $c\phi$ is the concentration of adsorbed fibrinogen, K is a constant of proportionality, and $E^*(\phi)_{ad}$ is the ratio of the effective energy of adsorption of the fibrinogen molecule with respect to the energy of adsorption of "tight" binding, that is, no desorption. The $E^*(\phi)_{ad}$ term can be expressed as,

$$E^*(\phi)_{ad} = E_{ad} + I_1 - I_2 \tag{2}$$

where E_{ad} is the energy of adsorption of a fibrinogen molecule to a surface, I_1 is the $\phi\cdot\phi$ intermolecular interaction on the surface (18), and I_2 is the ϕ·high molecular weight kininogen intermolecular interaction at the surface (all terms with respect to the energy of adsorption of "tight"-binding). Because the kininogen displaces fibrinogen on hydrophilic surfaces, we assume that $E^*(\phi)_{ad} < E^*$ (high molecular weight kinongen)$_{ad}$, whereas the reverse is true for certain hydrophobic surfaces.

Within this framework then, the SBS block copolymer adsorbs fibrinogen less tightly than hydrophobic glass, but more tightly than hydrophilic glass. Similarly, the protein adsorbed onto the mixed state is probably more loosely attached than that adsorbed onto the phase-separated state. Therefore, either one of the phases or the phase boundary region is apparently capable of binding fibrinogen more strongly. Since the transition boundary region between phases would be expected to exhibit behavior similar to the mixed state, the enhanced adsorption of fibrinogen is probably more likely associated with one of the phases, in particular, the PS phase. This conclusion is supported by evidence that the π-electrons of the phenyl group are available for bonding because the phenyl group can interact with hydroxyl groups in hydrogen-bonding liquids (19). In addition, in vitro assays of adsorbed proteins from plasma have demonstrated that fibrinogen rapidly reaches an equilibrium concentration on PS, as opposed to glass or polyethylene surfaces where the fibrinogen concentration reaches a maximum and then decreases with time (20).

Using data from the model for the fibrinogen molecule, the area of the molecule is much larger than the apparent area of the PS domains (Figure 2), where the sphere diameter is 190 Å. Thus, if this interpretation is correct, a model of fibrinogen interaction can be developed in the following way: the fibrinogen molecule might be expected to be adsorbed to the styrene domains in the "end-on" configuration. Such a configuration might be stabilized by interfibrinogen bonding (18), which could increase $E^*(\phi)_{ad}$ by adding a relatively large I_1 term (Equation 2). The fibrinogen molecule can readily adsorb in the "lying-flat" configuration in the region of phase separation that contains rods lying parallel to the surface.

Acknowledgments

This research was supported by Public Health Services Grant No. HL-15195 from the National Heart and Lung Institute. M. N. Helmus also acknowledges the support of the Timken Fellowship.

Literature Cited

1. Berger, S.; Salzman E. W. *Prog. Hemostasis Thromb* **1974**, *2*, 273–309.
2. Salzman, E. W. *Chem. Biosurfaces* **1972**, *2*, 489–522.
3. Vroman, L.; Adams, A. L. *Surf. Sci.* **1969**, *116*, 438.
4. Vroman, L.; Adams, A. L.; Fischer, G. C.; Munoz, P. C. *Blood* **1980**, *55*, 156.
5. Zucker, M. B.; Vroman, L. *Proc. Soc. Exp. Biol. Med.* **1969**, *131*, 318.
6. Nyilas, E.; Ward, R. S., Jr., *J. Biomed. Mater. Res. Symp.* **1977**, *8*, 69.
7. Picha, G. J.; Gibbons, D. F.; Auerbach, R. A. *J. Bioeng.* **1978**, *2*, 301.
8. Ostler, M. I., Ph.D. Dissertation, Case Western Reserve Univ., Cleveland, 1975.
9. Kaelble, D. H. *J. Adhes.* **1970**, *2*, 66.
10. Good, R. J.; Girifalco, L. A. *J. Phys. Chem.* **1960**, *64*, 561.
11. O'Malley, J. J.; Crystal, R. G; Erhardt, P. F. In "Block Polymers," Aggarwal, S. L., Ed.; Plenum: New York, 1970; pp. 179–193.
12. Lyman, D. J.; Brash, J. L.; Chatkin, S. W.; Klein, K. G.; Carini, M. *Trans. Am. Soc. Artif. Intern. Organs* **1968**, *14*, 250.
13. Van Kampen, C. L.; Jones, R. D; Gibbons, D. F. *Biomater. Med. Devices, Artif. Organs* **1978**, *6*, 37.
14. Hoffman, A. S.; Horbett, T. A.; Ratner, B. D. *Ann. N.Y. Acad. Sci.* **1977**, *283*, 372.
15. Weathersby, P. K.; Horbett, T. A.; Hoffman, A. S. *J. Bioeng.* **1977**, *1*, 395.
16. Vroman, L.; Adams, A. L.; Klings, M.; Fischer, G. C.; Munoz, P. C.; Solensky, R. P. *Ann. N.Y. Acad. Sci* **1977**, *283*, 65.
17. Ratnoff, O. D.; Saito, H. *Proc. Natl. Acad. Sci. U.S.A.* **1979**, *76*, 958.
18. Morrissey, B. W. *Ann. N.Y. Acad. Sci.* **1977**, *283*, 50.
19. Good, R. J. *J. Colloid Interface Sci.* **1977**, *59*, 398.
20. Brash, J. L.; Uniyal, S. *3rd Int. Conf. Plastics Med. Surgery, Plastics and Rubber Institute*, London, 1979; 29–1.

RECEIVED for review January 16, 1981. ACCEPTED April 27, 1981.

8
A Critical Study of Segmented Polyurethanes

E. W. MERRILL, VERA SA DA COSTA, E. W. SALZMAN,
D. BRIER–RUSSELL, L. KUCHNER, D. F. WAUGH, G. TRUDEL, III,
S. STOPPER, and V. VITALE

Massachusetts Institute of Technology, Departments of Chemical Engineering and Biology, Cambridge, MA, and Harvard Medical School and Beth Israel Hospital, Department of Surgery, Boston, MA 02139

> *The components of segmented polyurethanes having polyether "soft segments" and aromatic diisocyanate–diamine "hard segments" were studied separately and in the form of segmented polyurethanes. Platelet retention index (the capacity of the polymer to bind human platelets) was studied in relation to properties determined by scanning calorimety, Fourier transform infrared spectroscopy, gel permeation chromatography, and x-ray photoelectron spectroscopy. Carbon 1s spectra, which differentiate carbon bound to ether oxygen from other carbon in the outermost 30 Å of the surface, predicted platelet retention to a remarkable degree. In general, the hard segment analogues have high platelet retention. As a soft segment, poly(ethylene oxide) showed very low platelet retention.*

Segmented polyether polyurethanes are widely studied biomaterials that can be conceptualized (1–3) as a virtual network in which the continuous phase contains the polyether chain molecules. These chain molecules are tied at their ends to the molecular species (diisocyanate, diamine) which serve as junctions by associating into clusters. These clusters of high melting point form "the hard-segment phase" and are dispersed in the continuous polyether phase.

In global overview of what was discovered, we note the following:

1. Molecular models (2) of the hard-segment phase of segmented polyether polyurethanes tested in the in vitro bead column (4) show a high platelet retention index ($\bar{\rho} \cong 0.8$) regardless of molecular composition. The variable $\bar{\rho}$ is defined as the fraction of platelets in whole citrated human blood entering a test column that are retained on the bead surfaces, averaged for

several donors and five successive 1-mL aliquots of blood. Thus, to the extent that it appears at the surface of a finished polyurethane, the hard-segment phase will promote platelet activation.

2. Unambiguous testing of the soft segment only, that is, the polyether part, by the same procedure was more difficult, but important information was obtained. Each of the polyethers studied—poly(tetramethylene oxide) (PTMO), poly(propylene oxide) (PPO), and poly(ethylene oxide) (PEO)—are partially crystalline in the form of dry, α, ω diols after deposition on the bead surfaces from organic solvents.

   Upon contact with blood, polyethers absorb varying amounts of water and undergo partial dissolution while remaining partially crystalline. They show platelet retention index values around 0.2–0.3.

3. When polyethers are synthesized into polyurethanes, their melting points can be depressed sufficiently, depending on the choice of the molecular weight of the initial diol, so that when in contact with blood at 37°C, the polyether phase is totally amorphous. When amorphous, the substance is substantially more bland (lower $\bar{\rho}$) than when the polyether remains partially crystalline.

4. PPO and PEO both are more bland than PTMO, when compared as polyurethanes that remain amorphous during testing against blood.

5. Segmented polyurethanes having as soft segment content, mixtures of PEO, PPO, and diblocks of PEO–PPO, have very low $\bar{\rho}$, around 0.04, suggesting that molecular disorder, thereby created, is useful.

6. Increasing the molecular weight of α, ω diol PEO in the segmented polyurethane to 1500, systematically increases the water content of the segmented polyurethane, and produces one with with an usually low $\bar{\rho}$, about 0.04, in which the PEO remains amorphous.

7. X-ray photoelectron spectroscopy (XPS, also known as ESCA) is valuable in rationalizing these observations (3). The $\bar{\rho}$ correlates well with the percent of the C 1s signal that corresponds to carbon bonded to ether, this carbon belonging to the polyether component (no such carbon existing in the hard-segment components).

8. Parallel tests show that thrombin adsorption is minimal on well-prepared polyurethanes containing amorphous PEO, greater on PTMO, and very high on analogues of the hard segment (diisocyanate–diamine copolymers), thus paralleling the trends in platelet retention index $\bar{\rho}$. This result is consistent with the postulate that protein adsorption must precede platelet adsorption.

9. Evidence from these studies and from other laboratories (5–9) indicates that PEO is an unusually promising polymer, when properly formed into a network (as by segmented polyurethane formation, for example). We attribute this result to the following properties:
  • high water content without any ionic group or hydrogen bonding H
  • consequent balance between hydrophilic and hydrophobic nature, and thus relatively nonattractive to plasma proteins
  • capability of remaining amorphous if incorporated into a network

Experimental

Segmented polyurethanes were synthesized from the α, ω diol polyethers listed in Table I and the diisocyanates **IV**, **V**, and **VI** by the two-step process shown in Figure 1 or the three-step process in Figure 2. In all cases, chain extension of isocyanate-terminated prepolymers was accomplished with ethylenediamine. The synthesis took place in a 2:1 (v/v) mixture of dimethyl sulfoxide and 4-methyl-2-pentanone at 60°C.

$$HO[\overset{*}{C}H_2CH_2CH_2\overset{*}{C}H_2O]_n - \overset{*}{C}H_2CH_2CH_2\overset{*}{C}H_2OH$$

I

$$HO - (\overset{*}{C}H-\overset{*}{C}H_2-O)_n \overset{*}{C}H-\overset{*}{C}H_2-OH$$
$$||$$
$$CH_3CH_3$$

II

$$HO-(\overset{*}{C}H_2-\overset{*}{C}H_2-O)_n-\overset{*}{C}H_2-\overset{*}{C}H_2-OH$$
$$\bar{M}_n = 4500, 3500, 1500, 1000, 600$$

III

* = C 1s peak chemically shifted 1.5 eV in ESCA spectra.

Table I. Polyethers Used

Polyether	$\overline{M}_n$	n
Poly(tetramethylene oxide) (**I**)	2000, 1000, 650	27, 13, 8
Poly(propylene oxide) (**II**)	2000, 1200, 400	42, 27, 7
Poly(ethylene oxide) (**III**)	4500, 3500, 1500, 1000, 600	101, 79, 33, 22, 13

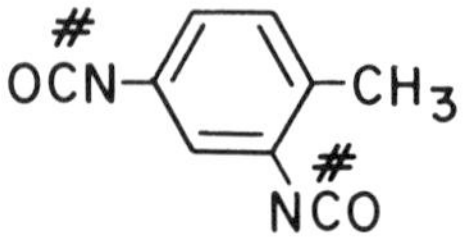

IV: 2, 4-Tolylene diisocyanate (2,4-TDI)

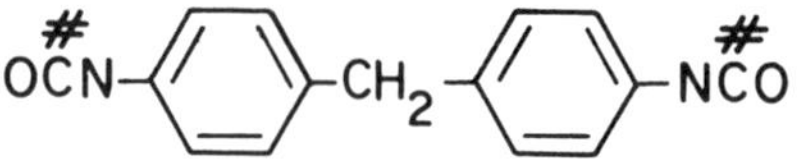

V: Diphenylmethane 4,4'-diisocyanate (MDI)

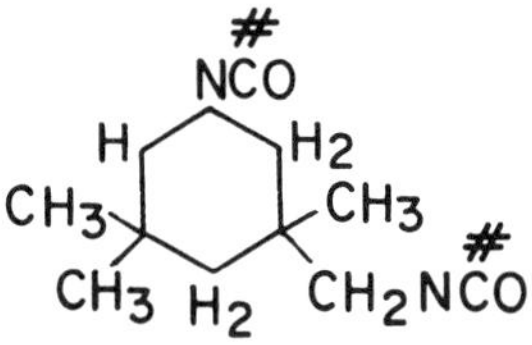

VI: 3-Isocyanatomethyl-3,5,5-trimethylcyclohexyl isocyanate (isophorone diisocyanate, IPDI)

*In Structures **IV–VI**, #, C 1s peak chemically shifted 3 eV when incorporated into urea or urethane bonds.*

To obtain a solution suitable for casting on test surfaces, the segmented polyurethanes after synthesis were precipitated by methanol (which also terminated excess isocyanate groups) and after drying were redissolved in dimethylformamide (DMF).

Using the two-step process (Figure 1), a Type I segmented polyurethane was created (Scheme I), whereas the three-step process created a Type II or Type III segmented polyurethane (Figure 2). Idealized, these polyurethanes are:

Type I. The soft segment consists only of polyether chains (of one kind) connected at each end to a hard-segment triad consisting of diisocyanate–diamine–diisocyanate, where the diisocyanate is either toluene diisocyanate (TDI) or isophorone diisocyanate (IPDI).

Type II. The soft segment consists of diblock polyether chains (of one kind) achieved by a connector diisocyanate (TDI) molecule between two α, ω diol precursors. The ends of this doubled chain are connected to hard-segment triads, but in this triad, the diisocyanate is diphenylmethane 4,4'-diisocyanate (MDI).

Scheme I. Segmented Polyurethanes According to Type and Composition

Generalized Sequence

Type I: PE–HSDI–ED–HSDI–
Type II: PE–CDI–PE–HSDI–ED–HSDI–
Type III: PE_1–CDI–PE_2–HSDI–ED–HSDI–(PE_2 different from PE_1)

Key: $PE_{1,2}$, polyether sequence (from α,ω—dihydroxy precursor) PTMO, PPO, or PEO, HSDI, diisocyanate residue in hard-segment phase (TDI, MDI, or IPDI); CDI, connector diisocyanate residue (TDI only); and ED, ethylenediamine residue.

Step 1: Prepolymer formation

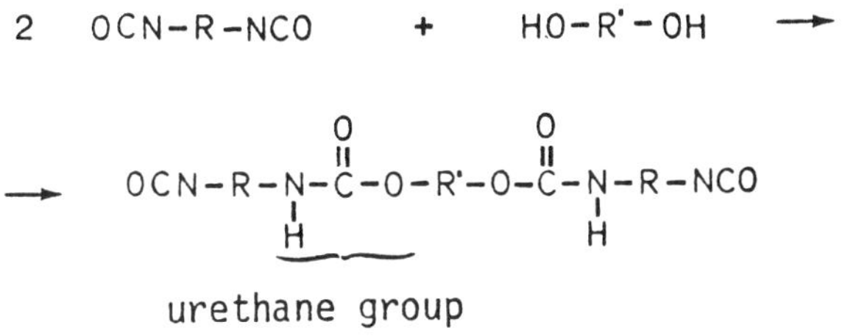

$$2 \ \text{OCN–R–NCO} + \text{HO–R'–OH} \longrightarrow$$

$$\longrightarrow \text{OCN–R–}\underset{H}{\text{N}}\text{–}\overset{O}{\underset{\|}{\text{C}}}\text{–O–R'–O–}\overset{O}{\underset{\|}{\text{C}}}\text{–}\underset{H}{\text{N}}\text{–R–NCO}$$

urethane group

Step 2: "Chain extension"

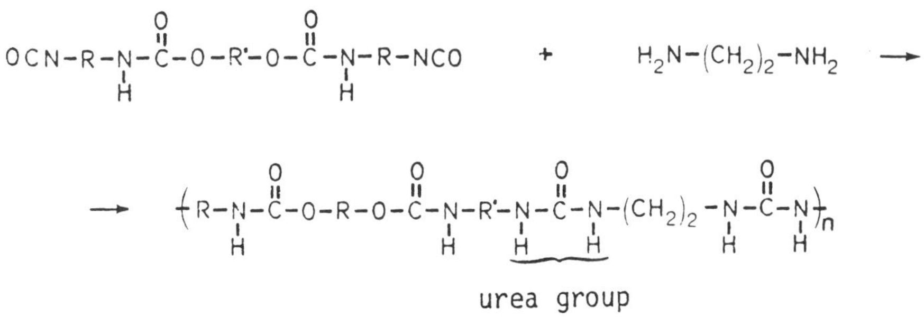

$$\text{OCN–R–}\underset{H}{\text{N}}\text{–}\overset{O}{\underset{\|}{\text{C}}}\text{–O–R'–O–}\overset{O}{\underset{\|}{\text{C}}}\text{–}\underset{H}{\text{N}}\text{–R–NCO} + H_2N\text{–}(CH_2)_2\text{–}NH_2 \longrightarrow$$

$$\longrightarrow \left\{ \text{R–}\underset{H}{\text{N}}\text{–}\overset{O}{\underset{\|}{\text{C}}}\text{–O–R–O–}\overset{O}{\underset{\|}{\text{C}}}\text{–}\underset{H}{\text{N}}\text{–R'–}\underset{H}{\text{N}}\text{–}\overset{O}{\underset{\|}{\text{C}}}\text{–}\underset{H}{\text{N}}\text{–}(CH_2)_2\text{–}\underset{H}{\text{N}}\text{–}\overset{O}{\underset{\|}{\text{C}}}\text{–}\underset{H}{\text{N}} \right\}_n$$

urea group

Figure 1. Two-step synthesis leading to Type I segmented polyurethanes.

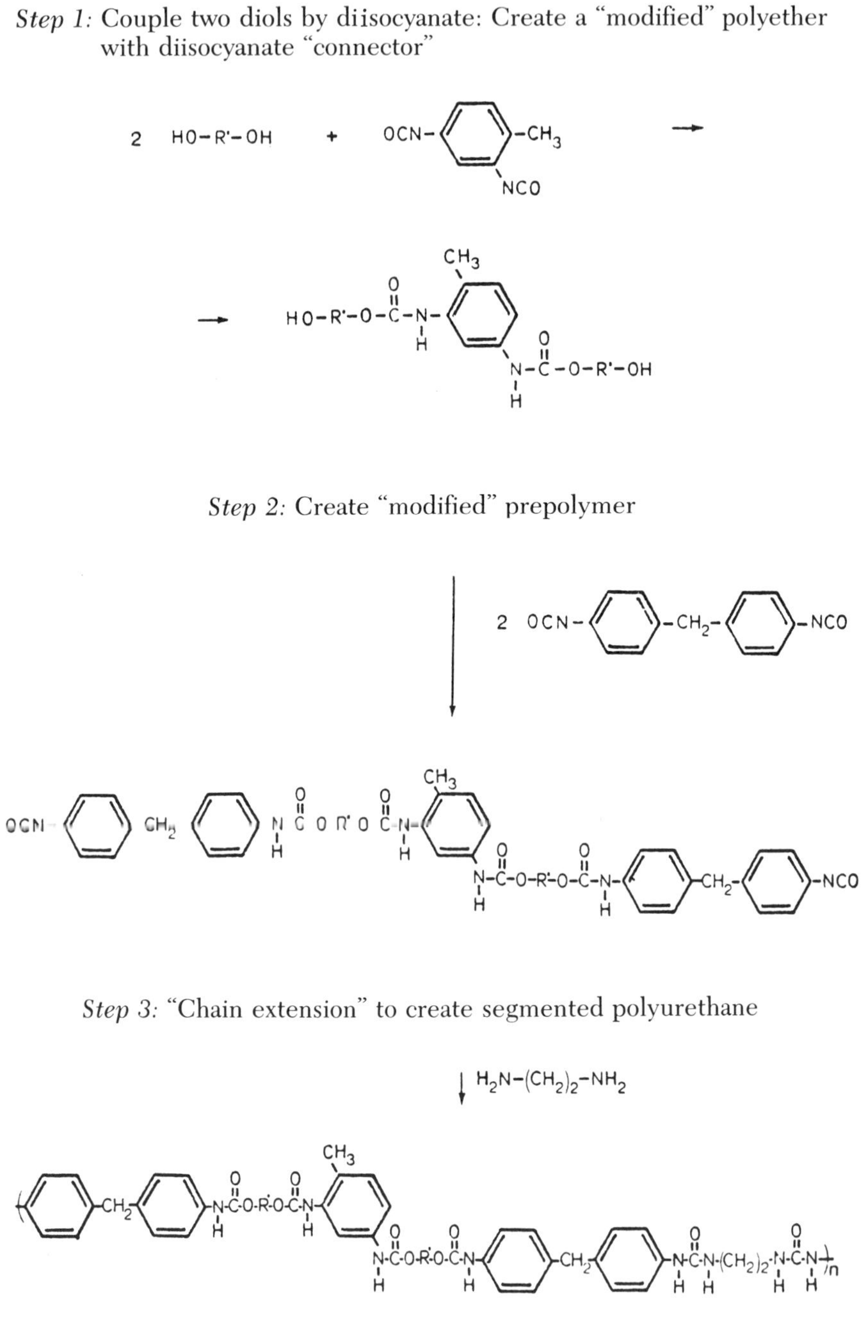
Step 1: Couple two diols by diisocyanate: Create a "modified" polyether with diisocyanate "connector"
2 HO–R'–OH
OCN–
–CH3
NCO
Step 2: Create "modified" prepolymer
2 OCN–
–CH2–
–NCO
Step 3: "Chain extension" to create segmented polyurethane
H2N–(CH2)2–NH2

Figure 2. Three-step synthesis leading to Type II and Type III segmented polyurethanes (cf. Table III).

Type III. The soft segment contains polyether chains that are diblocks, obtained by Step 1 of the three-step process (Figure 2), where two different polyether diols, for example PEO and PPO, are mixed in equimolar ratios. The ends of these diblocks are then connected to hard-segment triads, which, as in Type II, are composed of MDI–ethylene diamine–MDI.

Gel permeation chromatography (GPC) (Waters Model 244, with micro Styragel columns) of the diol polyethers and of the prepolymers created therefrom, in combination with data from the literature, confirms that these idealized types must be modified by the following considerations:

1. The intended stoichiometric ratios (e.g., of diisocyanate to diol, or diisocyanate to diamine) are never exactly achieved because of:
   - dimerization and trimerization of the diisocyanates
   - allophanate and biuret reactions (the $-NCO$ reacts not with the intended $-OH$ or $-NH_2$, but with urethane links $-NHCOO-$ or urea links $-NHCONH-$).

2. The hard-segment triad is accompanied by single diisocyanate residues, pentads, and heptads, in consonance with Flory's theory for step polymerization (10), when $A \sim A$ molecules react with $B \sim B$ molecules in a ratio of $r = \frac{1}{2}$, and all A groups are reacted. Thus, phase separation into "clusters" (which create network junctions) must involve, to varying degrees, isolated diisocyanate units (either the connector unit or from the prepolymer forming step), the triads, the pentads, etc. Therefore, the degree of phase separation achieved may vary widely, depending on synthesis conditions and subsequent casting from the solvent.

3. Most of the α, ω diol polyethers had the "most probable" distribution of molecular weight (1). Thus, weight-to-number average is around two, and the lengths of polyether chains between diisocyanate groups vary correspondingly.

4. When equimolal quantities of two different polyethers, for example, PEO and PPO, are mixed to create Type III segmented polyurethanes, three different diblock sequences of equal probability must be obtained: PEO–PEO, PEO–PPO, and PPO–PPO are the principal species. The same principles that govern the formation of 1-,3-,5-,-7... unit combination of diisocyanates and diamines in the hard segment, also predict that the reaction product of 2 mol of α, ω diol with 1 mol of diisocyanate after Step 1 of the three-step process (Figure 2) will consist mostly of the monomer (the diol), some of the desired trimer (diol -TDI-diol), but also some of the pentamer (diol–TDI–diol–TDI–diol), etc.

Thus, the actual substances produced as segmented polyurethanes (Scheme I and Table II) that were tested for thrombogenic potential, are peculiarly complicated in molecular structure.

These polyurethanes (and their precursors or analogues) were cast from an appropriate solvent, usually DMF, onto the glass bead surfaces used in the in vitro test for platelet retention (4), or for the thrombin absorption test used previously (2). Crystals of KBr for Fourier transform infrared (FTIR) spectroscopy and glass microscopic slides for examination by XPS (ESCA) served as supports for polymers cast from the same solvents. Concentration of polymer (5 wt %), temperature of casting

Table II. List of Segmented Polyurethanes Identified by Scheme I
Identification of Segmented Polyurethanes (SPU)

SPU No.	SPU Type	PE Type	PE Mol wt	CDI (if any)	HSDI Type	CDI/PE (if any)	HSDI/PE	ED/PE
24	II	PTMO	2000	TDI	MDI	0.58	1.01	0.45
25	I	PTMO	2000	None	MDI	—	1.39	0.36
26	I	PTMO	2000	None	MDI	—	2.25	1.32
39	II	PEO	600	TDI	MDI	0.61	0.86	0.48
40	II	PEO	1000	TDI	MDI	0.52	1.08	0.65
401	II	PEO	1000	TDI	MDI			
403	II	PEO	1000	TDI	MDI			
42	I	PPO	2000	None	TDI	—	2.16	0.05
44	I	PPO	1200	None	TDI	—	2.02	0.97
441	I	PPO	1200					
46	I	PPO	1200	None	TDI	—	2.16	1.17
48	II	PPO	1200	TDI	MDI	0.54	0.99	0.49
481	II	PPO	1200	TDI	MDI			
49	II	PPO	400	TDI	MDI	0.66	0.78	0.42
51	II	PEO	1500	TDI	MDI			
1500	I	PEO	1500	None	IPDI	—		
3500	I	PEO	3500	None	IPDI	—		
4500	I	PEO	4500	None	IPDI	—		
401/481	III	1 = PEO 2 = PPO	1 = 1000 2 = 1200	TDI				

(25°C), and subsequent slow evaporation conditions under argon gas (40°C, 21 days) were maintained as closely identical as possible in preparing surfaces for each test (FTIR, ESCA, and platelet retention). The air side of the film was the side exposed to platelets and examined by XPS. The other side (against the glass substrate) was not exposed.

Films of the segmented polyurethanes, and the precursor polyethers and hard-segment analogues (diisocyanate–diamine), stripped from glass plates, were compressed into pellets for analysis by differential scanning calorimetry (DSC) (Du Pont Model II). FTIR spectroscopy was performed with a Digital Model FTS-14, and XPS (ESCA) was performed with a Physical Electronics Industries Model 548 Auger/Leeds/ESCA spectrometer using 100-pass energy for C $1s$ and O $1s$, and 25-pass energy for N $1s$, through a solid angle of about 60° over a width of about 1 mm. In the XPS tests, as in the platelet tests, the films were *not* stripped from the surface on which they were cast.

DSC confirmed that in segmented polyurethanes formed with the aromatic diisocyanates TDI and MDI, phase separation was fair to good as judged by the appearance of transitions corresponding, respectively, to the diol and of the isocyanate–diamine copolymer (1). Furthermore, except for SPU 24, SPU 3500, and SPU 4500 (Table II), the polyether phase had its crystalline melting point depressed below the biological test temperature (37°C) as a consequence of copolymerization with the diisocyanate. That the unreacted diols (Table I), the hard-segment analogue (TDI–ethylenediamine copolymer), and the SPU 24, SPU 3500, and SPU 4500 were crystalline at 37°C in contact with water or blood, was confirmed also by their grossly observable turbidity. The other segmented polyurethanes were, to the contrary, transparent when equilibrated with isotonic saline at 37°C.

FTIR was used to determine if further judgment could be made about the extent of phase separation achieved, by analyzing for adsorption bonds corresponding to -NH interactions with ether –O– (hard–soft), -NH interactions with -NH and -C=O (hard–hard), etc. (1). Qualitatively, the FTIR results were consistent with the DSC interpretation, but neither method gave insight into the morphological characteristics of the phase separations achieved. FTIR was also used, more effectively, to determine the distribution of the forms of nitrogen in the bulk polymer as urethane nitrogen N_{ut} (i.e., -NHCOO-), urea nitrogen N_u (i.e., -NHCONH-), and amine nitrogen N_{amine}.

These data were used in conjunction with the experimentally fixed stoichiometric ratios of carbon, oxygen, and nitrogen, for comparison with the concentrations of these elements (C, O, N) in the outermost 30 Å of surface as determined by ESCA (XPS). Representative results are shown in Table III. No consistent relationship exists between the surface nitrogen content and the distribution of nitrogen among urethane, urea, and amine groups; furthermore, no apparent relationship exists between surface nitrogen/bulk nitrogen (N_S/N_B) and the polyether type, polyether molecular weight, or diisocyanate type.

The hard-segment analogues in Table III are the copolymer of TDI and ethylenediamine and the copolymer of MDI and ethylenediamine. Bulk and surface composition agree fairly closely, as do bulk and surface compositions for the soft-segment precursors, polyether diols PTMO 2000 and PEO 1000. In marked contrast, the polyurethanes derived from these materials show from about 34% to 60% of stoichiometric nitrogen in the ESCA-scanned surface layer of 30 Å deep. Clearly the surface is deficient in nitrogen and, therefore, in the hard segment, but whether the nitrogen is *at* the surface or buried to a depth less than 30Å, and whether the nitrogen is in clusters or dispersed (it could be both) (2), is impossible to determine from the XPS (ESCA) experiment, executed without angular-dependent resolution.

In contrast, the analysis of the C $1s$ spectra was particularly illuminating, as shown in Figure 3. The abscissa φ is the fraction of carbon at the surface in the form

Table III. Surface and Bulk Composition of Segmented Polyurethanes, Hard-Segment Analogues, and Soft-Segment Precursors

Sample	Polyether	Diisocyanate	Surface Composition				Bulk Composition					Surface N/ Bulk N
			C%	O%	N%		C%	O%	N%	%N Ureth.	%N Urea	%N Amine	
24	PTMO 2000	TDI,MDI	57.2	42.7	—	79.4	18.2	2.5	1.79	0.71	—	
25	PTMO 2000	MDI	73.5	25.2	1.3	79.6	18.3	2.1	1.56	0.54	—	0.62
26	PTMO 2000	MDI	73.0	25.5	1.5	78.9	17.3	3.8	1.64	2.05	0.11	0.39
31	PTMO 2000	MDI	74.0	24.0	2.0	79.0	17.5	3.6	1.62	1.67	0.31	0.57
39	PEO 600	TDI,MDI	70.2	27.2	2.6	69.3	24.5	6.2	4.19	1.97	0.04	0.42
40	PEO 1000	TDI,MDI	70.5	27.6	1.9	68.8	26.7	4.6	2.79	1.67	0.14	0.41
47	PPO 400	TDI	71.0	24.9	4.1	69.8	19.8	10.5	5.12	5.22	0.15	0.39
49	PPO 400	TDI,MDI	65.5	30.7	3.8	74.1	19.1	6.8	4.82	1.98	—	0.56
48	PPO 1200	TDI,MDI	70.9	27.3	1.8	74.7	21.7	5.3	3.60	1.70	—	0.34
44	PPO 1200	TDI	70.2	25.6	4.2	72.4	22.4	5.2	2.70	2.50	—	0.81
46	PPO 1200	TDI	70.1	26.9	3.0	72.2	22.2	5.7	2.63	3.05	0.02	0.53
Hard-segment analogues													
urea (1)		TDI	59.3	13.2	27.5	62.5	12.5	25.0	—	25.0	—	
urea (2)		MDI	67.7	9.8	22.5	73.8	8.7	17.5	—	17.5	—	
Soft-segment precursors													
PTMO 2000			78.3	21.7		80.0	20.0					
PEO 1000			69.5	30.5		66.7	33.3					

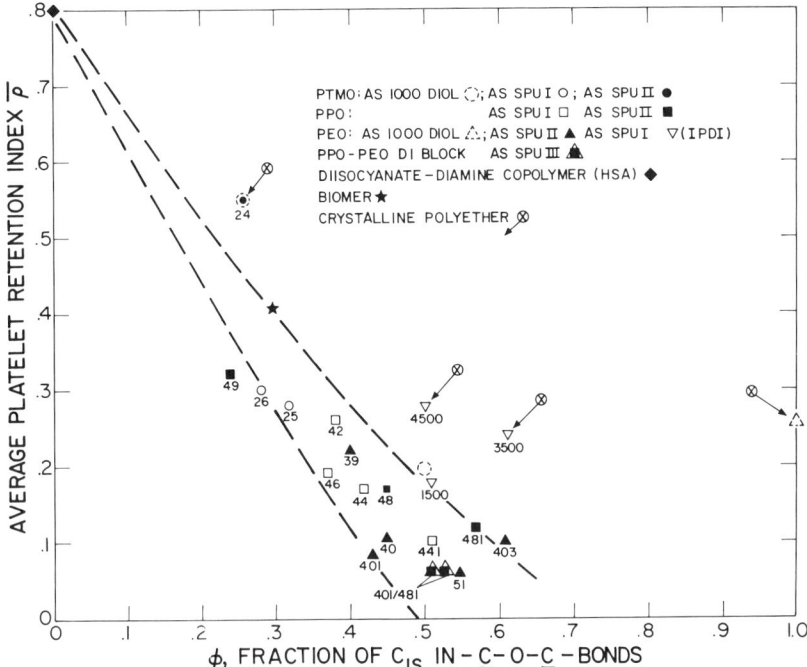

Figure 3. Average platelet retention index vs. ϕ, where ϕ = fraction of C 1s in -C-O-C- bonds.

of ethereal-bonded carbon, recognized as a peak downshifted 1.5 eV from carbon–carbon and carbon–hydrogen. For example, in segmented polyurethanes on PEO as the polyether, if all the carbon in the scanned layer belonged to PEO, ϕ would equal 1.0.

From Figure 3 we draw the following conclusions. First, data corresponding to a polyether that is crystalline when in contact with blood, denoted by the symbol ←⊗, lie well outside the range of the other data that pertain to amorphous polyether. The polyurethanes SPU 24 and SPU 26 are a particularly good test because they represent the same soft segment (PTMO 2000) manipulated so as to be both crystalline (SPU 24) and amorphous (SPU 26).

Second, the highly crystalline and hydrogen-bonding alternating copolymer of diisocyanate and diamine, an analog of the hard segment of polyurethanes, shows high platelet retention ($\bar{\rho} \sim 0.8$). Therefore, this molecular species will cause platelet retention, to the extent that it appears at the surface of polyurethanes.

Third, polyurethanes based on PTMO (Biomer, SPU 24, SPU 25, and SPU 26) tend to cluster with values of $\bar{\rho}$ from 0.28 to 0.42 (excluding the crystalline PTMO in SPU 24), whereas polyurethanes based on PPO are in a cluster with $\bar{\rho}$ ranging from about 0.1 to 0.32. Among PEO-containing segmented polyurethanes, the value of $\bar{\rho}$ ranges from 0.05 (SPU 51) to about 0.2.

Fourth, the nature of the diisocyanate affects the value of $\bar{\rho}$. For example, SPU

51 made with the aromatic diisocyanates TDI and MDI, and PEO 1500, shows a much lower $\bar{\rho}$ (0.05) than SPU 1500 made from the same PEO but from the aliphatic IPDI.

Finally, the mixed diblock copolymer SPU 401/SPU 481 containing PEO–PEO, PEO–PPO, and PPO–PPO soft segments is remarkably bland. In this polymer, the surface in contact with blood could very well be rich in PEO.

Thus, ESCA C 1s spectra present a remarkable correlation of platelet retention indices, provided that crystalline materials are excluded from the analysis. However, at any value of ϕ in Figure 3, a range of $\bar{\rho}$ exists.

Conclusions

Even without angular dependence, XPS (ESCA) appears to be a promising analytical technique, and angular-dependent measurements for nitrogen, carbon, and oxygen will be of great interest in resolving the distribution of hard-segment and soft-segment material in segmented polyurethanes containing polyethers.

Apart from any spectroscopic analytical evidence, PEO, when in the amorphous state and swollen by water (or isotonic saline) appears to be a potentially very bland material when contacted by platelets. Other methods should be used to ascertain whether PEO, appropriately rendered into a nondissolving network, represents a generally useful material as a container or conduit for blood. Our conclusions agree with results reported previously in References 5–9.

Note Added in Proof

Since preparation of this manuscript, subsequent studies were completed (11) on new segmented polyurethanes of type I made exclusively from polyethylene oxide diols, ethylene diamine, and 1,4-cyclohexane diisocyanate (CHDI) (no other diisocyanate was used). They were synthesized in toluene (not DMSO/pentanone) with dibutyltin dilaurate as catalyst (no catalyst was used to synthesize the polymers listed in Tables II and III) and eventually cast from hexafluroisopropanol or formic acid solutions (not DMF in which they were insoluble).

By XPS, much less nitrogen was found in their surfaces than in most of the polymers reported in Table III, and ϕ, the fraction of ethereal carbon, ranged upward from 0.8. When PEO 3500 was used as the diol, the XPS scans of the segmented polyurethane were identical with the PEO calibration standard; i.e., no nitrogen signal could be detected at any level of amplification, and the expanded C 1s scan corresponded to only carbon bonded to ether; i.e., $\phi = 1$. Platelet retention indices were 0.05 or less.

Acknowledgment

The support of the United States Public Health Services under Grant No. HL 20079 is gratefully acknowledged.

Literature Cited

1. Sa da Costa, V.; Ph.D. Thesis, Massachusettes Institute of Technology, Cambridge, MA, 1979.
2. Sa da Costa, V.; Brier-Russell, D.; Trudel, G., III; Waugh, D. F.; Salzman, E. W.; Merrill, E. W. *J. Colloid Interface Sci.* **1980**, *76*, 594–596.
3. Sa da Costa, V.; Brier-Russell, D.; Salzman, E. W.; Merrill, E. W. *J. Colloid Interface Sci.*, **1981**, *80*, 445–452.
4. Lindon, J. N.; Rodvien, R.; Brier, D.; Greenberg, R.; Merrill, E.; Salzman, E. W. *J. Lab Clin. Med.* **1978**, *92*, 904–915.
5. Gilding, D. K.; Reed, A. M. "Systematic Development of Polyurethanes for Biomedical Applications: I. Synthesis, Structure, and Bulk Properties," presented at the Trans. 11th Symp. Biomater., *Vol. III*, Society for Biomaterials, San Antonio, TX,
6. Reed, A. M.; Gilding, D. K.; Wilson, J.; Johnson, M. "Systematic Development of Polyurethanes for Biomedical Applications: II. Surface and Biological Properties," presented at the Trans. 11th Symp. Biomater., *Vol. III*, Society for Biomaterials, San Antonio, TX.
7. Furusawa, K.; Shimura, Y.; Otobe, K.; Alsomi, K.; Tsuda, K. *Konburshi Ronburshu* **1977**, *34* (4), 317–324.
8. Whicher, S. J.; Brash, J. L. *J. Biomed. Mater. Res.* **1978**, *12*, 181–202.
9. Brash, J. L.; Uniyal, S. *J. Polym. Sci. C*, **1979**, *66*, 377.
10. Flory, P. J., "Principles of Polymer Chemistry," Cornell Univ. Press: Ithaca, 1953, pp. 322–323.
11. Mahmud, N.A.; Wan, S.; Sa da Costa, V.; Vitale, V.; Brier–Russel, D.; Kuchner, L.; Salzman, E. W.; Merrill, E. W. "XPS Analysis of Segmented Polyurethane-ureas: Assessment of Surface Activity toward Blood Platelets," in press.

RECEIVED for review January 16, 1981. ACCEPTED May 7, 1981.

The Effect of Polyether Segment Molecular Weight on the Bulk and Surface Morphologies of Copolyether-Urethane–Ureas

K. KNUTSON and D. J. LYMAN

University of Utah, Department of Materials Science and Engineering, Salt Lake City, UT 84112

The degree of phase separation for the bulk and surface morphologies of a series of block copolyether-urethane–ureas with polyether segment molecular weights of 2000, 1000, and 700 was studied by Fourier transform infrared spectroscopy coupled with internal reflectance techniques. Band assignments were made using a series of model compounds and polymers. Shifts in band location and shape were determined for interactions between phases due to mixing under selected environments with homogeneous mixtures of the model compounds and polymers. In the bulk, the urea domains were well separated and completely hydrogen bonded. The urethane interface region narrowed with decreasing polyether molecular weight as determined from the percentage of hydrogen-bonded urethane Amide I. As the surface was approached, the interface region also narrowed as compared to the bulk.

Block copolyurethanes form a domain-matrix morphology due to the chemical and steric incompatibilities of the chemically different blocks or segments. The unusual range of physical and chemical properties associated with these copolyurethanes results from this morphological separation. Recently, several block copolyurethanes have shown blood compatibility properties needed for vascular implants. However, investigation of a series of copolyether-urethane–ureas in which the molecular weight of the polyether segment was varied to modify mechanical properties has shown that blood protein adsorption and subsequent reactions with platelets do vary in this series of chemically related block copolyurethanes (1–3). Detailed studies using Fourier transform infrared spectroscopy (FTIR) and electron spectroscopy for chemical analysis (ESCA) have shown that the bulk and surface chemical and morphological structures are affected by both synthetic alterations of the polymeric repeat unit and by fabrication variables (1, 4–6). This chapter discusses our progress in determining the chemical and morphological structures of the bulk and the surface for this series of block copolyurethanes.

Experimental

Polymer Syntheses. The block copolyether-urethane–ureas were synthesized from polypropylene glycol, methylene bis(4-phenylisocyanate), and ethylenediamine using a two-step solution polymerization (7). The repeat unit structure was:

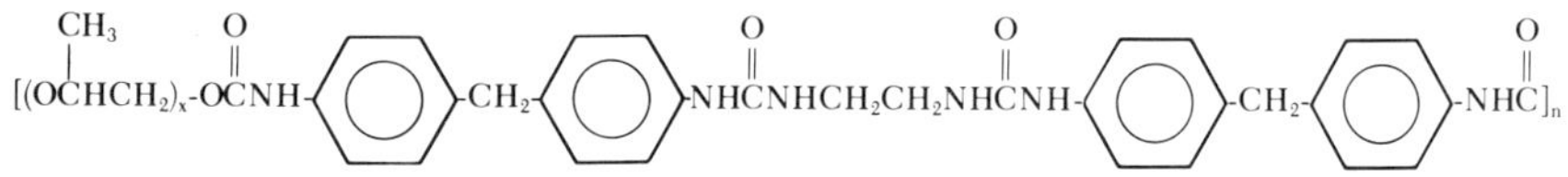

$$[(OCHCH_2)_x\text{-}OCNH\text{-}\langle\bigcirc\rangle\text{-}CH_2\text{-}\langle\bigcirc\rangle\text{-}NHCNHCH_2CH_2NHCNH\text{-}\langle\bigcirc\rangle\text{-}CH_2\text{-}\langle\bigcirc\rangle\text{-}NHC]_n$$
$$\overset{|}{CH_3}$$

Peuu

The polypropylene glycols used were of 700, 1000, and 2000 molecular weight (where x is approximately 12, 17, and 34, respectively). The copolymers are denoted as PEUU 700, PEUU 1000, and PEUU 2000. Inherent viscosities in N,N-dimethylformamide (0.5% concentration) at 30°C were 0.40 for PEUU 700, 0.65 for PEUU 1000, and 0.43 for PEUU 2000.

Films were prepared by solvent casting a filtered solution, 10% solids by weight of the polymer in distilled N,N-dimethylformamide, onto glass plates. The plates were placed in a forced air draft oven at 75°C for 1 h to evaporate the solvent. The films were then dried in a vacuum desiccator at 0.1 mm mercury for 24 h to insure complete removal of any residual solvent. The glass plates were washed with 0.1% aqueous Ivory soap solution, then rinsed with deionized water and absolute ethanol prior to use.

Model Compound Syntheses. The urea segments were modeled with two diurea compounds. Urea I was synthesized by reacting a 2:1 molar ratio of p-tolylisocyanate and ethylenediamine in anhydrous toluene to form:

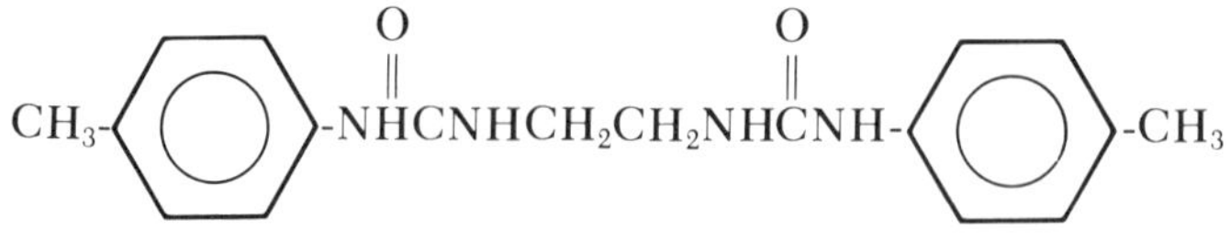

$$CH_3\text{-}\langle\bigcirc\rangle\text{-}NHCNHCH_2CH_2NHCNH\text{-}\langle\bigcirc\rangle\text{-}CH_3$$

Urea I

The white powder was recrystallized from hot N,N-dimethylformamide and the melting point was 233°–235°C. Urea II was synthesized by reacting a 2:1 molar ratio of hexylisocyanate and ethylenediamine in anhydrous ether to form:

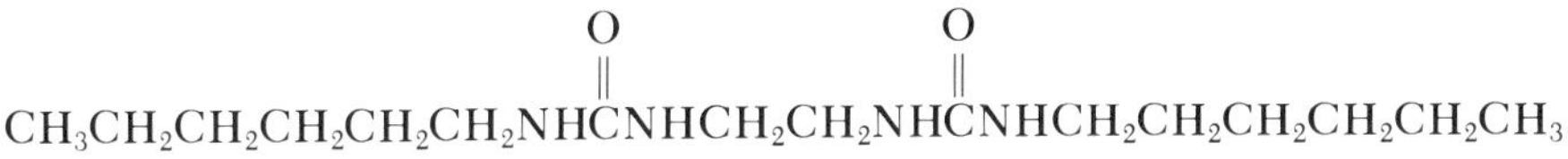

$$CH_3CH_2CH_2CH_2CH_2CH_2NH\overset{\overset{O}{\|}}{C}NHCH_2CH_2NH\overset{\overset{O}{\|}}{C}NHCH_2CH_2CH_2CH_2CH_2CH_3$$

Urea II

The white powder was recrystallized from hot N,N-dimethylformamide and the melting point was 203°–204°C.

The urea segment also was modeled with a polyurea homopolymer synthesized from methylene bis(4-phenylisocyanate) and ethylenediamine in dimethyl sulfoxide using a one-step polymerization technique (8). The repeat unit was:

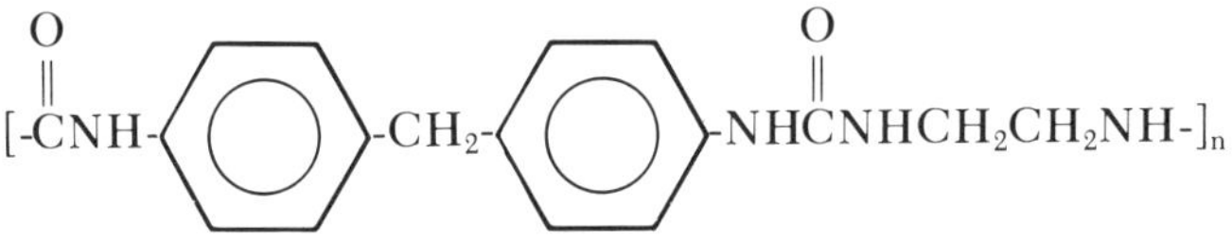

$$[-\overset{\overset{O}{\|}}{C}NH-\langle\bigcirc\rangle-CH_2-\langle\bigcirc\rangle-NH\overset{\overset{O}{\|}}{C}NHCH_2CH_2NH-]_n$$

Polyurea

The polymer was slightly soluble in *m*-cresol. Films were cast from a filtered solution, 5% solids by weight in *m*-cresol, and dried at 75°C in a forced air draft oven for 1 h. The films were then placed in a vacuum desiccator for 24 h (0.1 mm mercury) to remove residual solvent. The glass plates were cleaned prior to casting the films as described previously.

The urethane interfacing linkage was modeled with four model compounds. Urethane I was synthesized by reacting *p*-tolylisocyanate with 1-propanol in anhydrous toluene to form:

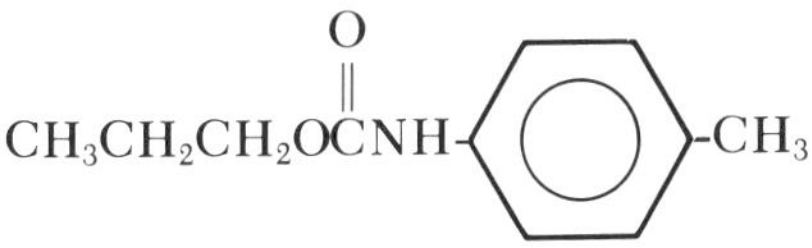

$$CH_3CH_2CH_2O\overset{\overset{O}{\|}}{C}NH-\langle\bigcirc\rangle-CH_3$$

Urethane I

The white powder was recrystallized from hot ethanol and the melting point was 55.5°–56.5°C. Urethane II was synthesized by reacting p-tolylisocyanate with 2-propanol in anhydrous toluene to form:

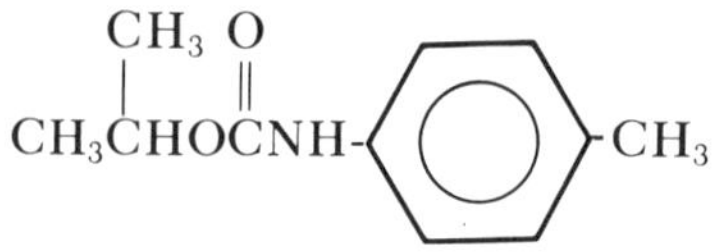

$$CH_3CHOCNH-C_6H_4-CH_3$$
(with CH_3 on the CH carbon and $\overset{O}{\underset{\|}{C}}$)

Urethane II

The white powder was recrystallized from hot ethanol, and the melting point was 54.5°–55.0°C. Urethane III was synthesized by reacting hexylisocyanate with 1-propanol in dioxane to form:

$$CH_3CH_2CH_2O\overset{O}{\underset{\|}{C}}NHCH_2CH_2CH_2CH_2CH_2CH_3$$

Urethane III

Excess isocyanate and dioxane were removed by distillation (as verified by infrared analysis) leaving a viscous liquid. Urethane IV was synthesized by reacting hexylisocyanate with 2-propanol in dioxane to form:

$$CH_3\underset{|}{\overset{CH_3}{C}}HO\overset{O}{\underset{\|}{C}}NHCH_2CH_2CH_2CH_2CH_2CH_3$$

Urethane IV

Excess isocyanate and dioxane were removed by distillation (as verified by infrared analysis) leaving a viscous liquid.

The urea segments and interfacing urethane linkage were modeled by an alternating copolyurethane–urea synthesized from methylene bis(4-phenylisocyanate), propylene glycol, and ethylenediamine in a two-step polymerization (7). The repeat unit of the copolyurethane–urea was:

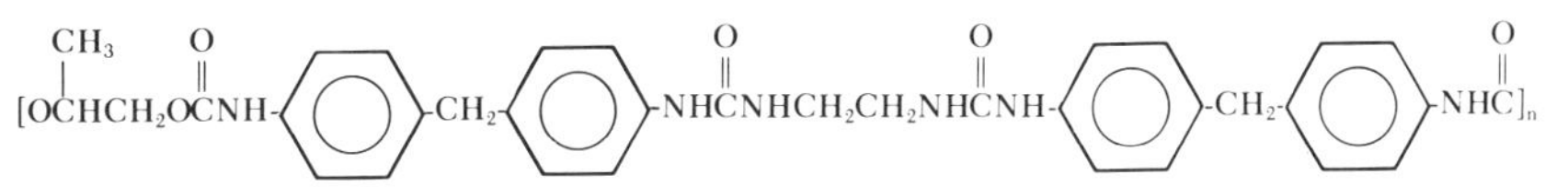

$$[\text{OCHCH}_2\text{OCNH}-\text{C}_6\text{H}_4-\text{CH}_2-\text{C}_6\text{H}_4-\text{NHCNHCH}_2\text{CH}_2\text{NHCNH}-\text{C}_6\text{H}_4-\text{CH}_2-\text{C}_6\text{H}_4-\text{NHC}]_n$$
(with CH$_3$ on the OCHCH$_2$ carbon and C=O groups as shown)

Polyurethane-Urea

Films were cast from a 5% solution of polymer in N,N-dimethylformamide onto glass plates (cleaned as described previously), dried in a forced air oven at 75°C for 1 h, and then placed in a vacuum desiccator (0.1 mm mercury) for 24 h to insure complete removal of any residual solvent.

The urethane interface region and polyether segments were modeled with a copolyether-urethane synthesized from polypropylene glycol (1000 MW) and methylene bis(4-phenylisocyanate) using a one-step solution polymerization technique (8). The copolymer has the following repeat unit structure:

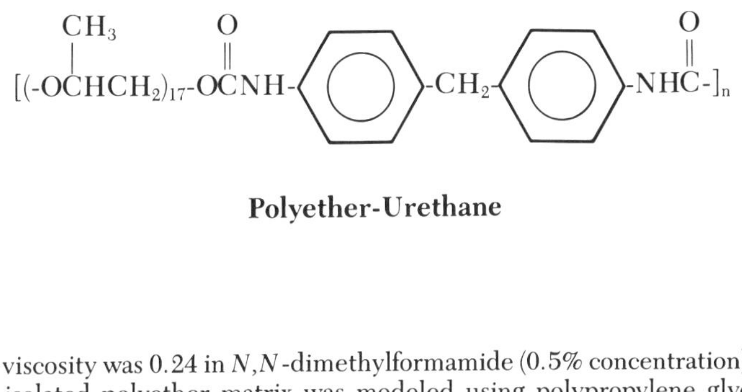

$$[(-\text{OCHCH}_2)_{17}-\text{OCNH}-\text{C}_6\text{H}_4-\text{CH}_2-\text{C}_6\text{H}_4-\text{NHC}-]_n$$
(with CH$_3$ substituent and C=O groups as shown)

Polyether-Urethane

Inherent viscosity was 0.24 in N,N-dimethylformamide (0.5% concentration) at 30°C.

The isolated polyether matrix was modeled using polypropylene glycol (2000 MW) and isotactic polypropylene oxide. The polypropylene glycol was degassed and placed over molecular sieves to remove residual water present in the polyol. The isotactic polypropylene oxide was isolated by repeated crystallization from acetone (9). Inherent viscosity was 1.85 in benzene (0.5% concentration) at 25°C. Films of the isotactic polypropylene oxide were cast onto glass plates (cleaned as described previously) from a 6% solution of the polymer in N,N-dimethylformamide, dried in a forced air draft oven for 1 h at 75°C, and then placed in a vacuum desiccator (0.1 mm mercury) for 24 h to insure complete removal of residual solvent.

Instrumental Methods. A Hewlett–Packard 595B ESCA spectrometer was utilized in the ESCA studies of the block copolyether-urethane–urea and model polymer films. The samples were allowed to come to equilibrium at 10^{-9} Torr at 300

K prior to data collection. The x-rays from the $Al(K_{\alpha 1,2})$ line at 1487 eV were used. Samples were scanned 10 times with a scan width of 20 eV centered around elemental spectra of interest: $C1s$ 290–270 eV, $N1s$ 405–385 eV, and $O1s$ 540–520 eV. Radiation damage was evaluated by overlaying the carbon spectrum obtained first for each sample on one obtained after all other elements of interest were scanned. Differences in spectra were within experimental error, so radiation damage was considered to be negligible for the qualitative studies. All bands were referenced to the 285-eV band of the $C1s$ spectrum for each sample. Peak areas were determined digitally and by a planimeter.

A Digilab 14B/D Fourier Transform infrared spectrometer was utilized to obtain 1-cm^{-1} resolution spectra over the 4000–400 cm^{-1} region for polyether-urethane–urea films. The sample chamber was allowed to come to equilibrium with a continuous nitrogen purge prior to data collection of 1000 scans per sample.

A Harrick variable-angle internal reflectance attachment and quadruple diamond polarizer were used to obtain spectra of the first 2000 Å of the surface of the films formed in contact with the glass plate. Germanium internal reflectance crystals (25 × 5 × 2 mm) having face cut angles of 60° were used at a 60° incident angle with perpendicular (90°) polarized radiation. Absorbance spectra of the internal reflectance crystals were obtained prior to placement of the sample films, and were stored in memory for later subtraction. Thus, only spectra of the sample films were obtained after the proper arithmetic operations.

Model polymers (polypropylene glycol, polyether-urethane, and polyurethane–urea) were studied by transmission using a Harrick transmission cell with 25 × 2-mm round ZnSe transmission crystals. The viscous polypropylene glycol and polyether-urethane were spread onto the crystals, with 0.005-mm spacers separating the crystals at a uniform thickness. Polyurethane–urea was solvent cast onto a single ZnSe crystal from a 5% solution (by weight) of the polymer in distilled N,N-dimethylformamide. The crystal was placed in a forced air draft oven at 75°C for 1 h to evaporate the solvent, and then placed in a vacuum desiccator (0.1 mm mercury) for 24 h to remove residual solvent. The transmission cell also was used to obtain spectra of homogeneous mixtures of polypropylene glycol or polyether-urethane with urea model compounds (Urea I or II) and/or urethane model compounds (Urethane I, II, III, or IV). The molar ratio mixtures studied included: 1:2 polypropylene glycol:urethane model compound; 1:4 polypropylene glycol:urethane model compound; 1:2 polypropylene glycol:urea model compound; 1:2:2 polypropylene glycol:urethane:urea model compound; 1:4:2 polypropylene glycol:urethane:urea model compound; and 1:2 polyether-urethane:urea model compound. Absorbance spectra of the ZnSe crystals were obtained prior to use, and were stored in memory for later subtraction, thus yielding only the spectra of the model polymers after the proper arithmetic operations.

Model compounds (Ureas I and II; Urethanes I, II, III, and IV) were studied in KBr pellets. KBr and model compounds were placed in a vacuum desiccator (0.1 mm mercury, 50°C) for 24 h prior to use to insure the absence of moisture. Absorbance spectra of the blank KBr pellet were obtained prior to model compound studies, and were stored in memory for later subtraction. Thus, only the spectra of the model compounds were obtained after the proper arithmetic operations.

Results and Discussion

While AB block copolymers are known to phase separate into relatively pure two-phase morphologies, multiple block copolymers such as these block copolyurethanes may not necessarily have such a complete phase separation.

Much literature is available concerning the degree of phase separation of copolyether-urethanes using infrared spectrscopy and other techniques (*10–14, 16, 18–20, 23–32*). However, much less information has been reported on the degree of phase separation for copolyether-urethane–ureas (*15, 17, 21, 22*). These studies indicate that phase separation occurs with the urethane groups forming domains in copolyether-urethane and with the urea groups forming the domains in polyether-urethane–ureas. However, the degree of phase separation, purity of the domains and polyether matrix, as well as mixing within the urethane interfacial region in polyether-urethane–ureas appear to be functions of the copolymer synthetic structure and thermal or mechanical history.

Our preliminary studies on copolyether-urethane–ureas based on polypropylene glycol, methylene bis(4-phenylisocyanate), and ethylenediamine also indicated a phase-separated morphology, but with mixing primarily between the urethane groups and the polyether matrix within the interface region (*4–6*). When the repeat structure of the copolyether-urethane–urea was modified by changing the molecular weight of the polyether segment, distinct changes occurred in the morphology of the three copolyurethane structures. In addition, the surface morphology changed as compared to the bulk. To understand these effects, the bulk morphology of the three copolyether-urethane–ureas was studied by transmission FTIR. The 3600–2500 cm^{-1} region of the spectra of PEUU 700, PEUU 1000, and PEUU 2000 are shown in Figure 1. Characteristic bands in this region include the N-H stretching band at 3320 cm^{-1} and the C-H stretching bands between 3000 and 2800 cm^{-1}. Because the free N-H stretching band near 3450 cm^{-1} was absent, the single symmetric band indicates complete hydrogen bonding of the urethane and urea N-H groups. The CH_3 asymmetric C-H stretching band absorbs at 2972 cm^{-1} and the symmetric stretching band at 2900 cm^{-1}; the CH_2 asymmetric C-H stretching band absorbs at 2932 cm^{-1} and the symmetric at 2872 cm^{-1}. The slight differences among the three polymers in the C-H stretching bands indicate the change in molecular weight of the polyether segment.

The 1800–900 cm^{-1} spectral regions of PEUU 700, PEUU 1000, and PEUU 2000 are shown in Figure 2. The characteristic bands include the urethane Amide I (C=O stretching) absorbing at 1730 cm^{-1}, with a 1712-cm^{-1} shoulder. The 1730-cm^{-1} band arises from the free urethane carbonyls, while the 1712-cm^{-1} shoulder arises from the portion of the urethane carbonyls in the hydrogen-bonded state. The single urea Amide I band at 1635 cm^{-1} illustrates essentially complete hydrogen bonding of the urea carbonyls. The 1600-cm^{-1} band is due to aromatic ring breathing vibrations. The Amide II bands of the urethane and urea groups absorb as a complex band between 1600 and 1510 cm^{-1}. Similarly, the urethane and urea Amide III bands overlap in the 1300–1210 cm^{-1} region, along with the asymmetric stretching band of the ester portion (O=C-O) of the urethane group. The broad ether stretching band absorbs at 1110 cm^{-1}.

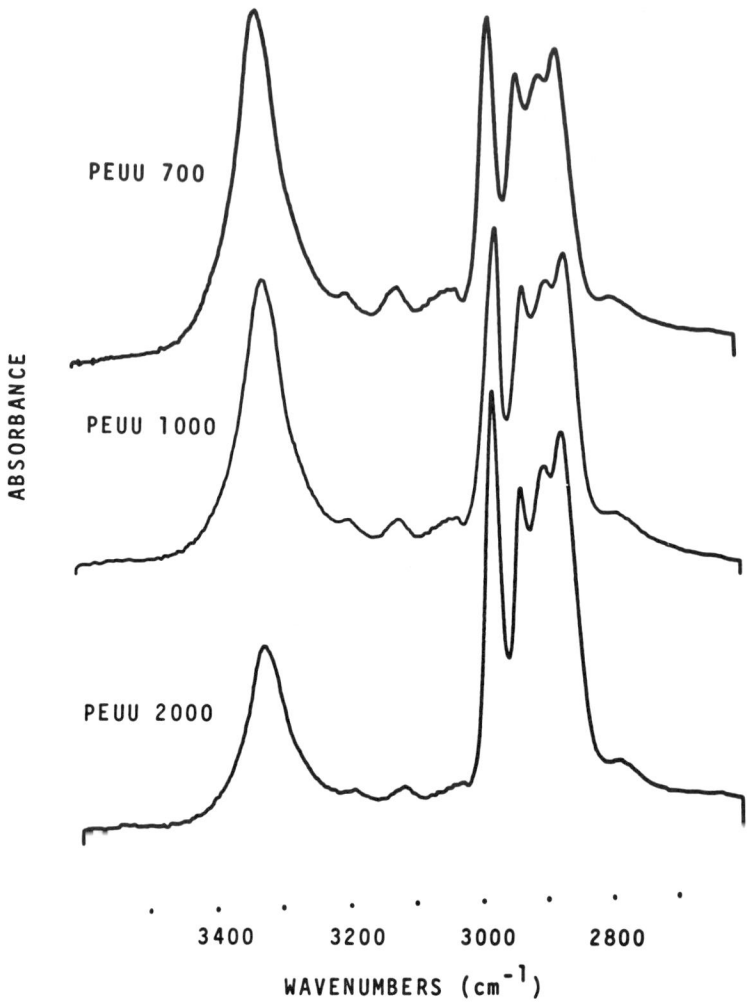

Figure 1. Transmission spectra (3600–2600 cm^{-1}) of copolyether-urethane–ureas.

Urethane and urea Amide bands coupled with the N–H stretching bands have been studied by many investigators to explore the relationship between intermolecular and intramolecular interactions and morphologies of polyether-urethanes (16, 18–20, 23–32) and polyether-urethane–ureas (15,17,21,22,33–37). The N–H groups serve as proton donors in the interactions. The possible proton acceptors in polyether-urethanes initially were assumed to be only the urethane carbonyls or polyether oxygens (16, 19, 23–27). Under these assumptions, complete phase separation characterized

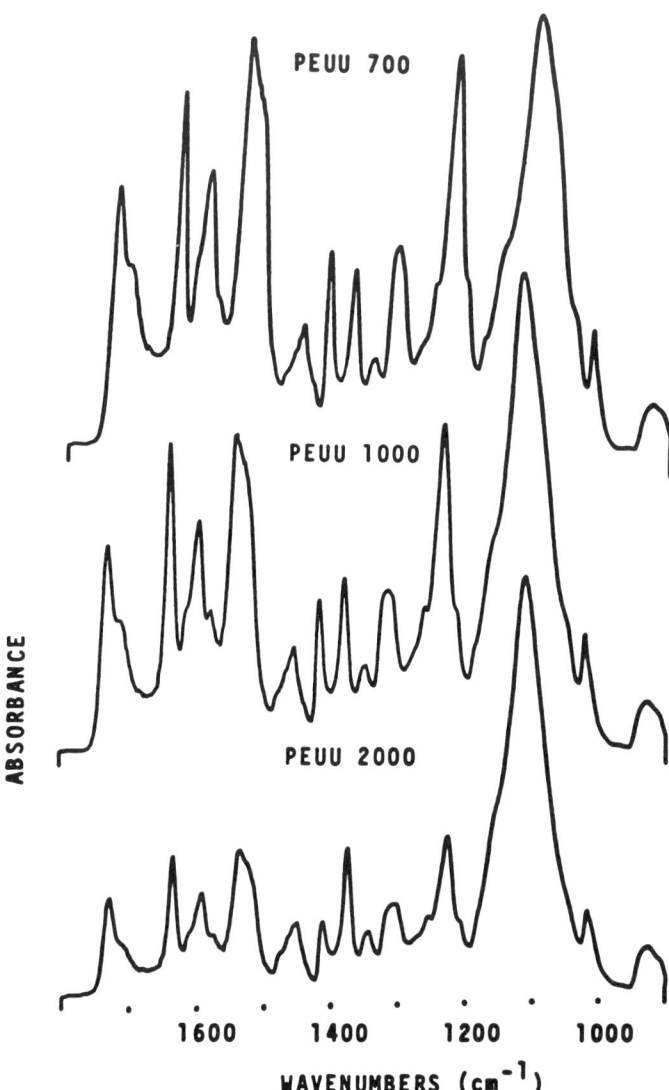

Figure 2. Transmission spectra (1800–900 cm^{-1}) of copolyether–urethane–ureas.

by pure urethane domains dispersed in a pure polyether matrix would be illustrated in the infrared spectrum by complete hydrogen bonding of the N–H groups to the urethane carbonyls. The presence of a free urethane Amide I band despite essentially complete hydrogen bonding of the N–H proton donating groups arises from interactions between the urethane N–H, and the polyether oxygen, thereby freeing the urethane carbonyl (*15–17, 19, 24–29*). Phase mixing and purity would be studied in terms of the degree of hydrogen bonding of the urethane Amide I carbonyl band. However, an additional proton acceptor was postulated by Boyarchuk et al. (*28*) and later by Sung et al. (*18, 22, 30–33, 37*). Interactions between the urethane alkoxy oxygen and the N–H group within the domain-interface region would result in a free urethane carbonyl, similar to the interactions involving the polyether oxygen. Therefore, the ratio of hydrogen-bonded to free urethane carbonyl with complete N–H hydrogen bonding results in a minimum estimation of phase separation. However, increased urethane carbonyl Amide I in the hydrogen-bonded state has been associated with polyether-urethanes having higher degress of phase separation (*10–37*).

Polyether-urethane–urea morphologies are different from those of polyether-urethanes in that the urea segments form domains interfacing through the urethane linkage to the polyether matrix. The urethane carbonyl Amide I indicates interface size and purity, while the urea Amide bands indicate degree of phase separation. The possible proton-donating groups are the urea and urethane N–H groups, and the possible proton acceptors include urethane carbonyl (*1–37*), urethane alkoxy (*18, 22, 30–33*), and polyether (*14–37*) oxygens.

A well phase-separated polyether-urethane–urea morphology would be reflected in the infrared spectrum by hydrogen bonding between urea groups and possibly urethane groups, as well as by limited interactions between the urethane groups and the polyether matrix at the interface. The urea segment has two possible proton-donating N–H groups per proton-accepting carbonyl; therefore, complete hydrogen bonding within the pure domain may exist despite the presence of free urea N–H stretching. However, Bonart et al. (*39*) and later Sung et al. (*22, 33*) postulated the ability of the single proton-accepting urea carbonyl to form a three-dimensional dihydrogen bond between two neighboring proton-donating N–H groups. We showed this type of dihydrogen bonding in an aromatic urea model compound (*4*).

A phase-mixed morphology would have urea segments dispersed throughout the polyether matrix. This structure would be evidenced by a large degree of free urethane and urea carbonyls due to interactions of the proton-donating N–H groups with the polyether oxygens.

A partially phase-separated morphology may be characterized by either segments of polyether dispersed within the domains and/or segments of urea dispersed in the polyether matrix. Another partially phase-separated morphology would involve relatively pure urea domains and polyether matrix separated by a wider urethane interface due to interactions with either the urea segments of the domain or polyether segments from the matrix. This structure would be reflected in the infrared spectrum by interactions between urea and urethane, as well as by a higher number of urethane carbonyls in the free state due to interactions between the urethane N–H groups and polyether oxygen. As in polyether-urethanes, the possibility of urethane alkoxy oxygens acting as a proton acceptor for either urethane or urea proton-donating N–H groups would result in low estimations of interfacial size and domain purity as determined by the free urethane Amide I carbonyl. Sung et al. (18) estimated that approximately 15% of the N–H groups participate in interactions with the urethane alkoxy oxygens in polyether-urethanes.

The infrared spectra of polyether-urethane–ureas are complex due to the varying chemical structure and possible morphological structures resulting in many different types of intermolecular and intramolecular interactions. To study how chemical and morphological structures might affect interactions involving the sensitive Amide and N–H stretching regions in our particular block copolyurethane systems, model compounds and model polymer systems were studied under selected secondary bonding environments in the pure state or in homogeneous mixtures. These selected bonding environments enhanced particular associations that would mimic various degrees of phase separation and purity possible within the copolyether-urethane–urea systems. In addition, the individual model compounds were used in band assignments and to distinguish between the overlapping bands of the urethane and urea Amide II and Amide III regions.

Aromatic urethane model compounds (Urethanes I and II) were studied in the crystalline form to identify the characteristic Amide bands in the interface region when freed of any interactions with urea or polyether segments. Aliphatic urethane model compounds (Urethanes III and IV) were studied to identify the influence of aromatic rings on particular bands. The 1800–1200 cm^{-1} regions of aromatic Urethane I and aliphatic Urethane III are shown in Figure 3.

The aromatic urethane carbonyl stretching Amide I bands were comprised of several shoulders. The aromatic urethane Amide I bands are dominated by an intense band absorbing at 1705 cm^{-1} for Urethane I (Figure 3) and at 1695 cm^{-1} for Urethane II. A distinct shoulder due to free carbonyls is emerging at 1720 cm^{-1} in the spectra of Urethane I and Urethane II. In addition, Urethane I has an N–H region comprised of an asymmetric band absorbing at 3320 cm^{-1} with a weak shoulder emerging at 3305 cm^{-1}. Urethane II has a symmetric band absorbing at 3300 cm^{-1}. Therefore, the N–H groups are essentially completely hydrogen bonded. Thus, these aromatic urethane model compounds show that the free carbonyl stretching shoulder must arise from N–H groups interacting with the alkoxy oxygen. The emerging shoulder at 1685 cm^{-1} in the spectrum of Urethane I (Figure 3) and at

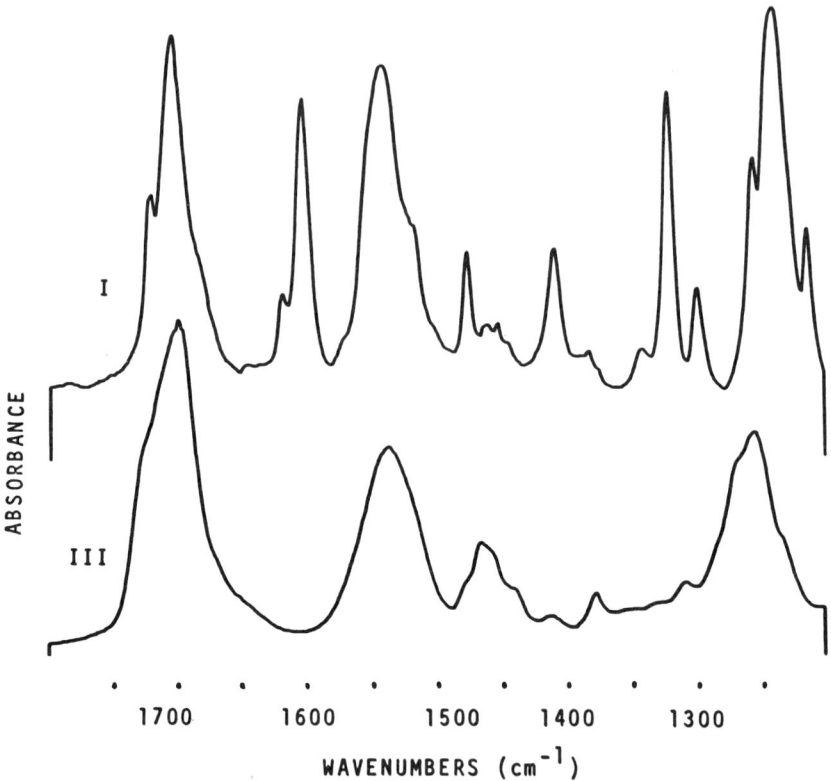

Figure 3 Transmission spectra (1800-1200 cm^{-1}) of Urethane I and Urethane III.

1675 cm^{-1} for Urethane II, coupled with the lower wave number N–H stretching shoulders, represents a portion of the hydrogen-bonded urethane carbonyls in a higher ordered state (4). The C–N stretching and N–H bending vibrations give rise to the complex Amide II bands. Both aromatic Urethane I (Figure 3) and Urethane II have the major Amide II band absorbing at 1540 cm^{-1} and an emerging shoulder at 1520 cm^{-1}. The 1510-cm^{-1} shoulder arises from aromatic ring breathing vibrations. The C–N stretching and N–H bending vibrations also contribute to the Amide III band overlapping with the O=C–O asymmetric stretching vibration. The Amide III band of Urethane I (Figure 3) absorbs at 1240 cm^{-1} with a weaker shoulder at 1255 cm^{-1}. Urethane II has a major band at 1250 cm^{-1} with shoulders at 1260 and 1280 cm^{-1}. The aromatic in-plane C–H bending vibration absorbs at 1210 cm^{-1} in both compounds. The aromatic urethanes also have an additional C–N stretching band that has been described in aromatic amines as being associated with the benzene ring (38).

The infrared spectra of the aliphatic Urethane III (Figure 3) and Urethane IV model compounds were more similar to each other than the spectra for the aromatic urethane model compounds. The amide region of the aliphatic model compounds had an intense hydrogen-bonded Amide I absorbing at 1700 cm^{-1} in the spectrum of Urethane III (Figure 3) and at 1695 cm^{-1} for Urethane IV. The spectra of both compounds have emerging shoulders at 1720 cm^{-1}. The N–H stretching region was comprised of a symmetric band at 3337 cm^{-1} and a very weak 3450-cm^{-1} band. The majority of the N–H groups are hydrogen bonded; however, unlike the aromatic urethane model compounds, a portion are in the free state. The portion of N–H groups in the unbonded state does not account for the intense free shoulder noted in the urethane carbonyl Amide I region. Therefore, a portion of the N–H groups are interacting with the urethane alkoxy oxygen, resulting in the high-frequency shoulder. The Amide II region is comprised of a single asymmetric band absorbing at 1537 cm^{-1} with an emerging low-frequency shoulder in the spectra of both aliphatic compounds. The Amide III region is more complex with the major band absorbing at 1255 cm^{-1}. Weaker shoulders are absorbing at 1265 and 1235 cm^{-1}.

Complete dispersion of the aromatic urethane model compounds in polypropylene glycol modeled interactions that might occur between the urethane linkages in the interface region and the polyether matrix without the influence of the urea domains. Aromatic Urethanes I and II and aliphatic Urethanes III and IV were in homogeneous 1:2 and 1:4 molar ratio mixtures with polypropylene glycol (2000 MW) to study the influence of increasing polypropylene glycol molecular weight on the intermolecular interactions between the urethane N–H group and the polyether oxygen. The 1:2 molar ratio homogeneous mixture represents 34 polyether repeats to 2 urethane groups as found in PEUU 2000, while the 1:4 molar ratio mixture represents the 17 polyether repeats to 2 urethane groups as found in PEUU 1000.

Figure 4 illustrates the 1800–1200 cm^{-1} regions of the 1:2 and 1:4 homogeneous mixtures of aromatic Urethane I with polypropylene glycol. The homogeneous mixtures with aromatic Urethane II were similar. The urethane Amide I bands in the mixtures are comprised of the free carbonyl stretching band at 1730 cm^{-1} and the less intense hydrogen-bonded shoulder at 1712 cm^{-1}. Because the N–H stretching band for the two aromatic mixtures absorbs as a single band at 3320 cm^{-1}, the N–H groups are essentially completely hydrogen bonded. The free carbonyls arise principally from interactions with the poly-ether oxygen; however, some N–H groups also could be interacting with urethane alkoxy oxygen (*18, 22, 28, 30–33, 37*). Absorbance ratios of the two shoulders show that 73% of the carbonyls are in the free state in the 1:2 mixtures and 68% are in the 1:4 mixtures. The Amide II region is similar to that for the pure aromatic urethane model compounds. However, the Amide III region is comprised of only the dominant 1225-cm^{-1} band and weaker 1210- and 1260-cm^{-1} shoulders.

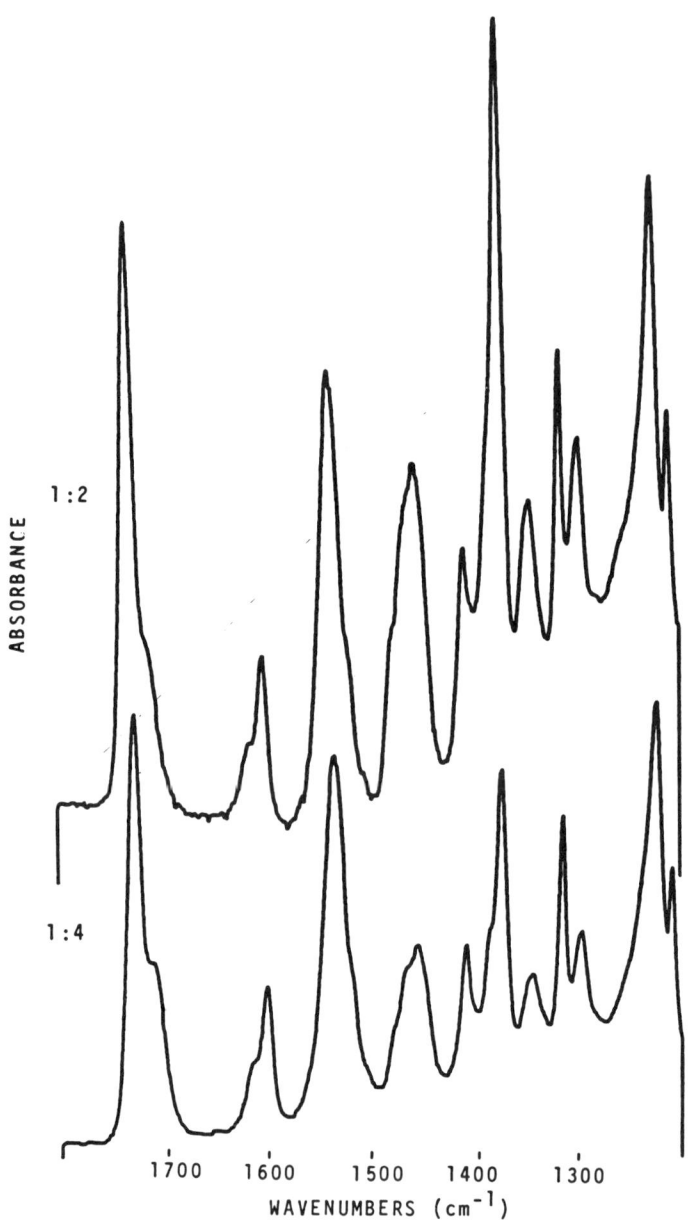

Figure 4. Transmission spectra (1800–1200 cm^{-1}) of 1:2 and 1:4 molar ratio mixtures of polypropylene glycol to Urethane I (4).

Homogeneous 1:2 and 1:4 molar mixtures of aliphatic Urethanes III or IV with polypropylene glycol (2000 MW) are similar to the aromatic Urethane I or II mixtures in the Amide I and II regions. However, the Amide III band absorbs at 1245 cm^{-1}, with a weaker 1260-cm^{-1} shoulder. The 1210-cm^{-1} shoulder due to vibrations of the aromatic ring is missing. Also, the 1320-cm^{-1} shoulder present in the aromatic mixtures is absent in the aliphatic mixtures.

Polyether-urethane having 17 polyether repeats to 2 urethane groups was studied also. The urethane Amide regions and N–H stretching regions were similar to the 1:4 mixtures of either aromatic Urethane I or II with polypropylene glycol (*4*). The urethane Amide region coupled with the N–H stretching region indicates that 68% of the urethane carbonyls are in the free state due to intermolecular interactions between the urethane N–H groups and either the polyether or urethane alkoxy oxygens.

Both model compound and polymer studies indicate that the urethane Amide region is particularly sensitive to the interactions between the urethane interface and the polyether matrix. Also, the steric and chemical incompatibilities between the urethane and polyether groups are not sufficient to promote significant phase separation of the urethane segments with the particular urethane segment length. The absorbance of the free urethane Amide I shoulder provides an indication of hydrogen bonding between the urethane N–H groups and the polyether or the urethane alkoxy oxygens. Although the ether oxygen is assumed to be the principal proton acceptor resulting in the free shoulder, only limited interactions occurred between the urethane alkoxy oxygen and N–H groups in the crystalline urethane model compounds.

The types of secondary bonding occurring within a pure urea domain due to complete phase separation were investigated with crystalline aromatic Urea I and aliphatic Urea II. The 1800–700 cm^{-1} regions of the urea model compounds are shown in Figure 5. The urea carbonyl stretching Amide I absorbs at 1635 cm^{-1} for atomatic Urea I and at 1620 cm^{-1} for aliphatic Urea II. Aromatic Urea I has aromatic ring breathing vibrations absorbing at 1610 and 1595 cm^{-1}. Aromatic Urea I also has Amide II bands absorbing at 1580 and 1525 cm^{-1}, while aliphatic Urea II has Amide II bands absorbing at 1590 and 1535 cm^{-1}. The 1590-cm^{-1} shoulder in the spectrum of aliphatic Urea II is not due to aromatic ring vibrations, as confirmed by the absence of the 820-cm^{-1} aromatic C–H bending band. A shift of the Amide I band to higher wave numbers (1635 cm^{-1}) in the aromatic Urea I spectrum, as compared to the Amide I band (1620 cm^{-1}) in the aliphatic Urea II spectrum, coupled with an opposing shift in the Amide II high wave number shoulder from 1580 cm^{-1} for aromatic Urea I to 1590 cm^{-1} for aliphatic Urea II, indicates that the high wave number Amide II shoulder arises from the N–H bending vibration. The aromatic Urea I Amide III region is comprised of a series of bands absorbing at 1290, 1270, 1257, and 1235 cm^{-1}. The aliphatic Amide III region is also comprised of a series of bands absorbing at 1290, 1275, 1265, 1245, and 1227 cm^{-1}. Both urea model compounds have complete hydrogen bonding of the urea carbonyl and N–H groups. Therefore, a single urea carbonyl must be capable of forming a dihydrogen bond with two N–H groups, as postulated by Bonart et al. (39) and Sung et al. (22, 35), and as evidenced in the spectra of the urea model compounds (Figure 5) by complete hydrogen bonding of both the N–H and carbonyl groups in the crystalline state.

The types of intermolecular and intramolecular interactions occurring with dispersion of urea segments in the polyether matrix were modeled with homogeneous 1:2 molar mixtures of aromatic Urea I or aliphatic Urea II, with polypropylene glycol having the same ratio of polyether repeats to urea groups as in the repeat unit of PEUU 1000. Neither mixture spectrum showed a shift in location nor a broadening of the urea Amide I bands; therefore, no interactions occurred between the urea proton-donating N–H groups and polyether oxygens, resulting in a free urea carbonyl Amide I shoulder. The Amide II band was not altered in the aromatic urea mixture;

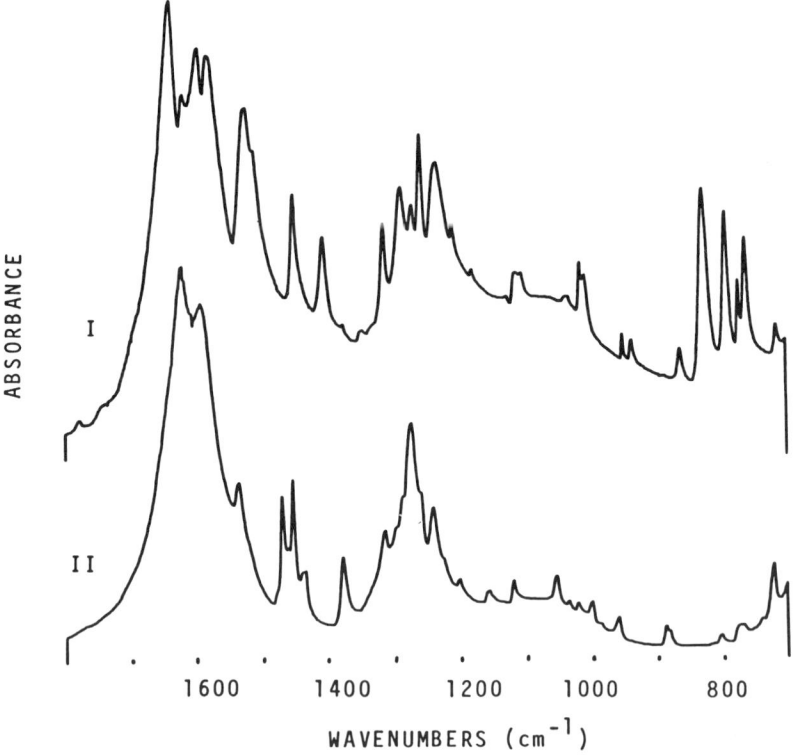

Figure 5. Transmission spectra (1800–700 cm^{-1}) of Urea I and Urea II.

however, the N–H bending Amide II shoulder in the aliphatic urea mixture did broaden toward 1600 cm^{-1}. Thus, the urea compounds remain essentially hydrogen bonded to ureas rather than interacting with the polypropylene glycol. Therefore, the aromatic urea segment does have a strong tendency to form domain-like aggregations due to strong secondary bonding and steric hindrances. The dihydrogen bonding between the single carbonyl and two N–H groups was maintained in the homogeneous mixtures.

Tri-mixtures of polypropylene glycol with urethane and urea model compounds were studied to investigate the interactions occurring when the three possible proton acceptors were present together. The 1:2:2 homogeneous molar ratio mixtures of polypropylene glycol (2000 MW) to aromatic Urethane I or Urethane II to aromatic Urea I have the same ratio of polyether, urethane, and urea groups as in PEUU 2000, while the 1:4:2 molar ratio has the same number of groups as in PEUU 1000. Similar mixtures of polypropylene glycol, aliphatic Urethane III or IV, and aliphatic Urea II were studied to investigate further the influence of the aromatic rings.

Spectra of the 1:2:2 and 1:4:2 mixtures involving aromatic Urethane I and Urea I are illustrated in Figure 6. The urethane Amide I bands absorb at 1730 and 1712 cm^{-1} for 1:2:2 and 1:4:2 mixtures with either aromatic Urethane I or Urethane II and aromatic Urea I. The 1:2:2 mixtures have approximately 74% of the urethane Amide I bands arising from urethane carbonyls in the free state, which is the same percentage as determined in the 1:2 mixtures with only polypropylene glycol and the aromatic urethane model compounds. The 1:4:2 mixtures have approximately 67% of the urethane carbonyls nonhydrogen bonded as compared to 68% in the 1:4 mixtures. The urea Amide I bands do not broaden or shift in frequency. The Amide II bands are broad and asymmetric, absorbing at 1530 cm^{-1} and having a weak shoulder at 1510 cm^{-1}. In addition, the aromatic ring breathing band absorbtion at 1600 cm^{-1} with a low-frequency shoulder previously associated with absorption at 1575 cm^{-1}. The Amide III bands are broad and asymmetric, absorbing at 1225 cm^{-1}.

Similar results were noted in a 1:2 homogeneous molar ratio mixture of polyether-urethane to aromatic Urea I. Also, mixtures with polypropylene glycol and aliphatic Urethane III or IV and aliphatic Urea II are similar to the trends noted in the aromatic tri-mixtures. The aliphatic mixture spectra do not have the 1320 cm^{-1} previously associated with the aromatic C–N stretching vibrations. The urea Amide bands also do not broaden or shift in frequency as compared to the 1:2 molar ratio mixture involving only polypropylene glycol and aliphatic urethanes or aliphatic ureas.

Therefore, negligible interactions, if any, occur between the urea proton-donating N–H groups and polyether oxygen due to the absence of a free urea carbonyl Amide I. Also, significant interactions occur between the urethane N–H groups and polyether oxygens, as evidenced by the significant free urethane Amide I band.

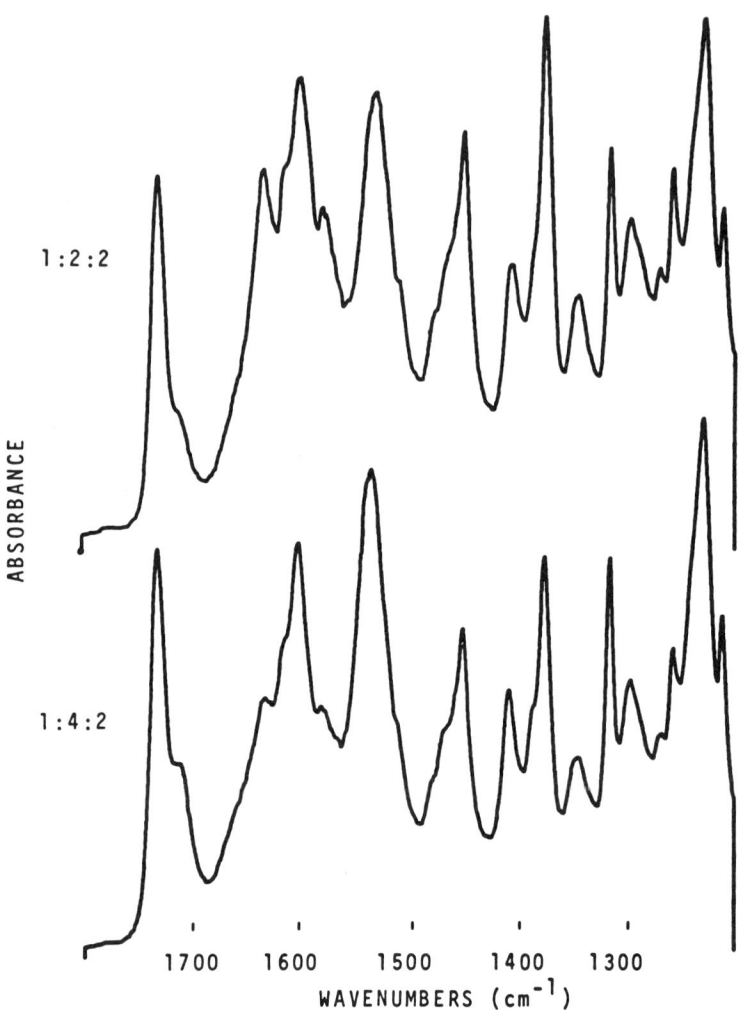

Figure 6. Transmission spectra (1800–1200 cm^{-1}) of 1:2:2 and 1:4:2 molar ratio mixtures of polypropylene glycol to Urethane I to Urea I.

Homogeneous mixtures of homopolymers and model compounds provide significant information concerning the possible intermolecular interactions occurring between the molecular groups in polyether-urethane–ureas, as long as the chemical and steric structures of the model compounds were chosen appropriately to model existing structures in the copolyurethane–urea. The reproducibility between model compound mixtures and the similar model polymer (polyether-urethane) indicates that mixing was occurring on the molecular level in the model compound mixtures. The modeling studies have demonstrated the ability of the urea segment to hydrogen bond completely with other ureas through three-dimensional interactions, thereby forming domain-like aggregates. Also, urethane groups are capable of significant interactions with the polyether matrix through the urethane N–H groups and polyether oxygens. The urethane model compounds do show the feasibility of the urethane N–H proton-donating groups to interact with the urethane alkoxy oxygen. Therefore, the absorbance ratio of urethane Amide I carbonyls in the free to hydrogen-bonded state provides a high estimation of mixing within the interface. The purity of the domains is illustrated through the absence of urea Amide I carbonyls in the free state.

The bulk morphology of PEUU 1000 has been described as having urea domains essentially completely phase separated and hydrogen bonded; the urethane interface is of moderate size (i.e., 10–15 Å rather than 3 Å), with 61% of the urethane carbonyls freed due to dipolar interactions between the urethane N–H proton-donating groups and either the polyether or urethane alkoxy proton-accepting oxygens (4–6). Alterations in the interface region have occurred as the molecular weight of the polyether segment decreased from 2000, 1000, to 700 molecular weight. The weight percent of the diisocyanate and ethylenediamine for the copolyether-urethane–ureas has a corresponding increase from 22% for PEUU 2000, to 35% for PEUU 1000, to 44% for PEUU 700.

A decrease in molecular weight of the polyether segment from 2000 to 700 molecular weight results in an increase in hydrogen bonding of the urethane carbonyls in the bulk as evidenced in the urethane Amide I. The percentage of the urethane Amide I in the hydrogen-bonded state increases progressively from 35% for PEUU 2000, to 39% for PEUU 1000, to 41% for PEUU 700 (Figure 2). This would imply a decreased mixing between the polyether matrix and urethane interface as the molecular weight of the polyether segment decreases. The decrease in mixing is representative of a narrower interface region.

The urea domains do remain completely hydrogen bonded and do not show evidence of mixing with the polyether matrix, that is, the N-H stretching and urea carbonyl Amide I bands do not broaden or shift in location. However, differences in the Amide II bands could indicate a change in order occurring within the domain or in the region between the urea domain and the urethane interface as the molecular weight of the polyether segment is decreased. The urea Amide II shoulder at 1575 cm^{-1} is a distinctive shoulder in PEUU 1000 and PEUU 2000, but it is a weaker emerging shoulder at 1580 cm^{-1} in PEUU 700. The other urea Amide II shoulder absorbing at 1525 cm^{-1} is more intense in PEUU 1000 and PEUU 2000 as compared to the 1522-cm^{-1} shoulder in PEUU 700. The shift of the higher wave number Amide II shoulder to higher wave numbers (1575–1580 cm^{-1}) in the copolyurethanes containing the lower molecular weight polyether segment also indicates an increase in the strength of the urea hydrogen bond due to less mixing between the urea and urethane groups with a narrower interface.

The surface morphologies of these block copolyurethanes differ from their bulk morphologies (4–6). Because the surface controls the interaction of a vascular implant with blood, the surface structure and its relation to the bulk structure of the same material was determined also. Originally, ESCA was explored to study the surface structure because the depth of penetration was within the first 100 Å. The low surface depth of penetration and subtle shifts in binding energies that result in peak splittings of the elemental spectra appeared to make this an attractive method to study the chemical and bonding environments of the elements (40).

Polyurethane–urea, polyurea, and isotactic polypropylene oxide were used to study the peak splittings occurring in the carbon 1s spectrum of the polyether-urethane–urea that are particular to either the domain, matrix, or interface regions. The carbons π-bonding to oxygen in either the urea or urethane segment form a shoulder at 289.5 eV, while those carbons σ-bonding to oxygen in the polyether matrix and the ester portion of the urethane interface form the 286.5-eV shoulder. The base carbon shoulder at 285 eV represents the remaining carbons bonding either to carbon or nitrogen atoms. Therefore, the 289.5-eV shoulder is characteristic of the urea domains and urethane interface, while the 286.5-eV shoulder is more characteristic of the polyether matrix.

The surfaces of polyether-urethane–urea films formed in contact with the glass plate or the air were studied using ESCA. The ratios of the peak areas for the three carbon shoulders are given in Table I, along with the theoretical ratios of the carbon atoms participating in the three types of bonds per repeat unit as a representative of a bulk sample. The glass and air surfaces of PEUU 700 and PEUU 1000 show an increase in ether on both surfaces compared to the theoretical ratios. PEUU 2000 surfaces show an increase in urethane and urea carbonyls as compared to ether oxygen. However, the information obtained using ESCA does not distinguish between complete phase separation or homogeneous mixing, since the two extremes could still have the same population of groups on the surface. All the information

Table I. Ratios of ESCA Carbon 1s Bands

Surface	C–O/C–O	C–O/C–C	C=O/C–C
PEUU 700 glass	11.18	0.91	0.08
PEUU 700 air	8.30	0.67	0.08
PEUU 700 theory	6.00	0.60	0.10
PEUU 1000 glass	11.41	1.09	0.10
PEUU 1000 air	16.55	1.07	0.06
PEUU 1000 theory	9.00	0.78	0.09
PEUU 2000 glass	10.62	1.32	0.12
PEUU 2000 air	13.63	1.12	0.08
PEUU 2000 theory	17.50	1.11	0.06

concerning the surface chemical and morphological structures concerns only the population of the various chemical structures present, and not the intermolecular and intramolecular interactions leading to various degrees of phase separation and purity.

FTIR coupled with internal reflectance allows the study of the chemical groups as well as the intermolecular and intramolecular interactions occurring with varying degrees of phase separation. The depth of penetration using a 60° germanium internal reflectance crystal at an incident angle of 60° is within the first 2000 Å of the surface (41). Previous studies of PEUU 1000 using different internal reflectance crystals and angles have shown an increase in hydrogen bonding of the urethane carbonyl Amide I with decreasing depth of penetration. Therefore, the interface region is narrower within the surface as implied by the increase in urethane carbonyls in the hydrogen-bonded state. The surface FTIR studies also confirmed the increase in ether on the surface of PEUU 1000 compared to the bulk determined in the ESCA studies (4–6).

The 1800–900 cm^{-1} spectral regions for the three polymers obtained with the 60° germanium internal reflectance crystal are shown in Figure 7. Table II tabulates the percentage of urethane Amide I in the hydrogen-bonded state, as well as the absorbance ratio of the urethane Amide I band to the asymmetric stretching ether for the three surfaces and the bulk structures. The percentage of urethane Amide I in the hydrogen-bonded state on the surface is higher compared to the bulk for all three polymers, thus indicating a narrower interface region on the surface. The degree of increase in hydrogen bonding between surface and bulk was greater as the molecular weight of the polyether segment increased (2% for PEUU 700, 5% for PEUU 1000, and 8% for PEUU 2000). The ratio of the urethane Amide I to ether asymmetric stretching (indicating the relative concentration of interface on the surface) decreases for the surface as compared to the bulk, as the molecular weight of the polyether segment increases (40% for PEUU 700, 21% for PEUU 1000, and 5% for PEUU 2000). The FTIR data confirm the trend suggested by the ESCA data.

The urethane interface has significant mixing with the polyether matrix, although a limited degree of mixing also may occur with the urea segment. The degree of mixing increases with the molecular weight of the polyether segment as indicated from the amount of hydrogen bonding for the urethane carbonyls. As the surface of each copolyurethane is approached, the interface region narrows, as shown by increased hydrogen bonding of the Urethane I. The urea segments remain essentially completely phase separated, as evidenced by the complete hydrogen bonding of the urea carbonyls reflected in the urea Amide I band. The interface region on the surface narrows with decreasing polyether molecular weight, compared to the bulk for each particular polyether-urethane-urea.

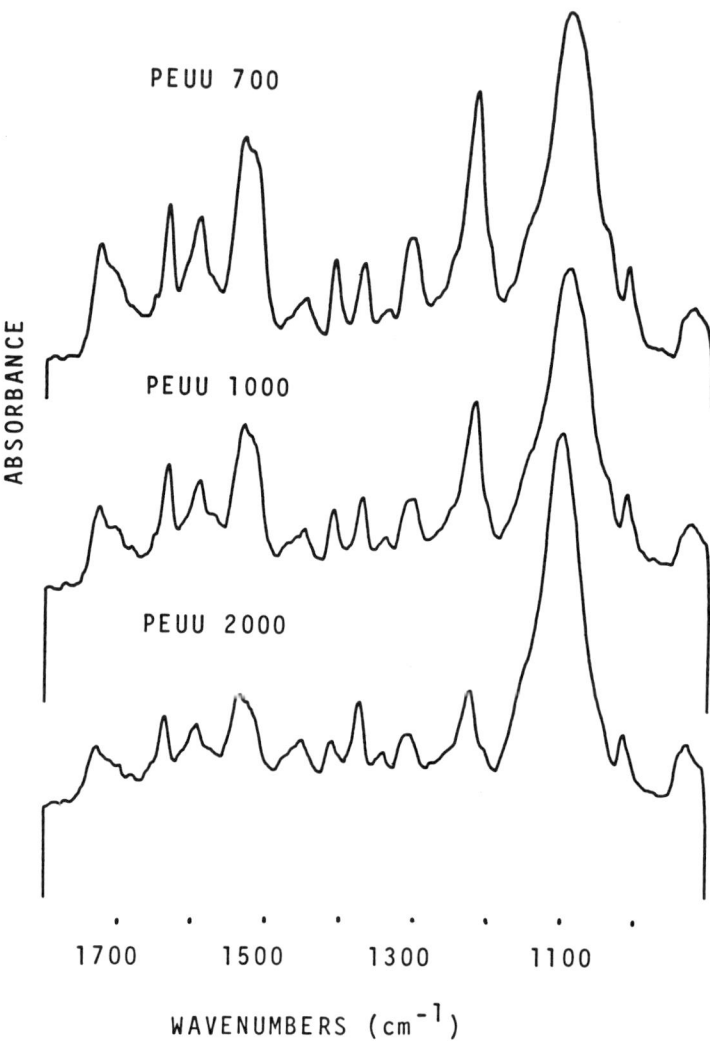

Figure 7. Internal reflectance spectra (1800–900 cm^{-1}) of copolyether–urethane–ureas.

Table II. Urethane Amide I Band

PEUU	% Hydrogen Bonded	Urethane/Ether
700 bulk	41[1]	0.98
700 surface	43	0.58
1000 bulk	39	0.72
1000 surface	44	0.51
2000 bulk	35	0.37
2000 surface	43	0.32

[1]Standard deviation is less than 0.3% hydrogen bonded.

In summary, the surface chemical and morphological structures of block copolyether-urethane–ureas may be determined by ESCA and FTIR coupled with internal reflectance techniques to probe the surface and bulk structures. These ESCA and FTIR data are being used to model the domain–interface structure of these copolyurethanes and their interaction with blood protein.

Acknowledgments

This work was supported by the National Science Foundation, Grant DMR 80–05499 A01, Polymer Program.

Literature Cited

1. Lyman, D. J.; Albo, D., Jr.; Jackson, R. T.; Knutson, K. *Trans. Am. Soc. Artif. Intern. Organs* **1977**, *23*, 253.
2. Lyman, D. J.; Knutson, K.; McNeill, B.; Shibatani, K. *Trans. Am. Soc. Artif. Intern. Organs* **1975**, *21*, 49.
3. Lyman, D. J.; Metcalf, L. C.; Albo, D., Jr.; Richards, K. F.; Lamb, J. *Trans. Am. Soc. Artif. Intern. Organs* **1974**, *20*, 474.
4. Knutson, K.; Lyman, D. J. "Biomedical and Dental Applications of Polymers," Gebelein, C. G., Ed., Plenum: New York, 1980; 173.
5. Lyman, D. J.; Knutson, K. "Polymeric Materials and Pharmaceuticals for Biomedical Uses," Nakajima, A.; Goldberg, E. P., Eds., Academic: New York, 1980; 1.
6. Lyman, D. J. "IUPAC Macromolecular Symposium," Ciardelli, C. F.; Giusti, P., Eds., Pergamon Press Ltd.: Oxford, 1980; p. 205.
7. Lyman, D. J.; Kwan-Gett, C.; Zwart, H. H. J.; Bland, A.; Eastwood, N.; Kawai, J.; Kolff, W. J. *Trans. Am. Soc. Artif. Intern. Organs* **1971**, *17*, 456.
8. Lyman, D. J. *J. Polym. Sci.* **1960**, *45*, 49.
9. Shibatani, K.; Lyman, D. J.; Shieh, D. F.; Knutson, K. *J. Polym. Sci. Polym. Chem. Ed.* **1977**, *15*, 1655.
10. Allport, D. C.; Janes, W. H., Eds. "Block Copolymers," John Wiley and Sons: New York, 1973.
11. Koutsky, J. A.; Hein, N. V.; Cooper, S. L. *J. Polym. Sci.* **1970**, *Part B–8*, 353.
12. Cooper, S. L.; Tobolsky, A. V. *J. Appl. Polym. Sci.* **1966**, *10*, 1837.
13. Bonart, R. L.; Morbitzer, L.; Rinke, H. *Kolloid Z.* **1970**, *240*, 807.
14. Huh, D. S.; Cooper, S. L. *Polym. Eng. Sci.* **1971**, *11*, 369.
15. Nakayama, K.; Ino, T.; Matsubara, I. *J. Macromol. Sci. Chem.* **1969**, *Part A–3*, 1005.

16. Tanaka, T.; Yokoyama, T.; Yamaguchi, Y. *J. Polym. Sci.* **1968**, *Part A–1*, 2137.
17. Ishihara, H.; Kimura, K.; Saito, K.; Ono, H. *J. Macromol. Sci. Phys.* **1974**, *Part B–10*, 591.
18. Sung, C. S. P.; Schneider, N. S. *Macromolecules* **1975**, *8*, 68.
19. Seymour, R. W.; Estes, G. M.; Cooper, S. L. *Macromolecules* **1970**, *3*, 579.
20. Tanaka, T.; Yokoyama, T.; Yamaguchi, Y. *J. Polym. Sci.* **1968**, *A-1*, 2153.
21. Sung, C. S. P.; Hu, C. B.; Wu, C. S. *Macromolecules* **1980**, *13*, 111.
22. Sung, C. S. P.; Smith, T. W.; Sung, N. H. *Macromolecules* **1980**, *13*, 117.
23. Trifan, D. S.; Terenzi, J. F. *J. Polym. Sci.* **1958**, *28*, 443.
24. Senich, G. A.; MacKnight, W. J. *Macromolecules* **1980**, *13*, 106.
25. Seymour, R. W.; Allegrezza, A. E., Jr.; Cooper, S. L. *Macromolecules* **1973**, *6*, 896.
26. Seymour, R. W.; Cooper, S. L. *Rubber Sci. Tech.* **1974**, *47*, 19.
27. Srichatrapimuk, V. W.; Cooper, S. L. *J. Macromol. Sci. Phys.* **1978**, *Part B-15*, 267.
28. Boyarchuk, Y. M.; Rappoport, L. Y.; Niktin, V. N.; Apukhtina, N. P. *Polym. Sci. USSR (Engl. Transl.)* **1965**, *7*, 859.
29. West, J. C.; Cooper, S. L. *J. Polym. Sci. Symp.* **1977**, *60*, 127.
30. Sung, C. S. P.; Schneider, N. S. *Macromolecules* **1977**, *10*, 452.
31. Schneider, N. S.; Sung, C. S. P. *J. Polym. Eng. Sci.* **1977**, *17*, 73.
32. Sung, C. S. P.; Schneider, N. S. *J. Mater. Sci.* **1978**, *13*, 1689.
33. Sung, C. S. P.; Hu, C. B.; Wu, C. S.; Smith, T. *Am. Chem. Soc., Div. Polym. Chem. Prepr.* **1978**, *19*, 692.
34. Sung, C. S. P.; Hu, C. B.; Merrill, E. W. *Am. Chem. Soc., Div. Polym. Chem. Prepr.* **1978**, *19*, 20.
35. Sung, C. S. P.; Hu, C. B.; Merrill, E. W.; Salzman, E. W. *J. Biomed. Mater. Res.* **1978**, *12*, 791.
36. Sung, C. S. P.; Hu, C. B. "Multiphase Polymers," Advances in Chemistry Series No. 176, Cooper, S. L.; Estes, G. M., Eds.; ACS: Washington, D. C., 1979; p. 69.
37. Hu, C. B.; Sung, C. S. P. *Am. Chem. Soc., Div. Polym. Chem. Polym. Prepr.* **1980**, *21*, 156.
38. Colthup, N. B.; Wiberley, S. E.; Daly, L. H. "Introduction to Infrared and Raman Spectroscopy," Academic: New York, 1975, p. 323.
39. Donait, R., Morbitzer, L.; Muller, E. H. *J. Macromol. Sci. Phys.* **1974**, *Part B–9*, 447.
40. Carlson, T. A. "Photoelectron and Auger Spectroscopy," Plenum: New York, 1975.
41. Harrick, N. J. "Internal Reflection Spectroscopy," John Wiley Interscience: New York, 1967.

RECEIVED for review January 16, 1981. ACCEPTED June 17, 1981.

10

Hydrogel Formation from Copolyether–Urethane–Ureas Salt Complex

Morphology Effects of Lithium Bromide

R. BENSON, S. YOSHIKAWA, K. KNUTSON, and D. J. LYMAN

University of Utah, Department of Materials Science and Engineering, Salt Lake City, UT 84112

> *Complexation of lithium bromide (LiBr) with copolyether–urethane–ureas led to the formation of hydrogels whose water absorption varied from 2 to 200%. Water absorption depended directly on the concentration of LiBr and the weight percent of the urethane–urea segment. Dynamic mechanical measurements, differential scanning calorimetry, and Fourier transform infrared spectroscopy were used to study the interaction of the LiBr with the copolyurethanes and the morphology of the resulting hydrogels. LiBr acted as a spacer through interactions with the urethane groups, thus freeing the urea segment from hydrogen bonding. The removal of LiBr led to a morphology that differed from films containing no LiBr in their casting solution.*

The addition of lithium salts can alter the melting, flow behavior, and mechanical properties of aliphatic polyamides (1–4). These effects have been attributed to the formation of a labile network resulting from the salt interacting with the amide group of the polymer. Subsequent work using polycaprolactam lithium chloride demonstrated a direct binding of the lithium ions to the carbonyl oxygen (5).

Earlier, we reported that complexes of lithium bromide (LiBr) with copolyether–urethane–ureas led to the formation of hydrogels (6). The water absorption curves for these hydrogels indicated the existence of two modes of absorption: an initial water absorption that depended on the concentration ratio of LiBr to the urethane–urea segment (hard segment) of the block copolymer, and the water uptake at higher salt concentration which was attributed to the formation of voids in the film.

In this chapter we discuss the nature of the interaction of LiBr with several segmented copolyether-urethane–ureas and the morphological changes resulting from these polymer–salt complexes.

Experimental

Materials. The copolyether-urethane–ureas were prepared from polypropylene glycol, methylene bis(4-phenylisocyanate), and ethylenediamine using a modified solution polymerization technique (7). The polypropylene glycols used had molecular weights of 700, 1000, and 2000; the resulting copolymers were coded PEUU 700, PEUU 1000, and PEUU 2000. Inherent viscosities in N,N-dimethylformamide at 30°C and 0.5% concentrations were 0.47, 0.65, and 0.50, respectively.

Hydrogel Preparation. Films were prepared by solvent casting 10% (by weight) solutions of the copolymers in N,N-dimethylformamide (with anhydrous LiBr added in varying concentrations to the solution) onto glass plates. The films were dried in a forced air draft oven at 75°C for 1 h and then dried for an additional 24 h under vacuum (0.1 mm mercury). The hydrogels were formed by immersing the solvent-cast films in water (which was changed daily) over a 2-week period.

Mechanical Properties. The stress–strain curves were determined with an Instron tensile tester (Table Model 1130). The crosshead speed was 50 mm/min. The measurements were performed on wet 1.3-cm × 0.4-cm dog bone samples at room temperature.

The dynamic mechanical measurements were made using a Vibron DDV-II. The determinations were carried out using samples dried at room temperature and 1 mm mercury at frequencies of 110, 11, and 3.5 Hz. The sample size was 3.0 cm × 0.5 cm × 0.01 cm, and the temperature ranged from $-170°$ to 200°C, with a heating rate of approximately 1°C/min.

Infrared Spectroscopy. Spectra over the 4000–700 cm^{-1} region were obtained at 1-cm^{-1} resolution and 1000 scans per sample using a DIGILAB 14B/D Fourier transform infrared spectrometer (FTIR). Spectra of the copolyurethanes with LiBr still incorporated within the films were obtained by transmission from films cast onto 25 × 2-mm round ZnSe crystals. The copolyurethane hydrogels with the LiBr extracted from the films were obtained by internal reflection using a 45° ZnSe crystal at a 45° incident angle. Blank crystal spectra were obtained and subtracted to give the spectra of the copolyurethane films.

Energy Dispersive Analysis of X-Rays (EDAX). Analysis for the presence of LiBr in slices of the dry extracted hydrogel was performed using a Cambridge scanning electron microscope (SEM) equipped with an EDAX attachment. Each sample was counted for over 200 s at a 200 × magnification.

Water Absorption Determination. The films to be measured for water absorption were soaked in deionized water for 48 h, then removed and placed on a dry paper towel. Another towel was immediately placed on top of the film, and a constant gentle pressure was applied. After placing the film on a second dry paper towel and repeating the procedure, the film was then weighed immediately. The wet films were dried in a vacuum desiccator for 24 h at 0.1 mm mercury and 55°C. The dry film was weighed and the water absorption was calculated as:

$$\frac{\text{wet weight} - \text{dry weight}}{\text{wet weight}} \times 100 = \% \text{ water (by weight)}$$

Differential Scanning Calorimetry (DSC). A Perkin-Elmer DSC-II was used to measure the temperatures at which various dissociations occurred in sections cut from nonextracted LiBr–PEUU 700 films. The temperature range examined was from −168° to 400°C, with a heating rate of 10°C/min.

The dissociation temperature of a urethane model compound based on p-tolylisocyanate and 2-propanol was studied also. One gram of the urethane model compound was dissolved in N,N-dimethylformamide containing 250 mg of anhydrous LiBr. An aliquot of this solution was transferred to a DSC sample pan and dried at 75°C in a forced air draft oven. The thermogram was then measured.

Results and Discussion

Preliminary studies have shown that hydrogels can be formed from hydrophobic copolyurethanes by incorporating inorganic salts into the casting solutions. Apparently, the hydrogel behavior of the films after removal of the salt resulted directly from changes in their bulk morphology. Water absorption curves for the extracted hydrogels demonstrated the magnitude of the increased sorption properties of the copolyurethanes resulting from these morphological changes (Figure 1). The water absorption properties depended directly on the concentration of LiBr in the casting solution, and the weight percent of the hard segment (urethane–urea segment) in the

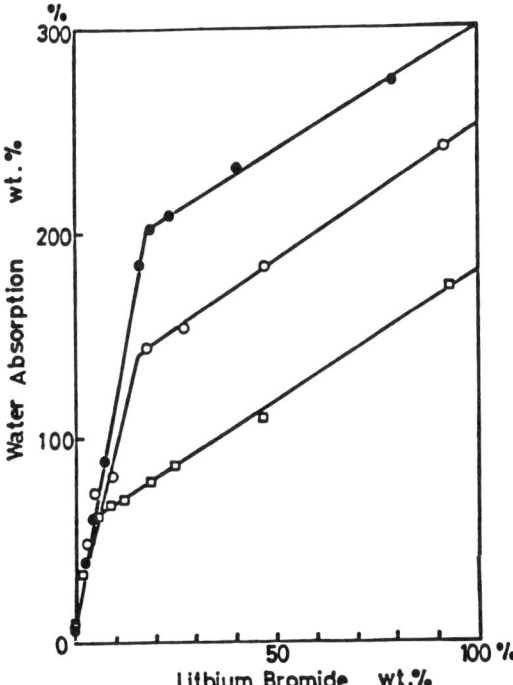

Figure 1. Water adsorption vs. concentration of LiBr for hydrogels (6). Key: ●, PEUU 700; ○, PEUU 1000; and □, PEUU 2000.

copolymer. The discontinuity in the curves occurring at LiBr concentrations of 18, 14, and 6 wt % for PEUU 700, PEUU 1000, and PEUU 2000, respectively, coincided with a 2:1 molar ratio of LiBr to copolymer hard segment (Table I).

Tensile strengths of PEUU 700, PEUU 1000, and PEUU 2000 hydrogels also decreased rapidly with increased concentrations of LiBr (Figure 2), with the decline being most pronounced for PEUU 700 hydrogels. The range in salt concentrations over which these maximum declines in tensile strength occurred coincided with the range in which maximum water absorption changes also occurred.

To understand the interaction of LiBr with the copolyurethanes and the resulting morphological changes, nonextracted samples of PEUU 700 were studied, because this copolyurethane exhibited the largest variation in water absorption and tensile strength as a function of salt concentration.

Dynamic mechanical measurements were performed on nonextracted PEUU 700 films in which salt concentrations ranged from 0 to 29 wt %. The loss tangent curves for samples containing LiBr had a peak at approximately 170°C. Figure 3 shows selected samples. The samples containing no LiBr did not have a peak in this region. The peak at 170°C was attributed to the dissociation of the complex formed from LiBr and the hard segment of the copolymer. The intensity of this dissociation peak increased as the salt concentration increased from 0 to 19 wt %, but beyond 19 wt % LiBr, no apparent increase was evident. To confirm the assignment of the 170°C peak to the dissociation of the LiBr–hard segment complex in the dynamic mechanical curves, the LiBr–PEUU 700 samples also were analyzed by DSC (Table II). The LiBr–PEUU 700 samples exhibited peaks in the 181°–188°C region. No increases in dissociation temperatures were observed from complexes having a salt concentration higher than 25 wt %. The slightly higher dissociation temperatures observed in the DSC experiments (188°C) as compared to 170°C in the dynamic mechanical experiments could be due partially to a faster heating rate. The DSC experiments were conducted with a heating rate of 10°C/min as compared to 1°C/min in the dynamic mechanical experiments. However, because the DSC test sample is under no stress, this heating rate would also contribute to a higher dissociation temperature in the

Table I. Water Absorption of PEUU at Saturation Point

Sample	% Hard Segment	LiBr Weight %	N^1	Water (%)
PEUU 700	44.1	18	2.65	200
PEUU 1000	35.3	14	2.65	140
PEUU 2000	21.7	6	1.82	62

[1] N is the molar ratio of LiBr to hard segment.

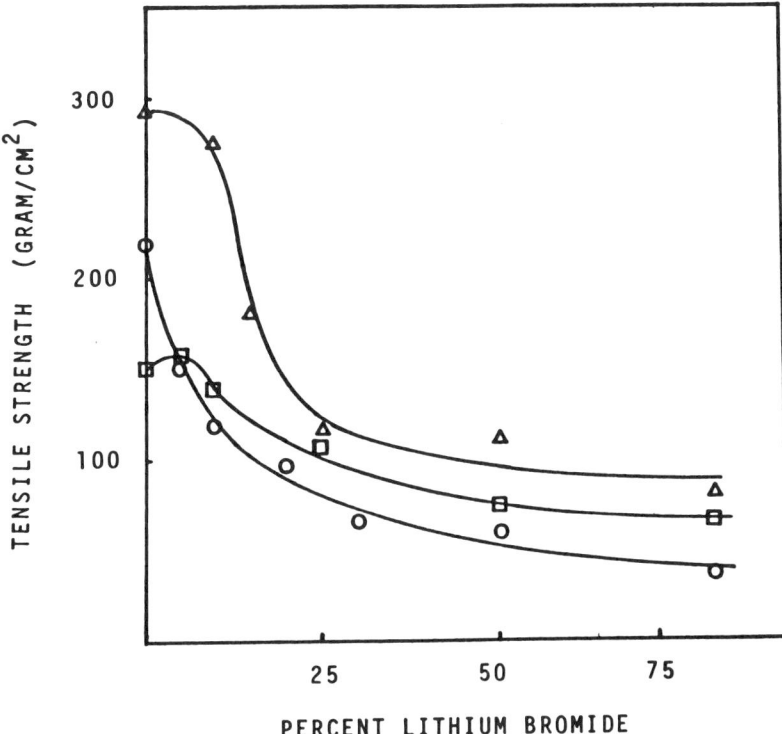

Figure 2. Tensile strength vs. concentration of LiBr for hydrogels. Key: △, PEUU 700; ○, PEUU 1000; and □, PEUU 2000.

samples. Since preliminary infrared studies (discussed later) indicated the LiBr interactions were with the urethane group as opposed to the urea group of the hard segment, a urethane model compound complexed with LiBr also was studied by DSC. The similar dissociation temperature for the urethane model compound complexed with 25 wt % LiBr and the PEUU 700 complexed with 25 wt % LiBr indicated that the LiBr was indeed interacting with the urethane groups of the hard segment.

FTIR was used to explore the dipolar interactions between the urethane and urea groups of the hard segments with LiBr. The 3600–2600 cm^{-1} regions of the infrared spectra of PEUU 700 with 5, 25, and 50 wt % LiBr are shown in Figure 4. Previous studies (8, 9) of PEUU 700 without LiBr assigned the hydrogen-bonded N–H stretching vibrational modes to the band absorbing at 3320 cm^{-1}. The symmetric and asymmetric stretching vibrational modes of the CH_3 and CH_2 groups form the bands absorbing in the 3000–2800 cm^{-1} spectral region. The urea and urethane groups are completely hydrogen bonded, with the N–H vibrational frequencies overlapping.

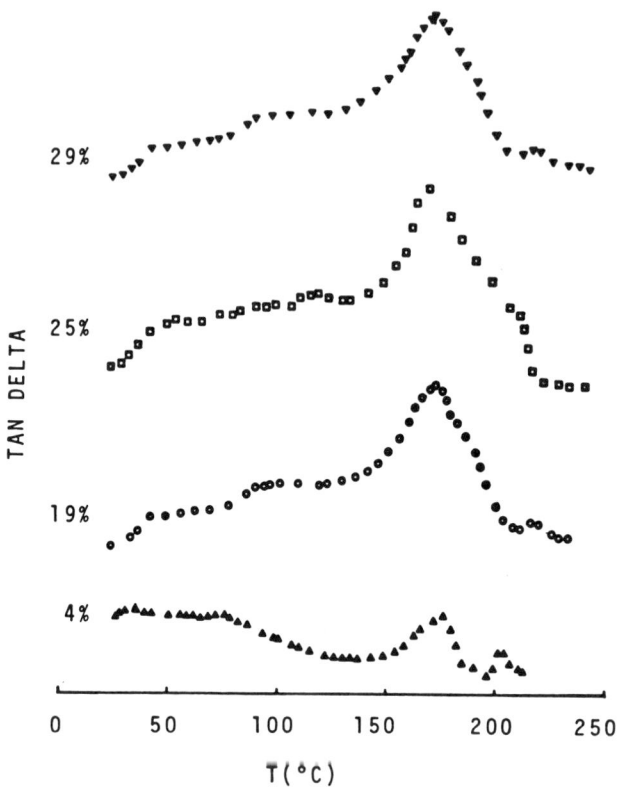

Figure 3. Loss tangent (tan delta) vs. temperature for LiBr–PEUU 700 complexes at 11 Hz.

Table II. DSC Dissociation Temperatures for LiBr–PEUU 700 Complexes

Sample	LiBr (Weight %)	Dissociation Temperature (T_D)
PEUU 700-4	4	181
PEUU 700-9	9	182
PEUU 700-25	25	188
PEUU 700-29	29	187
Urethane[1]–LiBr	25	189

[1] Urethane model compound CH$_3$–C$_6$H$_4$–NHCOCH(CH$_3$)$_2$

The effects of increasing concentrations of LiBr incorporated within the polymer films due to dipolar interactions with the hard segment are noted in the N–H stretching regions. At 5 wt % LiBr, the hydrogen-bonded N–H stretching band absorbing near 3300 cm^{-1} is asymmetric, with an emerging weak lower wave number shoulder. At 25 wt % LiBr, the 3250-cm^{-1} shoulder increased in absorbance, coupled with a broadening of the higher wave number shoulder between 3550–3350 cm^{-1}. At 50 wt % LiBr, the N–H stretching band split into two overlapping shoulders of nearly equal intensity absorbing near 3450 and 3250 cm^{-1}.

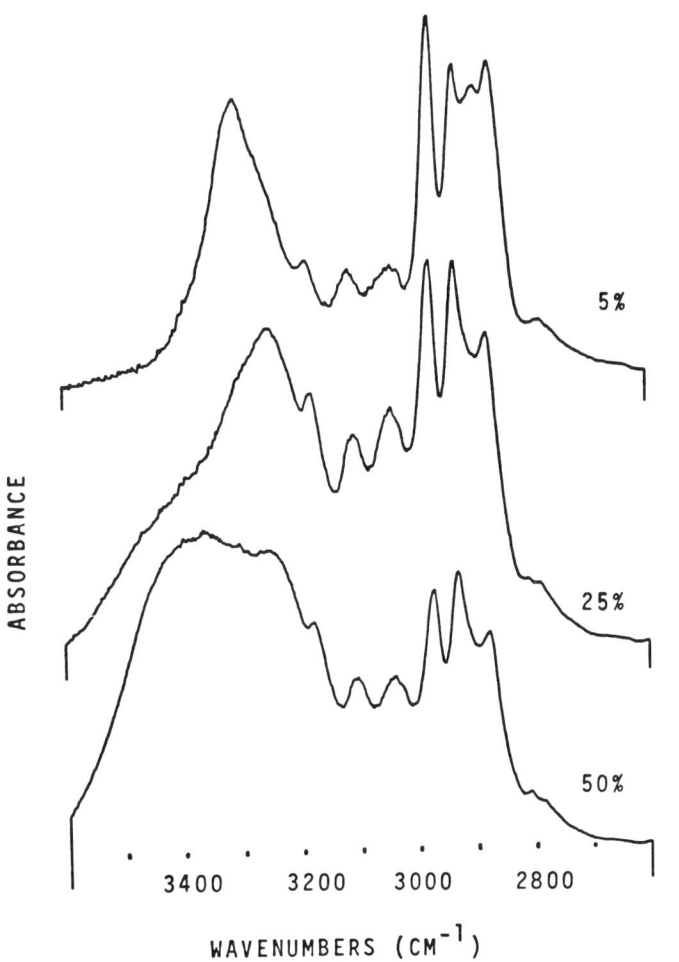

Figure 4. Transmission spectra (3600–2600 cm^{-1}) of LiBr–PEUU 700 complexes.

The 1800–1500 cm^{-1} regions of the infrared spectra of PEUU 700 with 5, 25, and 50 wt % LiBr are shown in Figure 5. While the N–H stretching vibrational modes of the urethane and urea groups in PEUU 700 overlap, the carbonyl stretching Amide I vibrational modes are well separated. Previous studies (8, 9) assigned the urethane carbonyl stretching vibrational modes in

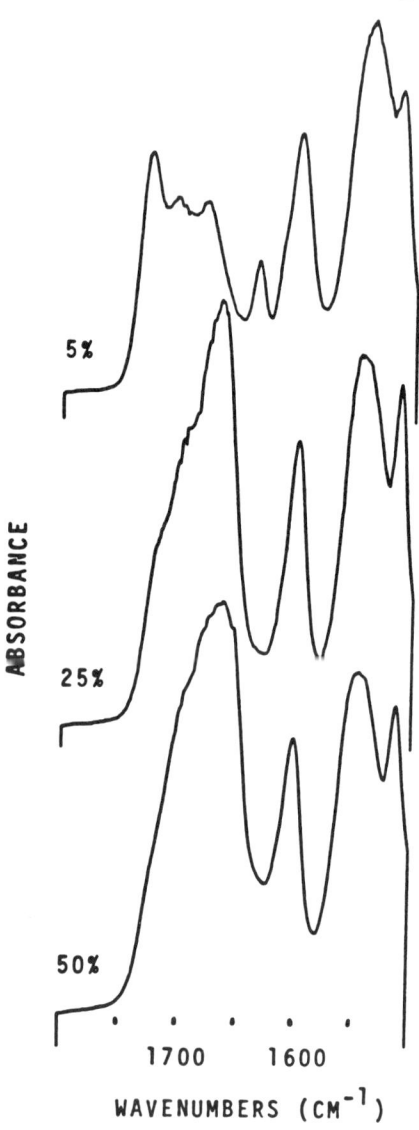

Figure 5. Transmission spectra (1800–1500 cm^{-1}) of LiBr–PEUU 700 complexes.

the nonhydrogen-bonded state to the band absorbing at 1730 cm^{-1}, with hydrogen-bonded vibrational modes absorbing as a weaker shoulder at 1712 cm^{-1}. The presence of free urethane carbonyls despite complete N–H hydrogen bonding results from a dipolar interaction between the urethane N–H groups and polyether oxygens. The urea carbonyls are completely hydrogen bonded, absorbing at 1635 cm^{-1}. The 1600-cm^{-1} band arises from ring breathing vibrations of the aromatic rings. The urethane and urea Amide II vibrations overlap to form the complex band absorbing between 1600–1500 cm^{-1}. The addition of 5 wt % LiBr resulted in a splitting of the hydrogen-bonded urethane Amide I shoulder to form two shoulders absorbing at 1705 and 1680 cm^{-1}. Increasing the salt concentration to 25 wt % LiBr further increased the absorbance of the hydrogen-bonded shoulders, and shifted the lower wave number 1680-cm^{-1} shoulder to 1665 cm^{-1}. The urea Amide I band at 1635 cm^{-1} was absent. Increasing the salt concentration to 50 wt % LiBr increased the absorbance of the 1665-cm^{-1} hydrogen-bonded band.

Previous model compound studies (8, 9) showed a lower wave number shift of the N–H bending hydrogen-bonded band, coupled with the splitting of the hydrogen-bonded urethane Amide I shoulder to form an additional 1680-cm^{-1} shoulder. This result indicated a stronger hydrogen bond between the urethane carbonyls and N–H groups. A dipolar interaction between the LiBr and the urethane groups might occur, as evidenced by the presence of the lower wave number urethane Amide I and N–H stretching shoulders. Increasing LiBr concentrations result in increased absorbances of these shoulders. Preliminary calculations of the repulsive forces between LiBr and the urethane groups as opposed to the urea groups, further support preferential interactions of the LiBr with urethane rather than urea groups. The size of the salts interacting with the urethane groups would preclude hydrogen bonding of the urea groups. This concept is supported by the absence of the hydrogen-bonded urea Amide I coupled with a higher wave number N–H stretching shoulder with increased salt concentrations. Free urea Amide I vibrational modes absorb at higher wave numbers that would overlap with the lower wave number hydrogen-bonded urethane carbonyl shoulder. The higher wave number shoulder in the N–H stretching region would be characteristic of free urea N–H groups.

We then determined if this spacing effect of the LiBr was retained after extraction of the salt to form the hydrogel. To eliminate the possibility that sufficient LiBr remained to prevent an altered morphology from developing, EDAX was performed on samples cut from the PEUU 700 hydrogels. Less than 0.2% of the salt was retained in the hydrogel following the extraction process. Therefore, the change in water absorption and decreased tensile strength properties resulted directly from the change in copolyurethane morphology rather than from the retention of LiBr.

Dynamic mechanical measurements were then made to determine if the extraction of LiBr caused an additional change in morphology. The storage modulus (E') and loss modulus (E'') curves for the hydrogels formed from solutions containing 10 and 25 wt % LiBr and the original hydrophobic copolyurethane are shown in Figure 6. The E'' curves for all samples exhibited two loss peaks. The peak at 0°C was designated as the β-relaxation that arose from the motion of the soft segments. The higher temperature α-relaxation peak was related to the relaxation of soft segments encountering more restriction to movement than those giving rise to the β-peak. The α-relaxation peaks shifted to higher temperature in the hydrogels, thus indicating that more restrictive motions were encountered by the soft segments in these materials. The glass transition region of the E'' curves broadened only slightly with increasing LiBr concentrations. Although no gross changes in morphology of the hydrogels occurred as compared to the PEUU 700 films cast from solutions without LiBr salts, sufficient minor changes caused an increase in the stiffening of the polyether segment. This stiffening was most likely in the interface region of the block copolymers.

The 1800–1500 cm^{-1} spectral regions of the PEUU 700 hydrogels formed after extraction of 10 and 25 wt % LiBr are shown in Figure 7. The urethane carbonyl Amide I vibrational modes absorb in the 1700 cm^{-1} region. The absorbance of the 1725-cm^{-1} shoulder indicates a significant portion of the urethane carbonyls returned to the nonhydrogen-bonded state with extraction of the LiBr; however, a higher percentage of carbonyls remained hydrogen bonded as compared to films cast from solutions without LiBr. In addition, a portion of the hydrogen-bonded carbonyls remained in a stronger hydrogen-bonded state than noted in the hydrophobic PEUU 700 films, as implied by the emerging 1680-cm^{-1} shoulder. The existence of a portion of urethane carbonyls participating in a stronger than normal hydrogen bond was confirmed by a lower wave number shoulder on the hydrogen-bonded N–H stretching band absorbing at 3300 cm^{-1}. The urea Amide I band absorbing at 1635 cm^{-1} coupled with the absence of a higher wave number shoulder on the N–H stretching band confirmed that ureas returned to essentially complete hydrogen bonding.

When LiBr is extracted, the urea groups close to each other re-form essentially complete hydrogen bonding. However, a small portion of urethane groups form a stronger hydrogen bond than noted in the original hydrophobic PEUU 700. Because the LiBr urethane complex is much less mobile, the hard segments cannot undergo the necessary reorientation with extraction of the LiBr to re-form the morphology seen in the original hydrophobic films.

Thus, the addition of LiBr to the copolyurethane casting solution does allow the formation of films having morphologies that cause these hydrophobic polymers to form hydrogels.

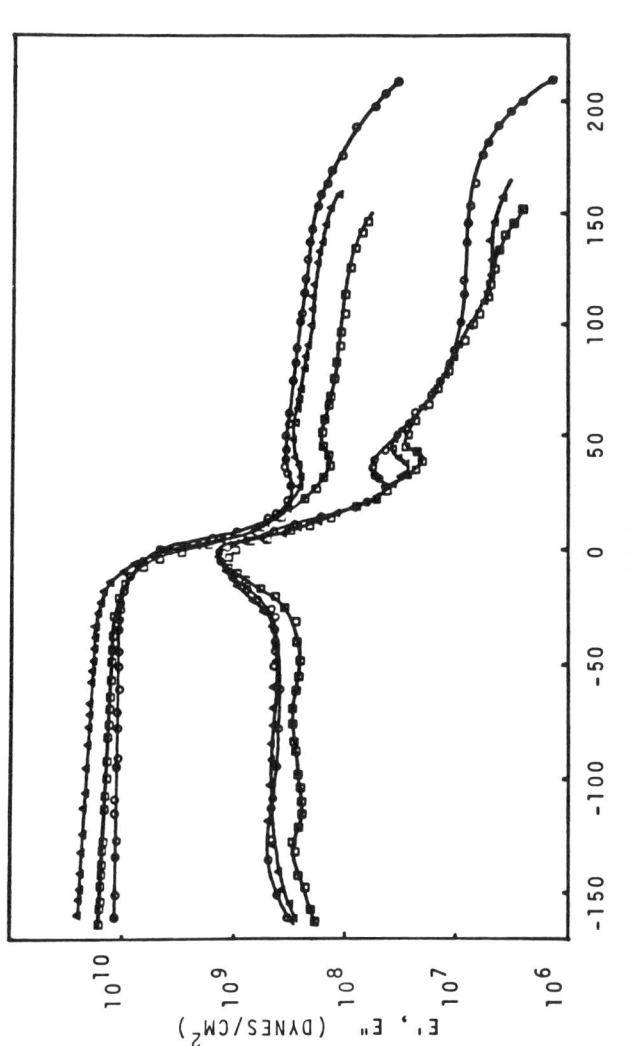

Figure 6. Loss modulus (E") and storage modulus (E') vs. temperature for extracted PEUU 700 hydrogels at 11 Hz. Key: ○, PEUU 700—0% LiBr (L); △, PEUU 700—10% LiBr (L); □, PEUU 700—25% LiBr (L).

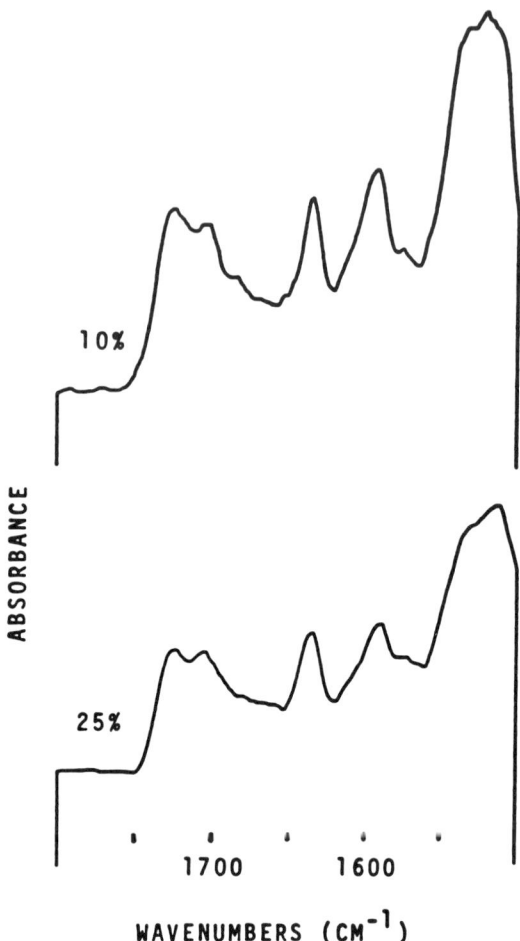

Figure 7. Internal reflectance spectra (1800–1500 cm^{-1}) of hydrogels (PEUU 700 without LiBr).

Acknowledgments

This work was supported by the National Science Foundation, Grant DMR 80–05499, Polymer Program, and by the National Institute for General Medical Science, Grant GM 24487.

Literature Cited

1. Acierno, D.; La Mantia, F. P.; Polizzotti, G. *J. Polym. Sci., Polym. Phys. Ed.* **1979**, *17*, 1903.
2. Bianchi, E.; Ciferri, A.; Tealdi, A.; Torre, R.; Valenti, B. *Macromolecules*, **1974**, *7*, 495.

3. Valenti, B.; Bianchi, E.; Tealdi, A.; Russo, S.; Ciferri, A. *Macromolecules,* **1976,** *9,* 117.
4. Acierno, D.; Bianchi, E.; Ciferri, A.; de Cindio, B.; Migliaresi, C.; Nicolais, L. *J. Polym. Sci., Polym. Symp.* **1976,** *54,* 259.
5. Ciferri, A.; Russo, S. *Polymer Prepr. Am. Chem. Soc. Div. Polym. Chem.* **1977,** *18,* 87.
6. Yoshikawa, S.; Lyman, D. J. *J. Polym. Sci., Polym. Letters,* **1980,** *18,* 411.
7. Lyman, D. J.; Kwan-Gett, C.; Zwart, H. H. J.; Bland, A.; Eastwood, N.; Kawai, J.; Kolff, W. J. *Trans. Am. Soc. Artif. Intern. Organs,* **1971,** *17,* 456.
8. Knutson, K.; Lyman, D. J., Chapter 9 in this book.
9. Knutson, K.; Lyman, D. J., In "Biomedical and Dental Applications of Polymers," Gebelein, C. G.; Koblitz, F. K.; Eds.; Plenum: New York, 1981.

RECEIVED for review January 16, 1981. ACCEPTED July 2, 1981.

11
The Fate of Surface Bound Heparin

M. F. A. GOOSEN and M. V. SEFTON

Department of Chemical Engineering and Applied Chemistry, University of Toronto, Toronto, Ontario, M5S 1A4, Canada

Displacement by plasma of radiolabeled thrombin and radiolabeled thrombin–antithrombin III inactive complex from a heparinized surface was measured and found to be significant; for example, removing 63% of the thrombin and 90% of the complex that could not be removed by phosphate-buffered saline alone. Heparin-poly(vinyl alcohol) (PVA) gel beads with a very low heparin release rate, prepared by acetal coupling of the heparin to the PVA, adsorbed thrombin and potentiated the inactivation of thrombin by antithrombin III, as measured by both thrombin time and chromogenic substrate assays. These results indicate that surface bound heparin retains its biological activity after immobilization and does not become saturated with inactive thrombin–antithrombin III complex. These results support the argument that heparinization can be an important means of preparing the materials needed for the development of improved cardiocirculatory-assist devices and blood handling procedures.

The National Heart, Lung, and Blood Institute (NHLBI) Task Force on Biomaterials has reiterated the need for the development of blood-compatible materials since "progress in this field is a condition for advances in the application of cardiocirculatory-assist devices and other procedures which require continuous or intermittent handling of blood" (1). For example, the task force has specifically identified the development of small-diameter blood vessel prostheses and chronic blood access catheters as priority applications of blood-compatible materials. Both of these devices are used in low-flow situations where red thrombus formation (i.e., intrinsic clotting system activation) predominates (2).

One of the techniques used with varying degrees of success to produce nonthrombogenic materials (and particularly to prevent intrinsic clotting system activation) has been heparinization.

Numerous methods have been used to couple heparin, ionically or covalently, to polymer surfaces. Ionic bonding, whether by direct quaternization of suitable functional groups on the polymer surface (3, 4), by the addition of quaternary ammonium–heparin complexes (5–7), or by the copolymerization of cationic or tertiary amine monomers (8, 9), results in materials with excellent short-term compatibility. Covalent coupling (10, 11), on the other hand, frequently has inactivated the heparin, resulting in only very limited thromboresistance. However, the covalent coupling of heparin to poly(vinyl alcohol) (PVA) through an acetal bridge has resulted in materials that appear to retain long-term blood compatibility in vitro (12, 13) and in arteriovenous (AV) shunts in dogs (14, 15). Similar thromboresistance without apparent heparin elution has been reported for heparinized polymethyl acrylate (16) and Ce^{4+}-initiated heparin–methyl methacrylate graft copolymers (17). The reported nonthrombogenic activity of cyanogen bromide–bonded heparin (18) may, however, be complicated by the continuous loss of heparin from this surface (19). The covalent binding of a modified heparin is reported elsewhere in this volume (20).

Ionically heparinized materials or materials with a steady leakage of heparin are suitable for and have been used with success in short-term applications [e.g., temporary shunts during vascular surgery (21) and others] (22, 23). However, the continuous loss of heparin from the surface of a heparinized material would preclude its use as a long-term implant. Unfortunately, this statement has been interpreted to suggest that in the absence of heparin loss and the corresponding absence of a heparin microenvironment at the blood–material interface, the surface-bound heparin should not be effective in preventing thrombogenesis. Our experiments with immobilized heparin (12, 13, 24) and the work of others (17, 25) have shown that such a conclusion is invalid. Some covalently heparinized materials, for example, heparin–PVA, can be effective in preventing thrombogenesis, like heparin in solution, by the accelerated inactivation of thrombin through the formation of surface-bound thrombin–antithrombin III inactive complex.

Careful examination of the possible fates of the bound heparin and the bound inactive complex suggests hypothetical mechanisms which, if effective, could limit the utility of heparinized materials (Table I). For example, either the surface may become saturated with a heparin complex that can no longer accelerate the inactivation of thrombin, or consumption of antithrombin, prothrombin, or other clotting factors may result, leaving the blood systematically hypocoagulable.

In this chapter we present the results of an in vitro investigation into the fate of surface bound heparin and bound inactive complex to assess the concerns with long-term use of heparin. Heparin was immobilized onto PVA using a covalent acetal coupling procedure (12) to produce a hydrogel (~77% w/w water) in which the heparin appears to be bound through the amino acid terminus of the molecule (26). Although the detailed structure of

Table I. Conceivable Fates of Surface-Bound Heparin

- Heparin is lost from surface to create a heparin microenvironment at the blood/material interface.
- Heparin remains on the surface, but becomes saturated with inactive complex.
- Heparin acts catalytically and does not become saturated, but a high production rate of inactive complex causes a systemic hypocoagulability.
- Heparin does not become saturated, and inactive complex formation is maintained to within tolerable levels.

the linkage can only be hypothesized, like other acetal bonds, it is stable at pH 7.4 (12): the elution rate of heparin from heparin–PVA films into phosphate-buffered saline (PBS) or 3M NaCl was on the order of 10^{-5} $\mu g/cm^2 \cdot min$ (12, 27). The gel has been used by itself as a film or ground into fine beads (27), or more importantly, as a coating on an appropriate substrate. The coating has been applied, for example, to the inside of surface-hydroxylated styrene–butadiene–styrene (SBS) block copolymer tubing, for the preparation of small-diameter prostheses (12), and to the inside of ultrafiltration hollow fibers used in an artificial endocrine pancreas (24).

Experimental

Heparin–PVA Beads. Heparin–PVA films were prepared (12) from an aqueous solution containing 10% (w/w) PVA (20% acetylated PVA, Gelvatol 20–60, Monsanto Canada Ltd.), 5% $MgCl_2 \cdot 6 H_2O$, 0.5% glutaraldehyde, 3% formaldehyde, 4% glycerol, and 1% sodium heparin (porcine mucosal, 176 USP U/mg, Canada Packers Ltd.). The films were ground at 77 K to form beads within a nominal particle diameter range of 105–250 μm (27). Control beads were prepared without heparin. The elution rate of heparin from the beads suspended in 0.05M phosphate-buffered 0.15M NaCl (PBS) was measured by adding toluidine blue to samples of the used wash solution and quantifying the absorbance change at 600 nm (26). The detection limit of this assay is 2 ppm heparin, which means that heparin elution rates as low as 1×10^{-2} μg/g wet gel·min can be determined conveniently.

In Vitro Clotting Tests. The plasma recalcification time of citrated human plasma was determined in the presence of heparin–PVA beads and control PVA beads without heparin. Various amounts (10–200 mg) of gel were incubated with 0.5 mL of plasma at room temperature for 5 min. After the addition of 0.5 mL of 0.025M $CaCl_2$, the time to clot was noted by tilting the test tube gently each minute, until the beads clumped together or were found to stick to the test tube wall.

The thrombin time was determined similarly by incubation of 2 IU of crude bovine thrombin (10 IU/mL, Miles Laboratories) with the beads for 5 min at room temperature in an albumin-coated glass tube, followed by 0.2 mL of citrated human plasma. The time to clot was noted by tilting the test tube gently every few seconds. PBS, after incubation with heparin–PVA beads for 5–60 min, was analyzed for the presence of heparin using both toluidine blue and the thrombin time test (PBS in place of gel beads).

Thrombin Affinity. The affinity of thrombin for heparin–PVA and PVA beads was analyzed by loading 62 IU of crude bovine thrombin in PBS (96 IU/mg, Park Davis Co.) on chromatography columns (1.6-cm diameter × 2.5 cm) packed with the beads. The columns were washed with 100 mL of PBS and/or 20% (w/w) bovine albumin in PBS (Miles Lab.). The residual thrombin activity bound to the columns was measured by loading 0.5 mg chromogenic substrate (0.5 mg/mL PBS; S2238, Ortho Diagnostics, or Chromozym TH, Boehringer–Mannheim) onto the column and measuring the change in effluent absorbance at 381 nm. In some experiments, 3 mg of crude antithrombin III (15 mL of citrated human plasma, heat defibrinated at 54°C for 5 min) was used to inactivate the bound thrombin. The effect of precoating the gel columns with 20 mL of 10% (w/w) bovine albumin in PBS on purified human α-thrombin binding (3.53 IU/mg, courtesy of J. W. Fenton II, N.Y. State Department of Health, Albany) also was determined. The residual thrombin activity is reported as color yield: the ratio of color produced by enzymatic action to the total color possible from the load of chromogen.

Bound Thrombin/Antithrombin III Exchange. To determine whether the surface bound heparin becomes saturated with inactive complex, the ability to displace bound inactive complex and thereby regenerate the heparin was assessed by measuring the elution of the appropriate radiolabeled protein from the heparin–PVA column. Two sets of experiments were performed: one with only radiolabeled thrombin loaded onto a heparin–PVA column and one with unlabeled thrombin followed by radiolabeled antithrombin III loaded onto an identical column. Unbound protein was eluted with 20 mL of PBS. Flow rates of 97 mL/min were used throughout. Then, "loosely" bound protein was removed with another wash for 4–6 h with PBS (400–600 mL), followed by the overnight recirculation of 20 mL of PBS (closed system) until no further increase in PBS radioactivity occurred. At that time, the system was reopened (i.e., the eluent was passed through the column in the conventional manner), the gel was washed with 50–60 mL of PBS followed by defibrinated plasma (containing antithrombin III), and the increase in radioactivity in the eluted plasma was measured. The system was closed again, and defibrinated plasma was recirculated overnight to end the wash cycle. The amounts of thrombin, antithrombin III, and defibrinated plasma used in the two experiments are listed in Table II; no effect of the quantities used has been noted in subsequent experiments. Recirculation of eluent (closed system) was used to attain equilibrium. Then, 100 mL of PBS was passed through the column, and residual radioactivity on the beads was measured by adding the beads directly into 10 mL of Aquasol (New England Nuclear). For the liquid samples, 0.1-mL aliquots were taken and added to 10 mL of Aquasol for liquid scintillation counting (Beckman LS 8000 liquid scintillation spectrometer). Proteins were labeled with ^{125}I using the standard Enzymobead method (Biorad Laboratories), and retained approximately 70% of their original biological activity after labeling.

Results

Stability of Immobilized Heparin. The amount of heparin eluting from the gel beads was calculated from the amount of heparin found in the wash solvent at any time (determined using the toluidine blue technique) and the amount of heparin initially present in the heparin–PVA solution. After the first 50 h of washing, the rate of elution decreased rapidly to a low, relatively constant value of 1.67×10^{-2} μg/g wet gel·min. A similar elution rate was obtained in plasma using ^{35}S-heparin (27). Assuming a particle diameter of 180 μm and a gel density of 1.05 g/cm^3, this release rate corresponds to 5.3×10^{-5} μg/cm^2·min. The rate is comparable to the release rate

Table II. Displacement of Bound Thrombin–Antithrombin III: Experimental Parameters

	Thrombin	Thrombin–antithrombin III
Loaded protein	18 IU of crude bovine ^{125}I-thrombin	100 IU of crude bovine thrombin (unlabeled) followed by 2000 IU of pure human ^{125}I-antithrombin III
moles antithrombin loaded/moles thrombin loaded	—	23
Heparin–PVA gel Displacement eluent	1g gel; 7 mg heparin/g gel heat-defibrinated plasma, 7 mL (open) followed by recirculation of 20 mL	1 g gel; 7 mg heparin/g gel heat-defibrinated plasma, 350 mL (open) followed by recirculation of 90 mL

Note: specific activities before labeling: crude bovine thrombin—96 IU/mg (Parke-Davis), pure human antithrombin III—1000 IU/mg (M. Wickerhauzer, American Red Cross, Bethesda, MD); "open" implies material used as eluent in conventional chromatographic mode; and ratio of loaded protein does not include antithrombin III content of defibrinated plasma.

determined earlier using ^{35}S-heparin for a heparin–PVA film on SBS (12). These release rates are approximately 1/1000 the 4×10^{-2} μg/cm^2·min minimum required for thromboresistance of ionically heparinized catheters (4). After washing for 500 h, 30% of the original heparin was left in the gel beads, giving a final heparin content of approximately 7 mg/g wet gel.

In Vitro Activity of Bound Heparin. The prolongation of the thrombin time caused by the addition of heparin–PVA beads to plasma is contrasted with the negligible effect of PVA beads without heparin in Figure 1a. A similar prolongation was observed for the plasma recalcification time (Figure 1b). In both cases, clumping or adhesion of the beads caused presumably by fibrin was the end point of the assay.

Figure 2 shows that thrombin binds to both heparin–PVA beads and PVA beads without heparin. After a load of crude bovine thrombin (62 IU) followed by PBS and chromogen, color yields of 89% and 81% were obtained for the heparin–PVA and PVA gel, respectively, indicating the presence of active thrombin on the columns. Passing 15 mL of 20% (w/w) bovine albumin through the same columns followed by chromogen lowered the color yield for

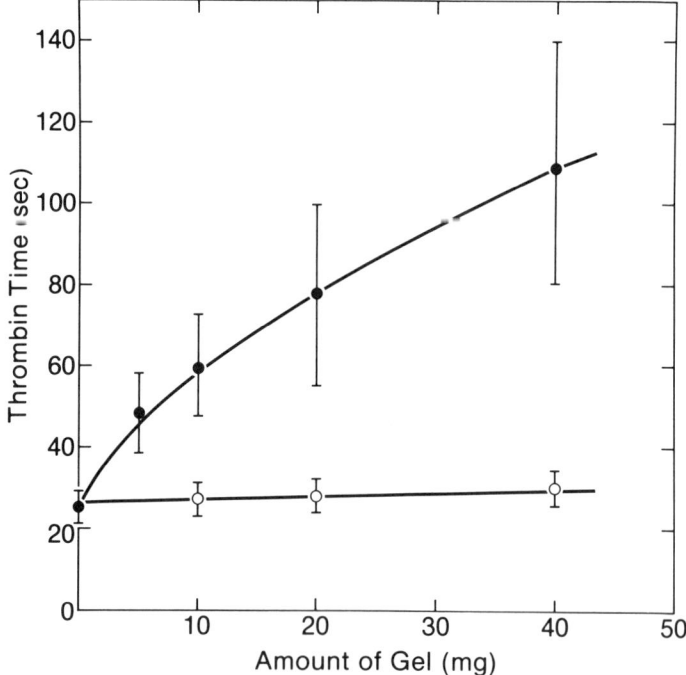

Figure 1a. Thrombin time of plasma in the presence of PVA (○) and heparin–PVA (●) beads. Thrombin incubated with beads prior to plasma addition (2 IU of crude bovine thrombin, 0.2 mL of citrated human plasma, and 7 mg of heparin/g gel) (13).

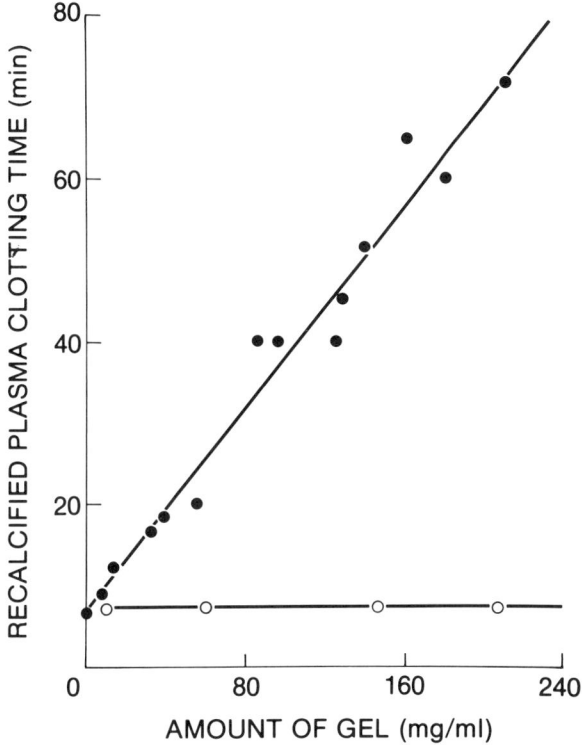

Figure 1b. Recalcification time of plasma incubated with PVA (○) and heparin–PVA (●) beads (0.5 mL of citrated human plasma, 0.5 mL of 0.025 M $CaCl_2$, and 7 mg of heparin/g gel) (13).

PVA to 54%, indicating that a substantial quantity of thrombin bound to PVA had been desorbed by bovine albumin. A similar color yield was obtained when 15 mL of defibrinated plasma (containing 3 mg of antithrombin III) were used in place of the bovine albumin. In contrast, crude bovine thrombin bound to heparin–PVA, while not being significantly inactivated (or desorbed) by 15 mL of 20% (w/w) bovine albumin, was almost completely inactivated by 3 mg of crude antithrombin III, as shown by the 24% color yield.

Precoating the gel columns with 20 mL of 10% (w/w) bovine albumin significantly reduced human thrombin binding to PVA, relative to heparin–PVA (Figure 2). Loading precoated columns with 1072 IU of purified human α-thrombin, followed by chromogen, gave a color yield of 78% with heparin–PVA and 38% with PVA alone. In contrast, 62 IU of crude bovine thrombin loaded on an untreated heparin–PVA column produced a slightly higher color yield, 89%, suggesting that precoating the gel column with albumin reduces the number of available thrombin binding sites on the heparin–PVA gel.

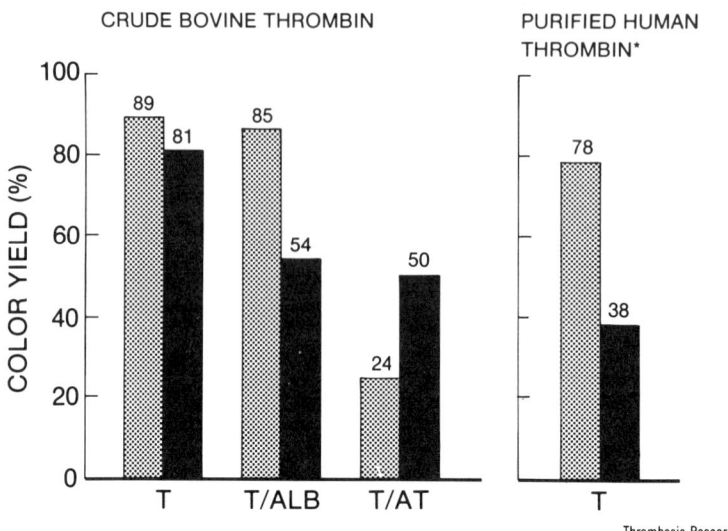

Figure 2. Inactivation of thrombin (T) by antithrombin III (AT) on heparinized beads in a chromatography column (27).

Thrombin (62 IU) loaded on the gel columns was followed by either 3 mg of crude antithrombin III or by 15 mL of 20% (w/w) bovine albumin (ALB). Key: * in the experiment with purified human thrombin (1072 IU), the gel columns were precoated with albumin; ▨, PVA–heparin; ■, PVA; and flow rate, 97 mL/h, 7 mg heparin/g gel, 3 g gel.

Exchange of Bound Thrombin/Antithrombin III. Displacement of bound radiolabeled thrombin or bound thrombin radiolabeled antithrombin III inactive complex from heparin–PVA by defibrinated plasma containing unlabeled antithrombin III, is shown in Figure 3. Approximately 8% of the loaded ^{125}I-thrombin and 14% of the loaded ^{125}I-antithrombin III were left on the column after the initial wash with 20 mL of PBS. These low percentages represent the limited purity of the radiolabeled proteins. Subsequent removals of radiolabeled protein from the columns are compared in Figure 3 on the same basis, by setting the bound fraction of protein after this 20-mL elution equal to 100%.

After washing the columns in an open-loop system for 4–6 h with PBS, and then overnight in a closed-loop system with 20 mL of PBS, a further 30% of the initially bound protein was removed, until an equilibrium had been established between the bound and unbound proteins. On changing the PBS eluent to heat-defibrinated plasma (containing antithrombin III), the desorption of both ^{125}I-thrombin and ^{125}I-antithrombin III from the column increased dramatically. In the experiments with radiolabeled antithrombin III, the column had been exposed previously to thrombin, therefore, the displaced radiolabeled antithrombin III should more properly be described as labeled inactive complex. Because defibrinated plasma contains antithrombin III, the eluted radiolabeled thrombin in the thrombin-alone experiment also may be in the form of inactive complex. Although further investigation is required to identify the form of the desorbed radioactivity (i.e., molecular weight, antithrombin III content) and mechanisms of exchange, binding of thrombin or thrombin–antithrombin III complex to immobilized heparin is not irreversible, and under some physiologically relevant circumstances (presence of plasma), thrombin alone or thrombin–antithrombin III inactive complex can be displaced from the heparinized surface. These results are consistent with experiments in rabbits that show that the heparin–thrombin–antithrombin III complex is readily dissociated in vivo (28), and the work of Griffith who showed that the thrombin–antithrombin III complex has a weaker affinity for heparin than uncomplexed thrombin or antithrombin III (29). Furthermore, Olsson et al. demonstrated that the sequence involving thrombin adsorption onto a heparinized surface

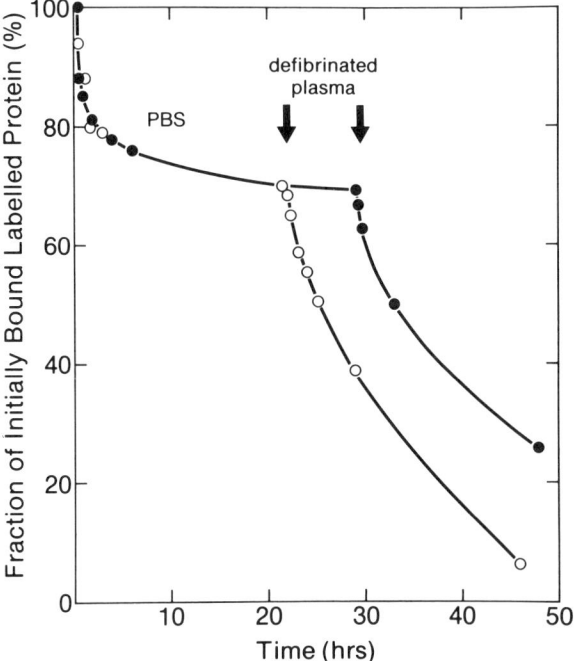

Figure 3. Displacement of bound radiolabeled protein from heparin–PVA.

After loading the labeled proteins on the column and eluting unbound protein with 20 mL of PBS, the amount of radioactivity remaining on the columns was taken as 100% (Time = 0). The columns were then washed with PBS, and at the indicated times, the eluent was changed to defibrinated plasma. Key: ●, labeled thrombin; ○, unlabeled crude bovine thrombin and labeled human antithrombin III.

and subsequent inhibition of the enzyme by circulating antithrombin III was regenerative (30).

Discussion

The results reported here, in addition to those reported earlier by ourselves and others, show that significant heparin elution is not necessary for bound heparin to retain biological activity. Prolonged partial thromboplastin times of greater than 1200 s were observed for plasma in contact with heparin–PVA–coated styrene–butadiene–styrene block copolymer films, despite a heparin elution rate on the order of 10^{-5} $\mu g/cm^2 \cdot min$ (12). Prolonged thrombin times also were observed for Ce^{4+}-initiated heparin methyl methacrylate graft copolymers, without measurable heparin release (17). The ability to inactive thrombin by reaction with antithrombin III also has been reported (25) for this latter material and for heparinized polymethyl acrylate without heparin release (16). The passivating effect of antithrombin III on platelet aggregation in Salzman columns was correlated with this ability to inactive thrombin (25). "Artificial Endocrine Pancreas," made from heparin–PVA–coated hollow fibers (0.5 mm i.d.), remained patent for longer than control shunts without heparin, when implanted as AV shunts in monkeys (24). Heparinized devices were patent for 2, 4, 5, or 6 days, while unheparinized shunts were patent for less than 1 h.

This chapter reported that thrombin times and plasma recalcification times were prolonged in the presence of heparin–PVA beads, despite the very stable binding of the heparin (elution rate of 1.67×10^{-2} $\mu g/g$ wet gel·min). Also, comparison of the chromogenic substrate activity of thrombin bound to heparin–PVA columns and PVA columns without heparin after loading antithrombin III (Figure 2) suggests that thrombin binding to heparin–PVA activates the enzyme, making it more receptive to antithrombin III. If, for example, binding of thrombin to heparin had not increased the affinity of enzyme for inhibitor, then the passage of crude antithrombin III through the columns followed later by chromogenic substrate would have produced similar color yields for both heparin–PVA and PVA. However, this result was not observed in these experiments, leading to the conclusion that the bound heparin was biologically active. Furthermore, the inactivation of thrombin observed here cannot be considered as a slow progressive inactivation of the thrombin by antithrombin III, because of the difference in behavior on heparin–PVA and PVA.

While direct comparison with the minimum elution rate suggested for ionically heparinized catheters may be misleading due to the different geometries involved, the measured elution rate is low enough to conclude that the heparin–PVA linkage is stable and that the observed biological activity cannot simply be attributed to the presence of a microenvironment of heparin around the beads. Thus, this primary conclusion of previous investigators with bound heparin is not necessarily valid. While this mode of action might account for the activity of loosely bound heparin, it is not sufficient to explain the activity of well-bound heparin such as heparin bound by acetal coupling. Therefore, bound heparin must be assumed to be effective in preventing thrombogenesis by the formation of a surface bound thrombin–antithrombin III inactive complex.

Concern over the fate of the bound complex appears unnecessary, since radiolabeled thrombin or thrombin–antithrombin III complexes were readily displaced from the surfaces by defibrinated plasma containing crude antithrombin III. Therefore, the bound heparin apparently does not become saturated with inactive complex, enabling the bound heparin, if it remains active, to act catalytically to potentiate the inactivation of thrombin as it is generated. Whether the consumption rate of antithrombin III or prothrombin, on the other hand, can be controlled, or whether it would result in a systemic blood defect, remains to be examined.

Other concerns regarding the practicality of surface bound heparin for the preparation of materials with long-term thromboresistance remain. Because the interaction of heparin with platelets is unclear (31), whether the immobilized heparin causes greater thrombosis under conditions where platelet deposition is more important than fibrin formation remains to be shown. The passivating effect of antithrombin III on platelet consumption caused by surface-bound heparin is a significant observation in this context (32, 33).

Conclusions

The results reported here, in conjunction with earlier results, indicate that immobilized heparin need not necessarily be lost from a surface in order to impart thromboresistance to that surface. For heparin–PVA, and perhaps for other covalent reactions that do not inactivate the heparin, the irreversibly bound heparin can accelerate the formation of a surface-bound inactive thrombin–antithrombin III complex. Furthermore, our results suggest that the inactive complex is not itself permanently bound to the surface, but rather can be displaced by a component or components in plasma.

While materials that lose heparin at a controlled rate can be clinically acceptable in short-term applications, the long-term use of heparinized materials requires materials that do not lose heparin, yet retain the biological function of the heparin. This investigation and others indicate that these requirements are not mutually exclusive, and that bound heparin can potentially retain its biological activity over the long term. Heparinization can be an important means of preparing the materials needed for the development of improved cardiocirculatory-assist devices and blood handling procedures.

Acknowledgments

The authors acknowledge the support of the National Heart, Lung, and Blood Institute, NIH, DHEW under Grant No. 5R01HL24020; the guidance of M. W. C. Hatton; and the technical assistance of B. A. Ramsoomair. M. F. A. Goosen thanks the Chemical Institute of Canada for having awarded him the Ogilvie Flour Mills–Kenneth Armstrong Memorial Fellowship.

Literature Cited

1. Galletti, P. M.; Brash, J. L.; Keller, K. H.; LaFarge, G.; Mason, R. G.; Pierce, W. S.; Reynolds, J. A. *Artif. Organs* **1978**, *2*, 189.
2. Leonard, E. F.; Friedman, L. I. *Chem. Eng. Symp. Ser.* **1970**, *66*(99), 59–71.
3. Merrill, E. W.; Salzman, E. W.; Lipps, B. J.; Gilliland, E. R.; Austen, W. G.; Joison, J. *Trans. Am. Soc. Artif. Intern. Organs* **1966**, *12*, 139.
4. Idezuki, Y.; Watanabe, H.; Hagewara, M.; Kanasugi, K.; Mori, Y.; Nagaoka, S.; Hagio, M.; Yamamoto, K.; Tansawa, H. *Trans. Am. Soc. Artif. Intern. Organs* **1975**, *21*, 435.
5. Gott, V. L.; Whiffen, J. D.; Koepke, D. E.; Daggett, R. L.; Boake, W. C.; Young, W. P. *Trans. Am. Soc. Artif. Intern. Organs* **1974**, *10*, 213.
6. Grode, G. A.; Anderson, S. J.; Grotta, H. M.; Falb, R. D. *Trans. Am. Soc. Artif. Intern. Organs* **1969**, *15*, 1.
7. Lagergen, H. R.; Erikssen, J. C. *Trans. Am. Soc. Artif. Intern. Organs* **1971**, *17*, 10.
8. Courtney, J. M.; Park, G. B.; Fairweather, I. A.; Lindsay, R. M. *Biomat. Med. Dev. Art. Organs* **1976**, *4*(3,4), 263.
9. Ferrutti, P.; Provenzale, L. *Transp. Proc.* **1976**, *7*(1), 103.
10. Grode, G.; Falb, R.; Anderson, S. Artificial Heart Program Conference Proceedings, p. 19 (1969).
11. Halpern, B.; Shirakawa, R. In "Interaction of Liquids at Solid Substrates"; Advances in Chemistry Series, No. 87, ACS: Washington, D.C., 1968; p. 197.
12. Goosen, M. F. A.; Sefton, M. V. *J. Biomed. Mater. Res.* **1979**, *13*, 347.
13. Sefton, M. V.; Goosen, M. F. A. In "Chemistry and Biology of Heparin"; Lundblad, R. L.; Brown, W. V.; Mann, K. M.; Roberts, H. R., Eds.; Elsevier North Holland: Amsterdam, 1981; pp. 463–474.
14. Merrill, E. W.; Salzman, E. W.; Wong, P. S. L.; Ashford, T. P.; Brown, A. H.; Austen, W. G. *J. Appl. Physiol.* **1969**, *29*(5), 723.
15. Merrill, E. W.; Wong, P. S. L., U. S. Patent 3658745, 1972.
16. Dincer, A. K., Ph.D. Thesis, Massachusetts Institute of Technology, 1977.
17. Boffa, M. C.; Labarre, P.; Jozefowicz, M.; Boffa, G. A. *Thromb. Haemost.* **1979**, *41*, 346–356.
18. Hoffman, A. S.; Schmer, G.; Harris, C.; Kraft, W. G. *Trans. Am. Soc. Artif. Intern. Organs A.S.A.I.O.*, **1972**, *18*, 10.
19. Schmer, G.; Teng, L. W. Y.; Vizzo, J. E.; Grefe, U.; Iutnovich, J. M.; Cole, J. J.; Scribner, B. H. *Trans. Am. Soc. Artif. Intern. Organs* **1977**, *23*, 177.
20. Ebert, C.; Lee, E. S.; Dineris, J.; King, S. W. Chapter 12 in this book.
21. Cox, J. L. In "Chemistry and Biology of Heparin"; Lundblad, R. L.; Brown, W. V.; Mann, K. M.; Roberts, H. R., Eds.; Elsevier North Holland: Amsterdam, 1981; pp. 449–462.
22. Leininger, R. I. *Chemtec.* **1975**, 172–176.
23. "Toray Antithrombogenic Catheter," Toray Industries Inc., Tokyo, Japan; 1977.
24. Sun, A. M.; Parisus, W.; Macmorine, H. G.; Sefton, M. V.; Stone, R. *Artif. Organs* **1980**, *4*(4), 275–278.

25. Salzman, E. W.; Silane, M.; Lindon, J.; Brier–Russell, E.; Dincer, A.; Rosenberg, R.; Merrill, E. W. In "Chemistry and Biology of Heparin"; Lundblad, R. L.; Brown, W. V.; Mann, K. M.; Roberts, H. R., Eds.; Elsevier North Holland: Amsterdam, 1981; pp. 435–448.
26. Goosen, M. F. A.; Ramsoomair, B. A.; Sefton, M. V., unpublished data.
27. Goosen, M. F. A.; Sefton, M. V.; Hatton, M. W. C. *Thromb. Res.* **1980**, *20*, 543–554.
28. Lam, L. S. L.; Regoeczi, E.; Hatton, M. W. C. *Br. J. Exp. Path.* **1979**, *60*, 151–160.
29. Griffith, M. J. In "Chemistry and Biology of Heparin"; Lundblad, R. L.; Brown, W. V.; Mann, K. G.; Roberts, H. R., Eds.; Elsevier North Holland: Amsterdam, 1981; pp. 237–248.
30. Olsson, P.; Larsson, R.; Lins, L.-E.; Nilsson, E. Abstracts, VIIIth International Congress on Thrombosis and Haemostasis, **1981**, *46*(1), 323.
31. Zucker, M. B. *Fed. Proc.* **1977**, *36*, 47.
32. Lindon, J.; Rosenberg, R.; Merrill, E. W.; Salzman, E. *J. Lab. Clin. Med.* **1978**, *91*, 47.
33. Salzman, E. W.; Rosenberg, R. D.; Smith, M. H.; Lindon, J. N.; Fabveau, L. *J. Clin. Invest.* **1980**, *65*, 65–73.

RECEIVED for review January 16, 1981. ACCEPTED October 15, 1981.

12

The Anticoagulant Activity of Derivatized and Immobilized Heparins

C. D. EBERT, E. S. LEE, J. DENERIS, and S. W. KIM[1]

University of Utah, Department of Pharmaceutics, Salt Lake City, UT 84112

> *Heparin anticoagulant activity decreases as the degree of carboxylic derivatization increases; however, partially derivatized heparin, both carboxylic and hydroxyl derivatives, retains anticoagulant activity. Heparin was immobilized via carboxylic groups to diaminoalkane agarose gels to provide coupling spacer groups of various lengths. Anticoagulant activity increased precipitously beginning with 10-carbon unit spacer groups, but heparin coupled with less than 10 spacer groups demonstrated only minimal anticoagulant activity.*

The complex interactions of blood upon contacting foreign surfaces resulting in thrombosis is an inherent problem in using blood-contacting biomedical devices. Although the precise mechanisms by which surface-induced thrombogenesis occurs are not fully understood, both cellular and molecular blood components participate, perhaps synergistically, in eventual thrombus formation. Biomedical device technology has experienced dramatic advances in the past two decades; however, the clinical means for thrombus prevention remains unchanged—anticoagulants are administered systemically concomitant with the operation of the device.

The anticoagulant most commonly used today is heparin. It is a highly polydispersed, acidic carbohydrate with a linear, helical structure composed of alternating sulfoglucosamine and hexuronic acid molecules joined by glycosidic linkages (1). The molecular weight of commercial heparin ranges from below 10,000 to well over 20,000 (2), and as a general rule, high molecular weight heparin has greater anticoagulant activity than low molecular weight heparin (3). In addition to a wide range in molecular weight, the chemical structure of heparin varies considerably. When high-activity (360 IU/mg) and low-activity (12 IU/mg) heparin fractions were analyzed chemically, the high-

[1]Author to whom correspondence shall be addressed.

activity heparin was composed predominantly of chains containing a unique tetrasaccharide with the following sequence:

L-iduronic acid →
N-acetylated D-glucosamine-6-sulfate →
D-glucuronic acid →
N-sulfate D-glucosamine-6-sulfate →

The low-activity fraction contained only 8.5% of this tetrasaccharide (4). Therefore, correlations between the chemical and physical structure and the anticoagulant activity must exist.

The mechanisms by which heparin exerts an anticoagulant function are controversial. When heparin is added to a solution of antithrombin III (AT-III), a naturally occurring inhibitor of the proteolytic enzyme thrombin, the rate of thrombin neutralization is essentially instantaneous as compared with a gradual thrombin neutralization rate in the absence of heparin (5). This result has led to the generally accepted scheme where heparin first binds to AT-III, greatly potentiating thrombin binding to AT-III binding sites in the heparin/AT-III complex. The heparin/AT-III complex not only binds to thrombin, but also to every active serine protease in the intrinsic coagulation pathway (6).

Only one-third of a commercial heparin preparation possesses anticoagulant activity as demonstrated by AT-III affinity chromatography (7). In view of the wide chemical–structural variance of heparin and the ability of heparin to bind with many enzymes and proteins, these observations are not overly surprising. Heparin has many pharmacological effects, of which anticoagulation is one. Many of these other functions manifest themselves as undesired side effects when heparin is administered systemically for anticoagulation purposes including: respiratory impairments, platelet cytopenia, increased fatty acid transport across biomembranes, inhibition of osteoblasts, and increased B-lymphocyte migration (1). These unwanted effects, in addition to the high danger of internal hemorrhaging from prolonged clotting times, which is especially critical to patients with hemophilic disorders and/or impaired hematopoietic function (such as kidney dialysis patients), make conventional heparin therapy a high risk to the great number of individuals who undergo daily treatment with blood-contacting biomedical devices.

To circumvent many of these undesired side effects associated with systemic heparin administration, many investigators have endeavored to immobilize heparin to blood-contacting polymers to form thromboresistant surfaces. Considering that heparin binds to the endothelium following systemic injection (1), this approach appears attractive.

Salzman et al. covalently coupled heparin to hydroxyl-bearing surfaces via an ethylene imide intermediate. Blood exposed to these surfaces exhibited prolonged clotting times, but platelet adhesion was substantially higher than untreated, controlled surfaces (8). The presence of heparin on the surface influenced the adsorption of plasma proteins, which subsequently caused platelet adhesion.

Other researchers (9, 10) immobilized heparin to polyethylene surfaces by prior adsorption of a cationic surfactant. Heparin was then ionically bound to the adsorbed surfactant and chemically stabilized by subsequent glutaraldehyde fixation. These surfaces provide approximately a 3% release of the total affixed heparin over a 10-h interval and essentially no release after that initial period. Blood exposed to such surfaces demonstrated variable prolonged clotting times dependent on the amount of heparin that could migrate through the resultant adsorbed protein layer, as revealed by Auger spectrosopy of the protein adsorbate surface. During the initial contact between the heparin-glutaraldehyde–stabilized surface and blood, the heparin was released from the surface and migrated through the adsorbed protein layer to the surface of the protein adsorbate where it was available for interaction with appropriate blood factors. If insufficient amounts of heparin penetrated the adsorbed protein layer, either due to inadequate amounts of surface heparin or to too strong of a surface/heparin interaction, the heparinized surfaces were ineffective in anticoagulation. Platelet adhesion was reduced dramatically for heparinized-glutaraldehyde–stabilized surfaces relative to untreated control polyethylene. This result was attributed to changes in the physiochemical nature of the heparinized surface influencing the adsorption of a platelet-compatible protein layer. A surface could be platelet compatible and thrombogenic if insufficient amounts of heparin penetrated the adsorbed layer (i.e., heparin tightly associated with the surface was ineffective).

Miura et al. (11) immobilized heparin on a variety of cyanogen bromide–activated surfaces. Although prolonged clotting times were observed, thrombin neutralization by immobilized heparin was indistinguishable in the presence or absence of AT-III, highly unlike solution heparin behavior. AT-III could not interact properly with surface-associated heparin or the heparin was immobilized via the AT-III binding sites. Perhaps heparin acts by first binding to thrombin, potentiating AT-III binding to a heparin/thrombin complex.

These studies indicate that heparin directly affixed to a surface does not provide optimal, solution-like, anticoagulant behavior. The immobilization of heparin directly to the polymer surface resulted in alterations of the surface properties relative to control surfaces, which greatly influenced the plasma protein adsorption characteristics, a controlling factor in platelet adhesion and overall blood compatibility (12).

Furthermore, the effects on the anticoagulant activity caused by covalent coupling via specific functional groups on the heparin molecule were not investigated. When these aspects are considered, the improved thromboresistance of the heparinized materials is not necessarily due to the biochemical interactions of heparin with the appropriate blood factors.

The strategy we adopted in developing thromboresistant, heparin-immobilized surfaces is:

1. To elucidate heparin anticoagulant effects caused by covalent coupling via specific functional groups, those heparin groups involved in immobilization reactions are first derivatized, and the effect of derivatization on anticoagulant activity is determined.
2. To circumvent alterations in the physiochemical properties of the surface caused by direct heparin coupling, heparin will be immobilized via a spacer intermediate group, thus removing immobilized heparin from the surface per se and locating the heparin in a more "bulk-like" plasma environment. The use of the spacer group not only aids in retaining physiochemical properties more similar to the original surface, but also places the heparin in a bulk solution phase where it can interact more with plasma factors as though it were in true solution (i.e., surface effects are reduced).
3. Having previously qualified the functional group or groups that least affect anticoagulant activity following derivatization, heparin is immobilized via spacer groups of various lengths utilizing reactions specific for noncritical heparin functional groups. The spacer group distance providing optimal heparin activity is then determined, and surfaces are immobilized using that specific reaction scheme.

This chapter focuses on the effects of anticoagulant activity caused by specific functional group derivatization of heparin, and on preliminary immobilization spacer group evaluations. The functional groups selected for immobilization are hydroxyl and carboxylic heparin groups.

Experimental

Free amine groups on porcine intestinal heparin (Sigma) were first blocked with acetic anhydride to form N-acetylated heparin (13). This blocking reaction was performed to insure against intermolecular or intramolecular cross-linking during heparin carboxylic activation reactions. The N-acetylated heparin was then dialyzed extensively and freeze-dried. This heparin preparation was used in all further derivatization and immobilization reactions.

Functional Group Derivatization. CARBOXYLIC DERIVATIZATION. Two grams of N-acetylated heparin and 2 mL of n-butylamine were dissolved in 40 mL of water, and the pH was adjusted to 4.75. A total of 0.8 g of 1-ethyl-3-(3-dimethylaminopropyl)carbodiimide hydrochloride was added to the heparin/n-butylamine solution in approximately 10-mg portions over a 6-h period while the reaction was maintained at 4°C and pH 4.75. Periodic samples were withdrawn from the reaction vessel, dialyzed, and freeze-dried. In a separate reaction, 0.5 g of N-acetylated heparin and 1.0 g of 2-aminoethyl hydrogen sulfate were dissolved in 10 mL of water and adjusted to pH 4.75. A total of 0.2 g of 1-ethyl-3-(3-dimethylaminopropyl)carbodiimide hydrochloride was added to the reaction vessel in approximately 10-mg portions over a 4-h period while maintaining the pH at 4.75 and the temperature at 4°C. The carboxylic-derivatized heparins were then dialyzed and freeze-dried. Carboxylic reaction schemes are illustrated in Figure 1.

HYDROXYL GROUP DERIVATIZATION. *Epichlorohydrin Activation.* One-half gram of N-acetylated heparin was dissolved in 10 mL of $1.0M$ Na_2CO_3 solution. One milliliter of epichlorohydrin and either 1 mL of n-butylamine or 1 g of glycine or 2-aminoethyl hydrogen sulfate were added to the heparin solutions and allowed to react at 40°C for 5 h. Reaction schemes are illustrated in Figure 2. The hydroxyl-derivatized heparins were then dialyzed and freeze-dried.

Divinylsulfone Activation. One-half gram of N-acetylated heparin was dissolved in 10 mL of $1.0M$ Na_2CO_3 solution. One milliliter of divinylsulfone and either 1 mL of n-butylamine or 1 g of glycine or 2-aminoethyl hydrogen sulfate were added to the heparin solutions which were allowed to react at 22°C for 3 h. The reaction schemes are illustrated in Figure 3. The hydroxyl-derivatized heparins were then dialyzed and freeze-dried.

Nuclear Magnetic Resonance (NMR) Spectrometry. Spectral verification of derivatization was provided by proton NMR of N-acetylated and carboxylic- and hydroxyl-derivatized heparins using a 300-MHz Varian SC 300 NMR spectrometer. Forty milligrams/milliliter of the respective heparin was dissolved in deuterium oxide with 1% 2,2-dimethyl-2-silapentane-5-sulfonate (DSS) and transferred to 5-mm NMR tubes. Spectra were obtained at room temperature with a spin rate of 20 rps and a gas flow rate of 13 ft^3/h.

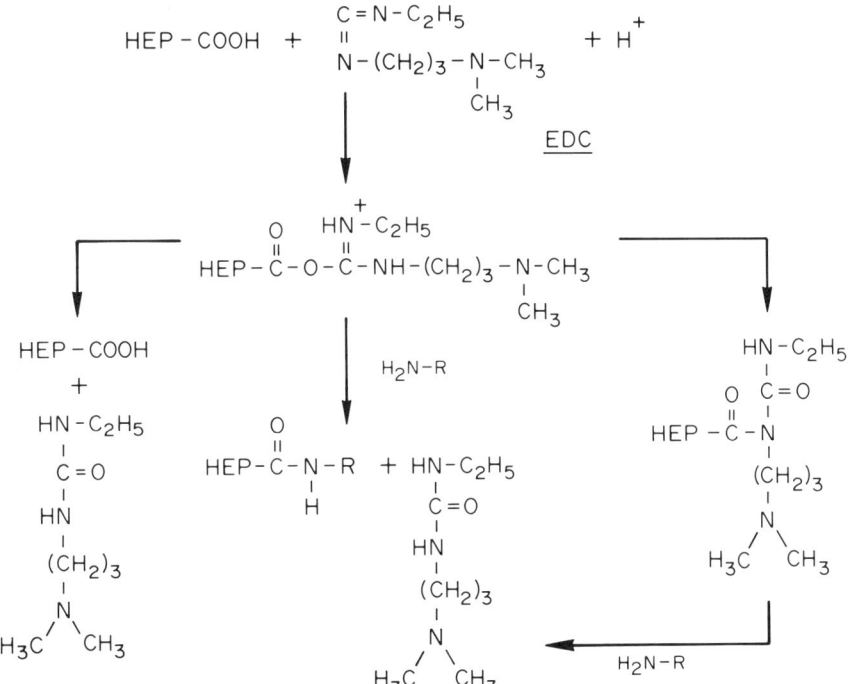

Figure 1. The 1-ethyl-3-(3-dimethylaminopropyl)carbodiimide–mediated N-acetylated heparin carboxylic group derivatization reaction scheme.

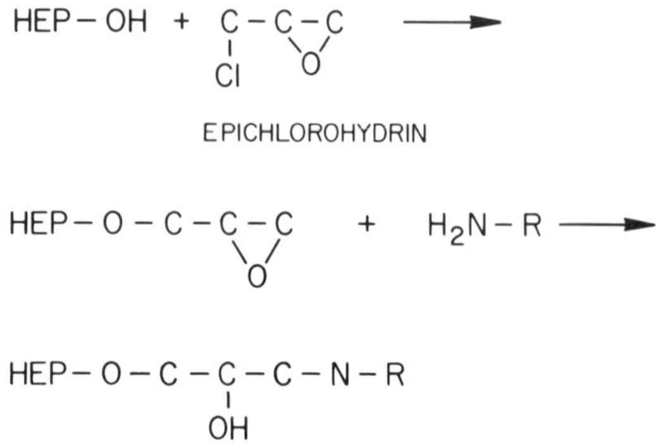

HEP−OH + C−C−C ⟶
         | \ /
         Cl   O

EPICHLOROHYDRIN

HEP−O−C−C−C + H_2N−R ⟶
       \ /
        O

HEP−O−C−C−C−N−R
         |
         OH

Figure 2. Epichlorohydrin-mediated N-acetylated heparin hydroxyl group derivatization reaction scheme.

Heparin Immobilization. Tritium-labeled heparin (New England Nuclear) was N-acetylated as described previously. All immobilization reactions were conducted with (^{3}H)N-acetylated heparin. Diaminoalkane-derivatized agaroses (1,2-diaminoethane agarose, 1,4-diaminobutane agarose, 1,8-diaminooctane agarose, 1,10-diaminodecane agarose, and 1,12-diaminododecane agarose) were purchased (Sigma) and used for immobilization substrates. Tritium-labeled, N-acetylated heparin was carboxylic-activated at 4°C in phosphate-buffered saline (pH 7.4) with N-ethyl-5-phenylisoxazolium-3′-sulfonate (Woodward's Reagent K) for 8 h. The Woodward's Reagent K was added in amounts to provide a maximum of 20% activation of the total carboxylic groups based on conductimetric titrations of the N-acetylated heparin (i.e., a minimum of 80% of the total carboxylic groups remains unmodified after immobilization on surfaces). A 10-mL aliquot of the activated heparin solution (8.0 mg activated heparin/mL solution) was added to 4 mL of each diaminoalkane derivatized gel, the resultant slurry being gently stirred at 4°C for 24 h. Woodward's Reagent K

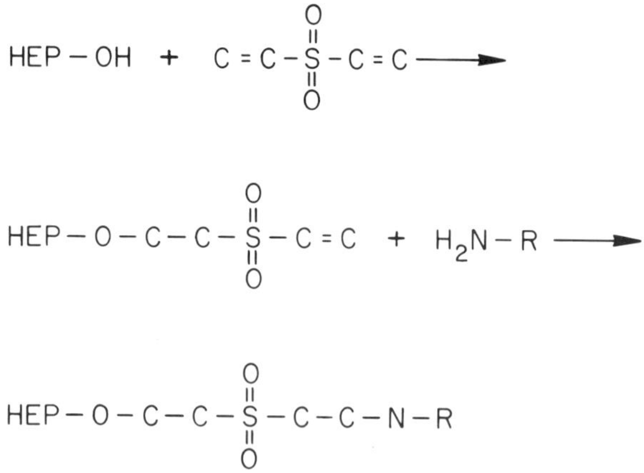

                O
                ‖
HEP−OH + C=C−S−C=C ⟶
                ‖
                O

              O
              ‖
HEP−O−C−C−S−C=C + H_2N−R ⟶
              ‖
              O

              O
              ‖
HEP−O−C−C−S−C−C−N−R
              ‖
              O

Figure 3. Divinylsulfone-mediated N-acetylated heparin hydroxyl group derivatization reaction scheme.

was used as the condensation agent during immobilization reactions because this reaction proceeds efficiently at pH 7.4. With carbodiimide reactions, acidic conditions must be used which, over a 24-h period, can lead to substantial desulfonation of the heparin. The reaction scheme is illustrated in Figure 4. Each gel was then collected by suction filtration with sintered-glass funnels and washed with phosphate-buffered saline (pH 7.4) in 50-mL increments, collecting each washing for heparin quantitation via liquid scintillation counting.

A 10-mL aliquot of 2 M 2-aminoethanol in phosphate-buffered saline (pH 7.4) was added to each gel to block all possible remaining activated carboxylic groups on immobilized heparin. The gels were then filtered and washed as described previously. Heparin was not detectable in any of these washings.

Carboxyl and Sulfate Group Determinations. Conductimetric titrations of heparin (14) provided a convenient measure of sulfate and carboxylic groups. Sodium heparin was first converted into the acid form by elution of a known quantity of heparin, dissolved in neutral deionized distilled water, through a column of previously washed Amberlite IR-120 (H^+) or bio-Rad AG 50W-X2 resin (i.e., 50–100 mg of heparin through a 7-mL column and diluted to a final volume of 150 mL to give a final concentration of 0.33 to 0.67 mg/mL heparin). The effluent was collected until only neutral water exited the column, and this then was diluted to a final volume of 150 mL.

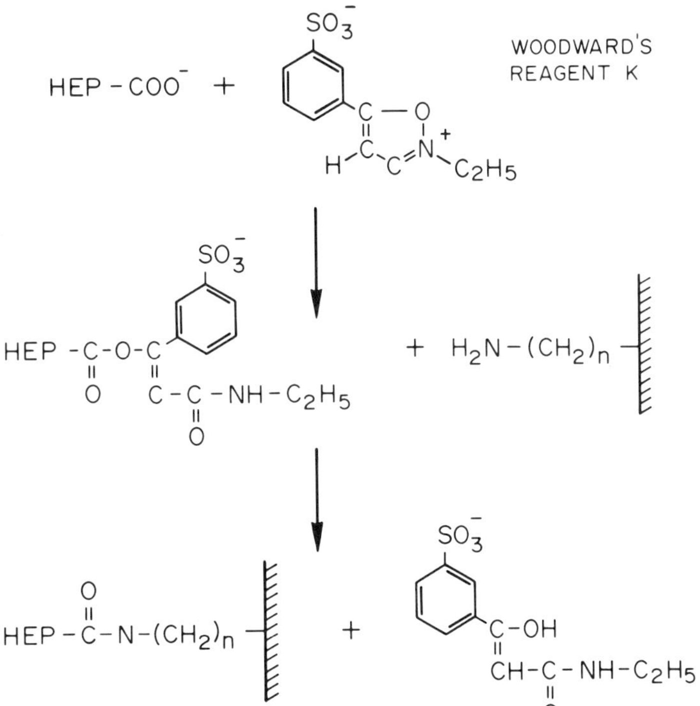

Figure 4. Immobilization of N-acetylated diaminoalkane agarose gels using N-ethyl-5-phenylisoxazolium-3'-sulfonate (Woodward's Reagent K) activated heparin carboxylic groups.

The solution was titrated with 0.1N NaOH while measuring solution conductivity vs. volume of NaOH solution added. The conductance of the sample solution, initially high mainly due to the contribution of mobile protons on the $-SO_3H$ groups from both N-sulfates and O-sulfates (specific conductance $\lambda_+ = 350$), decreased linearly as $-SO_3H$ protons were replaced by Na^+ ions ($\lambda_+ = 50$). After all of the $-SO_3H$ protons were neutralized, the curve leveled off. This plateau region corresponded to carboxylic group proton dissociation. Conductance barely changed in this region due to the compensatory effects from carboxylic proton neutralization and increased Na^+ ion concentration. After dissociation and neutralization of all carboxylic protons, conductance increased sharply primarily due to OH^- ion contributions ($\lambda_- = 198$). Extrapolation of the three branches of the conductimetric curves gave two intersection points, the first corresponding to the number of $-SO_3H$ groups while the second corresponded to the number of $-COOH$ groups (see Figure 5). Changes in the number of titratable carboxylic groups on derivatized heparins, relative to the N-acetylated heparin starting material, provide an accurate measure of the degree of carboxylic derivatization.

Anticoagulant Activity Assay. The anticoagulant activities of N-acetylated heparin and all further derivatized heparins were determined based on activated partial thromboplastin time (APTT) assay methods (15). Bovine blood was collected in 3.8% sodium-citrated (9 parts blood to 1 part citrate solution) and centrifuged at $5000 \times g$ for 15 min. The supernatant plasma was collected and pooled for subsequent APTT testing. Prior to testing plasma was kept refrigerated no longer than 6 h after

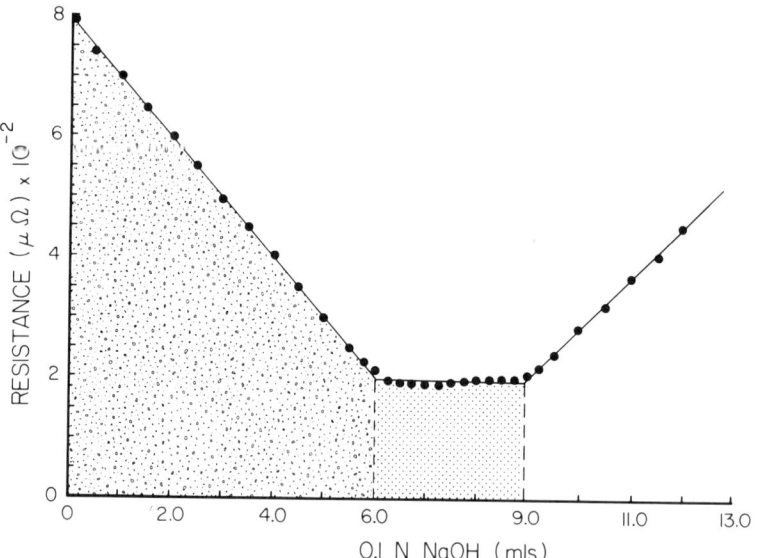

Figure 5. Conductimetric titration curve for epichlorohydrin-mediated 2-aminoethyl hydrogen sulfate N-acetylated heparin derivative $(R = N_{COO^-}/N_{SO_3^-} = V_2-V_1/V_1)$. Key: N_{COO^-}, and $N_{SO_3^-}$.

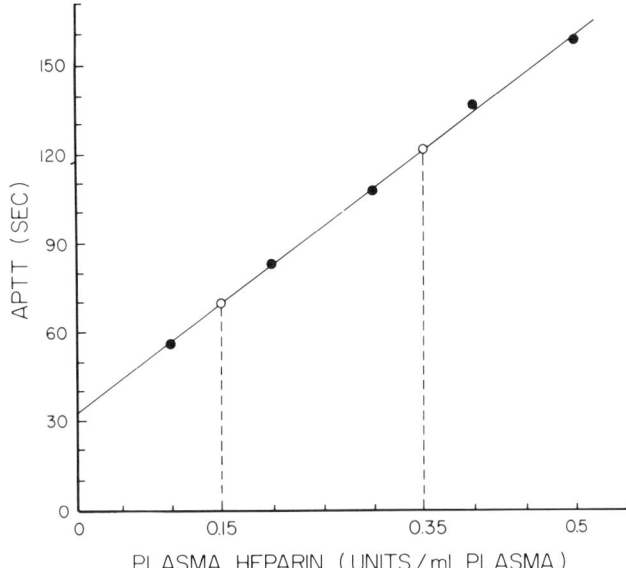

Figure 6. APTT heparin activity assay curve. Key: ●, *control heparinized plasma (units/mL plasma) calibration APTT and* ○, *derivatized heparin (at known weight concentrations, mg/mL plasma) APTT.*

collection. Bovine plasma was heparinized in 0.1 unit/mL plasma increments, and APTT was determined for each plasma heparin concentration using activated thromboplastin reagent (Ortho). A linear relationship exists between 0 and 0.5 unit/mL plasma (see Figure 6).

After determining the control heparin–APTT response curve, derivatized heparin was added to unheparinized bovine plasma (the same plasma used for preparing the control response curve) at known weight concentrations, and APTT was determined. Based on the interpolated heparin activity (units/mL plasma) of the derivatized heparin at known weight concentration (mg/mL plasma), the anticoagulant activity (units/mg) of the N-acetylated and hydroxyl- and carboxylic-derivatized heparins was determined.

Activated partial thromboplastin time assays also were used to evaluate heparin activity as a function of the spacer group distance with the heparin immobilized gels. The APTT vs. plasma heparin activity calibration curve was first prepared as described above. A 0.5-mL aliquot of each heparinized gel was added to 10 mL of the same plasma used in preparing the calibration curve. The gel and plasma were then gently rotated for 10 min at room temperature and centrifuged at 2500 × g for 5 min. The supernatant plasma was collected, and APTT was determined for each plasma. APTT was similarly determined for plasma exposed to substrate gels without heparin immobilization (i.e., 1,2-diaminoethane agarose, 1,4-diaminobutane agarose, etc.). Tritium-labeled free heparin levels in all gel-exposed plasma samples were determined by liquid scintillation counting using a Beckman LS 9000 scintillation counter.

Results and Discussion

Heparin Derivatization. Results from APTT activity assays and conductimetric titrations for carboxylic-derivatized heparins are presented in Table I. Hydroxyl-derivatized heparin results are listed in Table II. All conductimetric titration results are expressed as the ratio of the number of carboxylic groups over the number of sulfate groups ($R = N_{-COOH}/N_{-SO_3H}$). Activated partial thromboplastin time results for heparin derivatives are expressed as the mean activity (units/mg) ± 95% confidence limits (N greater than 10 for all derivatives). N-Acetylated heparin shows no significant alkane proton splitting patterns from 0 to 5 ppm (Figure 7), while derivatized heparins show characteristic alkane proton splitting patterns in that range (see Figure 8 for NMR spectrum of divinylsulfone-activated, 2-aminoethyl derivative).

The carboxylic derivatization experiments confirm previous findings (16), that derivatization leads to loss in anticoagulant activity. In that study, however, only fully derivatized compounds were evaluated. The degree of derivatization was evaluated in the n-butylamine/carboxylic derivatization series. Partial derivatization could be obtained (up to 45% derivatization) with minimal losses in anticoagulant activity. Considering that the average weight per heparin molecule had to increase after derivatization with the primary amines, the activity per initial amount of heparin remained nearly unchanged after partial derivatization. Further derivatization led to decreases in titratable $-SO_3H$ groups, as determined by conductimetric titrations, probably due to losses of 2-O-sulfates in L-iduronic acid residues under acidic conditions (17). Whether the loss in activity was strictly due to derivatization or to desulfonation cannot be determined at this time.

As with the carboxylic derivatives, hydroxyl derivatives showed minimal losses in activity under partial derivatization. In these experiments the substituted ligand end group, either a sulfate group (2-aminoethyl hydro-

Table I. Carboxylic Derivatives (Heparin–C–N–R) and Their Anticoagulant Activities

R (Alkyl Group)	% Derivatization	Activity[a] (units/mg)	COOH$^-$/SO$_3^-$
Control (N-acetylated)	0	157 ± 14	0.55
n-Butylamine	17.4	132 ± 8	0.50
n-Butylamine	24.4	126 ± 15	0.44
n-Butylamine	45.9	128 ± 8	0.30
n-Butylamine	100	0	0
2-Aminoethyl hydrogen sulfate	34.3	111 ± 10	0.40

[a]Not taking into account the weight increase above the initial amount of heparin due to derivatization.

Table II. Hydroxyl Derivatives (Heparin-O-Cross-linking Agent-R) and Their Anticoagulant Activities

Cross-linking Agent	−R (Alkyl Group)	Estimated Derivatization[a]	Activity[b] (units/mg)	COO^-/SO_3^-
Epichlorohydrin	n-butylamine	10–20	124 ± 11	0.58
Epichlorohydrin	2-aminoethyl hydrogen sulfate	10–20	132 ± 5	0.47
Epichlorohydrin	glycine	10–20	121 ± 8	0.43
Divinylsulfone	n-butylamine	10–20	113 ± 5	0.55
Divinylsulfone	2-aminoethyl hydrogen sulfate		133 ± 10	0.52
Divinylsulfone	glycine	10–20	180 ± 14	0.47

[a] Based on comparison of NMR spectra with carboxylic derivatized heparins where the % derivatization was measured.
[b] Not taking into account the weight increase above the initial amount of heparin due to derivatization.

gen sulfate), a carboxylic group (glycine), or a neutral methyl group (n-butylamine) had little to no effect on the activity of the derivatized heparin. This result was substantiated further by carboxylic-derivatization experiments where the 2-aminoethyl hydrogen sulfate derivative (34.3% derivatized) demonstrated anticoagulant activity comparable to n-butylamine derivates at a similar degree of derivatization.

These results indicate that, under partial derivatization, the chemical nature of the derivatized end group is not critical to anticoagulant activity within the limited number of derivatizing agents tested; however, the degree of derivatization is critical. Furthermore, both carboxylic and hydroxyl heparin groups can be utilized in heparin surface coupling reactions.

Heparin Immobilization. The amount of immobilized heparin per milliliter of each respective gel is listed in Table III. Results from APTT evaluations on plasma exposed to heparinized gels are presented in Figure 9. All heparinized surfaces produce prolonged clotting times relative to control surfaces and the baseline APTT. However, clotting times increase precipitously in an exponential fashion when at a spacer distance of 10 carbon atoms. None of the plasmas exposed to heparinized gels revealed free heparin via scintillation counting (specific activity of (^{3}H)N-acetylated heparin = 43,114 dpm/mg) at levels which could account for the increased clotting time. Free tritium-labeled heparin levels in plasma exposed to 10- and 12-carbon atom spacer gels were 15.05 and 22.52 dpm/mL, respectively. This corresponds to plasma heparin concentrations of 0.35 and 0.52 μg/mL, which are equivalent to 0.054 units/mL and 0.080 units/mL, respectively. Heparinized gels with 2-, 4- and 8-carbon spacer groups produced slightly prolonged clotting times relative to controls, which is insignificant compared

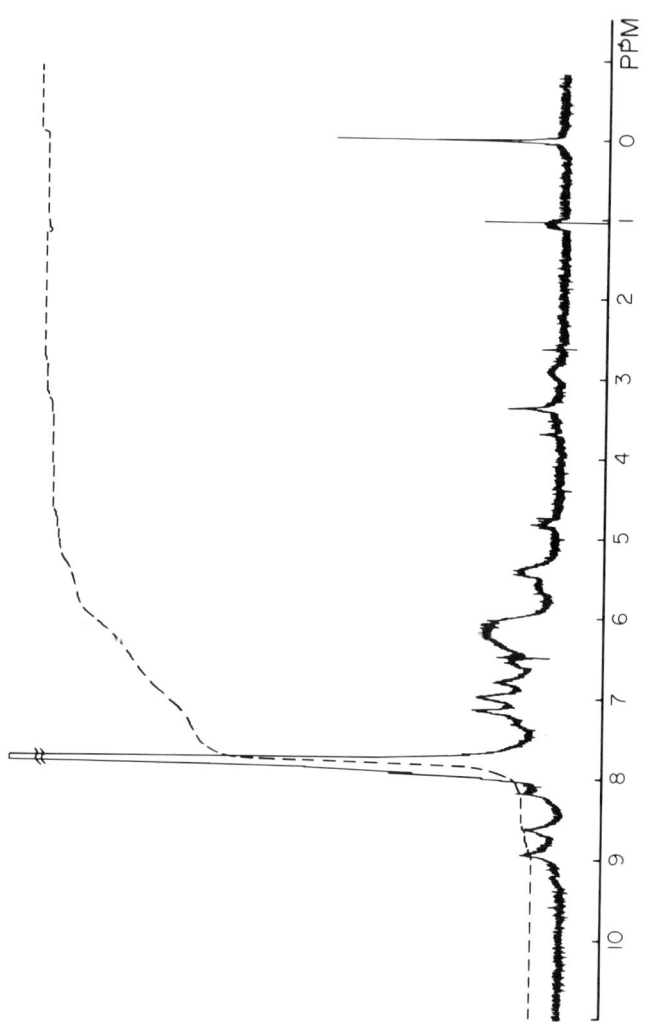

Figure 7. Proton NMR spectrum of N-acetylated heparin.

12. EBERT ET AL. *Derivatized and Immobilized Heparins* 173

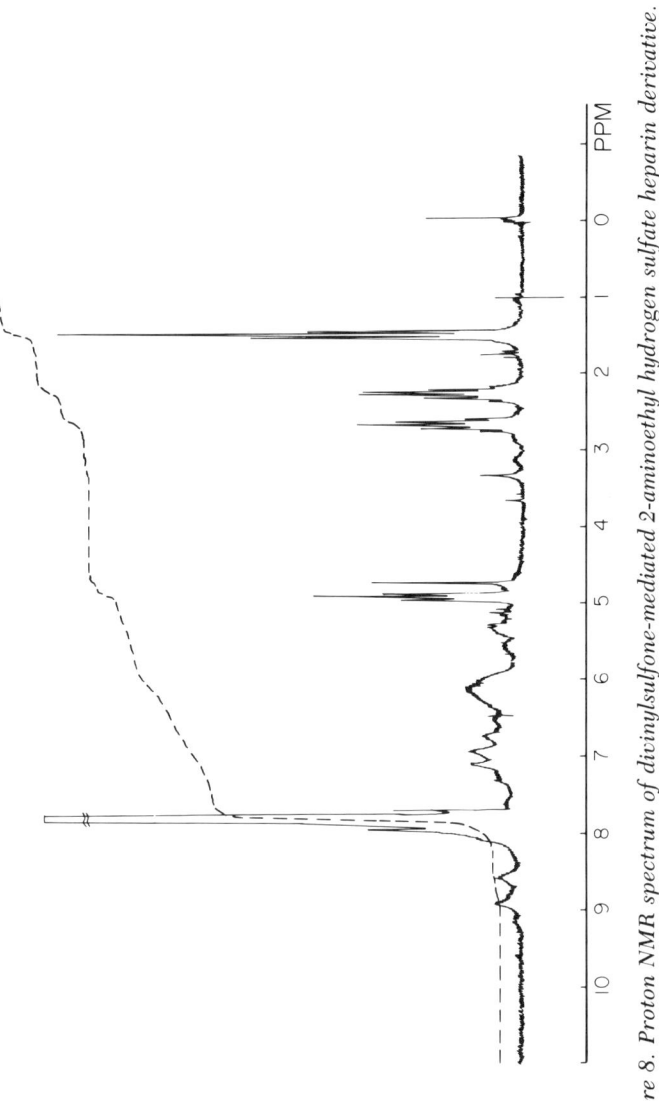

Figure 8. Proton NMR spectrum of divinylsulfone-mediated 2-aminoethyl hydrogen sulfate heparin derivative.

to 10- and 12-carbon spacer heparinized gels. These results would indicate that as the spacer group distance increases, the availability of surface-immobilized heparin to the binding sites on specific participating coagulation factors increases; however, because prolonged clotting times were observed for low spacer group distances, these heparinized surfaces are also binding coagulation factors (perhaps nonspecifically). Berg et al. (18) reported that thrombin, initially anionic in the prothrombin zymogen form, becomes cationic at normal blood pH following activation. The negatively charged heparin surfaces could readily adsorb thrombin nonspecifically from plasma. Thrombin adsorption from the test plasma could explain why only slightly elevated clotting times were observed for 8 or less carbon unit spacer groups, knowing that relatively few prothrombin enzymes would be activated into thrombin in the test plasma at that point.

The greatly elevated heparin activity associated with 10 or more carbon unit spacer groups may be due to specific heparin interactions with coagulation factors (i.e., specific binding of AT-III) more similar to solution heparin behavior. The mass transport of heparin binding factors to the heparinized surface is an important factor that must be considered in evaluating the efficacy of the immobilized anticoagulant. Utilizing the methods reported here for the immobilized heparin evaluations, this aspect cannot be addressed adequately at present, and further testing is necessary to resolve this question.

Irrespective of the anticoagulant mechanisms involved with immobilized heparins, the anticoagulant activity greatly increases as the immobilized heparin molecules are removed from the surface environment to a bulk-like plasma environment via spacer groups. The relative amount of unmodified carboxylic groups on immobilized heparin available for interaction with coagulation factors appears critical based on carboxylic derivatization results; therefore, the number of immobilization points per heparin molecule must be minimized for carboxylic immobilization reactions. The average number of immobilization points per heparin molecule due to the normal variation in chemical structure and molecular weight of commercial

Table III. Heparin Immobilization onto Agarose Gels

Gel	Spacer Distance (Carbon Number)	mg Immobilized/ mL Gel
1,2-Diaminoethane agarose	2	0.50
1,4-Diaminobutane agarose	4	1.00
1,8-Diaminooctane agarose	8	3.14
1,10-Diaminodecane agarose	10	2.33
1,12-Diaminododecane agarose	12	0.95

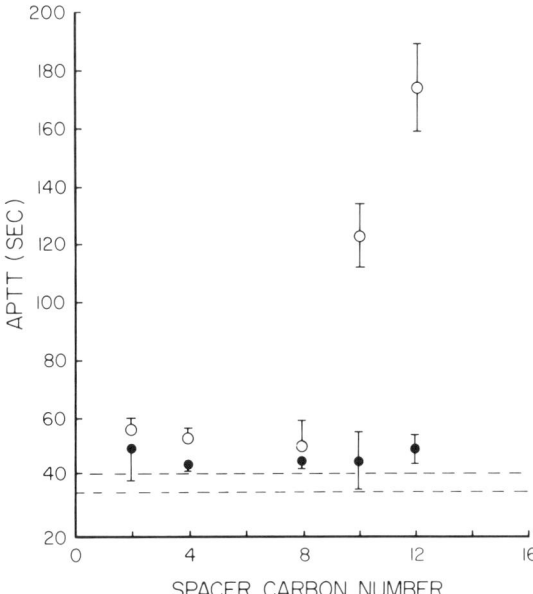

Figure 9. APTT vs. spacer unit carbon number results for heparin immobilized via carboxylic groups to diaminoalkane agarose gels. Key: ---, the baseline APTT (i.e., unheparinized plasma); ●, *respective control substrate APTT (i.e., untreated diaminoalkane agarose gels); and* ○, *respective heparin immobilized gels.*

heparin is difficult to estimate. However, a distribution of immobilization points per heparin molecule must exist, with the lowest molecular weight molecules probably being immobilized by a single bond and the higher molecular weight molecules being immobilized by several bonds.

Acknowledgments

The authors gratefully acknowledge the invaluable contributions to this work by Jan Feijen and Dennis Coleman. This work was supported by NIH Grant #HL-20251. S. W. Kim is an NIH Research Career Development Awardee (HL-00272).

Literature Cited

1. Jaques, L. B. *Science* **1979**, *206*, 528.
2. Horner, A. A. "Heparin Chemistry and Clinical Usage"; Kakkar, V. V.; Thomas, D. P., Eds.; Academic: New York, 1976; p. 37.
3. Barrowcliffe, T. W.; Johnson, E. A.; Eggleton, C. A.; Kemball-Cook, G.; Thomas, D. P. *Br. J. Haematol.* **1979**, *41*, 573.
4. Rosenberg, R. D.; Lam, L. *Proc. Natl. Acad. Sci. (U.S.A.)* **1979**, *76*, 1218.

5. Seegers, W.; Warner, E. D.; Brinkhous, K. M.; Smith, H. P. *Science* **1942**, *96*, 300.
6. Rosenberg, R. D. "Heparin Chemistry and Clinical Usage"; Kakkar, V. V.; Thomas, D. P., Eds.; Academic: New York, 1976; p. 101.
7. Rosenberg, R. D. *Semin. Hematol.* **1977**, *14*, 427.
8. Salzman, E. W.; Merrill, E. W.; Binder, A.; Wolf, C. F. W.; Ashford, T. P. *J. Biomed. Mater. Res.* **1969**, *3*, 64.
9. Lagergren, H.; Eriksson, J. C. *Trans. Am. Soc. Artif. Intern. Organs* **1971**, *17*, 10.
10. Larsson, R.; Eriksson, J. C.; Lagergren, H.; Olsson, P. *Thromb. Res.* **1979**, *15*, 157.
11. Miura, M.; Sadayoshi, A.; Kusada, Y.; Miyamoto, K. *J. Biomed. Mater. Res.* **1980**, *14*, 619.
12. Lee, E. S.; Kim, S. W. *Trans. Am. Soc. Artif. Intern. Organs* **1979**, *25*, 124.
13. Danishefsky, I.; Steiner, H. *Biochim. Biophys. Acta* **1965**, *101*, 37.
14. Casu, B.; Gennaro, U. *Carbohyd. Res.* **1975**, *39*, 168.
15. Cifonelli, J. A. *Carbohydr. Res.* **1974**, *37*, 145.
16. Danishefsky, I.; Siskovic, R. *Thromb. Res.* **1972**, *1*, 173.
17. Kosakai, M.; Yosizawa, Z. *J. Biochem.* **1979**, *86*, 147.
18. Berg, W.; Hillvarn, B.; Arwin, H.; Stenberg, M.; Lundstrom, I. *Thromb. Haemostas.* **1979**, *42*, 972.

RECEIVED for review January 16, 1981. ACCEPTED March 28, 1981.

13

Hemocompatibility Effect of Molecular Motions of the Polymer Interface

W. M. REICHERT—University of Michigan, Macromolecular Research Center, Ann Arbor, MI 48109

F. E. FILISKO—University of Michigan, Department of Materials and Metallurgy, Ann Arbor, MI 48109

S. A. BARENBERG[1]—University of Michigan, Department of Chemical Engineering, Ann Arbor, MI 48109

> *The effect and interrelationship between primary (segmental backbone) and secondary (side chain) molecular motions on thrombogenesis, independent of morphological order/disorder, crystallinity, and/or associated water, were elucidated using an amorphous hydrophobic polymer of poly[(trifluoroethoxy) (fluoroalkoxy)phosphazene]. The results indicated that for an amorphous hydrophobic polymer, thrombogenesis was sensitive, and depended on the degrees and types of primary and secondary molecular motions at the polymer interface.*

Surface charge, chemistry, topography, electrical conductivity, critical surface tension, morphology, and wettability have evolved as factors (1) in defining and correlating the surface properties of polymeric materials to thrombogenesis. However, these factors do not discriminate as to surface microcrystallinity, and/or lack thereof, and to surface hydrophobicity/hydrophilicity. In addition, the effect of primary (segmental backbone) and/or secondary (side chain) surface molecular motions on thrombogenesis has received limited attention (2, 3). Merrill (2) postulated that these molecular motions might influence the initial deposition of the blood plasma proteins. Subsequently, Barenberg (3) presented evidence indicating restricted and unrestricted side chain motions on thrombogenesis. However, in these studies and in others (4), the effect of substrate/surface molecular motions on thrombogenesis has been complexed by morphological order and/or disorder, crystallinity, and associated water. Subsequently, to date, no studies

---

[1]Present address: E. I. duPont de Nemours and Co., Inc., Experimental Station, Wilmington, DE 19898

have been presented researching solely the effects of primary and secondary molecular motions on thrombogenesis, independent of the above complexing factors.

Therefore, this chapter presents preliminary evidence indicating the effect and interrelationship between primary and secondary molecular motions on thrombogenesis, independent of morphological order and/or crystallinity. The polymer selected for this study was an amorphous elastomeric hydrophobic polymer of poly[(trifluoroethoxy) (fluoroalkoxy)phosphazene] (PNF) I (5, 6). The salient aspects of this polymer are that: (1) the onset of the secondary molecular motions occurs between $-160°$ and $-120°C$; (2) the side chain motion can be altered by irradiation (ultraviolet, electron beam, or gamma); (3) no apparent ultrastructure morphology exists; (4) the side chains can be derivatized (5); and (5) the polymer can be readily coated onto our extracorporeal test shafts (7) and irradiated accordingly. Additionally, contact angle measurements of the homopolymer (8) and the PNF (9), 19.7 and 15.0 dyn/cm^2, respectively, indicated that the fluorinated side chains comprised the surface to be interfaced in the extracorporeal blood studies.

$$\begin{array}{c} O(CH_2)(CF_2)xCF_2H \\ | \\ ---(P = N)_n--- \\ | \\ OCH_2CF_3 \end{array} \qquad x = 1, 3, 5, 7$$

Experimental

The polymer used in this study was PNF (Firestone Central Research).

The polymer was purified by dissolving the PNF in Freon TA (Miller Stephenson Chemical), followed by mixing in an equal volume of deionized distilled water with the Freon/polymer solution. The system was then allowed to phase separate. The Freon layer was eluted into hexane, causing the high molecular weight polymer to precipitate out. The polymer was then vacuum dried. Solutions of the purified polymer were prepared in reagent-grade acetone. All films were cast from solution in a closed environment to reduce surface contamination and retard the rate of solvent evaporation.

Ultraviolet irradiation of the PNF was done with a Hanovia 616 A high-pressure mercury vapor lamp with an output dosage of 70 $\mu W/cm^2$ at a distance of 50 cm. The time dosages used in this study ranged from 0 to 30 h.

The dielectric measurements were performed on an automated difference dielectric system (10, 11, 12). Thin films of the purified polymer (less than 1 mm) were cast at room temperature directly onto the cell from three successive 5-mL applications of a 1.0% (w/v) acetone solution. Each application was allowed to dry in a closed environment. After a suitable film was obtained, it was vacuum dried for 12 h. The original films were run, irradiated, and rerun, allowing us to observe the effects of irradiation on the same sample. The temperature range investigated was from $-200°$ to $100°C$, over a frequency range of 0.234–20.0 kHz. The thin films were used to increase the sample surface area, and therefore, increase the surface contribution to the spectra.

Difference dielectric measurements were obtained by placing the unirradiated PNF spectra in the memory of the dielectric system, and subtracting the unirradiated spectra from the irradiated.

Tensile stress–strain measurements were performed on solvent-cast (10% w/v) films using an Instron tensile tester.

The amount of bound water associated with the PNF was measured using a Perkin Elmer DSC II equipped with a subambient stage. The samples were scanned from 227 to 303 K at 10 K/min under dry nitrogen. The heats of fusion of the sorbed water were calculated relative to the heats of fusion of indium (12).

Mass spectroscopy of the gaseous by-products produced from irradiating the PNF was performed using a Finnigan 4000 mass spectrometer.

Critical surface tension and attenuated total reflectance infrared spectroscopy (ATR) of irradiated and unirradiated solution-cast PNF films was done in conjunction with R. Baier (9).

Angular resolved electron spectroscopy for chemical analysis (ESCA) of the irradiated and unirradiated PNF surfaces was done in conjunction with B. Ratner (13).

Morphological studies were done on thin films of the polymer as cast onto carbon-coated glass slides.

Thin films of the polymer were cast from acetone onto carbon-coated slides. The films were placed in contact with isotonic saline for 4 h, and then washed in deionized distilled water. A carbon film was subjected to the above saline/wash treatment to serve as the experimental control.

Conventional and scanning transmission electron microscopy (CTEM and STEM) were done on a JEOL 100C electron microscope. The scanning (secondary emission) electron microscopy was done on a JEOL U3.

The x-ray dispersion analysis was done on a JEOL 100C equipped with a Princeton Gamma Tech detector and Nuclear Data software. The count times were on the order of 20 min at magnifications of 20,000, 30,000, and 50,000 $\times$.

The extracorporeal shafts, 303 stainless steel and polypropylene, were prepared by dip coating the shafts into 1.0% (w/v) solutions of the copolymer and allowing the excess to drip off. The shafts were inverted and placed in a closed system to retard the rate of solvent evaporation. This technique resulted in an isotropic coating of the copolymer.

The animals used in these studies were conditioned male dogs of mixed breed. Access to the animals' circulatory systems was accomplished via an acute shunt surgically implanted in the neck of the dog. The shunt was constructed of 3/16 in. Silastic tubing anastomosed to the carotid artery and jugular vein. Blood flow through the shunt was on the order of 1 L/min.

Twenty-four hours prior to an experiment, 150 mL of blood were collected from the animal into a sterile Fenwal (450-mL) blood bag containing citrate–phosphate–dextrose. Aliquots were then transferred and centrifuged at 200 g for 15 min. The platelet-rich plasma supernatant was then centrifuged at 1000 g for 15 min. The platelet-poor plasma was transferred, leaving a residual 2 mL with each platelet pellet. The platelets were resuspended, to which 300–400 μc ^{111}In (Diagnostic Isotopes) was added. The system was incubated at ambient temperature for 60 min, after which 10 mL of platelet-poor plasma was added and the mixture was centrifuged at 1000 g for 15 min. The platelets were resuspended in platelet-poor plasma and reinfused into the animal. Additionally, human ^{125}I-labeled fibrinogen was injected into the animal 24 h prior to the experiment. The peak fibrinogen radioactivity after infusion was approximately 1×10^4 cpm/mL. No anticoagulants were used prior to or during the experiments.

The PNF-coated shafts were assembled into the test chambers. The test chambers were flushed with isotonic saline to displace the air interface. The blood flow through each of the chambers was adjusted to 200 mL/min using a Ward's doppler flow ultrasound cuff. The rotation of the shafts was maintained at 200 rpm. Under these conditions, a laminar flow regime was maintained with a shear rate of 150 s^{-1}. Experiments were carried out for time periods of 60 min. After completion of each of the experiments, the chamber was flushed with isotonic saline.

At the completion of the test, the test shafts were removed, and the relative radioactivity of each shaft was determined in a Nuclear Chicago well counter. The shafts were fixed by placing them into buffered glutaraldehyde, sucrose, and sodium cocadylate in deionized distilled water, followed by staining in a 1.0% solution of buffered osmium tetroxide. Afterwards, they were rinsed in distilled water, solvent exchanged, and critical-point dried. The shafts were coated with a 20-nm layer of gold using a pulsatile sputterer; this coating prevented any local heating of the sample.

Results

The PNF polymer morphology (Figure 1a) as cast from acetone exhibited a homogeneous morphology with no apparent indication of any form of ultrastructure, that is, nodules and/or microdomains. The x-ray disperson map (Figure 1b) of the unirradiated PNF exhibited a homogeneous distribu-

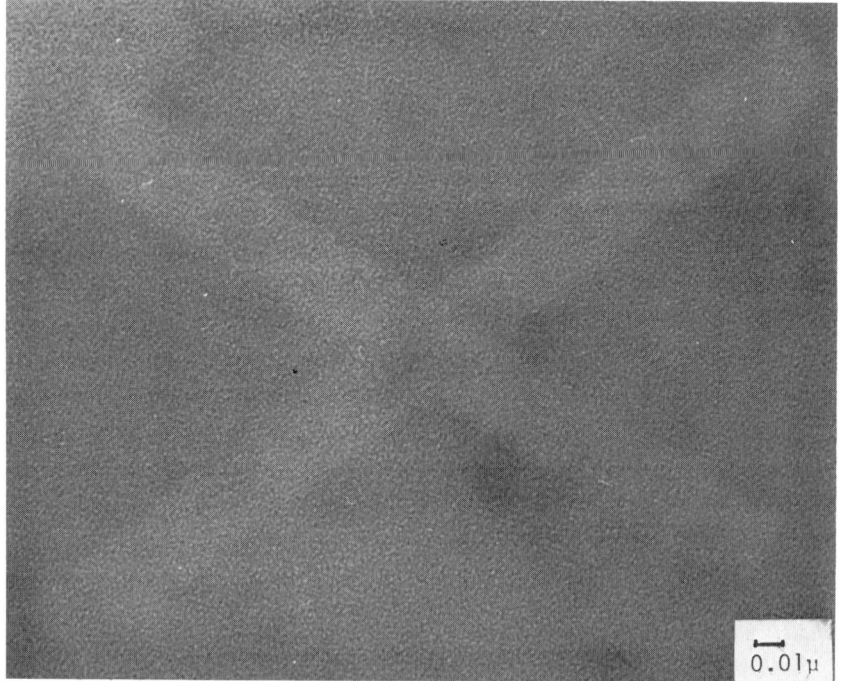

Figure 1a. TEM of the PNF as cast from acetone at 0 h irradiation.

Figure 1b. Phosphorus x-ray dispersion map of PNF as cast from acetone at 0 h irradiation.

tion of phosphorus with no apparent signs of aggregation or other impurities. The morphologies of the 1- and 30-h irradiated PNF's (Figures 2a and 3a) as above, exhibited homogeneous morphologies. The x-ray dispersion maps (Figures 2b and 3b) of the irradiated PNF's indicated no change in the phosphorus distribution. These results indicate that the blood interfacing surface of the PNF was homogeneous with respect to ultrastructure morphology and surface chemistry. Additionally, the PNF's appeared morphologically clean, that is, no residual catalysts, salts, etc.

When the polymers were exposed to isotonic saline and then washed (Figure 4), the PNF's sequestered the ions. The degree and amount of ion sequestering as a function of irradiation dose is currently under investigation.

The molecular motions of the PNF (i.e., primary and secondary molecular relaxations) were documented by dielectric and dynamic (Rheovibron) mechanical measurements (14) (Figure 5). The −160°C relaxation has been ascribed to the combined onset of the trifluoroethoxy, β', and fluoroalkoxy, β'', side chain motion (15, 16). The −50°C relaxation has been ascribed (15) to the glass transition (segmental backbone) of the PNF.

To study selectively the effect of primary and secondary molecular motions on thrombogenesis, the PNF was subjected to low-dose ultraviolet irradiation; the same dose rate as used in the extracorporeal studies. It was anticipated that this low-dose treatment would selectively cross-link the pendant side chains intramolecularly, followed by intramolecular/intermolecular cross-linking at higher dose rates.

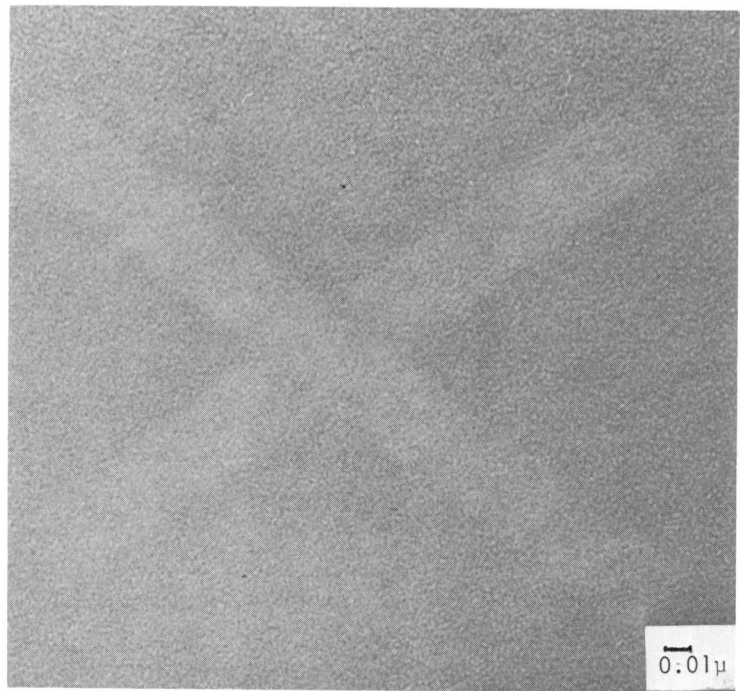

Figure 2a. TEM of the PNF as cast from acetone at 1 h irradiation.

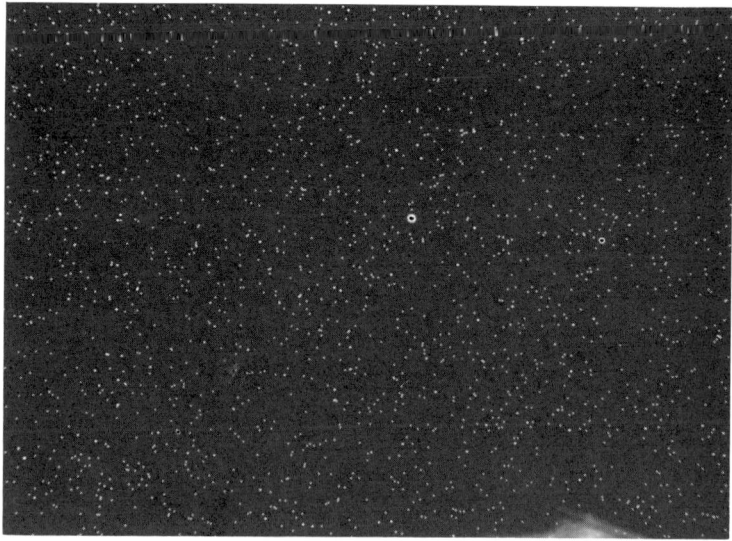

Figure 2b. Phosphorus x-ray dispersion map of PNF as cast from acetone at 1 h irradiation.

Figure 3a. TEM of the PNF as cast from acetone at 24 h irradiation.

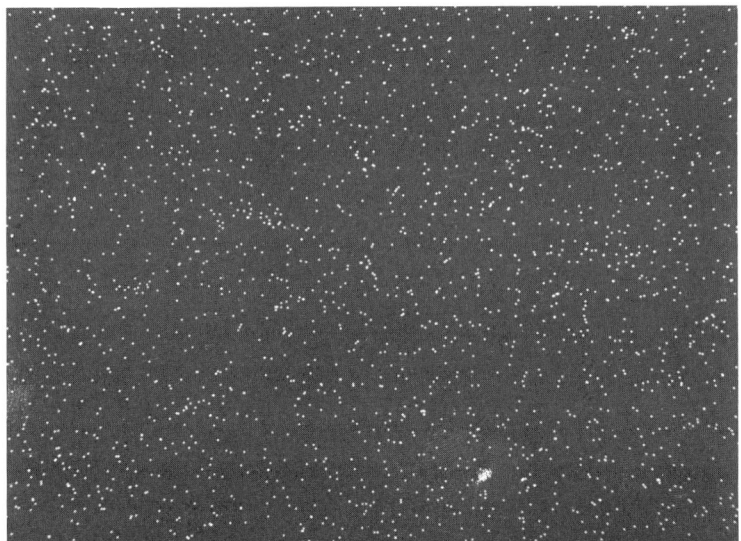

Figure 3b. Phosphorus x-ray dispersion map of PNF as cast from acetone at 24 h irradiation.

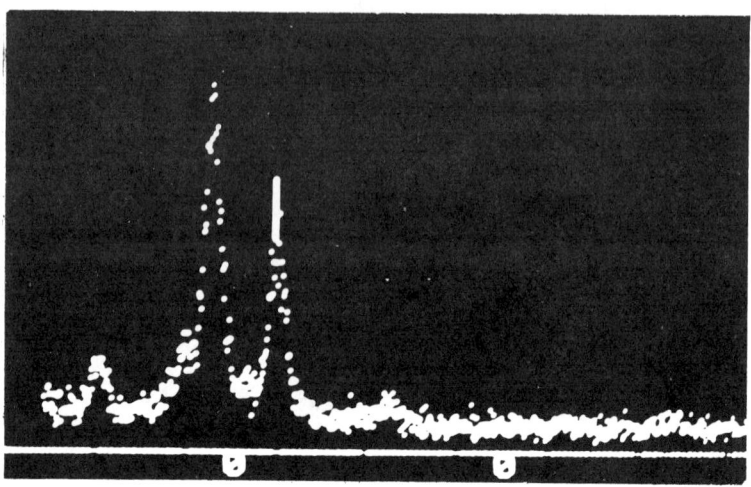

Figure 4. X-ray dispersion spectra of PNF exposed to isotonic saline, and washed. Dispersion peaks from left to right are sodium, phosphorus, and chlorine.

As can be observed in Figure 6, the magnitudes of the α- and β-relaxations increased at 1 h of ultraviolet irradiation, but then decreased at 30 h of irradiation. The difference dielectric spectra (Figure 7) indicate that the two side chains were not affected equally by the ultraviolet light. At low exposures to ultraviolet light (less than 6 h), the fluoroalkoxy side chains were selectively altered photochemically, while the trifluoroothoxy side chains remained relatively unaffected. Perhaps we are seeing either a backbiting mechanism as proposed by O'Brien (17) or the development of branch points as observed by Pineri (18), both of whom also observed a similar β-relaxation enhancement in their γ-irradiation studies of polyethylene. Upon further irradiation (greater than 6 h) (Figure 7), the pendant side chains underwent an intramolecular/intermolecular cross-linking, as evidenced by the β-decrease and α-shift in the difference dielectric spectra. This result is also supported by swelling studies (11) which showed the 30-h irradiated sample swelling in acetone while the 0- and 1-h irradiated samples did not. Therefore, the pendant side chain motions apparently are affected by ultraviolet irradiation.

The results of the contact angle measurements (Table I), ATR, and mass spectroscopy (11) of the irradiated and unirradiated PNF's indicate that neither a change in the surface chemistry, per se, nor irradiation-induced chain scission occurs.

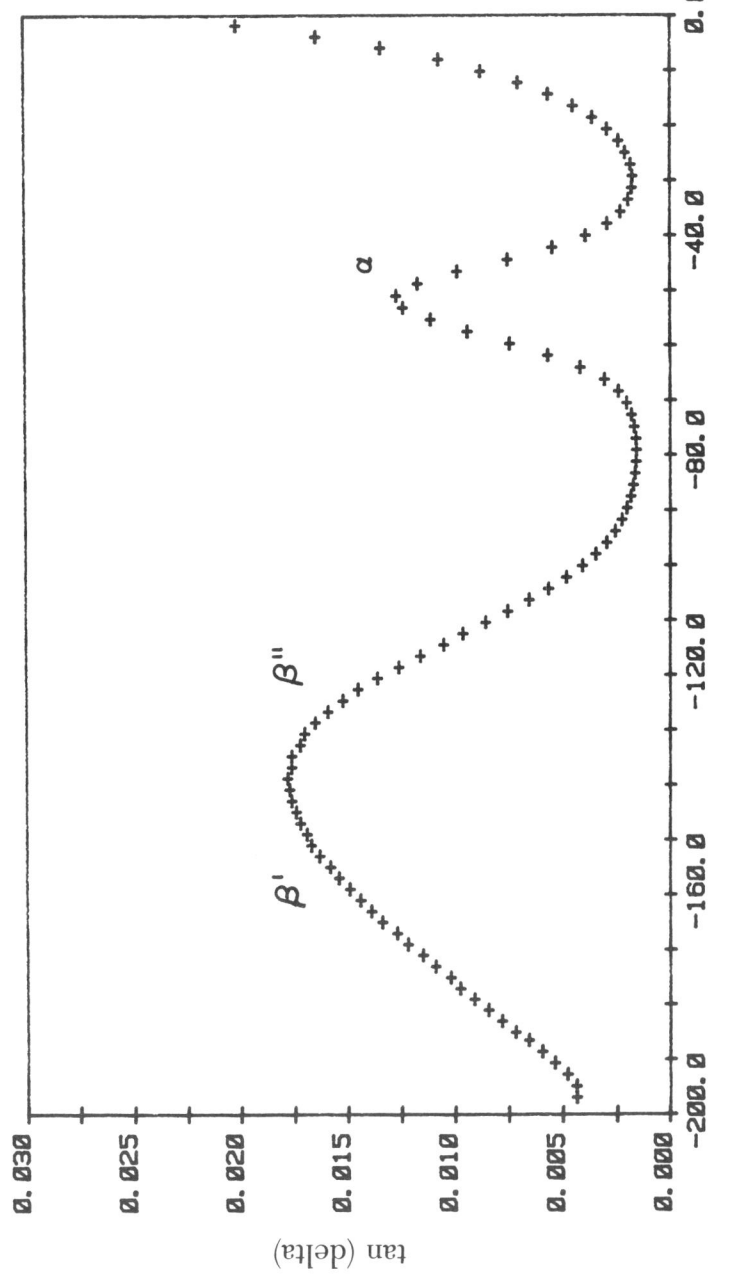

Figure 5. Dielectric spectra of unirradiated PNF polymer showing β'-, β''-, and α-relaxations.

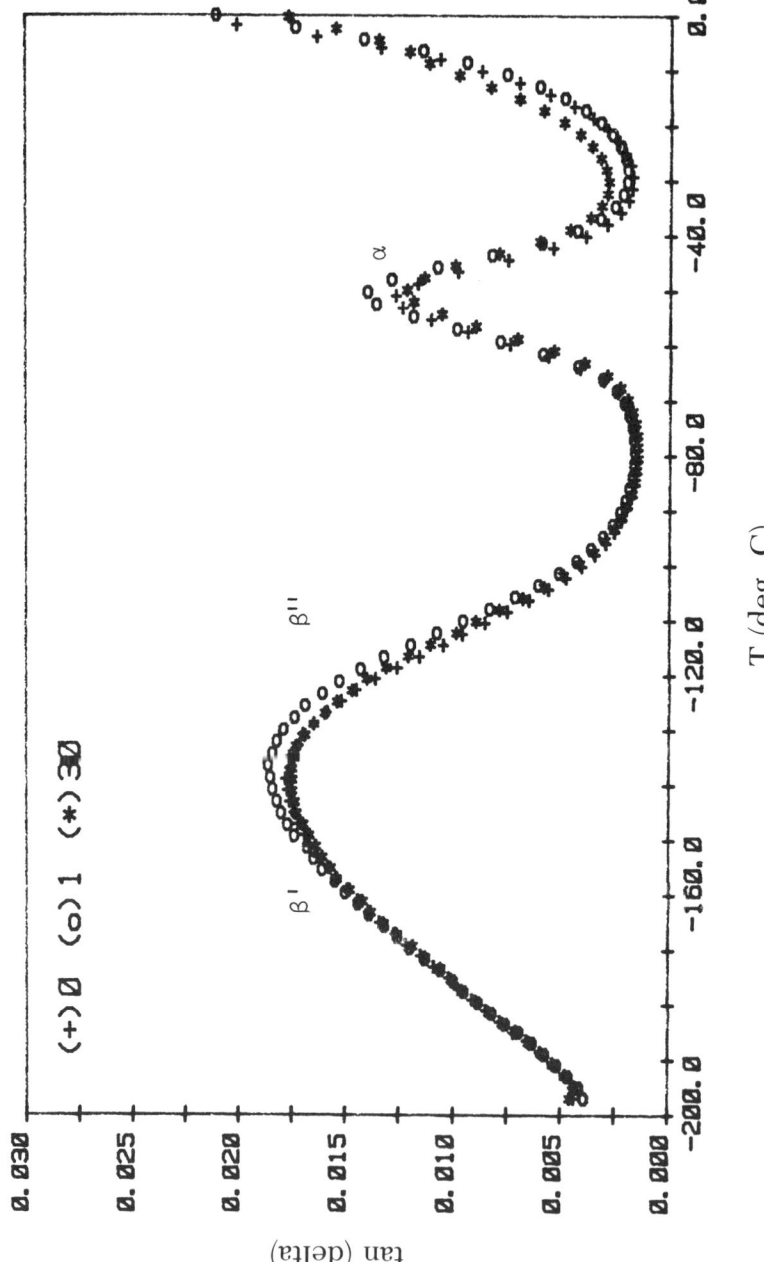

Figure 6. Dielectric spectra of 0-, 1-, and 30-h irradiated PNF. The magnitude of the β- and α-relaxations of the 1-h irradiated sample increases relative to the 0- and 30-h samples.

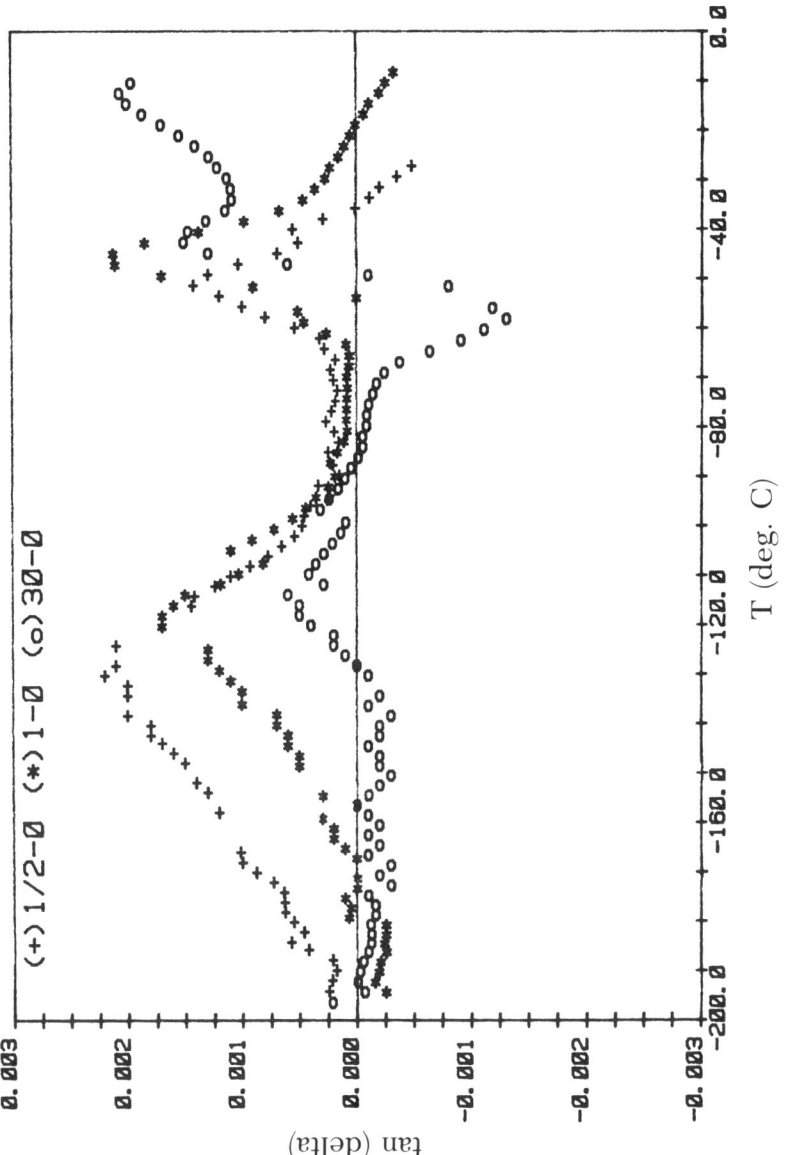

Figure 7. Difference dielectric spectra of the irradiated minus the unirradiated PNF's. The magnitude of the β-relaxation decreases as a function of irradiation dose.

Table I. Critical Surface Tension of PNF as a Function of UV Irradiation

Ultraviolet Light (time dose in h)	Critical Surface Tension (dyn/cm^2)
0	16.5
1	14.4
30	15.6

Preliminary analysis of the ESCA results (13) from irradiated and unirradiated PNF shows that the nitrogen/carbon (N/C) and the phosphorus/carbon (P/C) ratios remain relatively constant in the 0-, 1-, and 24-h irradiated samples. However, the fluorine/carbon (F/C) ratio increases continuously ($0 < 1 < 24$), and the oxygen/carbon (O/C) ratios of the 0- and 1-h irradiated samples are essentially the same, but slightly smaller than the O/C ratio in the 24-h irradiated sample. A more detailed analysis of this data, as well as Fourier transform infrared spectroscopy (FTIR) analysis of the PNF's, will be presented in a collateral paper (10).

The tensile stress–strain measurements (Figure 8) indicate that the PNF's are becoming cross-linked upon irradiation, as evidenced by the increase in the ultimate tensile properties.

Differential scanning calorimetry (DSC) was used to ascertain the degree, if any, of bound water associated with the PNF polymer. As seen in Table II, the virgin PNF contained 0.01 mg bound water/mg polymer, which increased to 0.05 mg bound water/mg polymer. The reasons for the increase in bound water content as a function of irradiation are currently under investigation (11). This change may be tied to the oxidation level of the polymer.

When the PNF polymers were exposed to canine blood for 60 min (Figures 9, 10, and 11, and Table III) as a function of irradiation time dose, the relative thrombogenic response was quite discernible. The virgin unirradiated PNF developed a large thrombus (Figure 9), with no apparent signs of becoming limited. In contrast, the 1-h irradiated PNF developed a limited thrombus, such that in given island areas, some platelet and leukocyte adhesion occurred. The 24-h irradiated PNF morphologically also exhibited a limited thrombogenic response like that of the 1-h irradiated sample. How-

Table II. Bound Water Content of PNF as a Function of UV Irradiation

Ultraviolet Light (time dose in h)	mg Bound Water/ mg Polymer
0	0.0105
1	0.0127
30	0.0514

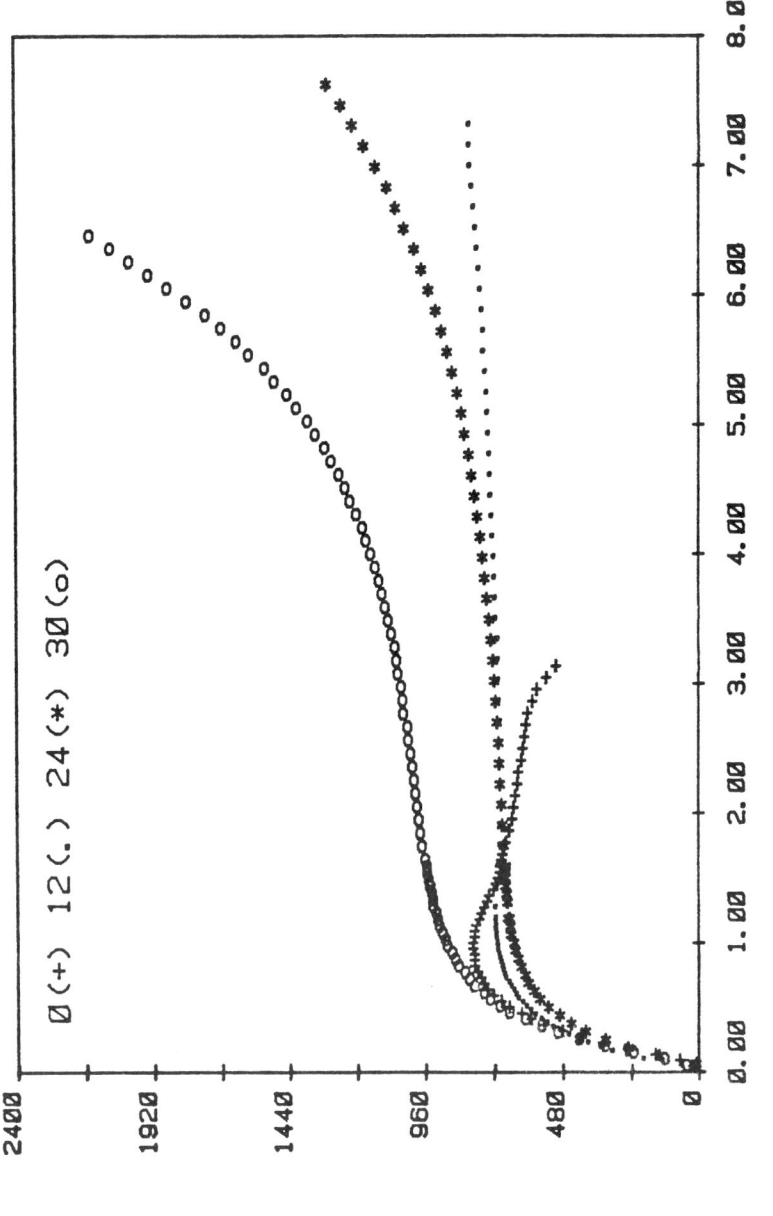

Figure 8. Tensile stress–strain plots of the PNF as a function of irradiation dose.

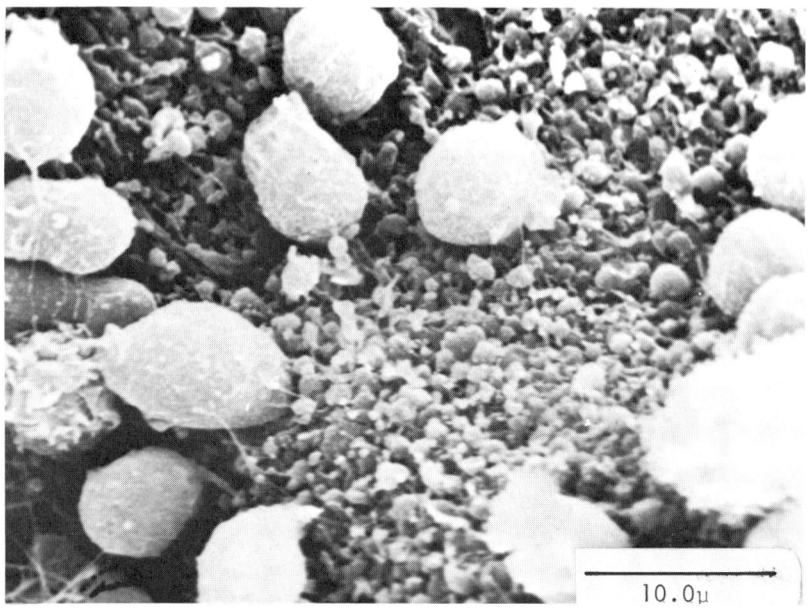

Figure 9. SEM of 0-h irradiated PNF exposed to canine blood for 60 min.

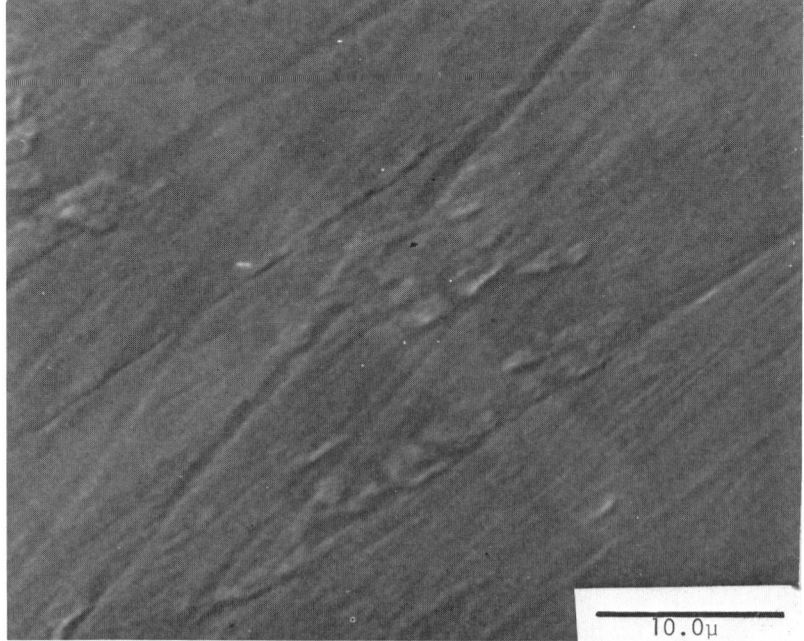

Figure 10. SEM of 1-h irradiated PNF exposed to canine blood for 60 min.

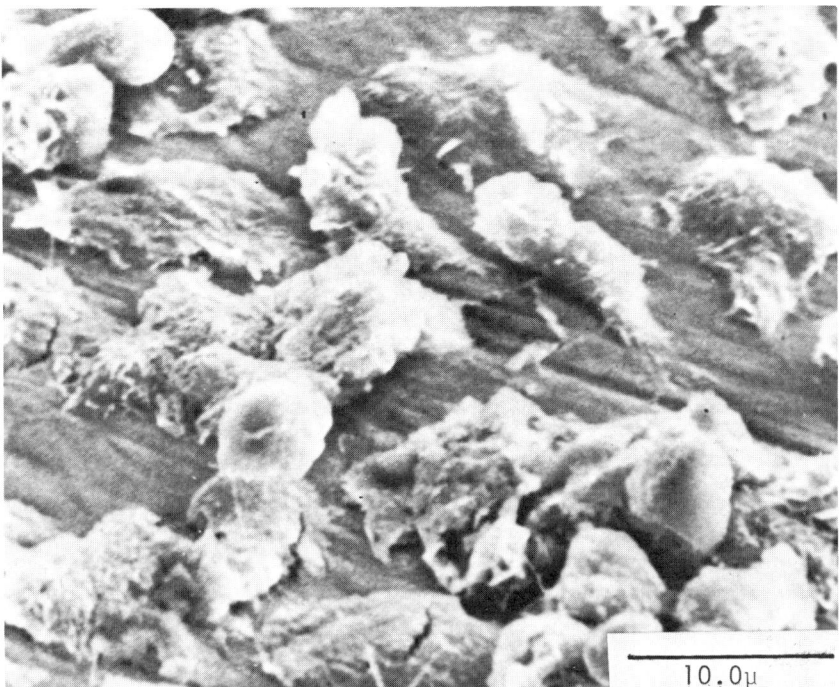

Figure 11. SEM of 24-h irradiated PNF exposed to canine blood for 60 min.

ever, the labeled studies (Table III) indicated that the thrombogenic response of the 24-h irradiated PNF polymer was not similar to that of the 1-h irradiated samples; the amount of fibrin and platelets in the 24-h irradiated samples increased relative to the 1-h samples. In addition, when the polymers were irradiated, the amount of labeled fibrin and platelets on the surface of the PNF polymers decreased substantially.

This decrease and subsequent increase in fibrin and platelet deposition appeared concurrently with the observed changes in the interfacial secondary molecular motions associated with the PNF polymers. This apparent interrelationship is addressed later.

Table III. Average Weight of Fibrin and Platelets per Clot on PNF-Coated Shafts Exposed to Canine Blood for 60 min

Ultraviolet Light (time dose in h)	[[fibrin]/Clot] (mg/Clot)	[Platelet]/ Clot x 10^{-8}
0	2.31	62.6
1	0.07	7.16
24	0.22	19.9

Discussion

The results of the difference dielectric measurements, in conjunction with the morphological and x-ray dispersion observations, tensile stress–strain, ATR, and contact angle measurements, indicated that in the extracorporeal studies, the blood is exposed to essentially the same surface; the only apparent change being the different degrees and types of surface molecular motions. The surface molecular motions of the unirradiated PNF consisted of both the trifluoroethoxy and fluoroalkoxy side chains in the unrestricted state, whereas the surface molecular motions in the 1-h irradiated PNF consisted of the trifluoroethoxy side chains in the dynamic state, with the fluoroalkoxy side chain motion being partially restricted. In the case of the 24- and 30-h irradiated samples, the surface molecular motions of both the trifluoroethoxy and fluoroalkoxy side chains were partially restricted.

The extracorporeal results indicated that the initial adsorption of the plasma protein(s) and/or cellular elements onto the surface of the PNF polymers was mediated, in part, given the above, by the relative degrees of surface molecular mobility associated with the fluoro pendant side chains. Specifically, when the PNF consisted of both the trifluoroethoxy and fluoroalkoxy side chains in an unrestricted state coupled with the backbone motion, a large thrombus occurred (Figure 9). However, when the PNF was irradiated for 1 h, resulting in the partial restriction of the trifluoroethoxy molecular motion, a limited thrombogenic response occurred (Figure 10). Upon further irradiation (24 h), where both the molecular motions of the trifluoroethoxy and fluoroalkoxy side chains became restricted, a limited thrombogenic response occurred (Figure 11). However, the radiolabeled studies (Table III) indicated an increased thrombogenic response for the 24-h irradiated sample relative to the 1-h irradiated PNF, but still showed a substantial decrease relative to the unirradiated PNF. The reason for the variance in the thrombogenic response between the 1- and 24-h irradiated samples may be attributed to the increased amount of associated bound water in the 24-h irradiated sample. In studies on hydrophilic and hydrophilic/hydrophobic polymers (19–21) the degree and type of associated water influenced hemocompatibility and platelet consumption. In this study, we are possibly observing the initial thrombogenic effects attributed to the presence of bound water (19–21), in conjunction with the variation in surface molecular mobility. The presence and increase in the bound water content as a function of irradiation time tend to infer that the PNF is undergoing chain scission as a function of irradiation, exposing carbonyl groups, and thus changing the surface chemistry of the surfaces being exposed in the extracorporeal studies. However, this result does not appear to be the case, because the infrared results do not show a carbonyl band nor do the mass spectroscopy results indicate any low molecular weight chain scission products being formed upon irradiation. In addition, the ESCA studies suggest that the surface may be oxidized by ultraviolet irradiation for only the 24-h irradiated samples, and not for the 0- and 1-h irradiated samples. This oxidation may then explain the change in the bound water content. The steady change in the F/C ratio as a function of exposure length indicates that the side chains on the surface are affected significantly by the ultraviolet irradiation. These results, in conjunction with the swelling studies (11), do indicate that the PNF's are undergoing intramolecular/intermolecular cross-linking as a function of irradiation, in opposition to chain scission. Furthermore, in both the virgin and 1-h irradiated samples, the amount of bound water (Table II) was approximately the same, but the thrombogenic response (Figures 9–11 and Table II) was grossly different. This result implies that the observed decrease in thrombogenicity between the virgin and 1-h irradiated samples was independent of water content, but dependent on the variation in molecular mobility of the surfaces. However, in the 24-h irradiated PNF, the bound water content increased to 0.05 mg water/mg polymer, suggesting that we could be observing the initial effect of bound water on thrombogenesis, complexed with the variation in molecular mobility between the 1- and 24-h irradiated samples.

Therefore, in conclusion, these results indicate that an initial effect of molecular motions on thrombogenesis occurs independent of morphological order/disorder, crystallinity, and/or associated water (at the 0.01 mg bound water/mg polymer level). At higher levels of bound water (0.05 mg bound water/mg polymer), the effect of molecular motions on thrombogenesis is complexed by the presence of the bound water, as evidenced by the increased thrombogenic response.

Acknowledgments

This work was supported by a grant from National Institutes of Health/National Heart, Lung, and Blood Institute, 1 RO1 HL 23288. In addition, the authors thank Richard Sicka and Firestone Research for their cooperation.

Literature Cited

1. Vroman, L.; Leonard, E. *Ann. N. Y. Acad. Sci.* **1977**, *283*.
2. Merrill, E. W. *Ann. N. Y. Acad. Sci.* **1977**, *283*, p. 6–16.
3. Barenberg, S. A.; Schultz, J. S.; Anderson, J. M.; Geil, P. H. *Trans. Am. Soc. Artif. Intern. Organs* **1979**, *25*, 159–162.
4. Salzman, E. W. Blood–Material Interaction Lecture, Devices and Technology Branch; presented at Annual Contractor's Meeting, Washington, D. C., December 1977.
5. Allcock, H. R. "Phosphorus Nitrogen Compounds;" Academic: New York, 1972.
6. Singler, R. E.; Schneider, N. S.; Hagnauer, G. L. *Polym. Eng. Sci.*, **1975**, *15*, 321–338.
7. Schultz, J. S.; Goddard, J.; Ciarkowski, A. A.; Penner, J. A.; Lindenauer, S. M. *Ann. N. Y. Acad. Sci.* **1977**, *283*, 494–523.

8. Allcock, H. R. "Phosphorus Nitrogen Compounds"; Academic: New York, 1972, 359.
9. Baier, R., personal communication,
10. Reichert, W. M.; Stuk, G. J.; Filisko, F. E.; Sicka, R.; Barenberg, S. A., unpublished data.
11. Reichert, W. M., Ph. D. Dissertation, Univ. of Michigan, Ann Arbor, Michigan, in preparation.
12. Garcia, C.; Anderson, J. M.; Barenberg, S. A. *Trans. Am. Soc. Artif. Intern. Organs*, **1980**, *26*, 294–298.
13. Ratner, B., personal communication,
14. Reichert, W. M., unpublished data.
15. Connely, T. M.; Gillham, J. K. *J. Appl. Polym. Sci.* **1976**, *20*, 473–488.
16. Reichert, W. M.; Filisko, F. E.; Barenberg, S. A. *Bull. Am. Phys. Soc.* **1980**, *25*, 400.
17. O'Brien, J. P.; Ferrar, W. T.; Allcock, H. R. *Macromol.* **1979**, *12* (1), 108–113.
18. Pineri, M.; Berticat, P.; Marchal, E. *J. Polym. Sci.* **1976**, *14*, 1325–1336.
19. Bruck, S. D. *Biomed. Mater. Res.* **1973**, *7*, 387–404.
20. Andrade, J. D.; Lee, H. B.; Jhon, M. S.; Kim, S. W.; Hibbs, J. B. *Trans. Am. Soc. Artif. Intern. Organs* **1973**, *19*, 1–7.
21. Ratner, B. D.; Hoffman, A. S.; Hanson, S. R.; Harker, L. A.; Whiffen, J. D. *J. Polym. Sci.* **1979**, *66*, 363–375.

RECEIVED for review January 16, 1981. ACCEPTED July 20, 1981.

14

Thrombogenesis: An Ionic Steric Phenomenon

S. A. BARENBERG[1]

University of Michigan, Department of Chemical Engineering, Ann Arbor, MI 48109

K. A. MAURITZ

52 Centenial Way, Geneva, OH 44041

A semiempirical/theoretical ionic model was derived to correlate and interrelate the ultrastructure morphology, surface charge, surface chemistry, and surface molecular motions of a model semicrystalline hydrophobic triblock copolymer to thrombogenesis. This chapter addresses the aspects of ultrastructure order vs. disorder, primary and secondary molecular motions, surface and side chain chemistry, thrombogenesis, and the resultant ionic model. This model can be extrapolated to predict the relative thrombogenic responses of various crystalline and semicrystalline hydrophobic polymeric substrates.

In defining and correlating the surface properties of crystalline and semicrystalline polymeric materials to thrombogenesis, the surface free energy, surface charge, ultrastructure morphology, surface chemistry, surface molecular motions, surface topography, critical surface tension, electrical conductivity, and water content have evolved as important factors (1, 2). Apparently, a complex interrelationship exists between the surface properties of a material and thrombogenesis. This chapter presents a semiempirical/theoretical epitaxial model that correlates and interrelates the ultrastructure morphology, surface molecular motions, and ionic and steric order of a model triblock copolymer to thrombogenesis.

We worked with the precept that morphologically ordered polymeric systems, of given side chain chemistry, can sequester ions, which can subsequently serve as an ionic array/template for ordered protein adsorption, for example, epitaxial crystallization. Additionally, we addressed the effect of side chain motion of the substrate on the epitactic process based, in part, on

[1] Present address: E. I. duPont de Nemours and Co., Inc., Experimental Station, Wilmington, DE 19898

our previous work (3, 4). A comprehensive review of polymer epitactic processes is given by Mauritz (5).

The polymeric system used in this study was a semicrystalline hydrophobic triblock copolymer synthesized and characterized in our laboratories (6). The salient aspects of this triblock copolymer are (1) the ultrastructure morphology of the copolymer (long-range order vs. no order) can be controlled through solution casting from selected solvents; (2) the onset of secondary side chain motion occurs between 12°–25°C; (3) the side chain motion can be restricted by casting the copolymers from a nonpreferential solvent; (4) the pendant side chain groups are projecting normal to the helical backbone, and (5) the copolymer can be extracorporeally evaluated with strict control of morphology and molecular motion.

Experimental

The polymer used in this study was a triblock copolymer $A_xB_yA_x$ of poly[(γ-benzyl-L-glutamate) (acrylonitrile/butadiene) (γ-benzyl-L-glutamate)], poly[(BLG)(ATBN)(BLG)] (6).

Solutions (0.1% and 1.0% w/v) of the copolymer were prepared from dioxane and chloroform, which were preferential and nonpreferential solvent systems, respectively.

The dynamic mechanical measurements were done using an inverted torsion (braid) pendulum (7).

Morphological and electron diffraction studies (not presented) were done on thin films of the copolymer as cast onto carbon-coated glass slides. The thin films were vapor-stained with osmium tetroxide.

Thin films of the copolymer were cast from dioxane and chloroform onto carbon-coated slides. The films were then placed in contact with isotonic saline for 4 h, and were washed in deionized distilled water. A carbon film was subjected to this same saline treatment to serve as the experimental control.

Conventional and scanning transmission electron microscopy (CTEM and STEM) were done on a JEOL 100C electron microscope. The scanning (secondary emission) electron microscopy was done on a JEOL U3.

The x-ray dispersion analysis was done on a JEOL 100C (in the STEM mode) using a Princeton Gamma Tech detector. The count times were on the order of 20 min at 30,000, 50,000, and 100,000 magnification.

The animals used in the extracorporeal studies (8) were conditioned male dogs. Access to the animals' circulatory system was via chronic shunts surgically implanted into the neck. The shunt was anastomosed to the carotid artery and jugular vein. Blood flow through the shunt was 1 L/min.

Twenty-four hours prior to the experiment, the platelets were labeled with ^{51}Cr and human ^{125}I-labeled fibrinogen, and were injected into the dog. No anticoagulants were used prior to and/or during the experiment. The morphological studies were done on unlabeled dogs.

Experiments were carried out for periods of 5, 10, and 60 min at a shear rate of 150 s^{-1}.

At the completion of the test the exposed shafts (not used in the radiolabeled studies) were placed in buffered glutaraldehyde. The shafts were post-fixed and critical-point dried (9). The critical-point–dried coatings were removed, embedded in

Spurr (via propylene oxide) and ultramicrotomed. The unstained (osmocated) thin sections were carbon-coated and examined by CTEM and STEM.

Results

The copolymer morphology (Figure 1), as cast from dioxane, exhibited a lamellar morphology, with the acrylonitrile/butadiene (ATBN) layers on the order of magnitude of 15 nm thick; the alternating benzyl-L-glutamate (BLG) layers were on the order of 50 nm thick. The copolymer morphology (Figure 2), as cast from chloroform, exhibited a homogeneous morphology with the ATBN midblock domains on the order of magnitude of 15 nm.

When the above copolymer cast films were exposed to isotonic saline and/or deionized distilled water, the above observed morphologies remained intact (Figure 3). When the copolymers were cast directly onto isotonic saline and/or deionized distilled water (Figure 4), the resultant morphologies were modified in that the dioxane-cast copolymer exhibited a phase-separated morphology complexed with the "salt," whereas the chloroform-cast exhibited a homogeneous "salt"-complexed morphology.

The x-ray dispersion analysis of the copolymers exposed to the saline solutions indicated (Figures 5 and 6) that the copolymers sequestered the sodium and chlorine ions. However, due to the low concentrations, given the limits of instrumental resolution, the location of the ions could not be mapped.

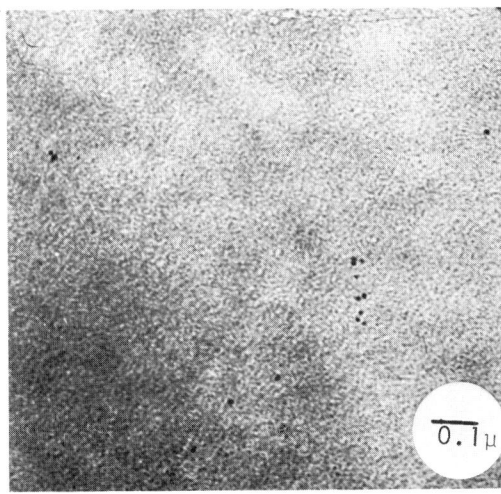

Figure 1. TEM of the phase-mixed, (chloroform-cast) osmium vapor–stained triblock copolymer. The stained (dark) regions are the ATBN midblock segments of the block copolymer and the unstained regions are the BLG portions of the block copolymer.

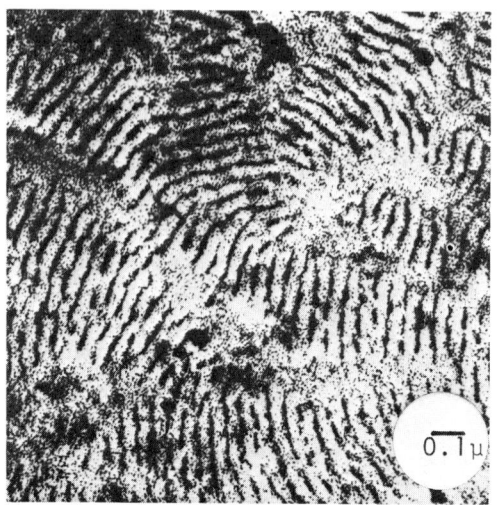

Figure 2. TEM of the phase-separated, (dioxane-cast) osmium vapor–stained triblock copolymer. The stained (dark) regions are the ATBN midblock segments and the unstained regions are the BLG segments of the block copolymer.

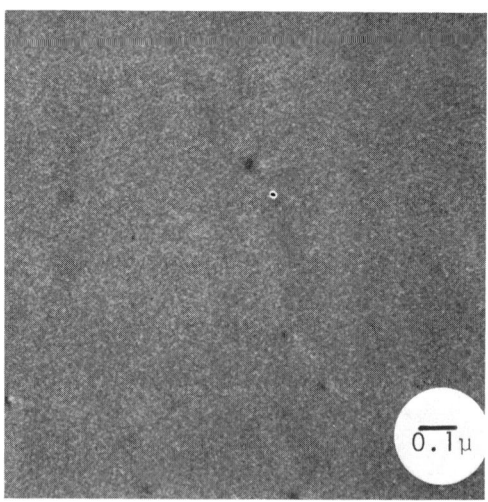

Figure 3. TEM of the phase-mixed (chloroform-cast) copolymer exposed to isotonic saline, washed and vapor-stained with osmium tetroxide.

Figure 4. TEM of the phase-mixed copolymer cast from chloroform directly onto isotonic saline and vapor-stained with osmium tetroxide.

The dielectric (6) and dynamic mechanical measurements (Figure 7) of the copolymer as cast from dioxane and chloroform revealed a dispersion maximum at 298 K and a split dispersion at 298 and 315 K, respectively. The 298 K dispersion maximum has been ascribed (10) to the onset of motion of the BLG side chains; the onset of molecular motion of the BLG backbone occurs at 408 K (11). Therefore, the only molecular motions occurring in the copolymers over the physiological temperature range affecting hemocompatibility are those that can be ascribed to the onset of side chain motion of BLG. The single dispersion maximum for the dioxane-cast copolymer infers unrestricted side chain motion (dynamic), whereas the split maxima (chloroform-cast) infers restricted side chain motion (static). This change, then, infers that at physiological temperatures, in conjunction with the morphological results, the motion of the side chains in the dioxane-cast phase-separated copolymer is unrestricted and occurs in an ordered steric array, whereas in the chloroform-cast copolymer the side chain motion is restricted in a disordered steric array. This type of side chain motion has been postulated previously by Merrill (12) and demonstrated by Barenberg (3) to influence the initial sorption of the plasma protein(s) and subsequent interaction with blood. These interaction effects in conjunction with the extracorporeal experiments and ion sequestering results are discussed in terms of the derived ionic model.

When the copolymers were exposed to canine blood (figures are not presented, *see* Ref. 4) for 5 min, the disordered copolymer surface

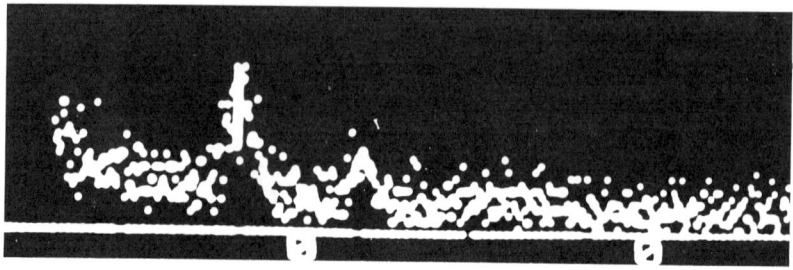

Figure 5. X-ray dispersion spectra of the phase-mixed (chloroform-cast) copolymer (Figure 3) exposed to isotonic saline and washed. The peaks correspond to sodium, osmium, and chlorine.

(chloroform-cast) consisted of platelets with no other type of observable deposition occurring. However, when the phase-separated copolymer (dioxane-cast) was exposed under the same conditions, a proteinaceous deposition was observed in addition to aggregates of adhering platelets. After 10 min exposure to canine blood, the platelets appeared to spread and flatten on the disordered copolymer surface forming a confluent type of sublayer. Whether these are in fact platelets has yet to be shown. In contrast, the phase-separated copolymer surface exhibited a large thrombus primarily composed of platelets, fibrin, and red blood cells. When the copolymers were exposed to canine blood for 60 min, the disordered surface developed a limited pseudoneointima, whereas the phase-separated copolymer surface developed a large thrombus, with no signs of becoming limited. These series of experiments were replicated using different dogs and substrate shafts (9), that is, stainless steel and polypropylene, with consistent reproducibility.

The above exposed copolymers were ultramicrotomed in cross section. The disordered surface exhibited a loosely bound 50-nm osmophilic layer,

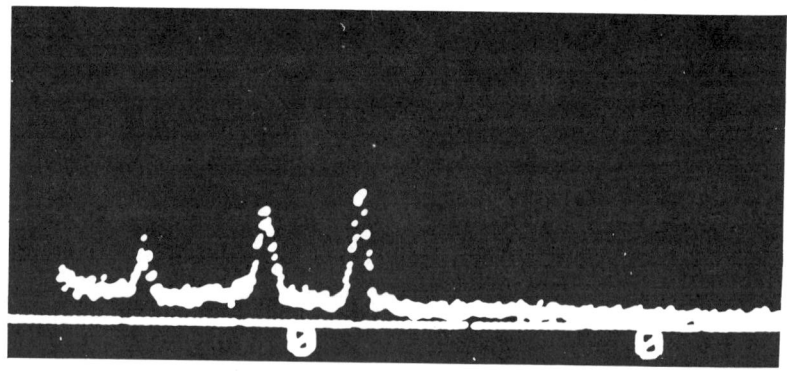

Figure 6. X-ray dispersion spectra of the phase-mixed copolymer (Figure 4) cast directly onto isotonic saline, washed, and vapor-stained. The peaks correspond to sodium, osmium, and chlorine.

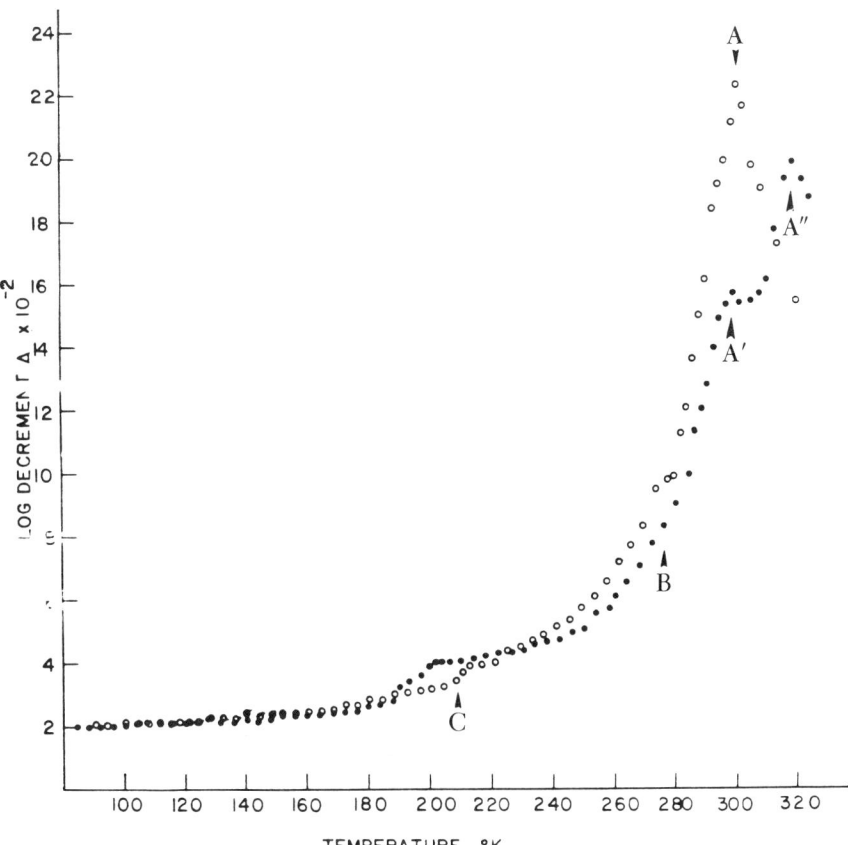

Figure 7. Dynamic mechanical spectra of the copolymer cast from dioxane (○) and chloroform (●) onto glass braids. Arrows A, A', and A" indicate the onset of side chain motion (10); B, interfacial relaxation (3); and C, the glass transition of the ATBN segment (3). The chloroform-cast copolymer is dispersion-split (A and A") relative to the single maxima for the dioxane-cast system, indicating restricted and unrestricted side chain motion, respectively.

whereas the phase-separated copolymer exhibited a tightly bound 10-nm osmophilic layer (Figures 8 and 9).

Discussion

These results indicate that an epitaxial model can be derived to correlate the above data. The model takes into account the differences between the two types of secondary molecular motions observed, the ultrastructural differences between the ordered (phase-separated) and disordered (phase-mixed) morphologies of the copolymers, the electronegativity of the side

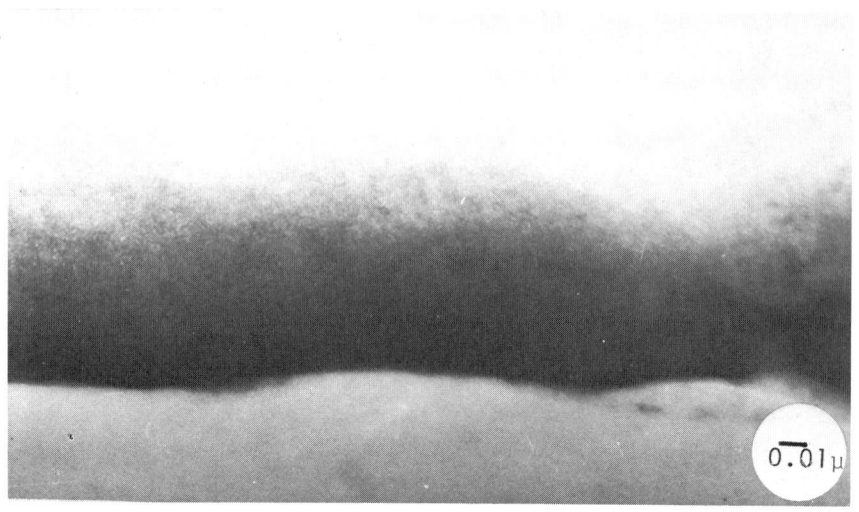

Figure 8. TEM of the phase-mixed (chloroform-cast) copolymer, in cross section, exposed to canine blood. Note the loosely bound osmophilic layer on the surface (250,000 ×).

Figure 9. TEM of the phase-separated (dioxane-cast) copolymer, in cross section, exposed to canine blood. Note the tightly bound osmophilic layer (345,000 ×).

chain carbonyl oxygens, the ionic clustering effects due to the above electronegativity, and the surface chemistry of the copolymers. The model does not take into account any effects due to streaming potential and/or local surface pH differences (13, 14), two very important areas that need to be addressed.

The model is divided into four parts: (1) the definition of the surface to be interfaced with blood, (2) the mode of the plasma protein(s) and/or electrolyte adsorption, (3) relaxation motion of the blood interfacing side chain groups, and (4) protein denaturation and/or liquid crystalline order.

The first aspect of the model is to define the surface that is to be interfaced with blood, that is, ordered vs. disordered. In the model system used in this study, the phase-separated (dioxane-cast) copolymer would be defined as a sterically ordered array, and the phase-mixed (chloroform-cast) copolymer as a sterically disordered array. The second aspect of the model incorporates the two types of adsorption occurring concurrently at the surface: (1) that of the plasma protein(s) and (2) that of either ions and/or polyelectrolytes. The sorption of the protein(s) occurs, in part, by a two-step process. The proteins would initially hydrophobically bond to the exposed phenyl groups in a metastable state, and subsequently surface-diffuse from this metastable state to a lower free-energy state located in the potential trough between the benzyl ester side chains (in the case for our model copolymers). These proteins would then align in an ordered fashion, in the case of the phase-separated copolymer, with the hydrophilic portion of the sorbed protein being exposed to the blood interface. In the case of a disordered surface, that is, the chloroform-cast copolymer, the sorbed protein would not sorb in an ordered fashion nor form an ordered type of surface. The third aspect of the model takes into account the relaxational motion of the side chains and the specific side chain chemistry. In our case, the BLG side chains contained an electronegative carbonyl oxygen and were in either a dynamic or static state, depending on the solvent system from which the copolymer was cast, dioxane or chloroform, respectively. The side chain mobility of the surface interface may facilitate ionic diffusion between the side chains, and the electronegativity of the carbonyl oxygens would, therefore, immobolize these cations. Additionally, since the side chains are in an ordered packing mode (15), the existence of a relatively ordered subsurface cationic array might be hypothesized (assuming that the cations are reasonably immobilized).

At this step, then, the differences between the effects of surface chemistry and secondary molecular motions as dictated by morphological order can be observed on thrombogenesis. In the case of the sterically ordered substrate, in conjunction with the subsurface cationic array, the sorbed protein(s) can assume a paracrystalline state, and subsequently be subjected to further pertubations. However, in the case of the disordered substrate, the sorbed proteins can not assume a paracrystalline state and, therefore, will not, per se, be subjected to any further conformational changes.

In the final state of the model two events may occur: (1) the adsorbed protein(s) may undergo denaturation as a result of the subsurface hydrophilic cationic array, causing the hydrophilic portion of the protein to partially bury itself in between the side chains, thus exposing the hydrophobic portion of the protein chain to the blood interface, and (2) the adsorbed protein(s) may be aligned on the substrate in an ordered paracrystalline and/or liquid crystalline fashion, which could serve as an ordered template to the other plasma proteins. This then would result in a developing ionomeric clot. Preliminary evidence (16) indicates that the latter does occur. In the final case of the nonthrombogenic model, neither a steric nor a subsurface cationic array exists; therefore, the adsorbed protein(s) will remain in their native conformation, presumably with the hydrophilic portions extending into the biological interface.

This model is depicted in Figure 10 for the model copolymer used in this study.

Additional evidence for this model recently has been reported by Filisko (17). In his studies on the heats of adsorption of proteins, Filisko observed an exothermic heat, indicative of surface ordering, rather than an endotherm

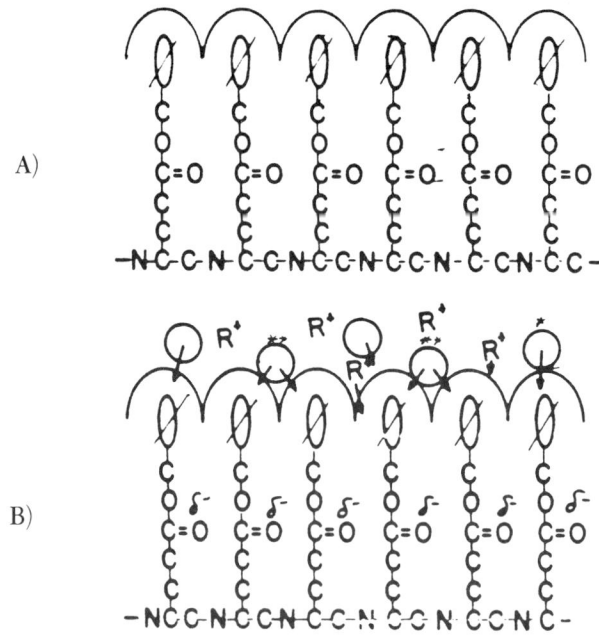

Figure 10. (A) Schematic of the BLG portion, in cross section, of the copolymer to be interfaced with blood and (B) initial mode of sorption upon contact with blood. Key: R^+, cations and/or electrolytes; ○, sorbing proteinaceous elements; *, metastable state of the initial sorption; and **, stable state. Continued on next page.

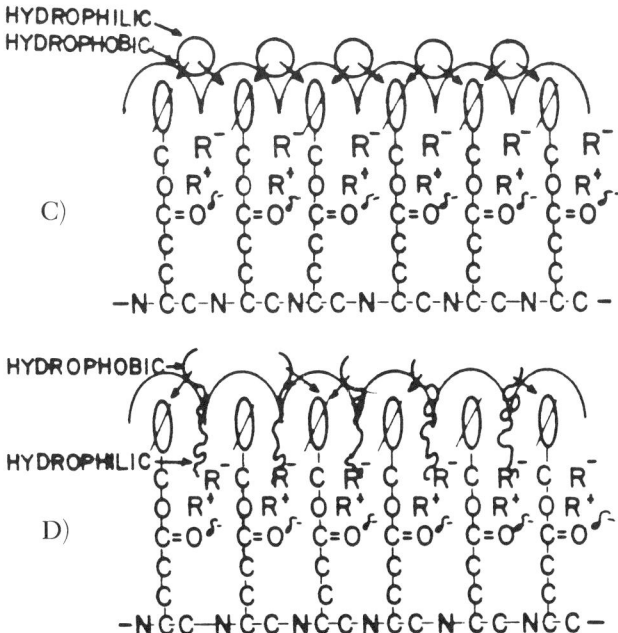

Figure 10. (C) Schematic of the hydrophobic bonding of the adsorbed protein(s) and the mode of ionic clustering. This ionic clustering the ionic subsurface template for surface ordering. Key: R, ions and/or electrolytes and ○, adsorbed protein(s). (D) Denaturation of the adsorbed layer. Continued on next page.

in the hydrated state. Additionally, Nyilas (18) reported similar calorimetric results in his hydrated adsorption studies. When Filisko and Nyilas did their studies in the dehydrated state, they both observed endotherms. Presumably, a priori, the differences between the exothermic and endothermic results can be attributed, in part, to the presence of the buffer that may have been substrate-sequestered and may have served as an ionic template.

The synopsis of the model is presented in Figure 11. In essence, the predicative flow chart works by defining (1) the polymer backbone and side chain chemistry and conformation in the hydrated and dehydrated solid state, (2) the surface crystallinity of the polymer, (3) the primary (segmental backbone) and secondary (side chain) molecular motions of the polymer relative to physiological temperatures, (4) the surface ultrastructure morphology, and (5) the ionic/steric order and/or disorder of the surface and its ability to develop an ordered and/or disordered array that may serve (or not) as a template for ordered protein adsorption. If the surface appears as an ordered ionic steric array, the model predicts that a thrombogenic response will result. However, if the surface appears as a disordered array, the model predicts that only a limited thrombogenic response will occur, given limited

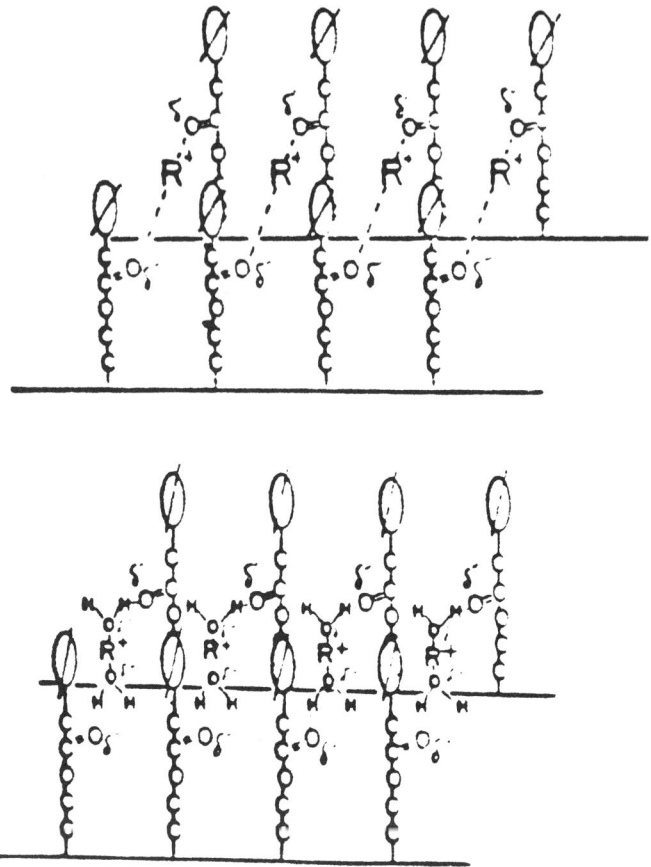

Figure 10. (E) Schematic of the immobilized cations forming the subsurface cationic array either ionically bonded directly to the carbonyl oxygens of the BLG side chains or through H-bonding of the bound water.

side chain mobility. The applicability of this model to other polymeric systems can be observed in the works of Picha (19), Helmus (20), and Lyman (21).

Therefore, in summary, the interaction between the immediate substrate surface and hydrophobic groupings appears to contribute to the overall adsorption process. However, the dynamic state of the side chains would

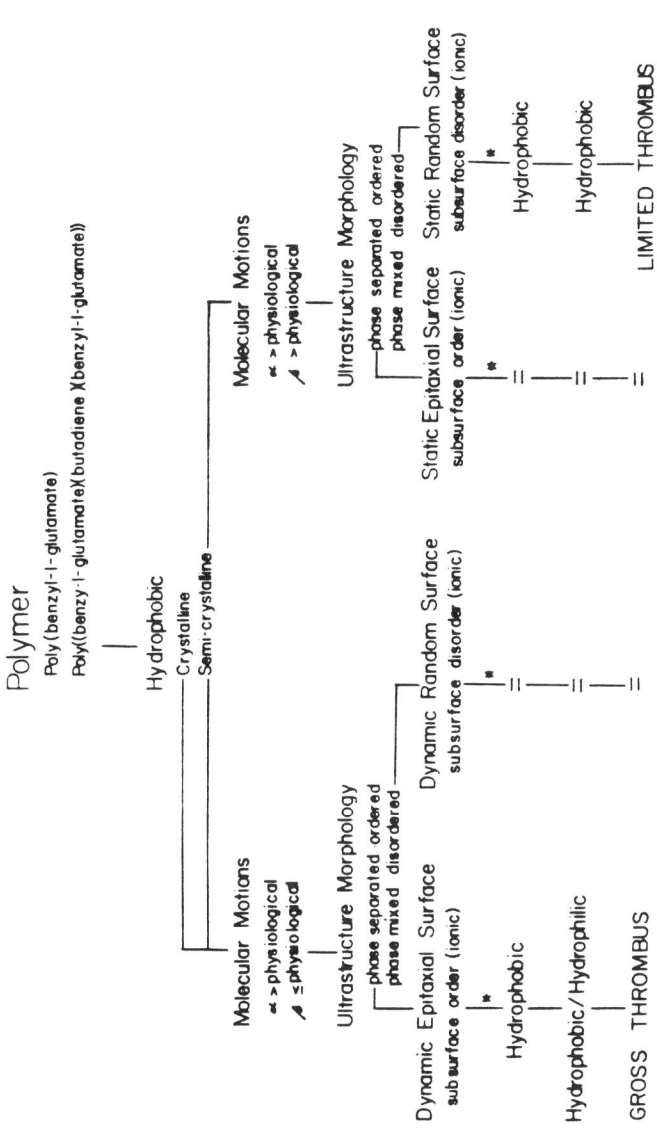

Figure 11. Synoptic flow chart of the proposed model indicating the complexity and interactive factors needed to consider in defining the surface to be interfaced with blood, followed by the proposed (Figure 10) mode of protein adsorption, and ultimately, the thrombogenic response. See text for a stepwise description of the model and flow chart.

present a dynamic "liquid" steric template rather than the conventional "solid" steric template, with an ill-defined periodic potential energy profile, in the near interfacial region. Whether this dynamic template would induce an orientational influence on incoming sections of proteins has yet to be proven. Therefore, given the assumptions of surface order and ionic distribution, an epitaxial adsorption orientation mechanism may be credible as the initial nucleation event in thrombogenesis on biomaterials having microstructural crystallinity.

Acknowledgment

This work was supported by a grant from NIH/NHLBI R01 HL 23288.

Literature Cited

1. Vroman, L.; Leonard, E., Eds. *Ann. N. Y. Acad. Sci.* **1977**, *283*.
2. "Guidelines for Physiochemical Characterization of Biomaterials," N.I.H.; 1980, No. 80–2186.
3. Barenberg, S. A.; Schultz, J. S.; Anderson, J. M.; Geil, P. H. *Trans. Am. Soc. Artif. Intern. Organs*, **1979**, *25*, 159–162.
4. Barenberg, S. A.; Anderson, J. M.; Mauritz, K. A. *J. Biomed. Mater. Res.* **1981**, *15*, 231–245.
5. Mauritz, K. A.; Baer, E.; Hopfinger, A. J. *J. Polym. Sci., Macromol. Rev.* **1978**, *13*, 1–61.
6. Barenberg, S. A.; Anderson, J. M.; Geil, P. H. *Int. J. Biol. Macromol.* **1981**, *3*, 82–90.
7. Armeniades, C. D.; Kuriyama, I.; Roe, J. M.; Baer, E. "Mechanical Behavior of Poly(ethyleneterephthalate) at Cryogenic Temperatures"; Serafini, T. T.; Koenig, J. L., Eds.; Dekker: New York, 1968; pp. 155–170.
8. Schultz, J. S.; Goddard, J.; Ciarkowski, A. A.; Penner, J. A.; Lindenauer, S. M. *Ann. N. Y. Acad. Sci.* **1977**, *283*, 494–523.
9. Schultz, J. S.; Lindenauer, S. M.; Penner, J. A.; Barenberg, S. A. "Evaluation of the Compatibility of Materials in Contact with Blood"; N.I.H./N.H.L.B.I., Annual Report 1981, No. N01-HV-4-2962-5.
10. Fukuzawa, T.; Uematsu, I. *Polym. J.* **1974**, *6*, 431–437.
11. McKinnon, A.; Tobolosky, A. *J. Phys. Chem.* **1968**, *72*, 1157–1161.
12. Merrill, E. W. *Ann. N. Y. Acad. Sci.* **1977**, *283*, 6–16.
13. Helmus, M. N., Ph.D. Dissertation, Case Western Reserve Univ., Cleveland, 1980.
14. Helmus, M. H.; Malhotra, O. D.; Gibbons, D. F., unpublished data.
15. Parry, D.; Elliott, A. *J. Mol. Biol.* **1967**, *25*, 1–13.
16. Barenberg, S. A., unpublished data.
17. Filisko, F. E.; Malladi, D.; Barenberg, S. A., unpublished data.
18. Nyilas, E.; Chiu, T.-H.; Turcotte, L. R. "Study of the Interaction of Plasma Proteins with Prosthetic Surfaces"; N.I.H./N.T.I.S., Annual Report 1977, N01-HV-3-2917-4, PB 284 092/AS.
19. Picha, G. J.; and Gibbons, D. F. *J. Bioeng.* **1978**, *2*, 301–311.
20. Helmus, M. N., M.S. Thesis, Case Western Reserve Univ., Cleveland, 1978.
21. Lyman, D. J.; Knutson, K.; McNeil, B.; Shibatani, K. *Trans. Am. Soc. Artif. Intern. Organs* **1975**, *21*, 49–54.

RECEIVED for review January 16, 1981. ACCEPTED July 27, 1981.

15

Alteration of Polymorphonuclear Neutrophil Leukocyte Response to Shear Stress Exposure In Vitro: Effects of Prostaglandin E_1 and Dipyridamole Derivative RA-233

DOUGLAS J. STOCKWELL and LARRY V. McINTIRE[1]

Rice University, Biomedical Engineering Laboratory, Department of Chemical Engineering, Houston, TX 77001

R. RUSSELL MARTIN

Baylor College of Medicine, Department of Internal Medicine, Houston, TX 77030

The effects of in vitro fluid mechanical trauma on buffered suspensions of polymorphonuclear neutrophil leukocytes (PMNs) were studied with and without preincubation with the platelet antiaggregating agents RA-233 (at 1×10^{-6}M) and prostaglandin E_1 (at 3×10^{-6}M). Total PMN counts were reduced by exposure to shear stress of 100 and 300 dyn/cm^2 for 10 min. The antiplatelet drugs diminished this reduction at the higher shear stress. Enzyme release, cell adhesion, and aggregation produced by mechanical trauma were all decreased by preincubation with the drugs, but the diminished generation of chemiluminescence following phagocytosis of opsonized zymosan by stressed PMNs was not affected. These results suggest a preservational effect of these "antiplatelet" agents on PMNs exposed to fluid mechanical trauma.

Increased margination of leukocytes in the circulation of the lung through adhesion to the pulmonary endothelium and formation of platelet microaggregates have been postulated as important components in the etiology of

[1]Author to whom correspondence should be addressed.

pulmonary and cardiovascular complications accompanying surgical procedures requiring extended extracorporeal circulation. In previous reports of the effects of fluid mechanical trauma, low to moderate levels of shear stress (100 to 300 dyn/cm^2) produced altered polymorphonuclear neutrophil leukocyte (PMN) morphology and function. Shear-related changes included increased adhesion, aggregation and cell lysis, moderate decreases in chemiluminescence accompanying phagocytosis, and substantial loss of lysosomal enzymes (1–4). These alterations, if they occur with mechanical trauma accompanying extended extracorporeal circulation, may contribute to the pathogenesis of post-perfusion reactions in the lungs.

Antiplatelet therapy, including dipyridamole (Persantin) and its derivatives and prostaglandins, has been effective in reducing microaggregate formation during hemoperfusion (5–7). This result prompted us to investigate the action of antiplatelet drugs on the leukocyte responses to in vitro shear stress. This chapter demonstrates that a derivative of dipyridamole, RA-233, and prostaglandin E_1 (PGE_1) have the capacity to preserve PMN integrity following exposure to low levels of shear stress in vitro. The use of these two drugs simultaneously is suggested by their complementary actions in raising intracellular cyclic adenosine monophosphate.

Experimental

Heparinized (10 units/mL) blood was obtained from normal volunteers after written consent was given according to the declaration of Helsinki. A portion of blood was retained to determine white blood cell counts (Coulter, Model ZBI), hematocrit values, and leukocyte alkaline phosphatase (LAP) levels. Leukocytes were separated from the blood by sedimentation in heparinized dextran, as described previously (8). Leukocyte-rich supernatant was collected and washed twice in sterile distilled water for 30 s, then restored to the isotonic state with an equal volume of 0.30M saline. The cell suspension was then layered on 5-mL volumes of Ficoll–Hypaque white cell separation fluid (Ficoll; Sodium Hypaque, Winthrop) in 15-mL conical-tip centrifuge tubes centrifuged at 400 × g for 20 min. The white blood cell pellets obtained in this manner were more than 95% granulocytes and were consistently more than 90% viable when tested by trypan blue exclusion. These leukocytes were suspended in phosphate-buffered saline containing 150 mg/100 mL glucose (PBS/G) at concentrations of 2 × 10^6 PMN/mL. PMN suspensions were used without further delay in incubations with drugs and in shearing experiments, as determined by the individual studies performed.

Incubation and Drugs. The RA-233 employed in this study was obtained from Wilbur Benson, Boehringer–Ingelheim, of Stamford, Connecticut. PGE_1 was provided by Joel Moake of the University of Texas School of Medicine at Houston. Cell suspensions were maintained at room temperature until addition of antiplatelet agents, at which time both drug-exposed suspensions and control suspensions were incubated at 37°C. Test samples contained 1 × 10^{-6}M RA-233 and 3 × 10^{-6}M PGE_1, while control samples received equal volumes of sterile saline. Both control and test suspensions were incubated for 10 min in a water bath at 37°C, then were sheared for 10 min in the Rice University ROM-8 viscometer which was maintained at 37 ± 1°C with warmed forced air.

Application of Shear Stress. The Rice University ROM-8 viscometer has been described previously (9). This apparatus permits volumes of 8 mL of fluid to undergo uniform shear stress exposure at readily quantifiable levels. For the present experiments, all surfaces coming into contact with leukocyte suspensions were coated with silicone (Siliclad), which had been demonstrated earlier to minimize or eliminate surface-mediated effects on PMNs (2). The surface-to-volume ratio in the viscometer could be varied by a factor of three using different bobs. Effectively, the fluid volume was varied at nearly constant surface area. Increasing the surface-to-volume ratio increased the accessibility of the surface to cellular elements in the sheared fluid. Shear stress levels were 100 and 300 dyn/cm^2 for the 10-min exposure, which had been documented previously to produce functional alterations in PMNs. Control samples were placed into the viscometer for 10 min, but were not subjected to rotational shear stress. After exposure to the viscometer, cell suspensions were assayed without further delay as described in the next section.

PMN Assays. Leukocytes in suspension were quantitated by electronic particle counting to determine the changes induced by mechanical trauma. Values obtained after incubation with drugs or with saline were the baseline values to which post shear values were related.

The assay for chemiluminescence has been described previously (4). Briefly, this procedure consists of measuring the light emitted following phagocytosis of opsonized zymosan particles, employing a model LS-100C Beckman liquid scintillation counter. Peak values for chemiluminescence were proportional to the total accumulated light emission over the 30-min test period, so tests were reported as peak chemiluminescence responses.

Measurement of β-glucuronidase released in the surrounding medium was performed using a modified Sigma assay as described previously (2). Alkaline phosphatase released from PMNs was assayed using the technique of DeChatelet and Cooper (10), employing a modification of Sigma assay Number 104 (Sigma Co.). A semiquantitative assessment of LAP activity was performed using a cytochemical assay (Sigma Co.). Azo dye staining of alkaline phosphatase–containing granules permitted grading of enzyme reactions from 0 to 4+. Values were reported as the total score for 100 cells evaluated microscopically.

Measurement of PMN adhesion was performed using serum-coated glass slides at 37°C. Two, four-chambered Lab-Tek slides were filled with 200 μL of autologous serum per chamber, and were placed in a 37°C incubator for 15 min to warm the slide and to preincubate the glass surface with the serum. A volume of 40 μL of PMN leukocyte suspension was added to each test chamber, and the suspension was distributed evenly by gentle rocking and swirling for 30 s. Slides were replaced in the incubator on a flat surface for 25 min. The slides were then removed, and each chamber was centered on the stage of an inverted light microscope, where five medium-powered (400×) microscopic fields were counted for PMN leukocytes in contact with the glass. The serum was poured off gently, and the chambers were washed by slowly refilling and pouring off PBS/G heated to 37°C. Chambers were refilled with 200 μL of PBS/G and recounted for the adherent cells. The percentage of adherent cells was calculated by dividing the counts after washing with the counts before washing × 100. Tests of PMN adherence were always performed in duplicate.

Results

The total number of leukocytes was counted on all samples after each step in the incubation and shearing protocol. The electronic particle counts are presented as percentages of the counts in the initial suspension, prior to the 10-min incubations at 37°C (Figure 1). In the control specimens which were not exposed to the drug and which were placed in the viscometer chamber but not sheared, the initial 10-min incubation at 37°C produced a drop to 92 ± 5% (mean ± SEM) in the electronic particle count with a further decrease to 89 ± 6% after 20 min at 37°C. In contrast to this gradual progressive aggregation, suspensions receiving the two antiplatelet agents demonstrated a marked transient aggregation, with the electronic particle count dropping to 82 ± 7% of the control after 10 min, and subsequently rising to 92 ± 8% after 20 min. The basis of the transient aggregation and disaggregation observed with PMNs incubated with drugs is not well understood.

Shearing control PMN suspensions (not exposed to drugs) for 10 min at 100 and 300 dyn/cm^2 produced a 25.5 ± 7% and 53.2 ± 3.5% drop, re-

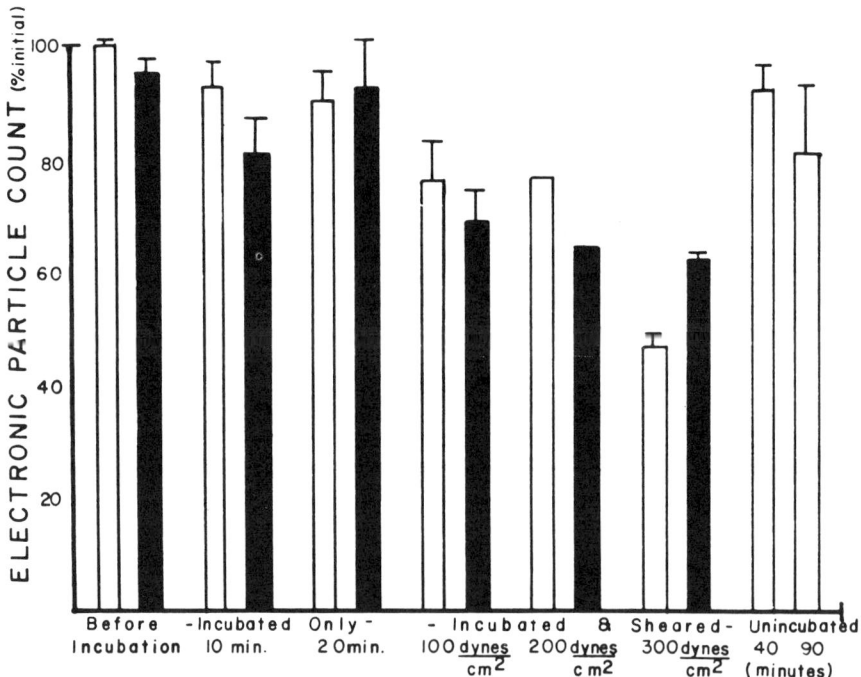

Figure 1. Bar graphs showing changes in electronic particle count in PMN suspensions with and without drugs (1×10^{-6}M RA-233 and 3×10^{-6}M PGE_1). All incubations and shearing were done at 37°C. The unincubated samples were maintained at room temperature for the time specified. The 200 dyn/cm^2 columns show no error bars as they represent the results of a single day's runs. Key: □, without drug (control) and ■, with drug.

spectively, in the electronic particle count. In contrast, samples receiving the antiplatelet drugs decreased 30.8 ± 6% following shear at 100 dyn/cm^2, but did not drop significantly farther after the higher shear stress exposure (36.8 ± 2.8%). This partial preservation of leukocyte counts after shearing at 300 dyn/cm^2 corresponded to the reduced numbers of lysed and aggregated cells in microscopic slides of the drug-treated suspensions, compared to sheared samples not exposed to drugs.

Adhesion of PMNs to serum-coated glass slides following shear stress exposure is presented in Figure 2. Increased PMN adhesion was noted after shear at 100 and 300 dyn/cm^2, both for drug-treated and untreated suspensions. For platen-exposed controls, adhesion was reduced significantly (13 ± 7%) in drug-treated samples compared to unincubated suspensions (30 ± 9.5%). The drug-treated leukocytes had lower levels of adherence following exposure to shear stresses of 100 dyn/cm^2 (21 ± 9%), compared to 42 ± 11% for control samples. The slight apparent reduction in adherence after exposure to 300 dyn/cm^2 probably reflected selection of a less adherent population of cells available for the assay, through selective loss of substantial numbers of adhesive-sheared PMNs to aggregation. By combining the adhesion assay with the particle counts and microscopic assessments of aggregates in suspension, we are able to estimate that more than 60% of the PMNs

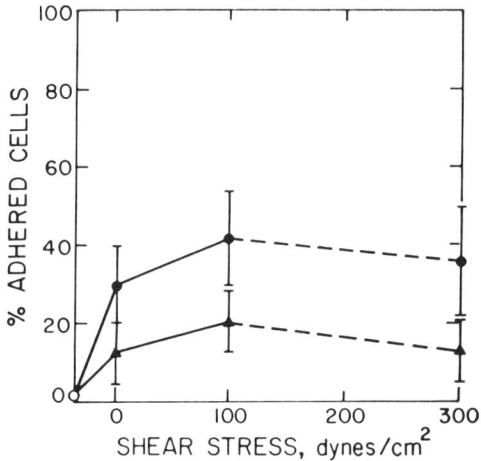

Figure 2. Adhesion to serum-coated glass slides of sheared and unsheared leukocytes was reduced significantly by 1×10^{-6}M RA-233 and 3×10^{-6}M PGE$_1$ (±SEM). Only a less adherent population of cells remained to be tested at shear stresses greater than 300 dyn/cm^2 because cell aggregates were removed during processing. Key: ●, without drug (control) and ▲, with drug.

remaining intact after 300 dyn/cm² demonstrated properties of adhesion. This observation corresponds to those made previously at similar shear stresses using a nylon fiber filtration technique for measuring adhesion (1). The filtration assay removes both cell aggregates and individual adhesive PMNs.

Phagocytosis of opsonized zymosan particles produced chemiluminescence in PMNs, which was reduced by shear stress exposures of 100 and 300 dyn/cm² (Figure 3). Peak chemiluminescence levels were reduced to $74.4 \pm 10\%$ of unsheared control values by exposure to 100 dyn/cm², and to $67 \pm 5\%$ of control values after exposure to 300 dyn/cm². Following preincubation with PGE_1 and RA-233, similar decreases in chemiluminescence with shear exposure occurred. However, although not shown in the graph, the cell suspensions receiving shear stress tended to achieve peak values of chemiluminescence somewhat more slowly than the unsheared sample.

Release of the lysosomal enzyme β-glucuronidase into media surrounding PMNs was studied with and without preincubation with drugs (Figure 4). This lysosomal enzyme is contained primarily in the azurophilic granules of PMNs, and may be a marker of the active release of these granules, and presumably of other enzymatic contents. Release may occur following lysis of cells, or as a result of sublytic trauma. A 10-min exposure to 100 dyn/cm² of shear stress produced release of $23 \pm 4\%$ of the total

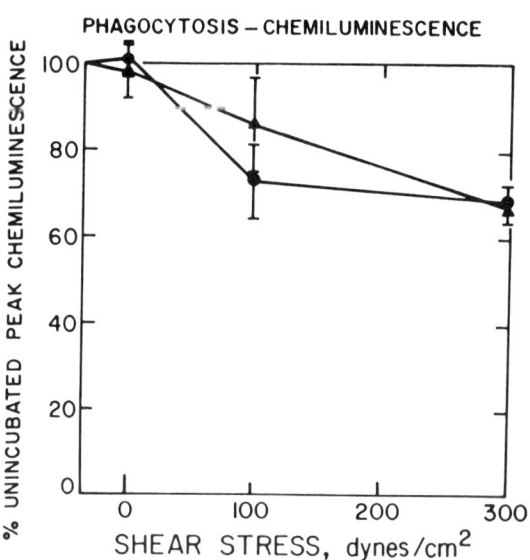

Figure 3. Leukocyte peak chemiluminescence, with $1 \times 10^{-6}M$ RA-233 and $3 \times 10^{-6}M$ PGE_1 showing only small preservational effects at 100 dyn/cm², diminishing at higher shear stresses (sheared in PBS/G at 37°C for 10 min). Key: ●, without drug (control) and ▲, with drug.

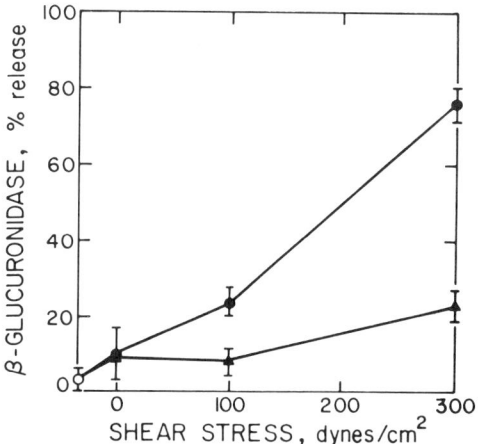

Figure 4. Leukocyte β-glucuronidase activity released into surrounding media after shearing in PBS/G at 37°C for 10 min (±SEM). Significant preservation of activity occurred with 1×10^{-6}M RA-233 and 3×10^{-6}M PGE_1 at all stress levels. Key: ●, without drug (control) and ▲, with drug.

β-glucuronidase content of PMNs, while release of 76 ± 5% of the enzyme occurred at 300 dyn/cm². Markedly lower levels of enzyme release occurred when cells were incubated and sheared in the presence of PGE_1 and RA-233. Drug-treated cells released only 8 ± 4% of total β-glucuronidase after 100 dyn/cm², and 22 ± 6% after 300 dyn/cm². Minimal release of only 9% of the enzyme occurred when incubations were performed for 20 min at 37°C without shearing, with similar degrees of release for both drug-treated and control suspensions.

The effects of mechanical shear stress on release of LAP were measured colorimetrically in supernatant fluids after shear, and cytochemically on blood films. LAP is contained principally in a different set of granules (the specific granules) than the acid hydrolases, such as β-glucuronidase. When placed in the viscometer but not sheared, both undrugged and drugged suspensions exhibited a 17% loss of LAP activity. Data at 200 dyn/cm² were limited to the results of a single experiment, which revealed slightly less release (31%) of LAP in supernatants from drug-treated cells compared to 38% LAP release in supernatants of untreated PMNs. At the higher shear stress level, 35% of the LAP was released from drug-treated samples, which was substantially less than the 66 ± 9% release occurring in supernatants of untreated PMNs (Figure 5).

The cytochemical assay for alkaline phosphatase activity is semiquantitative, and the absolute results were not expected to correspond to the direct measurement of enzyme activity in supernatants surrounding sheared

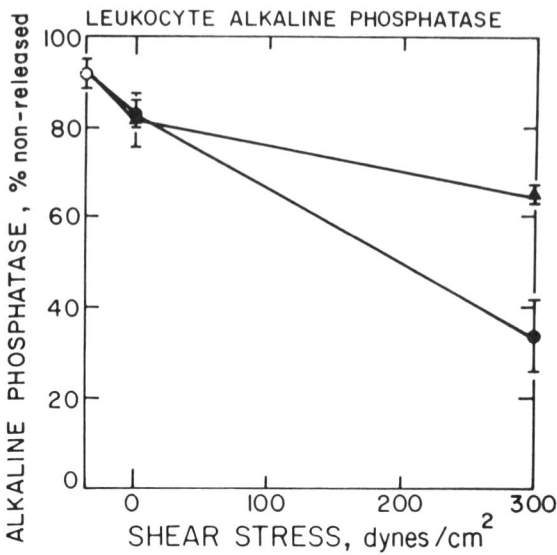

Figure 5. LAP activity released into surrounding media after shearing in PBS/G at 37°C for 10 min. Partial preservation of unreleased activity with 1×10^{-6}M RA-233 and 3×10^{-6}M PGE_1 (presented as % LAP not released to facilitate comparison with Figure 6). Key: ●, without drug (control) and ▲, with drug.

PMNs. Using this microscopic assay of enzyme activity, shear stress of 100 dyn/cm² produced a 40 ± 8% drop in LAP, with a modest increase to 50% loss within the intact cells remaining after 300 dyn/cm² of shear stress (Figure 6). In PMN leukocytes incubated with the two drugs, only a 17 ± 9% decrease occurred after 100 dyn/cm² and a 33 ± 10% decrease after 300 dyn/cm². Unsheared samples that were exposed to the viscometer surface for 10 min showed minimal changes in cytochemical values for LAP, decreases being about 5% of the total activity in PMNs that were not exposed to the viscometer surface.

Discussion

As the clinical use of blood-pumping devices has increased, and surgical procedures involving extended extracorporeal circulation have become widespread, the effects of these procedures on formed elements of the blood have become clinically important. Among the better studied trauma-induced effects on blood is that platelet microaggregates may form, sometimes in conjunction with small clumps of PMNs, followed by sequestering of these elements in the microvasculature (particularly that of the lung). The release of lysosomal enzymes and vasoactive substances from platelets and PMNs may produce increased vascular permeability to plasma components, and if these abnormalities persist unchecked, clinical degeneration and cardiopulmonary failure may occur.

Craddock et al. (11–14) documented that activation of the complement system leading to increased PMN adhesion may occur during hemodialysis and hemoperfusion. An additional mechanism that may be important in the pathogenesis of perfusion abnormalities is the contribution of the effects of trauma from bulk shear stress, which is considered in this study.

Shear stress levels encountered during hemodialysis and use of several common blood pumps range from 10 to 250 dyn/cm^2 for periodic exposures of between 1 s and 1 min. These levels are well within the range of shear stress exposures used in this investigation. In addition, extremely high shear stresses (4000 dyn/cm^2) of short (millisecond) duration may occur in the presence of mechanical valves, including artificial heart valves (15, 16).

Earlier work in this laboratory and others demonstrated in vitro dysfunction of both platelets and leukocytes following application of low-level shear stress (1–4). The effects of mechanical trauma can be attributed to bulk shear stress effects rather than surface-mediated ones, since changing the surface-to-volume ratio by a factor of three did not alter the leukocyte or platelet response to a given shear stress intensity and exposure duration (2). Platelet microaggregate formation and adhesion alterations occurred following shear stress exposure in the range of 150 dyn/cm^2 for 2 min, while

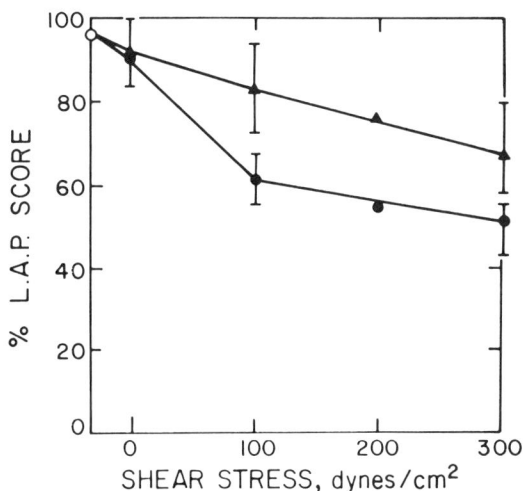

Figure 6. Loss of cytochemically assayed LAP activity after shearing in PBS/G at 37°C for 10 min. Partial preservation of activity with 1×10^{-6}M RA-233 and 3×10^{-6}M PGE$_1$ at all stress levels. The points at 200 dyn/cm^2 represent a single day's run. Key: ●, without drug (control) and ▲, with drug.

leukocytes showed increased adhesion, alteration in phagocytosis and chemotaxis, enzyme release, and decreased hexose monophosphate shunt activity after 150 dyn/cm^2 for 10 min (2–4).

The development and discovery of agents that affect platelet aggregation (antiplatelet agents) have contributed to the clinical control of this aspect of post-perfusion lung complications. One of the supposed actions of these agents is on the cyclic nucleotide system. Dipyridamole (Persantin) and its derivative RA-233 function, at least in part, as phosphodiesterase inhibitors, contributing to the elevation of intracellular cyclic adenosine monophosphate (cAMP) by reducing its degradation to AMP. On the other hand, PGE$_1$ is known to stimulate adenylate cyclase, increasing production of cAMP by that membrane-bound enzyme. Whether the in vivo effects of either of these antiplatelet agents are mediated by their action on intracellular cAMP remains to be shown. The complementary actions of the two chemical agents, however, make them a logical choice for the present study.

The action of PGE$_1$ and RA-233 upon granulocytes following shear stress trauma can only be surmised incompletely from the present in vitro study. Whatever interactive effects these agents have with blood proteins, complement, or other formed elements of the blood have been minimized to investigate their mode of action upon granulocyte function. Granulocyte release of lysosomal enzymes does involve multiple and complex processes. However, PGE$_1$ and RA-233 appear to have a definite preservational effect upon this process, due in part, to reduction of cell lysis following shear stress exposure. Increases in adhesion resulting from shearing PMN leukocytes also were greatly reduced by preincubation with the antiplatelet agents in a manner similar to the effect of these agents upon platelet response to shear stress (17). This similarity suggests possibly related actions upon PMN leukocyte adhesion during antiplatelet therapy after in vivo cardiopulmonary bypass. The fact that no effect of these agents upon chemiluminescence resulting from PMN leukocyte phagocytosis was found may reflect the lack of relationship between PMN chemiluminescence and the cyclic nucleotide system, or may be due to peculiarities within the assay. The chemiluminescence assay is performed on samples with the same adjusted PMN count. Thus, even though the activity per intact PMN is not changed by drug incubation, the fact that PMN counts are higher after shear stress (300 dyn/cm^2) in the drug-incubated samples implies that the total phagocytic ability of the treated PMN suspensions will be higher. PMN leukocytes have been shown to have reduced efficacy in combating bacterial sepsis following prostaglandin therapy, despite the lack of evidence of effects of elevated intracellular cAMP upon PMN leukocyte phagocytosis after either mechanical stress or inflammation (18).

The partial preservation of leukocyte numbers, following shearing of the suspension, in the presence of PGE$_1$ and RA-233 is most probably due to the combined effects of reduced adhesion and aggregation and minimization of cell lysis, as noted upon microscopic examination of slides made with the suspensions. Although the sharp drop in the white blood cell count during cardiopulmonary bypass and subsequent rebound proliferation of immature granulocytes might not be detrimental or pathological, preservation of granulocytes by the prevention of cell lysis and release can be considered significant if this action occurs in vivo. Therefore, the action of these antiplatelet agents may partly involve or be supplemented by amelioration of leukocyte functional changes resulting from fluid mechanical trauma.

Acknowledgments

This research was supported by NIH Grants HL 17437 and HL 18686. Computational assistance was provided by the Clinfo Project funded by the Division of Research Resources of NIH under Grant RR-00350. The authors thank Margaret Putman for her technical assistance in this project.

Literature Cited

1. Dewitz, T. S.; Hung, T. C.; Martin, R. R.; McIntire, L. V. *J. Lab. Clin. Med.* **1977**, *90*, 728–736.
2. Dewitz, T. S.; McIntire, L. V.; Martin, R. R.; Sybers, H. D. *Blood Cells* **1979**, *5*, 499–510.
3. Dewitz, T. S.; Martin, R. R.; Solis, R. T.; Hellums, J. D.; McIntire, L. V. *Microvasc. Res.* **1978**, *16*, 263–271.
4. Dewitz, T. S.; McIntire, L. V.; Martin, R. R. *Artif. Organs* **1980**, *4*, 311–316.
5. Woods, N. F.; Weston, M. J. "The Use of Antiplatelet Agents During Hemodialysis," *Dial. Transplant.* **1979** *8*, 958–960.
6. Addonizio, V. P.; Strauss, J. F.; Macarak, E. J.; Colman, R. W.; Edmunds, L. H. *Surgery* **1978** *83*, 619–624.
7. Richardson, P. D.; Galletti, P. M.; Born, G. V. R. *Trans. Am. Soc. Artif. Intern. Organs* **1976**, *22*, 22–28.
8. Martin, R. R.; Warr, G.; Gouch, R.; Knight, V. *J. Lab. Clin. Med.* **1973**, *81*, 520–526.
9. McCallum, R. N.; Lynch, E. C.; Hellums, J. D.; Alfrey, C. P. "Rheology of Biological Systems"; Thomas: New York, 1973; p. 70.
10. DeChatelet, L. R.; Cooper, M. R. *Biochem. Med.* **1970**, *4*, 61–68.
11. Craddock, P. R.; Fehr, J.; Dalmasso, A. P.; Brigham, K. L.; Jacob, H. S. *J. Clin. Invest.* **1977**, *59*, 879–888.
12. Craddock, P. R.; Fehr, J.; Bringham, K. L.; Kronenberg, R. S.; Jacob, H. S. *New Eng. J. Med.* **1977**, *296*, 769–773.
13. Craddock, P. R.; Hammerschmidt, D. E.; Moldow, C. F.; Yamada, O.; Jacob, H. S. *Semin. Hematol.* **1979**, *16*, 140–147.
14. O'Flaherty, J. T.; Craddock, P. R.; Jacob, H. S. *Blood* **1978**, *51*, 731–739.
15. Roschke, E. J.; Harrison, E. C.; Blankenhorn, D. H. *Proc. 28th Ann. Conf. Eng. Med. Biol.* **1975**, *17*, 269.
16. Roschke, E. J.; Harrison, E. C. "Fluid Shear Stress in Prosthetic Heart Valves," *J. Biomech.* **1977**, *10*, 299–308.
17. Hardwick, A., personal communication.
18. Deporter, D. A.; Dieppe, P. A.; Glatt, M.; Willoughby, D. A. *J. Pathol.* **1977**, *21*, 129.

RECEIVED for review January 16, 1981. ACCEPTED May 1, 1981.

16
A Method to "Count" Flow-Resistant Blood Microemboli

K. A. SOLEN and B. L. BETTERIDGE

Brigham Young University, Department of Chemical Engineering, Provo, UT 84602

> *A constant-pressure filtration (CPF) test was developed to "count" those blood microemboli in a blood sample that are likely to occlude arterioles and capillaries. For preliminary testing, blood microemboli were generated by shearing fresh heparinized human blood between parallel discs of Plexiglass, polystyrene, or polycarbonate for 15, 30, or 90 min (shear range: 0–1200 s^{-1}). CPF measurements were then made on the blood using a 40-mm mercury driving pressure and 15-μm pore filters. Filtration flow rate curves conformed to mathematical predictions from which "effective" microemboli concentrations were calculated. Microemboli production rates from the three materials were significantly different after 90 min of blood–material contact, with the order of increasing toxicity being polycarbonate < polystyrene < Plexiglass.*

The contact of blood with foreign materials or interfaces results in the formation of blood microemboli. Clinically, microemboli are generated by pump-oxygenators (1–7), hemodialyzers (8), ventricular assist devices (9), prosthetic heart valves (10), blood collection sets (11), and blood storage (12–21). When the microemboli are sufficiently large and rigid, blood flow through arterioles and capillaries is retarded or prevented, and the consequent blockage of vascular beds results in impairment of organ function. For example, with the use of pump-oxygenators for cardiopulmonary support, the presence of microemboli has been related to post-operative neurologic problems (22–25).

To improve biomaterials and blood-handling devices from the standpoint of blood microemboli production, the following questions must be answered:

　　1. What are the mechanisms of blood microemboli formation and the resultant microemboli compositions?

2. What are the flow properties of the various types of blood microemboli and their tendencies to retard or prevent microvascular flow?
3. What flow parameters and biomaterial surface characteristics promote the formation of the various types of blood microemboli?

While studies of platelet and thrombus accumulation on surfaces have provided important information concerning blood–material interactions, that accumulation is not a direct index of the rate of microemboli generation [e.g., kidney embolism induced by implanted aortic rings often was most severe from rings that remained "clean" (26, 27)]. Thus, analytical tests that directly quantify microemboli are needed.

The property of a blood microparticle that is clinically important is the flow resistance of that particle, that is, whether it will lodge in arterioles or capillaries and impede blood flow or, instead, break up or deform and thereby pass through the microvasculature. Unfortunately, present methods used to "count" microemboli, such as ultrasound (1, 4–6, 28), electronic counters (7, 19, 20, 29, 30), and filter collection at low, uncontrolled pressures (2, 31), do not distinguish between "occluding" particles (those that will impede flow) and "nonoccluding" particles (those that will pass through capillaries). The Kusserow kidney embolus test (25) does make that distinction by using the kidney of a dog to trap occluding microemboli that are produced by a ring of test material implanted in the suprarenal aorta; however, the resulting renal infarction is difficult to quantify and is obscured by biological variations and by compensatory and reparative processes of the kidney. The one existing quantitative test of flow-resistant microemboli is the screen filtration pressure (SFP) test (32), which measures the filtration pressure after imposed constant flow of the blood sample through a 20-μm pore filter for 10 s. The SFP test has been useful both clinically and in research (8, 33–39), but the test suffers from two significant drawbacks. First, the reading of the pressure at only one point along the pressure vs. time curve, namely, after exactly 10 s, ignores the rest of that curve; thus, a variety of completely dissimilar curves can produce identical final readings, and wide oscillations in pressure in that region of the curve can produce significant variability in the final reading. Second, the high, nonphysiological pressures sometimes generated during the SFP test (often as high as 1500 mm mercury or higher) cause the particle selectivity to be quite nonphysiological, that is, some microparticles that are forced through the filter at these high pressures might not pass through the filter under physiological pressures.

Considering this discussion, some features of an improved test to count flow-resistant microemboli might be that the test:

1. counts only those microemboli satisfying some flow-resistant criteria.
2. is based on physiological models and calibration.

3. yields quantitative data based on the entire sample.
4. is simple and reproducible (suggests an in vitro test).
5. is sufficiently sensitive to discriminate between microemboli generated by different surfaces.

This chapter describes the development and feasibility testing of a CPF system that has the potential to satisfy these requirements.

Experimental

The apparatus for the CPF test consisted of a vertical column [polyvinyl chloride (PVC) tubing] of saline solution with a Plexiglass filter assembly connected to the bottom of the column (Figure 1). The filter assembly supported a nickel-plated filter containing regularly spaced square pores of 15 ± 2 μm on a side (Buckbee–Mears Co.) across the flow channel, and the filter assembly and bottom 30 cm of the column were

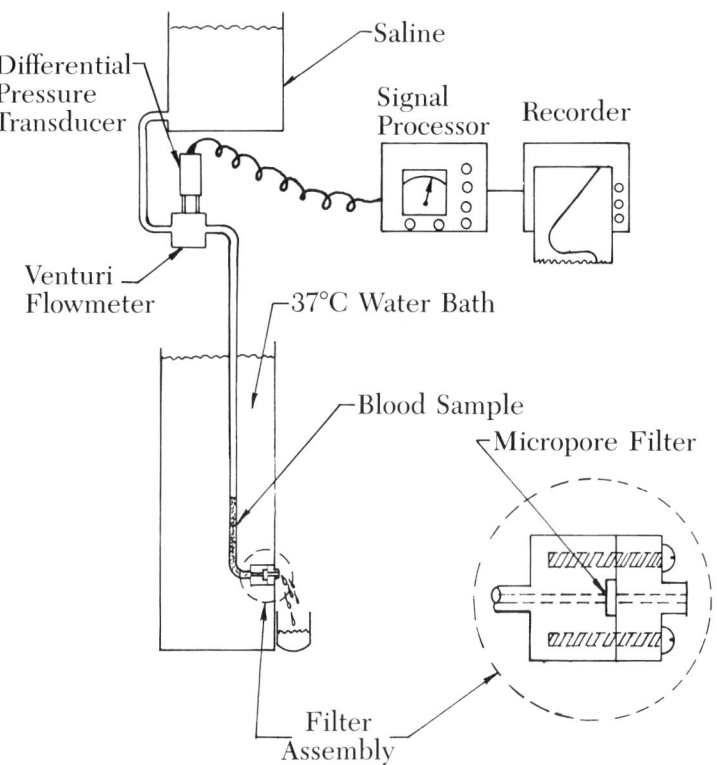

Figure 1. The CPF apparatus.

maintained at 37°C in a circulating water bath. A constant pressure difference was maintained across the filter by the fixed height of the saline solution column. To determine the embolic content of a blood sample, the blood was inserted into the bottom of the column, displacing the saline solution. A stopcock was then opened to allow flow through the filter. A custom-made, low-flow venturi flow meter was mounted in the column, and a sensitive differential-pressure transducer (Validyne Engineering Corp., DP–103/CD15–1383) and recorder monitored and recorded the flow rate.

For the tests described here, the pressure across the filter was set at 40 mm mercury. By comparison, pressure driving forces across microvascular beds range from approximately 20 mm mercury across capillaries to 80 mm mercury across arteriole–venule systems (40).

Biomaterial-induced microemboli were obtained as follows: ¼-in. sheets of Plexiglass G (Du Pont), polystyrene (Dow Resin F70502.00), or polycarbonate (Lexan, General Electric Co.) were cut, drilled, and mounted into the parallel-disc configuration shown in Figure 2. The surfaces were soaked in ethanol (95% for the polycarbonate and polystyrene and 50% for the Plexiglass) for at least 24 h, and then in saline solution for 12–18 h at 37°C just prior to exposure to the blood samples.

On the day of the experiment, 20 mL of whole blood was drawn into heparin (6 units/mL; Riker Laboratories) by venipuncture from normal healthy volunteers. The saline solution was removed from the parallel-disc apparatus, and 10 mL of blood was inserted between the discs. The top disc was then rotated at 200 rpm (shear rate range 0–1200 s^{-1}) for 15, 30, or 90 min, while the entire assembly was maintained at 37°C in a free-convection incubator. The space between the top disc and the collar was less than 2 mm, to minimize blood–air contact, and a cover over the discs (not shown in Figure 2) contained a water reservoir to humidify the air over the discs and prevent drying of the blood.

The remaining 10 mL of blood were filtered in the CPF apparatus to obtain a control curve, and after the prescribed period of disc rotation, the blood from the parallel-disc system was transferred to the CPF apparatus for the test run.

Fresh, previously unused discs were used for each test, and each type of material

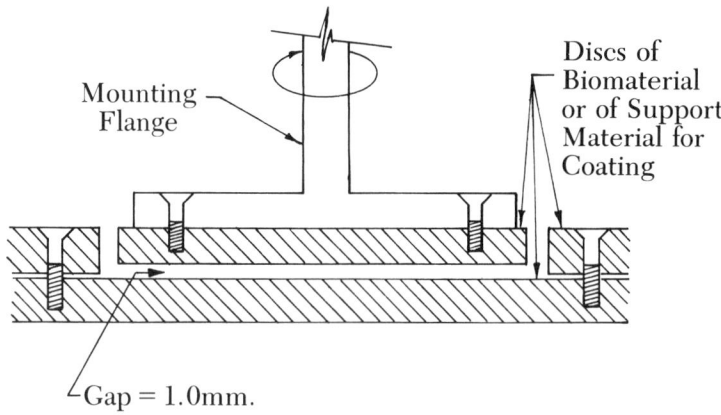

Figure 2. Parallel-disc apparatus for exposing blood to biomaterials.

(Plexiglass, polystyrene, and polycarbonate) was tested twice in 15-min tests, four times in 30-min tests, and four times in 90-min exposures. In addition, each donor was used twice on the same day for the testing of two different materials, so that all possible pairs of materials were tested with blood from a single donor.

Results and Discussion

The anticipated filtration curve for microemboli-laden blood is described as follows: The rate of obstruction of the filter pores by rigid particles would be

$$-dn/dt = cqn \qquad (1)$$

where n is the number of unblocked pores at a given instant; c, the concentration of particles in the blood that can occlude one pore each; q, the volumetric flow rate of blood through an unblocked pore; and t, the time. The solution to Equation 1 is

$$n = n_o e^{-cqt} \qquad (2)$$

where n_o is the total number of filter pores. The total flow rate at any instant is

$$Q = nq = n_o q e^{-cqt} \qquad (3)$$

$$Q = Q_o e^{-cqt} \qquad (4)$$

where Q is the total volumetric flow rate of blood through the filter at a given instant and Q_o, the volumetric flow rate when all the pores are unblocked.

Control blood (freshly drawn and not exposed to the biomaterial discs) should exhibit a constant flow rate, while blood from the parallel-disc exposure should produce an exponential filtration curve (Equation 4) from which the "effective" concentration of microemboli can be determined from a semilog plot of flow rate vs. time.

Fresh heparinized blood from the donor typically required 4–5 s to reach a steady filtration rate, and then exhibited a relatively constant flow rate through the micropore filter during the 10–15 s required to filter the entire sample (Figure 3a). In contrast, blood that had been exposed to the Plexiglass, polystyrene, or polycarbonate discs progressively occluded the filter with as much as 98% reduction in flow by the end of 30 s (Figure 3b). A semilog plot of flow rate vs. time for the latter sample was typically linear with excellent correlation (Figure 3c; correlation coefficients ranged from 0.994 to 1.000 for the 30 tests), indicating an exponential decline in flow rate, as predicted by the model just described.

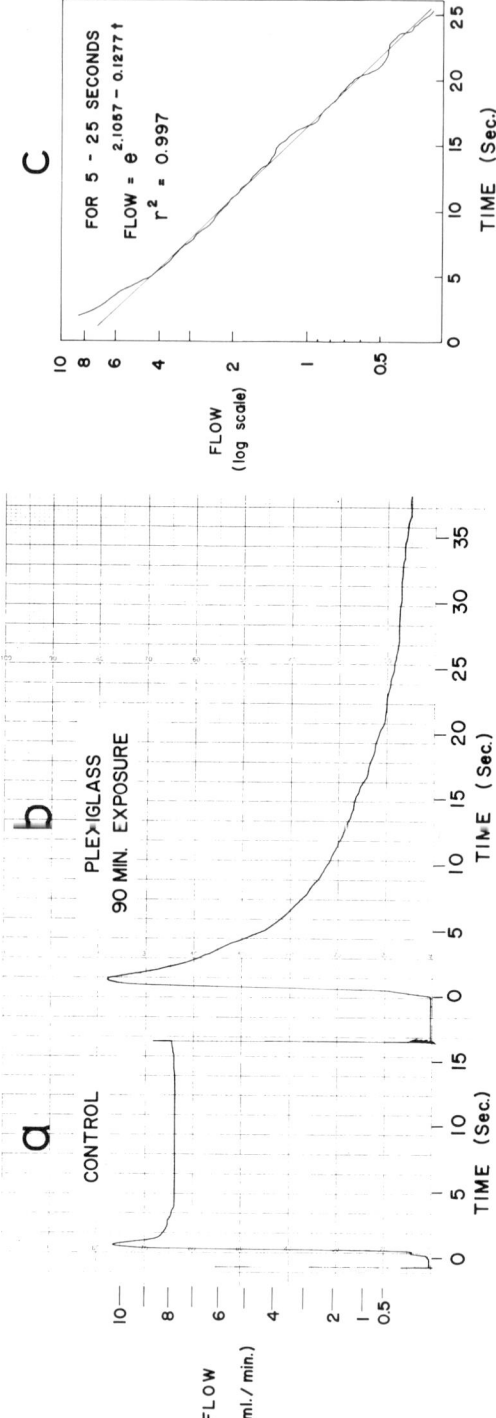

Figure 3. Typical results of the CPF test using a 15-μm pore size filter and fresh heparinized human blood. Key: a, control blood; b, blood exposed to Plexiglass discs (shear rates: 0–1200 s^{-1}) for 90 min; and c, semilog plot of the flowrate from Curve b.

Concentrations of microemboli were calculated from the slopes of the semilog plots of flow rate according to Equation 4. The concentrations produced by the three biomaterials were not significantly different after 15 or 30 min of blood–biomaterial contact (Table I). However, after 90 min of contact, each of the three materials produced significantly different microemboli concentrations (as determined by a paired-difference analysis), even with the small number of measurements made (*see* Table I). The order of increasing toxicity was polycarbonate < polystyrene < Plexiglass.

Conclusions

The CPF flow rate curves consistently conformed to Equation 4, with correlation coefficients from the semilog plots (*see* Figure 3c) ranging from 0.994 to 1.000 for the 30 curves generated. Therefore, nearly the entire curve (with the exception of an initial 4–5-s unsteady-state period) could be used to calculate an effective concentration of microemboli. The calculation itself is simple and reliable.

Because of the preliminary nature of this study, we did not use the steps of biomaterial surface preparation and characterization suggested as "Level One" (minimum level) tests by two recent study groups of the National Heart, Lung, and Blood Institute (*41, 42*). Neither bulk nor surface properties were analyzed, and the surfaces were not confined to a dust-free environ-

Table I. CPF Test Results for Three Biomaterials

Exposure Time (min)	Donor	Blood Emboli/Milliliter			Significance of Material Differences[a]
		Plexiglass	Polystyrene	Polycarbonate	
90	J.B.	1112	296		94.5%
90	V.J.	1928	770		
90	B.B.		824	156	99.9%
90	R.N.		957	292	
90	V.W.	1105		658	95.5%
90	V.B.	806		212	
	Ave.	1238	712	330	
	sem	241	144	113	
30	D.D.	217	263		Not Sig.
30	B.K.	76	396		
30	B.R.		923	290	Not Sig.
30	D.S.		132	54	
30	J.L.	883		320	Not Sig.
30	T.P.	209		162	
	Ave.	346	429	207	
	sem	182	173	61	
15	D.C.	407	367		
15	E.H.		263	360	
15	N.C.	221		155	
	Ave.	314	315	258	
	sem	93	52	103	

[a] Based on a paired-difference analysis.

ment. However, each type of material was purchased as a single batch to insure uniformity. Also, care was taken in handling of the surfaces to avoid contact with any type of oil or grease, and the surfaces were soaked in ethanol and saline solution to extract leachable impurities. With these minimal precautions and with the small numbers of tests conducted, the differences between microemboli production by the three types of materials were detected by the CPF test and were statistically significant after 90 min of blood–biomaterial contact. Using greater precautions against chemical variation and surface contamination would likely produce results of greater uniformity and more significance between test groups. These considerations strongly suggest that the CPF test has potential as a standard test to screen biomedical materials and devices, and to evaluate surface treatments in terms of microemboli potential.

Tests are needed (and are planned) to evaluate the effect of any blood–filter interaction on the test results. Even though freshly drawn blood exhibits constant flow through the filter (Figure 3a), blood that has been exposed to biomaterials (particularly in high surface/volume configurations) may be more "reactive" and capable of reacting as individual cells to form thrombi on the filter during the 30 s of the test. Possible methods of examining this question include microscopic examination of the filter during the test and comparison of the test results with and without antithrombogenic filter coatings.

A vital element in the establishment of a standard measure of "physiologically significant" microemboli is the calibration of the test with physiological systems. Tests are underway in our laboratory in which microemboli-laden blood is perfused through cat hind limbs under controlled pressure. The resulting flow curves will be modeled, and microvessel blocking will be compared with filter blocking by the same blood samples. Filter pore size and filtration pressure may then be varied to match the CPF test characteristics to the in vivo system. The net result will be a rapid, sensitive, in vitro test to detect physiologically significant blood microemboli.

Literature Cited

1. Carlson, R. G.; Lande, A. J.; Landis, B.; Rogoz, B.; Baxter, J.; Patterson, R. H., Jr.; Stenzel, K.; Lillehei, C. W. *J. Thorac. Cardiovasc. Surg.* **1973**, *66*, 894–904.
2. Dutton, R. C.; Edmunds, L. H., Jr.; Hutchinson, J. C.; Roe, B. B. *J. Thorac. Cardiovasc. Surg.* **1974**, *67*, 258–265.
3. Gervin, A. S.; McNeer, J. F.; Wolfe, W. G.; Puckett, C. L.; Silver, D. *J. Thorac. Cardiovasc. Surg.* **1974**, *67*, 237–242.
4. Lande, A. J.; Carlson, R. G.; Patterson, R. H., Jr.; Baxter, J.; Lillehei, C. W. *Trans. Am. Soc. Artif. Intern. Organs* **1972**, *18*, 532–537.
5. Patterson, R. H., Jr.; Kessler, J. *Surg. Gynecol. Obstet.* **1969**, *129*, 505–510.
6. Simmons, E.; MaGuire, C.; Lichti, E.; Helvey, W.; Almond, C. *J. Thorac. Cardiovasc. Surg.* **1972**, *63*, 613–621.
7. Solis, R. T.; Kennedy, P. S.; Beall, A. C., Jr.; Noon, G. P.; DeBakey, M. E. *Circulation* **1975**, *52*, 103–108.
8. Bischel, M. D.; Orrell, F. L.; Scoles, B. G.; Mohler, J. G.; Barbour, B. H. *Trans. Am. Soc. Artif. Intern. Organs* **1973**, *19*, 492–497.

9. Peters, J. L.; McRea, J. C.; Fukumasu, H.; Kolff, W. J. *Trans. Am. Soc. Artif. Intern. Organs* **1976**, *22*, 357–366.
10. Moggio, R. A.; Hammond, G. L.; Stansel, H. C., Jr.; Glenn, W. W. L. *J. Thorac. Cardiovasc. Surg.* **1978**, *75*, 296–299.
11. Jaques, L. B. In "Blood Coagulation, Hemorrhage, & Thrombosis;" Tocantins, L. M.; Kazul, L. A., Eds.; Grune and Stratton: New York, 1964.
12. Bennett, S. H.; Aaron, R. K.; Geelhoed, G. W.; Hoye, R.; Solis, R. T. *J. Surg. Res.* **1972**, *13*, 295–306.
13. Connell, R. S.; Swank, R. L. *Ann. Surg.* **1973**, *177*, 40–50.
14. Jenevein, E. P., Jr.; Weiss, D. L. *Am. J. Pathol.* **1964**, *45*, 313–325.
15. McNamara, J. J.; Boatright, D.; Burran, E. L.; Molot, M. D.; Summers, E.; Stremple, J. F. *Ann. Surg.* **1971**, *174*, 58–60.
16. McNamara, J. J.; Burran, E. L.; Larson, E.; Omiya, G.; Suehiro, G.; Yamase, H. *Ann. Thorac. Surg.* **1972**, *14*, 133–139.
17. Moseley, R. V.; Doty, D. B. *Ann. Surg.* **1970**, *171*, 329–335.
18. Solis, R. T.; Gibbs, M. B. *Transfusion* **1972**, *12*, 245–250.
19. Solis, R. T.; Goldfinger, D.; Gibbs, M. B.; Zeller, J. A. *Transfusion (Philadelphia)* **1974**, *14*, 538–550.
20. Solis, R. T.; Noon, G. P.; DeBakey, M. E. *Trans. Am. Soc. Artif. Intern. Organs* **1974**, *20*, 499–503.
21. Swank, R. L. *N. Eng. J. Med.* **1961**, *265*, 728–733.
22. Branthwaite, M. A. *Thorax* **1972**, *27*, 748–753.
23. Brennan, R. W.; Patterson, R. H., Jr.; Kessler, J. *Neurology* **1971**, *21*, 665–672.
24. Lee, W. H., Jr.; Brady, M. P.; Rowe, J. M.; Miller, W. C. *Ann. Surg.* **1971**, *173*, 1013–1023.
25. Witoszka, M. M.; Tamura, H. J.; Indeglia, R.; Hopkins, R. W.; Simeone, F. A. *J. Thorac. Cardiovasc. Surg.* **1973**, *66*, 855–864.
26. Kusserow, B.; Larrow, R.; Nichols, J. *Trans. Am. Soc. Artif. Intern. Organs* **1970**, *16*, 58–62.
27. Bruck, S. D. *Ann. N.Y. Acad. Sci.* **1977**, *283*, 332–355.
28. Kessler, J.; Patterson, R. H. *Ann. Thorac. Surg.* **1970**, *9*, 221–228.
29. Solis, R. T.; Wright, C. B.; Gibbs, M. B. *J. Appl. Physiol.* **1975**, *38*, 739–744.
30. Dewitz, T. S.; Martin, R. R.; Solis, R. T.; Hellums, J. D.; McIntyre, L. V. *Microvasc. Res.* **1978**, *16*, 263–271.
31. Dutton, R. C.; Edmunds, L. H., Jr., *J. Thorac. Cardiovasc. Surg.* **1973**, *65*, 523–530.
32. Swank, R. L.; Roth, J. G.; Jensen, J. *J. Appl. Physiol.* **1964**, *19*, 340–346.
33. Ashmore, P. G.; Svitek, V.; Ambrose, P. *J. Thorac. Cardiovasc. Surg.* **1968**, *55*, 691–697.
34. Ashmore, P. G.; Swank, R. L.; Gallery, R.; Ambrose, P.; Prichard, K. H. *J. Thorac. Cardiovasc. Surg.* **1972**, *63*, 240–248.
35. Rittenhouse, E. A.; Hessel, E. A.; Ito, C. S.; Merendino, K. A. *Surg. Forum* **1970**, *21*, 142–144.
36. Rittenhouse, E. A.; Hessel, E. A.; Ito, C. S.; Merendino, K. A. *Ann. Surg.* **1972**, *175*, 1–9.
37. Solen, K. A.; Whiffen, J. D.; Lightfoot, E. N. *J. Biomed. Mater. Res.* **1978**, *12*, 381–399.
38. Solen, K. A.; Whiffen, J. D.; Lightfoot, E. N. *Biomat. Med. Dev. Artif. Org.* **1980**, *8*, 35–48.
39. Solen, K. A.; Whiffen, J. D.; Lightfoot, E. N. *J. Lab. Clin. Med.* **1981**, *98*, 206–216.
40. Burton, A. C. "Physiology and Biophysics of the Circulation"; Yearbook Med.: Chicago, 1965; p. 87.
41. Keller, K. H. "Final Report of the Working Group on Physiochemical Characterization of Biomaterials to the National Heart, Lung, and Blood Institute, National Institutes of Health," 1979.
42. Mason, R. G. "Final Report of the Working Group on Blood-Material Interactions to the Devices and Technology Branch, National Heart, Lung, and Blood Institute, National Institutes of Health," 1979.

RECEIVED for review January 16, 1981. ACCEPTED October 6, 1981.

PROTEIN ADSORPTION ON BIOMATERIALS

17
Protein Adsorption on Biomaterials

THOMAS A. HORBETT

University of Washington, Department of Chemical Engineering, BF-10, Seattle, WA 98195

The problem of finding acceptable materials for use in contact with tissue is highly relevant to present day clinical practice. The difficulty of this problem reflects the complex nature of tissue–material interactions which are influenced by properties of the tissue, properties of the material, and by the transport of fluids around the implant. Implants designed with each of these aspects in mind may produce a "biocompatible environment," analogous to the nonthrombogenic environment thought to be required for blood compatibility (1).

The foreign body reaction occurring around soft tissue implants and thrombosis on surfaces in contact with blood are the major reactions encountered with implants. Both reactions involve the interaction of cells with the implant, especially in the later stages, and much previous study has therefore emphasized cellular events in the biocompatibility process. However, cells encounter foreign polymer implants under conditions that ensure the prior adsorption of a layer of protein to the polymer interface. The properties of the adsorbed layer are therefore important in mediating cellular response to the material.

Adsorbed proteins are important in a variety of biological processes, as illustrated in Table I. The length and diversity of this list suggest that all biological processes occurring at interfaces will be greatly affected by proteins. Unfortunately, many major questions concerning adsorbed proteins remain unanswered because of the difficulty of studying proteins at interfaces. For example, why are certain proteins present at interfaces rather than other proteins? What properties of proteins and surfaces regulate the localization of proteins at surfaces? Why are proteins at interfaces often more influential than they are in the bulk phase? The mediating layer of adsorbed protein is present on all materials, yet cellular responses are not the same—how does the implied difference in the organization of the adsorbed layer occur?

The sensitivity of cellular interactions to interfacial proteins probably is due to the presence of cell surface receptors for specific proteins and to the enhancement of receptor–protein interaction by the concentration of proteins at interfaces. To illustrate the role of specific proteins at interfaces,

Table I. Biological Processes Influenced by Proteins at Interfaces

- *Biocompatibility of synthetic polymers*
  — Thrombosis on catheters and replacements, arteries, and heart valves
  — Foreign body reaction to soft tissue implants
  — Other processes such as contact lens fouling
- *Cell adhesion*
  — Tissue cells are anchorage dependent for growth
  — Platelet and white cells require adhesion for function
  — Bacterial cell adhesion is involved in tooth decay and marine fouling
- *Blood coagulation*
  — The intrinsic system: factor XII activation on surfaces
  — The extrinsic system: phospholipid vesicles accelerate prothrombin activation
  — Platelet activation by collagen and other proteins
- *Immunology*
  — Antibody binding to foreign cells ("opsonization")
  — Complement protein activation and attack on foreign cells
  — Phagocytic processes aided by membrane receptors for proteins
- *Other*
  — Membrane receptors
  — Tumor cells may differ in surface proteins (?)
  — Protein separation by hydrophobic or affinity chromatography; enzyme immobilization

Table II summarizes the effects of five common plasma proteins on the response of a variety of cells to foreign materials. The examples in this table show that cellular response to materials is influenced strongly by adsorbed proteins. For example, adsorbed cold insoluble globulin enhances the adhesion of fibroblasts, the phagocytosis of particles by macrophages, and thrombus formation on polyvinyl chloride (PVC) exposed to blood. However, the response is specific, since not all cells react the same to a given protein: fibrinogen enhances platelet adhesion but decreases red-cell adhesion. Only a few of the proteins in plasma elicit a positive response from a given cell, providing further specificity. The strong and frequently specific influence of adsorbed proteins on cellular reactions with materials is the major reason for studying the nature of protein adsorption. This chapter describes the general behavior of proteins at interfaces and the specific questions regarding protein adsorption from complex mixtures which appear to be most important.

General Properties of Adsorbed Proteins

Certain general properties of proteins and their behavior at interfaces are important to remember when trying to comprehend the widespread influence of the interfacial protein layer. Most basic is the fact that the proteins are intrinsically surface active and tend to concentrate at interfaces, due partly to their polymeric structure and partly to their amphoteric nature (15). Thus, multiple contact points with the interface are possible for each protein molecule because of its large size, an effect that greatly increases the tendency for the molecule to remain at the interface. The presence of polar, charged, and nonpolar amino acid side chains in proteins provides the opportunity for multiple modes of binding with many different types of surfaces. The general tendency for nonpolar residues to be internalized in the native protein (16) may require structural alterations upon adsorption in order to maximize the number of contacts with the surface (17). For example, protein adsorption on a hydrophobic surface could involve conformational changes to optimize the various bonding interactions between the protein's hydrophobic and hydrophilic sites with the surface and water phases, respectively.

The adsorption of proteins at interfaces can lead to enormous local concentrations, far in excess of the bulk phase value. A 100-Å-thick albumin

Table II. Plasma Proteins Affecting Cellular Interactions with Foreign Materials

Protein	Plasma Concentration (mg/mL)	Material	Cell Type	Response
Complement C3	1.2	cellophane	granulocytes	acute leukopenia (2)
		mineral oil	neutrophils	phagocytosis enhanced (3)
		S. aureus	neutrophils	attachment enhanced (4)
Immunoglobulin G	10–30	glass	platelets	adhesion and release enhanced (5)
		polyvinyl toluene	leucocytes	phagocytosis enhanced (6)
		PHEMA–PEMA	fibroblasts and red cells	adhesion prevented (7)
Cold insoluble globulin	0.1–0.3	falcon dishes	fibroblasts	adhesion enhanced (8)
		RE-test emulsion	macrophages	phagocytosis enhanced (9)
		PVC	platelets	thrombus enhanced (10)
Fibrinogen	3–5	polystyrene	platelets	adhesion and release enhanced (11)
		silicone rubber	fibroblasts	adhesion enhanced (12)
		glass	red cells	adhesion prevented (13)
Albumin	40–60	glass	platelets	adhesion and release decreased (5)
		polyethylene	red cells	strength of adhesion decreased (14)
		falcon dishes	fibroblasts	adhesion prevented (8)

layer at 1 μg/cm² has a concentration at the surface of about 1000 mg/mL, not far below the theoretical maximum of 1400 mg/mL corresponding to the local concentration in the domain of the protein molecule itself. Interfacial concentrations of 1 μg/cm² are typical for many surfaces exposed to protein solutions that are 1 mg/mL or less in the bulk phase. The consequences of such extreme local concentration in terms of effects on protein properties have yet to be determined clearly, but in general, most chemical reactions are affected strongly by concentration of the reactants. Thus, many of the reactions that proteins can undergo in the bulk phase might be strongly enhanced in the surface phase. For example, modification by traces of enzyme might occur much more readily in the surface phase than in the bulk, and the normally weak tendency for most proteins to aggregate or form complexes might be greatly enhanced on the surface. Finally and most importantly, the concentration and localization of proteins at interfaces may greatly facilitate the ability of cells to react with the proteins, since interaction with closely spaced protein molecules by the cell could enhance binding. Examples of the special role of interfaces in the properties of proteins include activation of clotting factor XII (18, 19), enhancement of complement C3 activation (20), and activation of the alternate pathway of complement by adsorbed immunoglobulin G (IgG) (21).

Organization of the Adsorbed Protein Layer

The exposure of any material to a mixture of proteins such as plasma should lead to enrichment of certain proteins at the surface relative to the bulk phase. Therefore, the composition of the surface phase should differ from the bulk phase. The composition should also be different on each material because the chemical properties leading to enrichment vary significantly between various materials. Furthermore, the site density of any protein in the layer (expressed as molecules per square centimeter), and the accessibility or reactivity of the protein to larger probes such as cells should vary on different surfaces. The wide range in affinity of proteins for surfaces, which is the basis for most of these expectations, is evidenced by the routine separation of proteins by column chromatography using ionic and hydrophobic matrices (22, 23). Composition, site density, and reactivity of the proteins are the key organizational aspects of the adsorbed layer formed from complex media such as plasma. Surprisingly, few studies of these aspects of the adsorbed protein layer have been made.

The differences in affinity of proteins for surfaces is not readily discerned from the extensive literature on adsorption of proteins to surfaces from pure protein solutions (24). The typical result of such studies is the adsorption isotherm, but determination of the strength of interaction or surface affinity from such measurements is not possible because the adsorption is essentially irreversible. The surface activity of the plasma proteins has not been studied systematically as yet, nor have the structural properties of proteins that control this activity. However, an empirical study of the competition of various plasma proteins for surfaces from simple mixtures does provide information about the affinity of proteins for surfaces. For example, the adsorption of fibrinogen to several polymers is reduced to half its original value by an approximately tenfold weight excess of albumin or γ-globulin (25). Hemoglobin (in the ferric form) competes much more effectively than any other protein yet tested; at one-tenth the fibrinogen concentration, hemoglobin reduces the adsorption of fibrinogen to polyethylene by 50% (26). In a three-way mixture simulating the competition of the three major plasma proteins, fibrinogen forms 55 to 70% of the protein adsorbed in the first 2 min of exposure (depending on the polymer), but at steady state (2.5 h later), each material had approximately the same composition of adsorbed protein: 43–45% fibrinogen, 17–24% γ-globulin, and 32–39% albumin (27, 28).

Adsorption studies using whole plasma provide the most relevant in vitro approach to the composition of the adsorbed protein layer. Several observations not predictable from simpler systems have been made in the plasma studies. For example, surfaces exposed to plasma for 10 s or less bind fibrinogen antibodies, while longer exposure results in loss of antifibrinogen binding (29, 30). This process of "conversion" apparently involves high molecular weight kininogen, since loss of antifibrinogen binding does not occur with plasma deficient in this material (31). Large differences in the uptake of fluorescent antibodies against albumin, fibrinogen, and immunoglobulin by various types of hemodialysis membranes after exposure to blood have been attributed to overlaying of antigenic protein with other plasma proteins (32). The unequal availability of the proteins in the adsorbed layer suggested by both studies may be extremely important in understanding why some surfaces are able to elicit more intense cellular reactions than others.

Examination of the adsorbed protein layer formed from plasma by electrophoretic separation of the proteins in a detergent eluate of the surface has revealed the complexity of the layer (33–35). As many as nine separate proteins have been detected, including fibrinogen, IgG, albumin, and hemoglobin, as well as several unidentified proteins present in smaller amounts (35). These studies emphasize the fact that the adsorbed layer is *not* dominated by any particular protein. The composition of the adsorbed layer appears to reflect differences in surface activity and bulk concentration of the various proteins in the plasma. Thus, proteins with high surface activity such as fibrinogen and hemoglobin are present in the layer despite their relatively low bulk-phase concentration. Conversely, although albumin is not particularly surface active, its high bulk-phase concentration gives a competitive edge to this protein.

The presence of the major plasma proteins on all polymers exposed to plasma, and the lack of dominance by fibrinogen or other proteins in this layer, pose the question of what differences in the adsorbed layer are sufficient to elicit differences in cellular responses. Since a cellular response may require the close spacing of similar molecules on the interface to bind properly or otherwise trigger the cell, the site density or molecules per unit area of a particular protein may be a key parameter. Variations in the site density of specific proteins in the adsorbed layer formed from complex media have been demonstrated in several studies, using ^{125}I-labeled proteins added to plasma. The amounts of fibrinogen, γ-globulin, and albumin adsorption from the plasma seem to vary a great deal, depending on both material and protein. For example, albumin adsorption varied from about 0.2 μg/cm^2 on Teflon FEP to 3.0 μg/cm^2 on Biomer, while fibrinogen adsorption was generally much lower: 0.03 μg/cm^2 on Teflon to 0.06 μg/cm^2 on Biomer (36). In other studies, albumin adsorption from plasma to polyethylene, poly-(2-hydroxyethyl methacrylate) (PHEMA) and poly(ethyl methacrylate) (PEMA) varied over a narrower range (0.14–0.21 μg/cm^2), while fibrinogen adsorption was similarly lower (0.019–0.044 μg/cm^2) (37, 38).

Another unexpected aspect of plasma protein adsorption revealed by studies with complex media has been the rapid rearrangement of the adsorbed layer early in the adsorption process. The kinetics of adsorption of proteins from plasma either in vivo or in vitro were studied recently in three separate laboratories, and, surprisingly, each observed the same major result: fibrinogen adsorption was initially high on some surfaces but then decreased within an hour to lower, "steady-state" values (39–41). This effect appears to depend on the nature of the surface: in one study, the initially high fibrinogen value has been observed on PVC but not on Biomer (38), while in another study fibrinogen adsorption was initially high on PEMA but not on PHEMA (41). Similar transient adsorption maxima for albumin which varied with polymer type also were observed in two of these studies (39, 41). Hemoglobin and IgG adsorption from plasma increased rapidly and regularly to the saturation value on PEMA and PHEMA, so the high initial adsorption is specific to fibrinogen and albumin (41). The transient, initial maximum in fibrinogen adsorption may be related to Vroman's earlier observation of rapid conversion of adsorbed fibrinogen to a form unreactive with antifibrinogen. The conversion also appears to occur more on some surfaces than on others (42). Iodination of fibrinogen in the adsorbed state on surfaces exposed to plasma for various times also is unusual (43). On hydrophobic surfaces adsorbed for 150 min and then iodinated, little iodine uptake into fibrinogen was observed. After a 0.5-min plasma exposure, however, most of the iodine incorporated into adsorbed proteins was in fibrinogen. On hydrophilic surfaces, surfaces exposed to plasma showed increasing amounts of iodine in fibrinogen as adsorption time increased. Removal of preadsorbed fibrinogen on exposure to plasma has been observed (44). Taken together, the various kinetic studies of the structure of the adsorbed protein film formed from plasma to surfaces suggest a rapid rearrangement of the adsorbed layer, depending on the nature of the substrate, and point to the existence of a unique organization on each type of material. Furthermore, the major differences in the kinetics of fibrinogen adsorption and iodine uptake by fibrinogen adsorbed from plasma to different polymers suggest the possibility of differences in the structure or accessibility of adsorbed fibrinogen on the polymers.

Structure of Adsorbed Proteins

Proteins are known to become extensively "denatured" or unfolded at the air/water interface (15). Similar but perhaps less extensive perturbation of a protein's structure by the aqueous/solid interface is therefore often a reasonable but unproven assumption. The idea that proteins unfold to different extents on different polymers, thus eliciting differences in cellular response by the polymers, is a major alternative hypothesis to the possible compositional variation in the adsorbed layer. Therefore, the structure of proteins at solid interfaces has been the subject of many studies.

The degree of denaturation of adsorbed proteins is currently open to question. The fraction of the carbonyl groups in proteins adsorbed to silica surfaces that are in contact with the silica, determined with differential infrared spectroscopy, has been used to detect conformational changes (45, 46). Albumin and prothrombin adsorbed to silica appear to retain their native structure, while adsorbed γ-globulin appears to unfold at lower surface coverage (45, 46). Unfolding of γ-globulin during adsorption to polystyrene also was indicated by the release of protons occurring during adsorption (47). In the γ-globulin glass system, very high molar heats of adsorption indicative of substantial conformation changes occur at lower degrees of adsorption, but the heat of adsorption (per mole of adsorbed species) decreases markedly, and multilayer adsorption occurs at higher bulk concentrations (48). The calorimetry results suggest differences in the degree of denaturation as the distance from the surface increases. The results of the infrared and calormetric studies suggest that initially arriving platelets would encounter proteins denatured to quite different extents, because a model with denatured proteins underlying more loosely held native molecules is presumably quite different from a uniform layer of denatured molecules (49). Structural changes in factor XII upon adsorption to quartz have been detected with circular dichroism (18). Such perturbation may facilitate the proteolytic activation of factor XII on the surface (19), a mechanism possibly important for all the surface-bound proteins.

A variety of other techniques has been used to examine the structure of proteins at surfaces, including electron microscopy (50, 51), ellipsometry (52), electrophoretic mobility (53), and total internal reflection fluorescence (TIRF) (54). Several new techniques are being applied at present, including Fourier transform infrared spectroscopy (FTIR) and TIRF (see next section), and electron spectroscopy for chemical analysis (ESCA) (55). These techniques promise to enhance greatly our presently rather meager stock of knowledge about the structure of proteins at interfaces.

Current Research

The protein adsorption studies described in this volume provide a representative cross section of the current research in this area. The compositional and structural aspects of proteins at interfaces continue to receive major attention. Both new and previously developed techniques are being applied to these problems.

The use of FTIR (56) and the development of an internal reflection technique capable of detecting intrinsic fluorescence from tryptophane residues in protein (57) represent powerful new approaches to the structure of proteins adsorbed to interfaces. The speed, sensitivity, and high frequency resolution of the FTIR technique have permitted studies at very short adsorption intervals and discrimination among proteins in mixtures due to their slightly different infrared spectra. The TIRF technique monitors tryptophane residues, which are often buried in the protein structure, and thus provide a natural marker for changes in protein structure at interfaces. However, the signal utilized in both techniques is not solely due to protein molecules at the interface, because the light emanating from the substrate penetrates much further than the diameter of a typical protein. Some degree of averaging of events away from the interface is therefore intrinsic in these methods. Structural changes in adsorbed proteins using improved circular dichroism methodology indicate relatively slow rearrangements (58). Microcalorimetric studies of adsorbed proteins indicate differences in the denaturation behavior of proteins on various polymers (59). Use of prewetted polymer-coated alumina particles in this study represents a technical advance in the use of microcalorimetry, which is likely to make this technique of greater interest in the near future.

The rapid conversion of surface-bound fibrinogen to a form unreactive with antifibrinogen was reported originally some time ago (29, 30). From more recent studies, high molecular weight kininogen may be involved in the fibrinogen conversion reaction, perhaps by direct replacement of fibrinogen by the kininogen (31). Because high molecular weight kininogen might be necessary for the contact activation of coagulation (60), these results are potentially very important. The ability of narrow spaces between adjacent surfaces to somehow modulate the conversion reaction, as reported in this volume, may be important in understanding the influence of surface geometry in blood coagulation (e.g., the importance of surface imperfections). The ability of red cells to influence the composition of the layer by reducing fibrinogen adsorption from plasma (61) is an unexpected phenomenon, and is difficult to rationalize in view of the rapid transport of proteins to surfaces relative to cells. If the composition of the adsorbed layer reflects both cellular and protein interactions with the surface, a much more complex series of events than heretofore imagined must be involved in the response of blood to foreign materials. The visualization of proteins on surfaces with gold nucleation electron microscopy also appears to indicate behavior different than previously expected; protein deposition often was irregular and reticulated instead of being a regular monolayer often envisioned for proteins at interfaces (62). It would seem impossible, however, to eliminate the possibility of fixation or drying artifacts in the preparation of samples for electron microscopy. Results of ESCA analysis of frozen, undried hemoglobin on Teflon also suggest incomplete coverage (55).

The influence of specific proteins in the complex mixture in the adsorbed layer on cellular reactions has yet to be demonstrated directly, but purified proteins preadsorbed to surfaces and then exposed to blood provide information on the potential of various proteins to influence cellular events. A much more comprehensive study of this type which includes proteins such as von Willebrand factor and α_2-macroglobulin is presented in this volume (63). The ability of proteins to enhance or repress cellular reactions when used as pure preadsorbates does not indicate the magnitude of the role played by the protein when present in the complex layer adsorbed from plasma. The protein may be present in very small amounts in the plasma-derived adsorbate relative to the purified preadsorbed layer. For example, von Willebrand factor is present at very low concentrations in plasma (10–15 μg/mL) and is therefore probably present at very low levels in the absorbed layer formed on polymers exposed to plasma. Thus, although von Willebrand factor undoubtedly could be an important factor in surface thrombosis, its influence at the very low adsorption levels likely to exist in vivo must be demonstrated. However, the knowledge of which proteins are potentially important, derived from preadsorption studies, is extremely useful in focusing attention on specific proteins to study in the actual adsorbed layer.

Conclusions

Adsorbed proteins can greatly influence cellular reactions with synthetic materials. The sensitivity to adsorbed proteins, the variation in cellular response to specific proteins, and the rapid adsorption of proteins to all surfaces exposed to the biological environment, have led to the idea that the cellular response to implanted polymers is the result of specific interactions between components of the adsorbed protein layer on the polymer and the cell periphery. These observations, in turn, have led to the hypothesis that cellular interactions with foreign materials are controlled by the presence at the surface of specific proteins at sufficiently high surface density and degree of reactivity to elicit a response. Each of these factors constitutes an important aspect of the organization of the adsorbed protein layer.

Of the large number of proteins in plasma, probably only those with specific cellular receptors can elicit intense and specific responses from a given cell type (e.g., fibrinogen platelets), while the other proteins (e.g., albumin) inhibit cellular reactions. The proportion of activating and passivating proteins in plasma for a given cell type is not known at present, but most plasma proteins probably are passive in this sense. The particular balance between "reactive" and "nonreactive" proteins is determined by the biomaterial surface chemistry, and is due mainly to affinity differences among the proteins in much the same way that it occurs in affinity chromatography of proteins. The ability of material composition to influence the proportion of various proteins on the surface has been demonstrated clearly in several studies. The materials by themselves may elicit little or no active cellular response, but they become reactive by selecting and interfacially concentrating specific proteins from the bulk phase onto the surface phase. The cellular reactivity of the proteins in the layer also may be influenced by the accessibility and configurational state of the adsorbed proteins. These factors also may be influenced by surface chemical properties of the polymers underlying the proteins. Thus, both the specific composition of the adsorbed layer and the reactivity of the proteins in the layer may affect the cellular response elicited when materials are used as implants. This concept constitutes a major hypothesis about biocompatibility and merits further testing.

Literature Cited

1. Litwak, R. S.; Silvay, G.; Shiang, H.; Leonard, E. F. *Ann. N.Y. Acad. Sci.* **1977**, *283*, 542–549.
2. Craddock, P. R.; Fehr, J.; Dalmasso, A. P.; Brigham, K. L.; Jacob, H. S. *J. Clin. Invest.* **1977**, *59*, 879–888.
3. Stossel, T. P.; Field, R. J. *J. Exp. Med.* **1975**, *141*, 1329.
4. Scribner, D. J.; Fahrney, D. *J. Immunol.* **1976**, *116*, 892–897.
5. Packham, M.; Evans, G.; Glynn, M.; Mustard, J. *J. Lab. Clin. Med.* **1969**, *73*, 686.
6. Hallgren, R.; Jansson, L.; Venge, P. *J. Lab. Clin. Med.* **1977**, *90*, 786–795.
7. Horbett, T. unpublished material.
8. Grinnell, F.; Feld, M. K. *Cell* **1979**, *17*, 117–129.
9. Saba, I. M.; Blumenstock, F. A.; Weber, P.; Kaplan, J. E. *Ann. N.Y. Acad. Sci.* **1978**, *312*, 43–55.
10. Ihlenfeld, J. V.; Mathis, T. R.; Barbers, T. A.; Mosher, D. F.; Riddle, L. M.; Hart, A. P.; Updike, S. J.; Cooper, S. L. *Trans. Am. Soc. Artif. Intern. Organs* **1978**, *24*, 727–735.
11. Salzman, E. W.; Lindon, J.; Brier, D.; Merrill, E. W. *Ann. N.Y. Acad. Sci.* **1977**, *283*, 114.
12. Ratner, B.; Horbett, T.; Hoffman, A. S.; Hauschka, S. *J. Biomed. Mater. Res.* **1975**, *9*, 407.
13. George, J. N. *J. Cell Physiol.* **1972**, *79*, 457.
14. Mohandas, N.; Hochmuth, R.; Spaeth, E. *J. Biomed. Mater. Res.* **1974**, *8*, 119.
15. Macritchie, F. *Adv. Protein Chem.* **1978**, *32*, 283.
16. Wertz, D. H.; Scheraga, H. A. *Macromolecules* **1978**, *11*, 9–15.
17. Hoffman, A. S. *Biomed. Mater. J. Res. Symp.* **1974**, *5*, 77.

18. McMillan, C. R.; Saito, H.; Ratnoff, O. D.; Walton, A. G. *J. Clin. Invest.* **1974**, *54*, 1312–1322.
19. Cochrane, C. G.; Revak, S.; Wuepper, K. D. *J. Exp. Med.* **1973**, *138*, 1564–1583.
20. Schreiber, R. D.; Pangburn, M. K.; Lesavre, P. H.; Muller-Eberhard, H. J. *Proc. Natl. Acad. Sci. U.S.A.* **1978**, *75*, 3948–3952.
21. Miekka, S. I.; Gozze, I. *Vox Sang.* **1975**, *19*, 101–123.
22. Jennissen, H. P.; Heidmeyer, L. M. G. *Biochemistry* **1975**, *14*, 754–760.
23. Kissing, W.; Reiner, R. H. *Chromatographia* **1978**, *11*, 83–88.
24. Brash, J. L.; Lyman, D. J. In "The Chemistry of Biosurfaces," Hair, M. O., Ed.; Dekker: New York, 1971; pp. 177–232.
25. Horbett, T. A.; Hoffman, A. S. In Applied Chemistry at Protein Interfaces," Baier, R. E. Ed.; *Advances in Chemistry Series*, No. 145, ACS: Washington, D.C., 1975; pp. 230–254.
26. Horbett, T. A.; Weathersby, P. K.; Hoffman, A. S. *J. Bioeng.* **1977**, *1*, 61–78.
27. Lee, R. G.; Adamson, C.; Kim, S. W. *Thromb. Res.* **1974**, *4*, 485–490.
28. Kim, S. W.; Lee, R. G.; Oster, H.; Colemen, D.; Andrade, J. D.; Lentz, D. J.; Olsen, D. *Trans. Am. Soc. Artif. Intern. Organs* **1974**, *20*, 449–455.
29. Vroman, L.; Adams, A. *J. Biomed. Mater. Res.* **1969**, *3*, 669–671.
30. Vroman, L.; Adams, A. L. *Surf. Sci.* **1969**, *16*, 438–446.
31. Vroman, L.; Adams, A. L.; Fischer, G. C.; Munoz, P. C. *Blood* **1980**, *55*, 156–159.
32. Rubin, J. E.; Faui, K.; Friedman, E. A.; Berlyne, G. M. *Trans. Am. Soc. Artif. Intern. Organs* **1978**, *24*, 471–473.
33. Limber, G. K.; Mason, R. G. *Thromb. Res.* **1975**, *6*, 421.
34. Lyman, D. J.; Metcalf, L. C.; Albo, D.; Richards, K. F.; Lamb, J. *Trans. Am. Soc. Artif. Intern. Organs* **1974**, *20B*, 474.
35. Weathersby, P. K.; Horbett, T. A.; Hoffman, A. S. *Trans. Am. Soc. Artif. Intern. Organs* **1976**, *22*, 242.
36. Kim, S. W.; Wisniewski, S.; Lee, E. S.; Winn, M. L. *Biomed. Mater. Symp.* **1977**, *8*, 23–31.
37. Horbett, T. A.; Weathersby, P. K.; Hoffman, A. S. *Thromb. Res.* **1978**, *12*, 319–329.
38. Horbett, T. A. *J. Biomed. Mater. Res.*, **1981**, *15*, 673–695.
39. Ihlenfeld, J. V.; Cooper, S. L. *J. Biomed. Mater, Res.* **1979**, *13*, 577–591.
40. Brash, J. L.; Uniyal, S. *Proc. 52nd Colloid and Surface Sci. Symp.* 68, Knoxville, Tennessee, June 1978, NTIS Conf. No. 780601.
41. Horbett, T. A. *ACS Organic Coatings and Plastics Chemistry, Preprints*, (Honolulu, April, 1979) *40*, 642–646.
42. Vroman, L.; Adams, A. L.; Klings, M.; Fischer, G. In "Applied Chemistry at Protein Interfaces," Baier, R. E., Ed.; *Advances in Chemistry Series*, No. 145, ACS: Washington, D.C., 1975; pp. 255–289.
43. Horbett, T. A.; Weathersby, P. K. *J. Biomed. Mater. Res.* **1981**, *15*, 403–423.
44. Kochwa, S.; Litwak, R. S.; Rosenfeld, R. E.; Leonard, E. F. *Ann. N.Y. Acad. Sci.* **1977**, *283*, 37–49.
45. Morrissey, B. W. *Ann. N.Y. Acad. Sci.* **1977**, *283*, 50–64.
46. Morrissey, B. W.; Stromberg, R. R. *J. Colloid Interface Sci.* **1974**, 152–164.
47. Kochwa, S.; Brownell, M.; Rosenfield, R. E.; Wasserman, L. R. *J. Immunol.* **1967**, *99*, 981–986.
48. Nyilas, E.; Chieu, T. H.; Herzburger, G. A. *Trans. Am. Soc. Artif. Intern. Organs* **1974**, *20*, 480–490.
49. Baier, R. E. In *"Polymers in Medicine and Surgery,"* Oser, Z.; Martin, E. Eds.; Plenum: New York, 1975; p. 139–159.
50. Gorman, R. R.; Stoner, G. E.; Catlin, A. *J. Phys. Chem.* **1971**, *75*, 2103–2107.
51. Eberhart, R. C.; Prokop, L. D.; Wissenger, J.; Wilkov, M. A. *Trans. Am. Soc. Artif. Intern Organs* **1977**, *23*, 134–140.
52. Morrissey, B. W.; Smith, L. E.; Stromberg, R. R.; Fenstermaker, C. A. *J. Colloid Interface Sci.* **1976**, *56*, 557–563.
53. Chattoraj, D.; Bull, H. *J. Am. Chem. Soc.* **1959**, *81*, 5128.

54. Watkins, R. W.; Robertson, C. R. *J. Biomed. Mater. Res.* **1977**, *11*, 915–938.
55. Ratner, B. D.; Horbett, T. A.; Shuttleworth, D.; Thomas, H. R. *J. Colloid Interface Sci.* **1981**, *83*, 630–642.
56. Gendreau, R. M.; Leininger, R. I.; Winters, S.; Jakobsen, R. J. Chap. 24 in this book.
57. Van Wagenen, R. A.; Rockhold, S.; Andrade, J. D. Chap. 23 in this book.
58. Walton, A. G.; Koltisko, B. Chap. 18 in this book.
59. Filisko, F. E.; Reichert, W. M.; Barenberg, S. A. Chap 13 in this book.
60. Griffin, J. H.; Cochrane, C. G. *Proc. Natl. Acad. Sci. U.S.A.* **1976**, *73*, 2554–2558.
61. Uniyal, S.; Brash, J. L.; Degterev, I. A. Chap. 20 in this book.
62. Eberhart, R. C.; Lynch, M. F.; Bidge, F. H.; Wissinger, J. F.; Munro, M. S.; Ellsworth, S. R.; Qualtrone, A. J. Chap. 21 in this book.
63. Young, B. R.; Lambrecht, L. K.; Cooper, S. L.; Mosher, D. F. Chap. 22 in this book.

RECEIVED for review April 6, 1981. ACCEPTED July 14, 1981.

18

Protein Structure and the Kinetics of Interaction with Surfaces

ALAN G. WALTON[1] and BERNARD KOLTISKO

Case Western Reserve University, Department of Macromolecular Science, Cleveland, OH 44106

> *Adsorption of proteins onto surfaces involves a complex interplay of reversibility, exchange, conformational change, irreversible attachment, and denaturation. Several of these processes may be followed by measurement of the circular dichroism of adsorbed species and of desorbed material. The profile of chromatographically adsorbed material also contains, in principle, the details of the complex kinetics. Some aspects of each of these processes are examined.*

Although the adsorption of small molecules from solution onto solid surfaces represents a classic problem in surface science that is fairly well understood, the adsorption and desorption of proteins from surfaces possesses an added component of complexity because of the ability of adsorbed proteins to change structure.

In previous publications *(1–4)* we have shown that several of the blood plasma proteins (albumin, γ-globulin, fibrinogen, Hageman factor) undergo structural changes as a function of the period spent in the adsorbed state. The hypothesis was that the propensity of such proteins to undergo structural change is a function of the stability of their three-dimensional (tertiary) structure, which may be represented by the internal volume free energy and which is a function of the denaturation temperature. Thus, proteins such as ribonuclease and many of the hydrolytic enzymes are likely to undergo relatively little damage when adsorbed on a polymer surface for a given period of time, whereas very sensitive and unstable structures such as that of Hageman factor, which may depend highly on its hydration state, rapidly change structure on adsorption. Since the structural change is invariably in the direction of decreased structural integrity, a large entropic component is present in the adsorption process.

[1]Current address: University Genetics Company; 537 New Town Avenue, P.O. Box 6080, Norwalk, CT 06852.

By the same token, the chemical composition of the substrate may play a major role in protein adsorption, since highly hydrophilic (hydrogel) surfaces tend to adsorb plasma proteins reversibly with little damage, whereas hydrophobic surfaces cause strong and partially irreversible adsorption leading to extensive damage of adsorbed proteins.

However, adsorption/desorption kinetics are difficult to follow, particularly when simultaneous structural observations are being made. In this chapter we present information pertaining to two different techniques. The first method extends our previous measurements of surface circular dichroism, indicating structural changes as a function of contact time between a plane surface and protein solution. The second technique is based on a chromatographic method that allows us direct access to the kinetics of adsorption/desorption with a subsequent assessment of structural damage.

Circular Dichroic Observation of Structural Changes

In our initial work on the circular dichroism of adsorbed proteins (4), several inherent problems were encountered in obtaining and interpreting a signal. The sensitivity of instruments in that period was such that significant signals were produced only from 20 to 30 monolayers, thus requiring the design and development of a multisurface cell in which successive parallel disks were arranged in series with coated material.

Observations of adsorbed Hageman factor on quartz (5) showed that the protein underwent considerable structural modification; however, quantitative structural deductions were not made. Furthermore, no attempt was made to follow time-dependent changes in conformation.

More recently, using more sensitive equipment (JASCO J40A) and on-line computer processing (Ohio Scientific Challenger II Microprocessor), it has been possible to follow more subtle aspects of structural change.

Structure Determination by Circular Dichroism Spectroscopy

Most approaches to the interpretation of protein structure based on circular dichroism spectra assume that the conformational contributions from α-helix, parallel ($\|$) and antiparallel (a$\|$) β-sheet, β-bend, and irregular regions are additive such that

$$\Delta\epsilon_\lambda \propto [\theta]_\lambda = f_\alpha{}^a[\theta]_\lambda^\circ + f_{\beta_\|}{}^{\beta\|}[\theta]_\lambda^\circ + \ldots \qquad (1)$$

where $[\theta]_\lambda^\circ$ is the ellipticity at wavelength λ, $^x[\theta]_\lambda^\circ$ is the ellipticity of 100% of conformation x at wavelength λ, and f_x is the fraction of conformation x such that

$$f_\alpha + f_{\beta_\|} + f_{\beta a\|} + f_{\beta t} + f_I = 1 \qquad (2)$$

where α is the α-helix, $\beta_\|$, the parallel β-sheet; $\beta a_\|$, the antiparallel β-sheet; β_t, the β-turns; and I, the irregular structure.

Early attempts by Greenfield and Fasman (6) centered around the derivation of $[\theta]_x^\circ$ from model polypeptides, and by assuming only three conformations common to polypeptides and proteins (α-helix, a∥ β-sheet, and coil), it was possible to obtain structural parameters relatively consistent with x-ray data using ellipticity values at two wavelengths:

$$f_\alpha = -\left[\frac{[\theta]_{208} + 4{,}000}{29{,}000}\right] \quad (3)$$

Then, by solving Equation 1 at λ_2, and Equation 2, the fractions f_β and f_c could be obtained.

Subsequent methods included more model peptide conformations (7) or used proteins to form a basis set (8, 9). We have been particularly interested in resolving unique, irregular structures found in proteins (10). This method involves transposing peptide rotation angles ψ,ϕ into cylindrical space η, ι, correlating with known protein structures to provide unique values of $^x[\theta]_\lambda^\circ$ corresponding to irregular structures. Figures 1a and b show how this is done for the protein bacterial nuclease. Now, several fairly sophisticated methods are available for interpreting the structure of a wide range of proteins (at least in terms of secondary structure).

Although the detailed structures of the serum proteins albumin, globulin, fibrinogen, etc. are not known from x-ray crystallography, various studies including circular dichroism spectroscopy were combined to provide a picture of some of these species. Figure 2 shows such reconstructions in which albumin and fibrinogen contain α-helices as their main structural element, and γ-globulin contains antiparallel β-sheets. The structure of albumin is based on our computer predictions of conformation using the Chou/Fasman method (11) as described recently for thrombin and related proteins (12). The γ-globulin structure is based on a computer/microscope imaging process (13), and the fibrinogen structure is that predicted by Doolittle et al (14).

Table I contains data pertaining to the secondary structure of these three proteins desorbed from a silated surface as reported previously (3). The structural assessments were made using a modified Greenfield/Fasman approach (6) and may be in considerable error. Nevertheless, the trend is very clear: proteins become denatured as a function of their residence time on the surface.

Fibrinogen, which in these particular experiments showed almost complete surface denaturation, is not stable in the solution phase. The protein undergoes aggregation and may precipitate after long periods in aqueous solution, particularly if polymerizing contaminants are present. However, aggregation and even polymerization do not affect the secondary structure (conformation) to any large degree, but may introduce artifacts into the interpretation of circular dichroism spectra because of anomalous scattering of nonuniform concentration. Aggregation probably does occur with desorbed fibrinogen, but it is almost certainly denatured also.

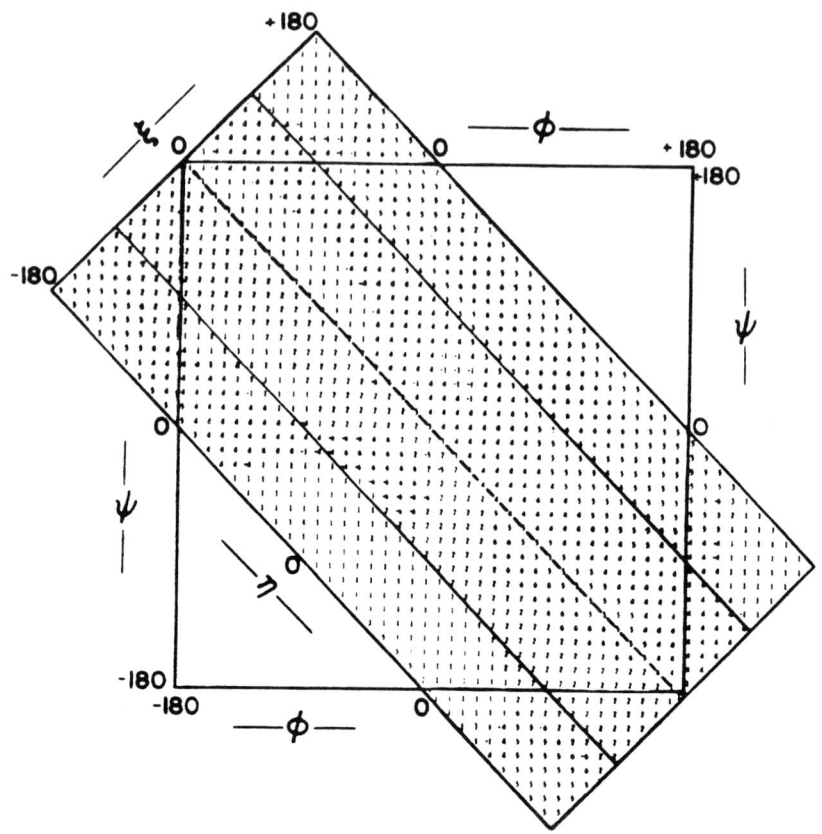

Figure 1a. Representation of protein bacterial nuclease in ϕ, φ space ($\phi = C-N$ and $\varphi = C_\alpha-C$).

Problems Associated with Circular Dichroism of Adsorbed Proteins

Reliable circular dichroism spectra cannot be obtained from crystalline, oriented polypeptide material that is birefringent or scatters light. However, monolayers of protein do not appear to provide anomalous spectra (4, 15), probably because of the relative uniformity of the film and the minimal refractive index increment at the protein/water interface. Nevertheless, previous results from this and other laboratories (3, 16, 17) have shown that albumin and fibrinogen molecules tend to lie "flat," that is, with their long axes parallel to the surface, whereas globulins lie perpendicular to the surface.

This surface orientation provides a peculiar problem in detailed interpretation of circular dichroism spectra, since a component of the interactive spectrum is plane polarized.

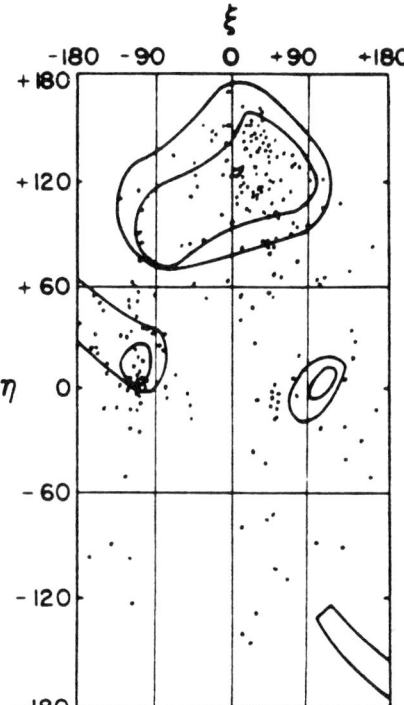

Figure 1b. Representation of the same protein as in Figure 1a in η, ξ space where $\eta = (\phi_{i+1} - \varphi_i)/2$ and $\xi_i = (\phi_{i+1}^+ + \varphi_i)$.

The problem of the interaction of circularly polarized light with an α-helix lying flat on a surface is depicted in Figure 3.

The intensity of ultraviolet light absorption is given by

$$I = \int \psi_g^{el} \mathbf{M} \psi_{ex}^{el} d\tau \qquad (4)$$

where ψ's are the appropriate wavefunction and **M** is an electric vector operator.

In Dirac notation Equation 4 is

$$I = <\psi_g|\boldsymbol{\mu}|\psi_{ex}> \qquad (5)$$

Now electronic transitions in the polypeptide are associated with the delocalized carbonyl electron. If the carbonyl group alone is considered in C_{2v} symmetry, the $n-\pi^*$ (symmetry forbidden transition) is a_2 and $\pi-\pi^*$ is b_1; in C_s symmetry one has a'' and a' allowed transitions. Neither is precisely correct, but for present purposes we can treat the $n-\pi^*$ transition as polarized perpendicular to the carbonyl bond and in the plane of the peptide group, and $\pi-\pi^*$ as in the plane of the peptide group and nearly parallel to

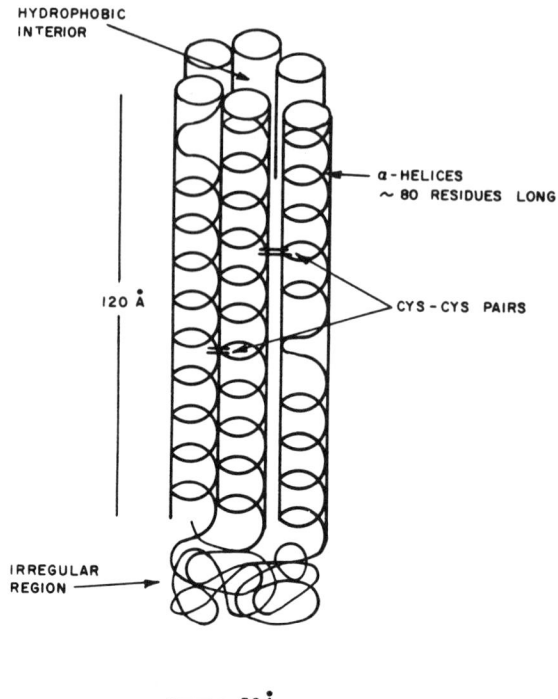

Figure 2a. Representation of albumin.

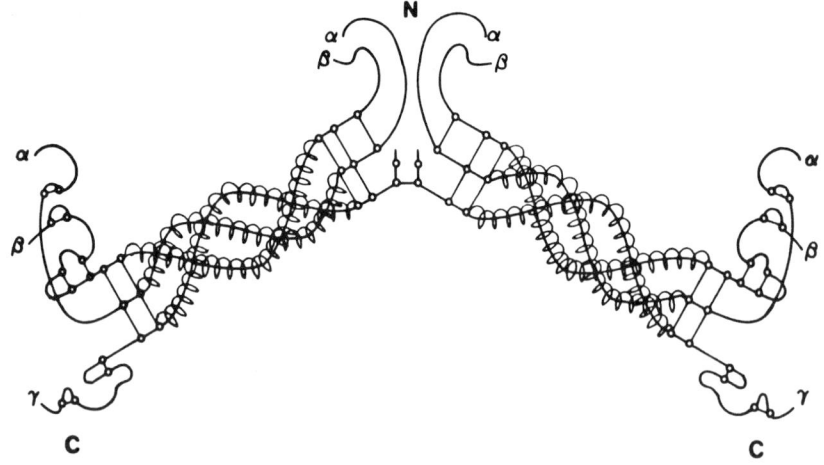

Figure 2b. Representation of fibronogen.

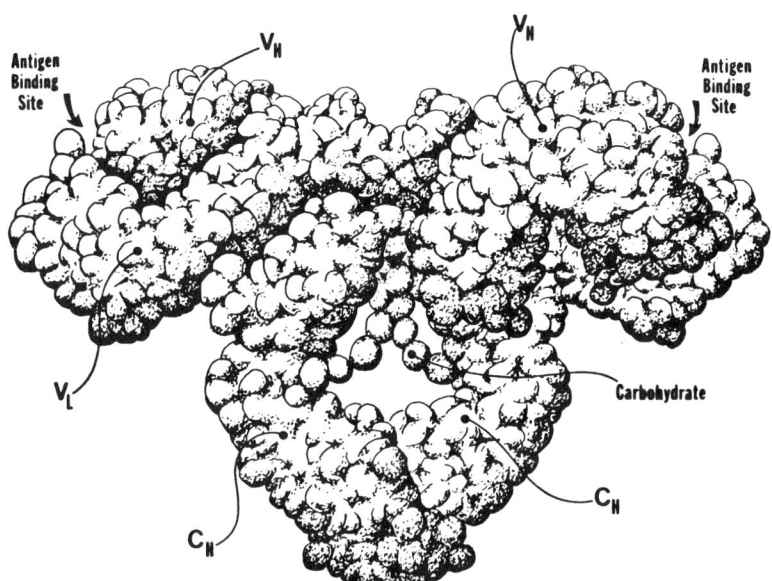

Figure 2c. Representation of γ-globulin.

Table I. Change of Desorbed Protein Structure on Tetradecane–Trimethylsilane–Coated Glass

Protein	Time (h)	% Desorbed	% Native Structure
Albumin	15	12	86
(pH 4.7, 0.13M)	22	21	29
	40	38	23
γ-Globulin			
(pH 7.4, 0.26M)	34	37	100
	106	66	78
	274	78	62
Bovine fibrinogen			
(pH 7.4, 0.26M)	36	7	42
	84	86	24
	128	100	2

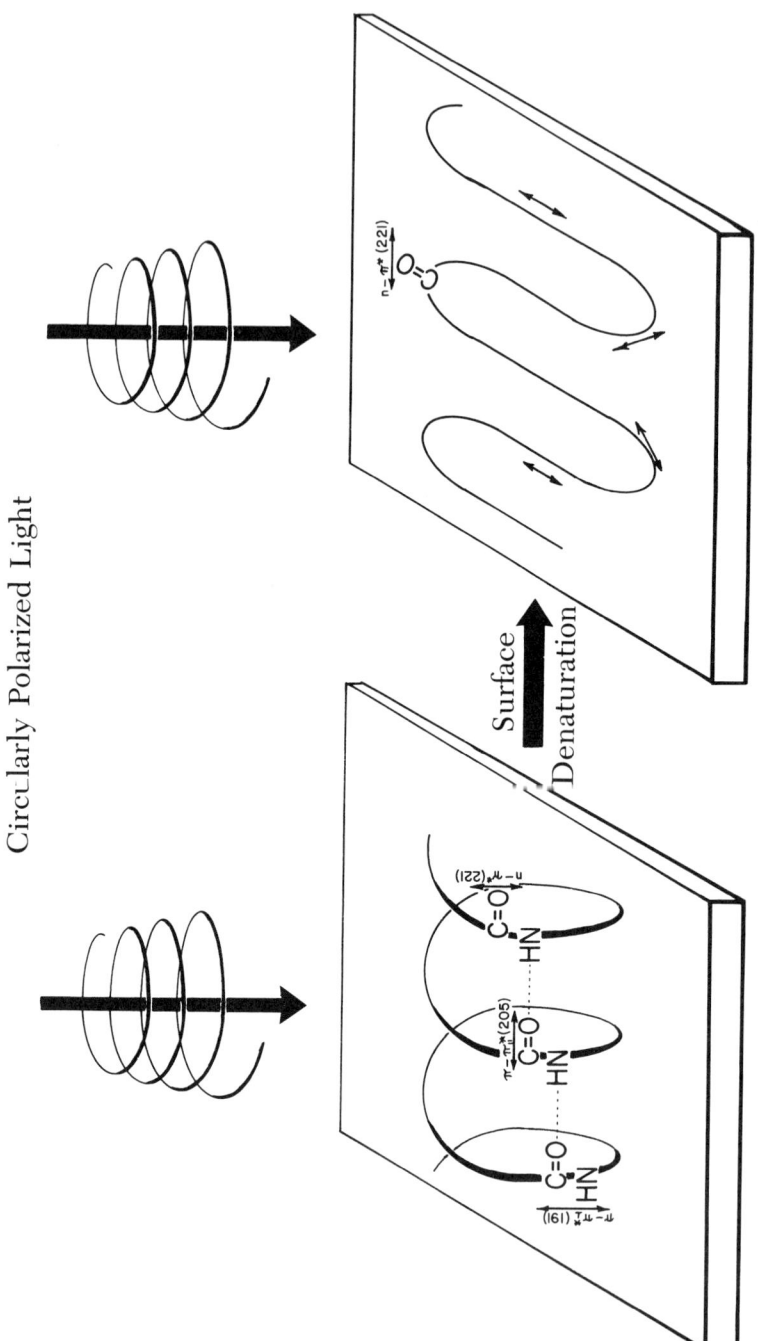

Figure 3. Polarization of electronic transitions in a flat α-helix vs. a flat irregular structure.

the carbonyl bond. Since the helix involves a rotation of the peptide group about the axis, absorption of linearly polarized light might be absorbed preferentially by the $\pi-\pi^*(\|)$ transition compared with the random orientation in solution.

In circular dichroism spectra the absorption intensity is given by

$$I = <\psi_g|\boldsymbol{\mu}|\psi_{ex}><\psi_g|\mathbf{m}|\psi_{ex}> \tag{6}$$

where **m** is the magnetic dipole operator. Whereas $\boldsymbol{\mu}$ transforms as x, y, z, **m** transforms as R_x, R_y, R_z, and thus weak vibronic $n-\pi^*$ coupled transitions are amplified. Without detailed calculations it is difficult to estimate a priori whether the magnitude of the magnetic or electric dipole components predominate; however, experimentally, the $n-\pi^*$ ($\lambda = 208$) band is amplified preferentially in two-dimensionally oriented helical films.

We can now examine the behavior of albumin adsorbed on quartz. Albumin was coated onto the four surfaces of a double compartment cell allowed to incubate for about 15 min, rinsed, filled with doubly distilled water, and then examined by accumulation circular dichroism spectroscopy. The spectra are shown in Figure 4. Although the protein cannot definitely be

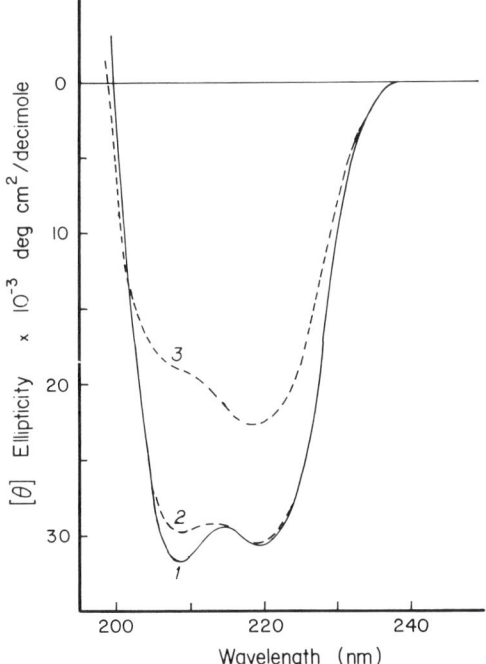

Figure 4. Successive averaged circular dichroism spectra of BSA on quartz: (1) solution spectrum; (2) adsorption spectrum at 15 min; and (3) adsorption spectrum at 6 h.

placed on the surface throughout the experiment, the bathing solution showed no detectable protein present at the end of the experiment. The thickness of the film, and protein ellipticity, can be calculated essentially by reverse use of Equations 1–3, although the modified shape of the spectrum creates some ($\pm 5\%$) uncertainty. The spectrum at early time resembles the solution spectrum with a modified band ratio that we ascribe to protein orientation, and subsequently, the ellipticity decreases in accord with our previous observations (3). The decreased structure in the protein does not appear to correlate with the normal denaturation process in which a band at 205 nm usually predominates. Since the outside of the albumin helices consists of ionic residues typically in the 1,4,7 . . . sequence of helices with one hydrophobic side, the helices would probably unwind to present the more hydrophobic interior of the protein to the surface. The unusual nature of the denatured albumin spectrum would then correspond to an irregular two-dimensional structure in which the $\pi-\pi^*(\|)$ component has been minimized by the loss of the oriented helices.

The problem with detailed assessment of the structure of surface adsorbed proteins is that the two-dimensional orientation of structural features gives a linear component to the resultant spectrum. Nevertheless, in the surface denaturation of adsorbed albumin, the helices appear to unfold such that the $n-\pi^*$ transition is amplified at the expense of the $\pi-\pi^*$ transition. This situation suggests binding of the carbonyl group of the peptide to the surface, or at least orientation of the carbonyl group perpendicular to the surface.

Chromatographic Examination of Protein Adsorption

Application of a quantity of solution, in this case protein solution, to a column filled with appropriate substrate, leads to an exchange between the solute and the surface, and movement with the solvent front such that the emerging solute profile contains complete information concerning the kinetics of adsorption/desorption. Apart from the interaction of solute with surface, concurrent three-dimensional diffusion often occurs, and perhaps occlusion, if the substrate is porous. Nevertheless, the option of deducing interfacial kinetics from the elution profile in a flowing system has a certain elegance and relevance to the performance of blood plasma proteins in vivo.

The details of the system are presented elsewhere (18), but in brief: an adsorbate consisting of 0.14-mm glass spheres coated with various silane coupling agents was packed into 50×0.7–cm glass columns (total surface area 2400 cm^2). Constant flow rate and temperature were maintained using a peristaltic pump and a temperature-controlled water jacket. The protein solution of concentration c_o was pumped through the column, and the emerging effluent profile was monitored by ultraviolet light absorbance at 280 nm. Proteins have a tendency to aggregate and the adsorption characteristics may well be different for different aggregation states. Consequently, both input and effluent protein aggregation were monitored by high pressure liquid chromatography (HPLC).

The chromatographic profile was evaluated using the following mass balance equation:

$$D_{ax}\frac{\delta^2 c}{\delta x^2} - v\frac{\delta c}{\delta x} - \frac{\delta q}{\delta t} = \frac{\delta c}{\delta t} \tag{7}$$

Where D_{ax} is the axial diffusion coefficient, x is the position of the profile along the flow direction, v is the linear flow velocity, t is the time variable, and c and q are the concentrations of the solute in solution and the adsorbed state, respectively (19).

Experimental interest lies in the value of q that depends on the applied concentration, that is, where $q = f(c)$, which thus describes the isotherm of the adsorbate. Application of protein solution to the column produced an effluent profile of the type shown in Figure 5. The amount of protein adsorbed may be calculated by integrating the area between the void volume and the actual effluent profile (lateral diffusion, D_{ax}, does not modify the integrated area). A series of runs using different c_o values thus establishes a "dynamic" isotherm.

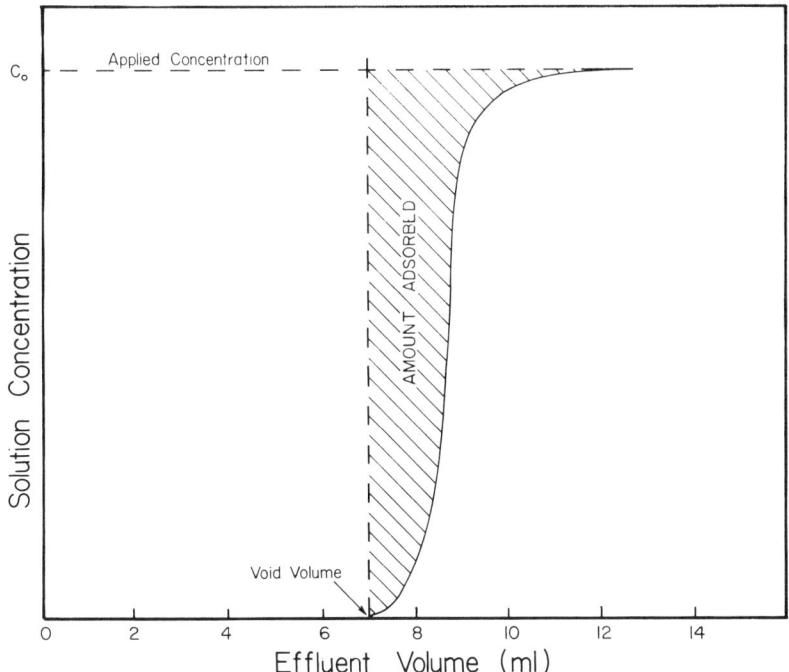

Figure 5. Emergent front of BSA on aminopropyltriethoxysilane-treated glass beads. The shape of the front should represent the adsorption process and diffusion broadening.

Using this method, we constructed a number of dynamic adsorption isotherms for several proteins on different surfaces. Here we present information for two proteins. The adsorption isotherm for bovine serum albumin (BSA) (87% monomer, 13% dimer; described by the supplier as 100% monomer) is shown in Figure 6. A plateau concentration for BSA on an amine/silane surface was 3.5 mg/m^2, which is comparable with monolayer adsorption reported previously in a static system (3). [The effect of flow rate, ionic strength, and temperature is reported elsewhere (18).] Perhaps more interesting are the data for plasma fibronectin (produced and purified extensively in our laboratory), because adsorption characteristics of this protein have not been reported elsewhere. Since it is a protein intimately involved in cellular adhesion, its surface behavior is particularly relevant to implant biocompatibility. We found a plateau uptake of approximately 7.0 mg/m^2 on both amine and dimethyldimethoxymethylsilane, and based on the assumption of monolayer coverage and a published axial ratio (20), we calculated that the molecule has dimensions of approximately $130 \times 80 \times 100$ Å.

Aside from the relative position of the profile, the shape of the effluent profile contains information concerning the kinetics of the adsorption process. All concentrations of protein from zero to c_o are brought into contact with the column surface as the protein solution flows through the column, as a function of the position of the profile, and therefore as a function of time. Working with small molecules, previous researchers have shown that compounds exhibiting Langmuir isotherms produce sharp fronts, and diffuse "tails," if pure solvent is used to desorb the column (21, 22). However, Equation 7 shows that both diffusional and adsorption effects can alter the shape of the effluent profile. The former effect includes both normal molecular diffusion, and also diffusion due to flow properties in the column (eddy diffusion), which broadens (decreases the slope) the affluent profiles. To examine the adsorption processes, apart from the diffusional effects, the following technique can be applied.

If the surface is first saturated with a monolayer of protein exposed to steady-state concentration c_o, and then is exposed to a second treatment at concentration $2c_o$, a second front emerges. The second profile represents the situation where no net protein is adsorbed and thus, in principle, is representative of the diffusion-shifted flow pattern of the nonadsorbed protein. Figure 7 shows both the initial (c_o) and second ($2c_o$) fronts and the subtraction curve which is very close to the ideal "step function." If the data are interpreted as solution-borne molecules passing over an inert surface, then (a) adsorption must be essentially instantaneous and (b) the surface must become covered by exhausting the concentration of solute at the front as it moves down the column. The slope of the difference profile should represent the rate of uptake of material on the column, and that is essentially infinite on the time scale of the experiment. The point of inflection of the subtracted front indicates the slowing of the sorption process due to filling of sites on the surface.

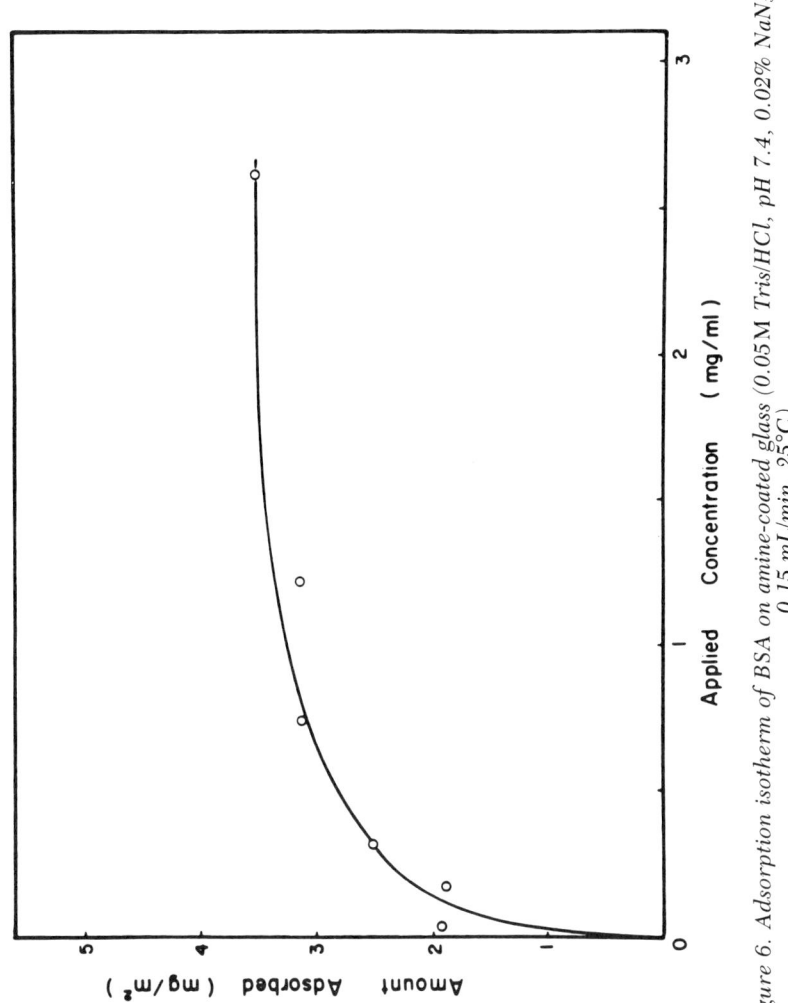

Figure 6. *Adsorption isotherm of BSA on amine-coated glass (0.05M Tris/HCl, pH 7.4, 0.02% NaN$_3$, 0.15 mL/min, 25°C).*

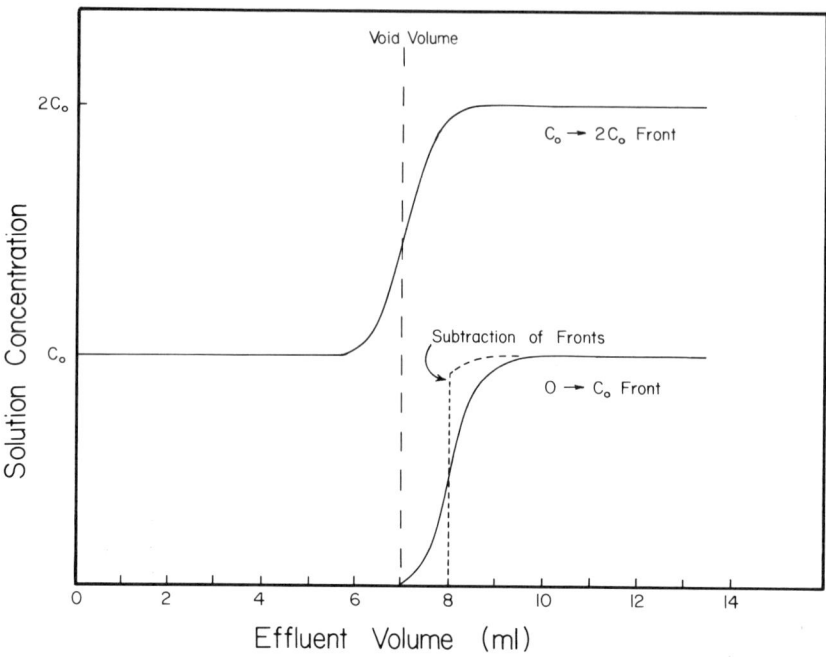

Figure 7. Two-step adsorption experiment with c_o great enough to form monolayer coverage. Then, $2c_o$ is applied and the resultant frontal profiles are subtracted as shown (- - -).

Alternatively, the saturated substrate may not be inert to new solution-borne protein molecules, but may exchange with such molecules (23). The result of such a process, which does indeed occur as will be shown later, does not appear to alter adsorption effluent profiles.

In some ways, analyses of these profiles are disappointing since they indicate that the adsorption portion of the elution profile does not provide a great deal of information concerning the adsorption kinetics. However, analysis of these frontal profiles has allowed us to examine protein–protein exchange processes that occur as the protein solution passes through the column. This has been accomplished by collecting and analyzing fractions by HPLC (Waters Associates I–250 protein column).

Initial experiments had indicated that the monomer standard BSA powder used in our experiments contained 13% dimer. Previous studies have shown that the different molecular weight species of human serum albumin exhibit varied affinities for surfaces (24). We were interested in elucidating the effect of dimer species in our adsorption experiments. The molecular weight differences of the monomer and dimer allowed us to follow the relative concentrations of each species in the effluent profile. Figure 8 illustrates the data obtained from a run in which 1.0 mg/mL BSA was applied to a methyl-coated column. Both the amount of BSA adsorbed in an effluent fraction (0.1 mL) and the percentage dimer adsorbed in this fraction are plotted against the number of void volumes eluted. This figure indicates that while the BSA dimer may in fact diffuse to the surface more slowly than the monomer (no initial dimer preference), as the adsorption process continues, monomer is replaced preferentially with dimer on the surface. This is shown by the increasing percentage of dimer adsorbed. Apparently, a surface equilibrium is reached because the adsorbed percentage of dimer decreases to the applied stock solution value. If the area under the percentage dimer curve is integrated, 19% of the adsorbed surface layer contains BSA dimer, which is 6% greater than the applied value. Similar results were found on the amine surface (21% dimer), but in contrast, a much greater dimer preference was found on a surface coated with N-(trimethoxysilylpropyl)ethylenediaminetriacetic acid (carboxyl), indicating that preferential adsorption and exchange depend on surface chemistry.

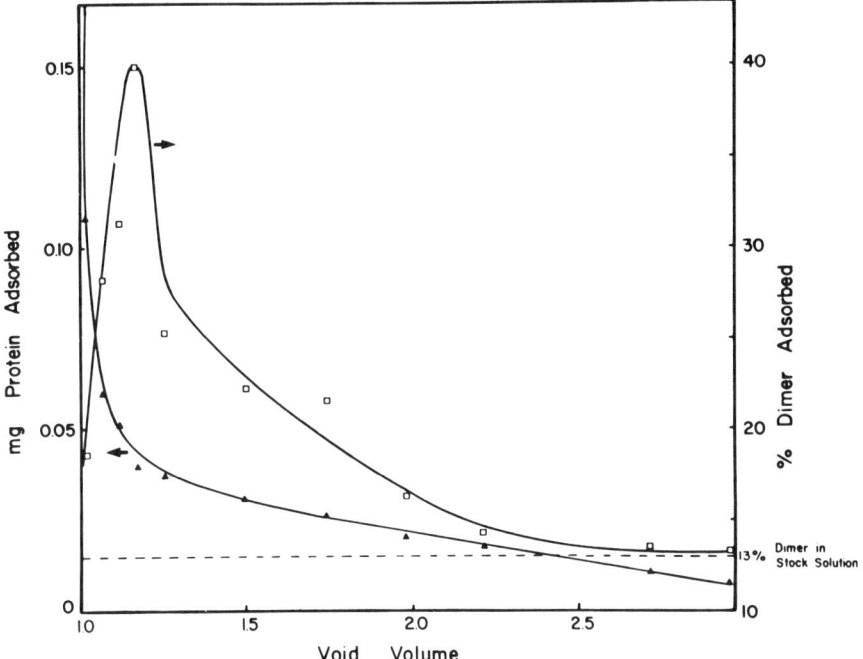

Figure 8. *Instantaneous adsorption of BSA on a methyl-coated surface. The stock solution of BSA contained 13% dimer* (0.05 M Tris/HCl, pH 7.4, 0.02% NaN_3, 0.15 mL/min, 37°C, c_o=1.0 mg/mL). Key: ▲, *the amount of BSA adsorbed from a single effluent volume;* □, *the percentage of dimer adsorbed in the same effluent volume.*

Similarly, the exchange of one protein for another on a surface was examined. Experiments were performed in which BSA was precoated on an amine-coated column to which a solution of pure fibronectin was subsequently applied. Figure 9 shows the relative concentration of BSA monomer, dimer, and fibronectin in the column effluent. Fibronectin displaced the BSA monomer but not the dimer. A similar effect was observed on the methylsilane surface.

Desorption Processes

The desorption behavior of BSA was investigated by first applying a solution of BSA to the column, obtaining equilibrium ($c = c_o$), and then eluting the column with buffer solution. While the aforementioned two-step procedure can be used to subtract diffusional effects from the profile, an additional mixing effect at the detector precluded exact analysis of the desorption profile shapes. We estimated the amount of desorbable BSA by integrating the concentration area after the void volume to obtain the total amount of BSA desorbed from the column. A series of experiments were conducted in which both applied concentration and flow rate were varied, and both the amount of BSA adsorbed and desorbed were calculated. Data obtained from the amine-coated columns are given in Figure 10. At each datum point, the same flow rate was used for both adsorption and desorption. Furthermore, the point indicating the lowest flow rate and the lowest applied concentration required the longest time to reach adsorption equilibrium (13.6 h), whereas the point indicating the highest flow rate and the highest concentration required the shortest equilibrium time (15 min). In the former case, only 20% of the adsorbed BSA desorbed, while in the latter case, 58% BSA desorbed. These data are in accordance with previous experiments, which have shown that as protein molecules are allowed more time to interact with a surface, they tend to change conformation and become more resistant to desorption (3). While shear effects certainly contribute to the amount of protein capable of being desorbed, the upward trend of the data at each flow rate indicates an applied concentration dependence, which is also an important contributing term to the equilibrium time.

Interpretation of Adsorption/Desorption Information

Previously we have postulated several stages in the interfacial behavior of proteins (3).

Initial Fast Reversible Adsorption. The chromatographic profiles indicate that protein is adsorbed almost instantaneously on coated glass surfaces, and at short adsorption times, the contact points of the protein with the surface are limited and the kinetic energy of colliding solvent molecules is sufficient to cause desorption, that is, the desorption rate is a function of the surface adsorbed concentration.

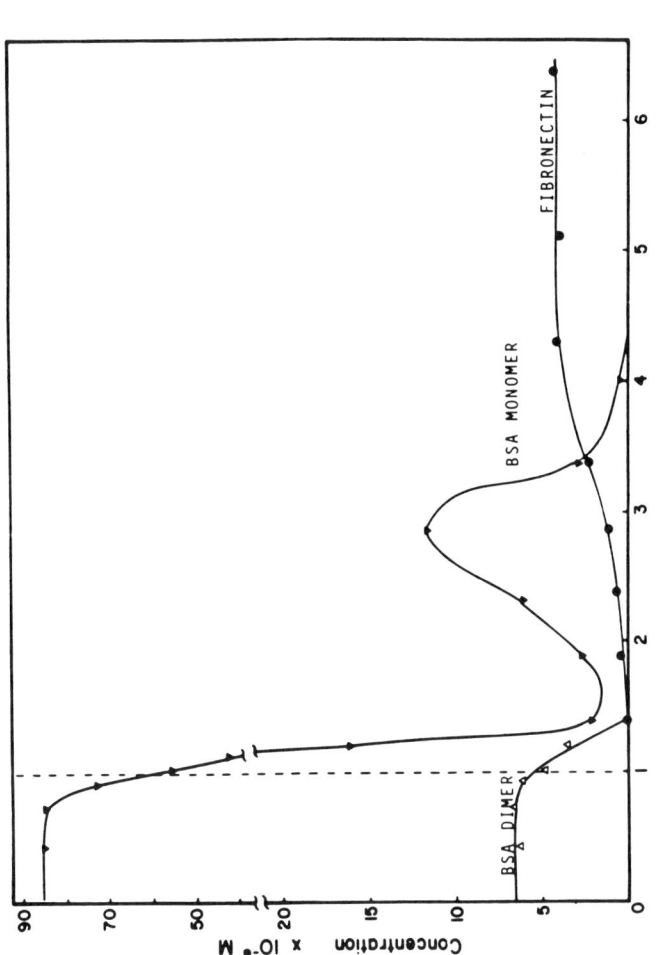

Figure 9. Exchange of BSA by fibronectin on amine-coated surface. Profiles illustrate the molar concentrations of each protein in the column effluent. The dashed line indicates the void volume, or the point at which the BSA solution is just displaced from the column by the fibronectin solution (0.05 M Tris/HCl, 0.02% NaN$_3$, pH 7.4, 0.15 mL/min, 37°C). Key: ●, fibronectin; ▼, BSA monomer; and △, BSA dimer.

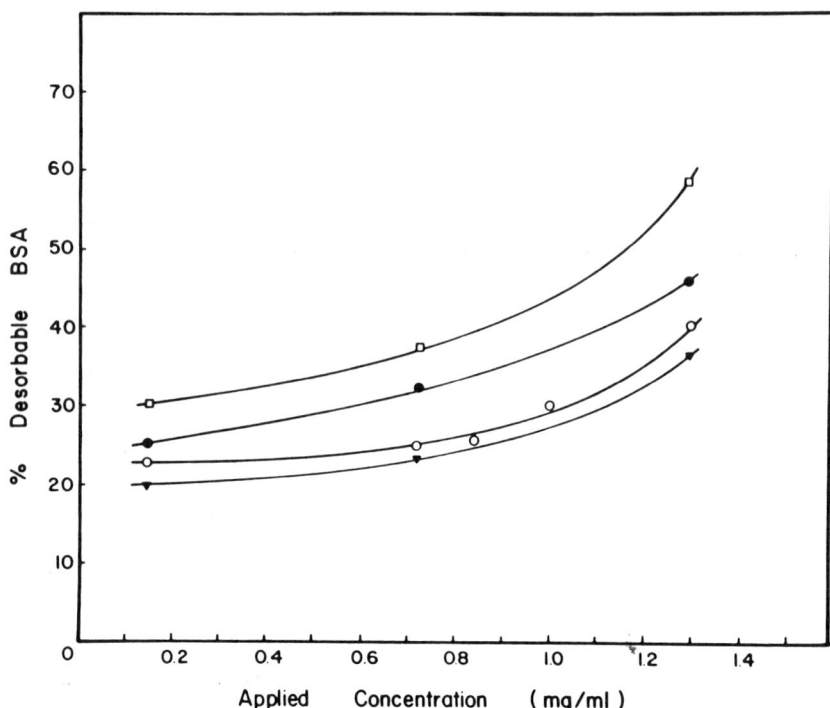

Figure 10. Desorption plot of BSA on amine-coated surface showing the relationship between the percent of desorbable protein as a function of applied concentration and flow rate (0.05 M Tris/HCl, pH 7.4, 0.02% NaN_3, 25°C). Key of flow rates: □, 0.672 mL/min; ●, 0.277 mL/min; ○, 0.150 mL/min; and ▼, 0.087 mL/min.

Induced Desorption. As the protein prolongs its stay on the surface, three phenomena occur—the protein molecule becomes partially desolvated and increases its interaction with the substrate, time-dependent conformational changes occur, and surface spreading is evident. Under the first of these circumstances, simple collision with solvent molecules no longer provides the momentum transfer for desorption; however, collision with the larger protein molecules does provide sufficient momentum exchange, and exchange of surface and solution molecules results. As the denaturation process occurs and the surface binding increases, more kinetic energy is required and may only be achievable by a combination of shear energy and collision exchange.

Desorption of Denatured Protein. The energetics of protein binding to hydrophobic surfaces probably involves the unfolding of protein to achieve optimal hydrophobic bonding, but is undoubtedly entropically driven. In our experience, previously denatured protein does not adhere significantly to polymer surfaces, probably because no further entropic contribution to binding can be obtained.

Since we have shown previously that at very long periods (days) significant portions of almost completely denatured albumins, γ-globulin, and fibrinogen are desorbed from hydrophobic surfaces, this effect also is probably related to entropic considerations.

Summary

The kinetics of the adsorption/desorption process are complex and consist of an initial period where equilibrium is achieved essentially in a few seconds.

Subsequently, desorption slows because of protein convolutions, and thus, in principle, the surface should take up more material. However, several factors contribute to decreased adsorption efficiency:

(1) Collision of one molecule with the surface may displace one or more surface adsorbed species.
(2) The surface area available for adsorption may decrease due to expansion of surface adsorbed material. This feature can be observed by successive adsorptions of material where surface saturation may be achieved at $2.5 mg/m^2$ or less of BSA.
(3) Collision of previously adsorbed molecules may have diminished efficiency.

The interrelationship of these processes appears to depend on the nature of the protein and substrate. If the protein is a typical plasma protein and the surface highly hydrophobic, the surface denaturation is accelerated, and the binding is strong and mainly irreversible in the second and subsequent stage. If, however, the protein has a particularly stable tertiary structure and the surface is highly hydrated, the first, reversible phase may be maintained almost indefinitely.

Acknowledgment

This work was supported in part by an Institutional Biomedical Sciences Grant from the National Institutes of Health.

Literature Cited

1. Walton, A. G. In "Biomedical Polymers"; Goldberg, E., Ed.; Academic: New York, 1980.
2. Walton, A. G.; Soderquist, M. E. *Croat. Chem. Acta* **1980**, 363.
3. Soderquist, M. E.; Walton, A. G. *J. Colloid Interface Sci.* **1980**, 75, 386.
4. McMillin, C. R.; Walton, A. G. *J. Colloid Interface Sci.* **1974**, 48, 345.

5. McMillin, C. R.; Saito, H.; Ratnoff, O. D.; Walton, A. G. *J. Clin. Invest.* **1974**, *54*, 1312.
6. Greenfield, N.; Fasman, G. D. *Biochemistry* **1969**, *8*, 4108.
7. Brahms, S.; Brahms, J. *J. Mol. Biol.* **1980**, *138*, 149.
8. Saxena, V. P.; Wetlaufer, D. B. *Proc. Natl. Acad. Sci. U.S.A.* **1971**, *68*, 969.
9. Hennessey, J. P.; Johnson, W. C., *Biochemistry*, in press.
10. Walton, A. G.; Solomon, D. D.; Rao, S. P.; Hurwitz, F. *Polym. Prep., Am. Chem. Soc., Div. Polym. Chem.* **1979**, *20*(2) 82.
11. Fasman, G. D.; Chou, P. Y. *Biophys. J.* **1976**, *16*, 1202.
12. Walton, A. G. *Proc. Int. Symp. Biomol. Struct.* **1980**, 76.
13. Fox, J. L. *Chem. Eng. News* **1979**, *57*, 22.
14. Dolittle, R. F., *Polym. Prep., Am. Chem. Soc., Div. Polym. Chem.* **1979**, *20*(2), 47.
15. Akaike, T. *Polym. Prep., Am. Chem. Soc., Div. Polym. Chem.* **1979**, *20*(1), 581.
16. W. Norde, Ph.D. Thesis, Agr. Univ., Wageningen, Netherlands, 1976.
17. Norde, W.; Lyklema, J. *J. Colloid Interface Sci.* **1978**, *66*, 257.
18. Koltisko, B. M.; Walton, A. G., M.S. Thesis, Case Western University, Cleveland, Ohio, 1981.
19. Giddings, J. C. "Dynamics of Chromatography, Chromatographic Science Series"; Dekker: New York, 1966; Vol. 1.
20. Alexander, S., Jr.; Colonna, G.; Edelhoch, H. *J. Biol. Chem.* **1979**, *254*(5), 1501.
21. Habgood, H. W. In "The Solid–Gas Interface"; Flood, E. A., Ed.; Dekker: New York, 1967; Vol. 2.
22. Locke, D. C. *Adv. Chromatogr.* **1976**, *14*, 87.
23. Brash, J. L.; Samak, Q. M. *J. Colloid Interface Sci.* **1978**, *65*, 495.
24. Smith, L. E., Natl. Bur. Stand. Report, Devices and Tech. Branch, Div. of Heart and Vascular Diseases, Gaithersburg, MD; 1976.

RECEIVED for review January 16, 1981. ACCEPTED May 21, 1981.

19
Proteins, Plasma, and Blood in Narrow Spaces of Clot-Promoting Surfaces

LEO VROMAN, ANN L. ADAMS, GENA C. FISCHER,
PRISCILLA C. MUNOZ, and MICHAEL STANFORD

Veterans Administration Medical Center, Interface Laboratory, Brooklyn, NY 11209

> *Blood plasma deposits fibrinogen on many surfaces. On those able to activate clotting, high molecular weight kininogen and factor XII supplant the adsorbed fibrinogen. Platelets adhere only where fibrinogen remains adsorbed. In recent studies we found that, in spaces of less than about 10 μm wide, plasma contains insufficient high molecular weight kininogen and factor XII per surface area to supplant the fibrinogen; here platelets will adhere. Between a glass convex lens and a glass or anodized tantalum slide, plasma will leave a central disc of fibrinogen; diluted plasma will leave a larger ring of which the center—where the thin plasma layer lacks sufficient fibrinogen—may contain a ring of albumin. Whole blood leaves a ring of platelets corresponding to that of fibrinogen; in absence of erythrocytes the ring of platelets deposited is smaller.*

When blood plasma comes into contact with a solid, it will deposit proteins at the interface within 1 s. Fibrinogen dominates the proteins adsorbed onto many materials (1). On surfaces such as glass, which is known to activate clotting, plasma will quickly supplant its own fibrinogen deposit by high molecular weight kininogen and by factor XII (2). High molecular weight kininogen carries factor XI and prekallikrein to the surface (3), and the interactions among these factors (4) probably complete the surface activation of the intact plasma clotting system.

Where high molecular weight kininogen and factor XII in intact form are limited, for example, in plasma congenitally deficient in this kininogen (5), and in activated plasma, much less fibrinogen is supplanted. Even in normal intact plasma, the concentration of fibrinogen is greater than that of high molecular weight kininogen and factor XII by an order of magnitude. On the other hand, the affinity of high molecular weight kininogen for glass is very high (5). Consequently, in a thin layer of blood, factor XII and high molecular weight kininogen may be depleted by adsorption on the activating surface before all adsorbed fibrinogen is supplanted. Since platelets only adhere where they find adsorbed fibrinogen (6), they should adhere in narrow spaces, rather than on more open areas where the activating surface will have supplanted all fibrinogen before the platelets arrive.

In the present study we allowed normal intact plasma to fill spaces of varied thickness on anodized tantalum–sputtered glass (TaO) or on glass, and then rendered the resulting pattern visible by subsequent exposure to antisera. The most suitable configuration of solid surfaces was a convex lens placed on a slide: it allowed us to compute and correlate liquid film heights with the radii of circular concentric patterns resulting from the experiments. Fibrinogen solutions, heparinized blood, and citrated plasma were used in this arrangement of interfaces.

Our methods for detecting and identifying adsorbed proteins were tested further with known proteins, matching and nonmatching antisera in recent years (1, 7, 8), and proved to be specific.

Experimental

Materials. Anodized tantalum–sputtered glass slides (TaO). Tantalum-sputtered glass slides, 1×3 and 3×4 in., were kindly supplied by N. Schwartz and D. Gerstenberg, Bell Telephone Labs; others were purchased from Millis Research. Slides were anodized at approximately 20 V in 0.01% nitric acid, to obtain a deep-bronze, first-order interference color at nearly vertically incident natural light (7). Glass slides (borosilicate glass, 1×3 in. or larger) (A.H. Thomas); Kimwipes (Kimberly–Clark Corp.); Sparkleen detergent (Fisher Scientific Co.); antisera to human fibrinogen (Behring Diagnostics, and M. Mosesson, SUNY at Downstate); and Coomassie Brilliant Blue R or G (2), were purchased from the suppliers indicated. Veronal-buffered saline, pH 7.4, was prepared as described in Ref. 1. Normal human intact citrated plasma obtained from freshly donated blood by centrifugation (2) at 20°C was stored in aliquots in polystyrene test tubes at -75°C. Red cell poor blood was prepared by collecting blood into 100 U of heparin (Lipohepin of Riker Labs. or heparin from K&K Labs. Inc.) per approximately 10 mL of blood, allowing it to settle in polystyrene tubes, and then collecting the red cell poor, but platelet and white cell rich, supernatant. Curved surfaces were provided by several objects: a 1-in. diameter stainless steel ball bearing ball (radius 12.7 mm), and several plano-convex lenses with a diameter of 42 mm and radii of curvature ranging from 44 to 2000 mm.

Handling and Cleaning of Test Solids. Slides and curved objects were handled with forceps. Kimwipes wound around applicator sticks were drenched in concentrated Sparkleen, and were used to brush all materials. The materials were then rinsed with large amounts of distilled water, dried in a clean air current, and passed five times across the colorless section of a gas flame. All materials were used within 10 min after cleaning and cooling; all were highly wettable for water.

Procedure. All experiments were carried out at room temperature (about 20°C). The lens was placed on a glass or TaO slide. Then, 0.2 to 0.4 mL of intact plasma that had been thawed at 37°C was deposited with an automatic plastic pipet between curved surface and slide so that it spread rapidly between the two surfaces. The preparation was placed in a moist chamber, and after 10 to 30 min (effects of time within a range of 10–60 min having proved minimal), the slide was flooded with large amounts of Veronal-buffered saline, slightly tilted to allow the lens to float off (a technique that proved not to damage significantly the adsorbed protein film under it), rinsed with more Veronal-buffered saline and then covered with 0.1 mL of an antiserum while wet with the saline. Then, 4 min later, the slides were rinsed with Veronal-buffered saline followed by water. The TaO slides were dried in a flow of clean air, while the glass slides were covered with a solution of one of the Coomassie Blues (250 mg of dye in 50 mL of methanol and 10 mL of glacial acetic acid, diluted to 100 mL with distilled water). Four min later, these slides were flooded and rinsed with water, and then air dried. In other experiments, red cell poor and whole heparinized blood were used. Blood was applied like the plasma and rinsed off with Veronal-buffered saline, after 10 min, but these preparations were then fixed with 2.5% glutaraldehyde in the saline, and stained (if on glass) with Wright's stain or a Coomassie Blue. Preparations on TaO substrates were not stained, but rinsed with water and observed with a vertically illuminating microscope. Experiments with protein solutions were carried out as were those with plasma. When a steel ball was used, it was held in a holder that allowed it to be moved only normal to the plane of the slide, so that it could be lifted off vertically after the first Veronal-buffered saline rinse. Diameters of the resulting circular patterns were measured with calipers, and if small, with a microscope provided with a calibrated grid in the ocular.

In previous studies, we avoided creating an air/solution/solid interface, where a protein film on the advancing fluid could otherwise be transferred to the solid. In the present arrangement, prewetting either the lens or slide with Veronal-buffered saline would introduce unpredictable flow and dilution effects when the protein-containing reagent was added. In several tests the following sequence of reagents was applied. Lens and slide were wetted with Veronal-buffered saline, a large amount of plasma was allowed to flow over the lens with its convex side up, and then the plasma-wetted lens was placed rapidly on the buffer-wetted slide. The results of these tests correspond to those of the experiments carried out on the wettable surfaces without prewetting. Data reported here refer to the latter technique.

Results

Where plasma had resided for 10 min to several hours, it left little or no immunologically detectable fibrinogen, except as a tiny disc around the point of contact between curved and planar surface. Figure 1 shows patterns of fibrinogen left in a space between a convex lens and a glass slide by increasingly diluted normal intact plasma (top row) and by fibrinogen (bottom row). Curvature of the lens was approximately 95 mm. Results were obtained with undiluted plasma (top, left), plasma diluted 1:10 with Veronal-buffered saline (top, center), and plasma diluted 1:50 (top, right). Dark areas indicate deep staining due to the presence of antifibrinogen on fibrinogen. Little fibrinogen remained where plasma had been injected (upper left corners of each photograph). The large circles correspond to the areas between lens and slide that were filled with plasma; only the center of the circle left by undiluted plasma contains fibrinogen. Beyond this circle, the plasma deposited some fibrinogen during its brief contact with the surface while being rinsed off. Little or no fibrinogen was deposited by the diluted plasma samples in the narrowest spaces, the plasma that had been diluted 1:50 showing the most notable central "empty" hole. At this dilution, the plasma

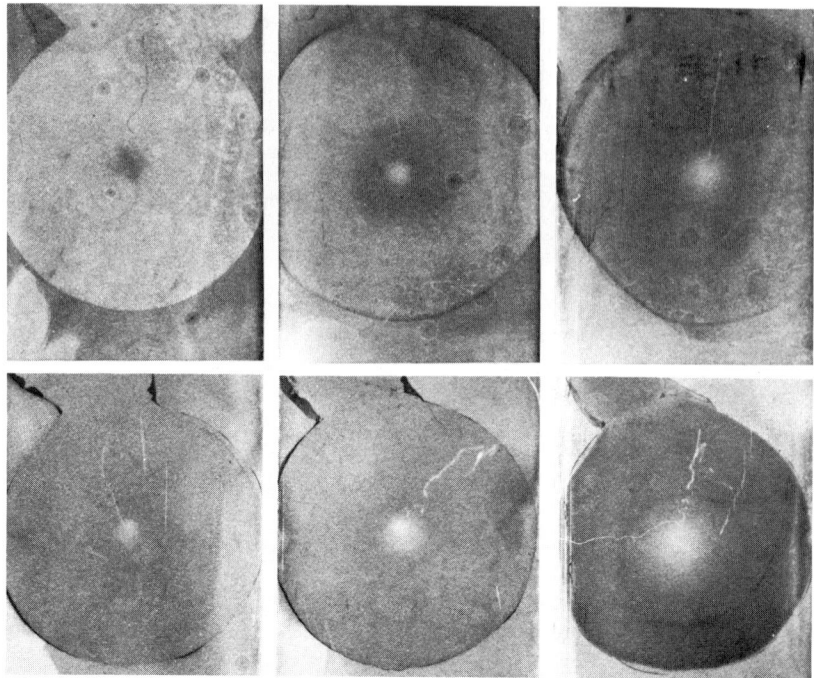

Figure 1. Fibrinogen left between convex lens and glass slide by various dilutions of plasma (top row) and of fibrinogen solutions (bottom row) (see text).

left fibrinogen wherever it had resided beyond this "hole", but was apparently too diluted to leave fibrinogen during its brief contact while washed beyond the area of prolonged residence.

Identical experiments were performed with solutions of fibrinogen (M. Mosesson, SUNY at Downstate, Brooklyn, NY; protein more than 90% clottable) at concentrations of 6 (Figure 1, bottom, left), 3 (center), and 0.3 (right) mg/mL of Veronal-buffered saline. The empty center increased with increasing dilution. Measurements and calculations (see equation below) are given in Table I.

In several experiments, only half of the pattern left by plasma was exposed to antiserum (*see* Figure 2). A lens with a curvature of approximately 147 mm was used on a TaO surface, and plasma was applied as described. The right half of the treated, air-dried surface was then covered with antiserum to human fibrinogen, and rinsed off 5 min later with Veronal-buffered saline followed by water. After air drying, the interference pattern (purple; darkest in the photograph, indicating thickest protein layer) showed a central dark semicircle only on the right (antiserum) side, indicating the presence of fibrinogen. Also on the antiserum-treated side, beyond the large circle where plasma had resided for 10 min, a darker area (right top and bottom of Figure 2) showed that, here again, brief contact with plasma during rinsing had caused it to deposit but not yet to remove fibrinogen.

The radius A_1 of the small central fibrinogen disc left by the plasma depended on the radius R of the curved object that had been used (*see* Table II) in such a way that the height of the plasma layer at the outer edge of the fibrinogen disc, being $H_1 = R - \sqrt{(R^2 - A_1^2)}$, was more or less constant, that is, about 10 μm (*see* Table II and Figure 3). Some normal plasma samples yielded slightly higher values.

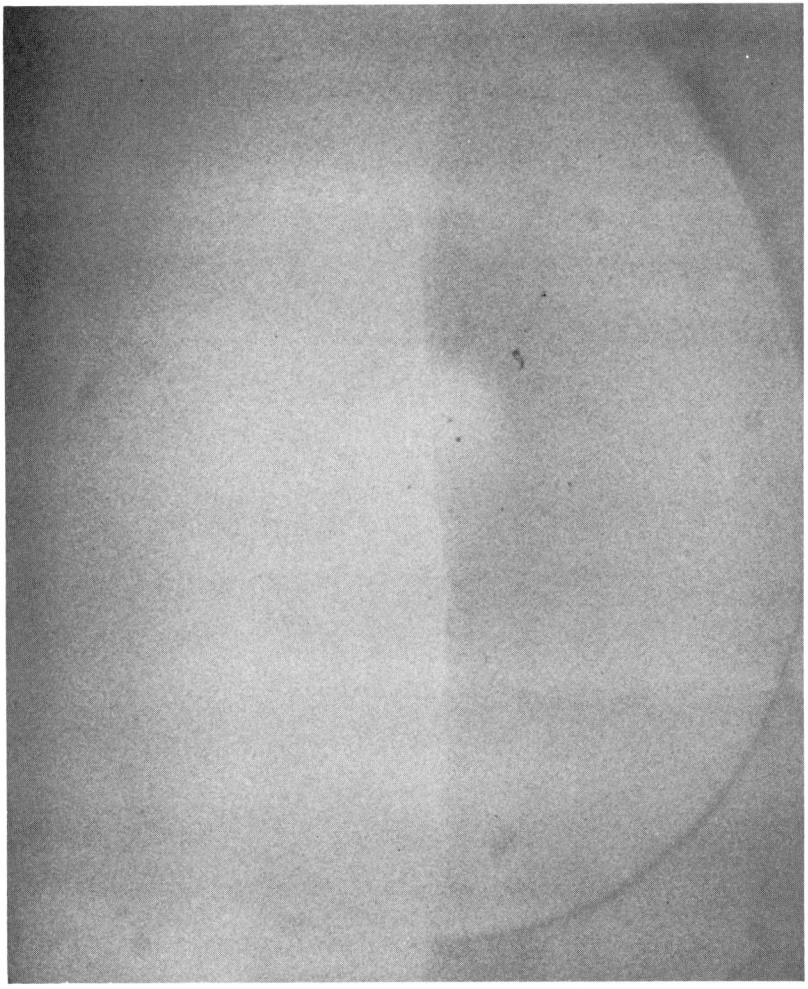

Figure 2. Fibrinogen left by intact plasma between convex lens and anodized tantalum–sputtered glass slide. Only right half of pattern was exposed to antiserum to fibrinogen (see text).

The very small "blank hole" at the center of the fibrinogen disc, increasing in size with dilution of plasma and fibrinogen solution used, had a radius A_2 corresponding to a liquid layer height of $H_2 = R - \sqrt{(R^2 - A_2^2)}$ (see Figure 3 and values in Tables I and II). The significance of H_2 is discussed later.

On TaO, rather than on glass, plasma diluted with 100 or more volumes of Veronal-buffered saline left a ring of albumin within the "empty hole" that lacked fibrinogen. A lens with a radius of curvature of approximately 2000 mm was used. The experiments were carried out as described, but antiserum to human albumin rather than to fibrinogen was used. The slide was rinsed with Veronal-buffered saline 2 min after its application, and 0.1 mL of goat antiserum to rabbit gamma globulins was applied; 2 min later the slide was rinsed with the buffered-saline, rinsed with water, and then air dried. The

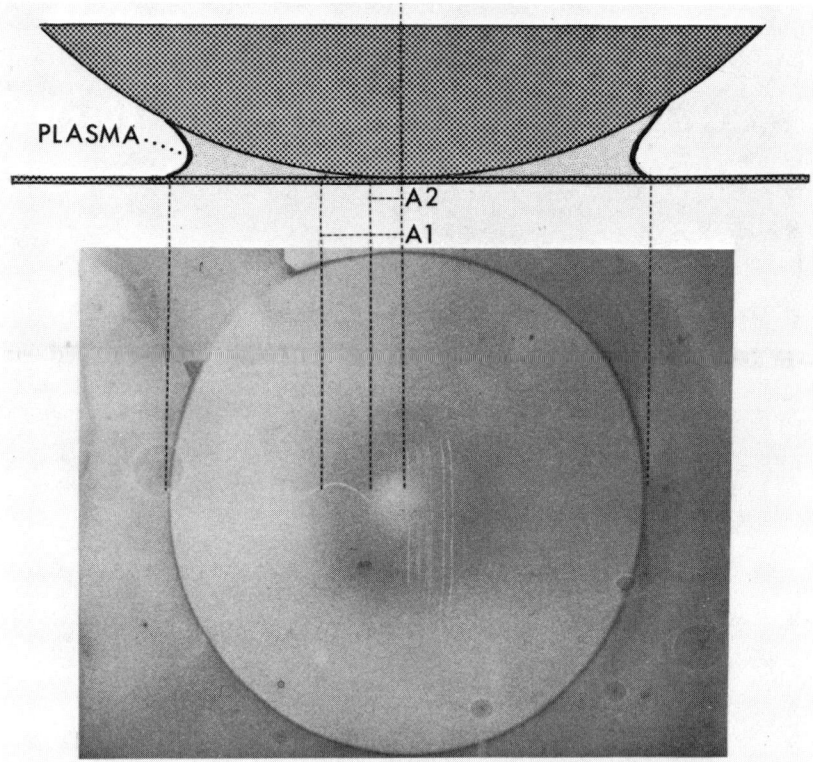

Figure 3. Top: Diagram showing outer and inner edge of the fibrinogen ring (radii A_1 and A_2) left by plasma. Outer vertical lines indicate diameter of area where plasma had resided. Bottom: Pattern of residual fibrinogen created as shown in Figure 1 but on TaO (plasma diluted 1:15). The pattern indicating antibody deposition is created by interference colors (see Figure 2).

Table I. Radii of Clear Centers Left by Fibrinogen Solutions of Various Concentrations (Under Lens of $R = 95$ mm) and Computed Heights of Solutions

Fibrinogen mg/mL	Radius $(A_2)^a$	Height $(H_2)^b$	$2/H_2^c$
6	0.7	2.6	.77
3	0.5	1.3	1.5
0.3	1.75	16	.1
0.06	2.75	40	.05

$^a A_2$ in mm.
$^b H_2$ in μm derived from values A_2 and R.
^{c}Expected values for mg of fibrinogen/mL on the basis of presumptions are described in the text.

Table II. Radii of Areas of Residual Fibrinogen Left by Intact Plasma, and Its Computed Heights^a

Dilution		Steel Ball	Lenses			
	R^b	12.7	44	95	147	2095
Undiluted	A_1	0.46	1.0	1.5	2.0	8.5
	H_1	8	11	12	14	17
1:1	A_1				2.5	
	H_1				21	
1:10	A_1	1.6		5.0		
	H_1	101		131		
	A_2	0.36		0.75		
	H_2	5		3		

$^a A_1$ and A_2 in mm, H_1 and H_2 in μm derived from values of A and R.
$^b R$ in mm; curvatures of lenses were calculated (a) from diameter and height of edge, (b) from focal length and presumed refractive index of lens, and (c) from Newton ring diameters.

resulting pattern (*see* Figure 4) indicated that albumin had been deposited well within the area where no fibrinogen deposit had been found. The direction of the teardrop shape of the deposited albumin ring depended on the direction in which the plasma had been injected (Figure 4, arrow).

Experiments with blood and erythrocyte-poor blood, as described in the Experimental section, using the 95-mm radius lens, produced a ring of platelets on the slide. In the absence of significant amounts of erythrocytes, this ring was much smaller than the ring deposited in the presence of erythrocytes (*see* Table III). Beyond and inside these rings, few platelets adhered to the glass under these conditions. Granulocytes adhered mostly beyond the ring of platelets.

Some experiments were carried out with normal intact plasma, but in addition to antiserum to fibrinogen, antiserum to kininogens (kindly provided by R. W. Colman, Temple University School of Medicine, Philadelphia, PA) was applied. A lens with an approximately 147-mm radius of

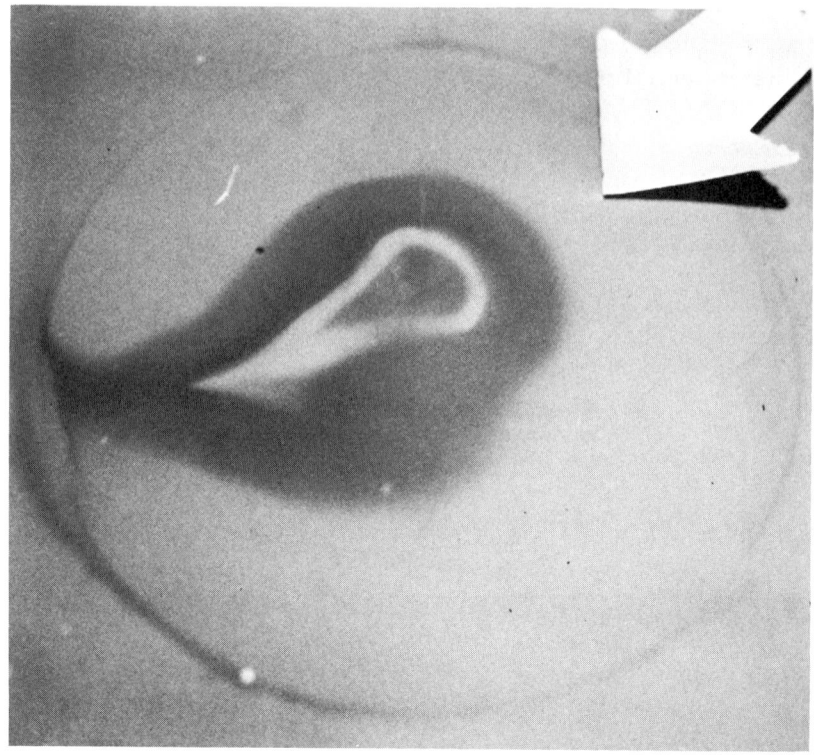

Figure 4. Albumin left by intact plasma diluted 1:100 between lens and anodized tantalum– sputtered glass slide (see text).

Table III. Outer Radii of Rings of Platelets Left by Heparinized Blood and by Its Erythrocyte-Poor Supernatant Between Glass Side and Lens of $R = 95$ mm[a]

Sample No.	Whole Blood		Supernatant	
	A_1	H_1	A_1	H_1
1	2.22	26	1.32	9.2
2	1.86	18	0.96	4.8
3	5.00	132	2.00	21
4	1.90	19	0.96	4.8
5	2.04	22	0.84	3.7

[a] Radii of platelet rings A_1 in mm; H_1 in μm.

curvature was used. Undiluted plasma resided between the lens and slide for 10 min. The two antisera were each applied to one-half of the dried surface (*see* Figure 5, antiserum to kininogens on right half). Where plasma had resided for 10 min, little or no fibrinogen remained (Figure 5, Area B), but kininogen was present (Area F). In the narrow, central space, fibrinogen was present (Area C), but kininogen was not (Area G). Where contact of the plasma with the glass had occurred only briefly, during rinsing, fibrinogen was deposited (Area A), but kininogen had not yet been adsorbed (Area E). A faintly dark area was seen in the center between the two antiserum sites (Area D), and this residual protein, presumably fibrinogen, was removed by the antiserum to kininogens (Area G being lighter than Area D). This removal can be explained as follows. Most sera, and even their purified globulins, contain intact surface-activatable clotting factors that can displace fibrinogen. Because fibrinogen molecules are much larger than kininogen or factor XII molecules, the replacement of fibrinogen causes a decrease in film thickness (*1*), so that even without exposure to antifibrinogen, the pattern created by this process may be detected. While exposure to an antiserum to fibrinogen will merely enhance the fibrinogen pattern, exposure to any other antiserum may cause its high molecular weight kininogen and factor XII to remove the residual fibrinogen and thus destroy the pattern.

Discussion

The contrast between patterns obtained with antisera to fibrinogen and those obtained with antiserum to kininogens indicates that normal plasma deposited fibrinogen, and within 10 min, replaced it on these activating substrates, by high molecular weight kininogen (and probably by factor XII), except in spaces of less than about 10 μm. Proportionally wider spaces were required for this replacement by plasma that had been diluted. In much narrower spaces, even the deposition of fibrinogen is restricted, as shown in patterns created by fibrinogen solutions as well as by dilute plasma. A few presumptions may suffice to interpret all results qualitatively as well as quantitatively.

1. For most proteins, about 1 mg tends to be adsorbed on a substrate area of 1 m^2 (*9*).
2. The "critical height" of a protein solution spread beyond its capacity of forming a complete protein monomolecular layer on the substrate is the value H_1 or H_2 described previously. A plasma layer of more than H_1 μm thick contains enough high molecular weight kininogen (and factor XII) to displace the fibrinogen that this plasma layer had deposited. A thinner layer will contain insufficient high molecular weight kininogen (and factor XII) to displace the entire fibrinogen coating, but will still contain enough fibrinogen to create this fibrinogen coating, unless the plasma layer is less than H_2 μm thick.

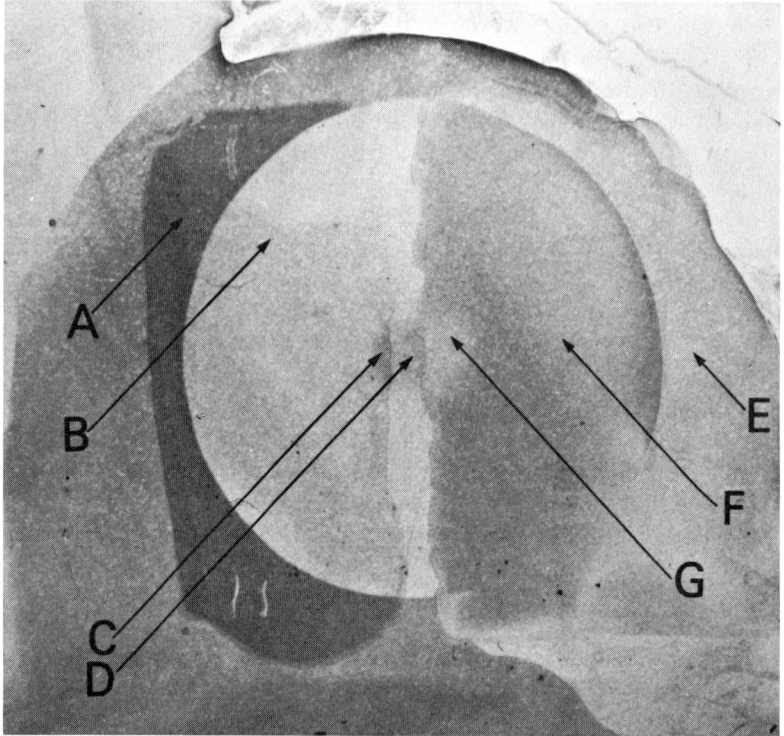

Figure 5. Fibrinogen (left) and kininogen (right) left by normal plasma between lens and glass slide (see text).

Then, even the fibrinogen in this thin plasma layer is insufficient to create a "carpet without holes." However, albumin, being much more abundant than fibrinogen, may then fill these holes.

3. From presumptions (1) and (2), C mg of a protein in 100 mL of solution can cover C m², so its critical height H, where a single substrate surface would be involved, is $100/(10,000 \times C)$ cm or $100/C$ μm. Twice as high a layer of solution will be needed between two surfaces. Because the surface of the curved objects within the narrow ranges of significance to this study is nearly planar, H_1 and H_2 have to be approximately $200/C$ μm, where C represents the concentration of high molecular weight kininogen (+ factor XII) derived from H_1, and the concentration of fibrinogen derived from H_2.

4. Platelets adhere where they find adsorbed fibrinogen (6).

Plasma normally contains about 10–30 mg of combined high molecular weight kininogen and factor XII per 100 mL, and about 300 mg of fibrinogen in the same volume. For undiluted plasma, H_1 should then be about 200/20 μm, and for plasma diluted 1:10, H_1 should be 200/2 μm. Actual values were about 10 and 120 μm, respectively (see Table II).

In undiluted plasma, or in fibrinogen solutions of physiological concentrations, H_2 (the height below which the solution cannot form an unbroken fibrinogen coating) should be about 200/300, or 0.66 μm, corresponding to a central "empty hole" with a diameter of only about 0.4 mm with our lenses. A fuzzy circle that small cannot be measured easily, so our data of A_2 and the calculated H_2 vary considerably (see Table I, upper lines) when undiluted plasma is used. When diluted serially, solutions of fibrinogen yielded reasonable values of H_2 (see Tables I and II): at 30 mg/100 mL, the expected value for H_2 is 200/30, or about 7 μm, while the actual value was 16; at 6 mg/100 mL the expected value is 200/6, or 33 μm, while a value of 40 was found.

Heparinized erythrocyte-poor blood left a ring of platelets between the lens and slide that was about as large as the ring of fibrinogen left by undiluted citrated plasma (compare A_1 in Tables II and III). The samples of whole heparinized blood left a larger ring of platelets than did their matching samples of erythrocyte-poor blood. This result suggests that the erythrocytes acted as a diluent of the plasma, reducing the amount of high molecular weight kininogen (and factor XII) available to displace adsorbed fibrinogen in areas of less than about 20 μm, so that platelets could find a wider ring of fibrinogen to adhere to in the presence of, rather than in the absence of erythrocytes. This explanation contrasts those proposed by others in the past; namely, that erythrocytes leak a substance such as ADP which stimulates platelet adhesion (10), or that erythrocytes under conditions of flow usually associated with tests for platelet retention in glass wool wicks (11) or glass bead columns (12), mechanically force platelets into contact with the glass surface (13). Under the conditions of our present experiments, flow was minimal, and preliminary tests indicated that the fibrinogen deposited by plasma in narrow spaces may remain for several hours, suggesting that diffusion of high molecular weight kininogen into these areas has not occurred to a measurable extent.

Whether the removal of fibrinogen by intact plasma represents physical or enzymatic displacement by high molecular weight kininogen and factor XII, or an indirect result of activation of plasminogen to the fibrino(gen)olytic enzyme plasmin via the activation of factor XII (14), remains to be studied.

Acknowledgment

This work was supported in part by the National Heart, Lung, and Blood Institute Grant No. 1 R01HL2389901.

Literature Cited

1. Vroman. L.; Adams, A. L.; Klings, M.; Fischer, G. C. In "Applied Chemistry at Protein Interfaces," *Advances in Chemistry Series*, No. 145; ACS: Washington, D.C., **1975;** p. 255–289.
2. Vroman, L.; Adams, A. L.; Fischer, G. C.; Munoz, P. C. *Blood* **1980,** 55, 156–159.
3. Wiggins, R. C.; Bouma, B. N.; Cochrane, C. G.; Griffin, J. H. *Proc. Natl. Acad. Sci. USA* **1977,** 74, 4636–4640.
4. Ratnoff, O. D.; Davie, E. W.; Mallet, D. L. *J. Clin. Invest.* **1961,** 40, 803–819.
5. Schmaier, A. H.; Colman, R. W.; Adams, A. L.; Fischer, G. C. Munoz, P. C.; Vroman, L. *Circulation* **1980,** 62, III-57.
6. Zucker, M .B.; Vroman, L. *Proc. Soc. Exp. Biol. Med.* **1969,** 131, 318–320.
7. Vroman, L. *Thromb. Diath. Haemorrh.* **1964,** 10, 455–493.
8. Adams, A. L.; Klings, M.; Fischer, G. C.; Vroman, L. *J. Immunol. Methods* **1973,** 3, 227–232.
9. Langmuir, I.; Waugh, D. F. *J. Am. Chem. Soc.* **1940,** 62, 2771–2793.
10. Hellem, A. J. *Scand. J. Clin. Lab. Invest. Suppl.* **1960.**
11. Moolten, S. E.; Vroman, L. *Am. J. Clin. Path.* **1949,** 19, 701–709.
12. Salzman, E. W. *J. Lab. Clin. Med.* **1963,** 62, 724–735.
13. Goldsmith, H. L. *Fed. Proc.* **1971,** 30, 1578–1588.
14. Goldsmith, G. H., Jr. *J. Lab. Clin. Med.* **1980,** 96, 222–231.

RECEIVED for review January 16, 1981. ACCEPTED March 3, 1981.

Influence of Red Blood Cells and Their Components on Protein Adsorption

S. UNIYAL, J. L. BRASH,[1] and I. A. DEGTEREV[2]

McMaster University, Departments of Chemical Engineering and Pathology, Hamilton, Ontario, Canada

Earlier observations from this laboratory showed that red blood cells have an inhibitory effect on adsorption of albumin and fibrinogen to polyethylene surfaces. The present work extends observations of this "red cell effect" to the glass–fibrinogen system. Adsorption in the presence of red cells was inhibited up to 50%, the inhibition increasing with increasing hematocrit at constant protein concentration in the free fluid volume. Since some hemolysis occurs in these experiments, the effect of deliberately added hemolysate was investigated, but found to be negligible. Adsorption in the presence of red cell ghosts was inhibited strongly. These results suggest that the red cell effect is not attributable to leakage of cell contents, but rather is a membrane-related effect.

Adsorption of proteins is the primary event upon contact between blood and foreign surfaces (*1*), and subsequent cellular interactions leading to thrombus formation are determined by these adsorbed proteins (*2*). Much of the early work on the study of adsorption was done in buffered solutions of single proteins or relatively simple mixtures (*3–7*). More recently, studies have been conducted using more "realistic" media, particularly plasma (*8, 9*). These studies have shown that the plasma interacts subsequently with the initially adsorbed proteins, causing some unexpected effects. For example, initially adsorbed fibrinogen is desorbed rapidly from several surfaces in the presence of plasma (*8*).

The question might well be asked whether the red cells, another major component of blood, have any effect on protein adsorption. The effect of red cells on platelet sticking has been noted widely, causing an augmentation of the rate of adhesion, probably by a combination of physical and biochemical mechanisms (*10*). However, studies of protein adsorption in the presence of

[1]To whom correspondence should be addressed.
[2]Soviet Union–Canada exchange scientist from Institute of Chemical Physics, Moscow.

red cells are, surprisingly, almost entirely lacking. In a previous study from this laboratory (11), the addition of red blood cells to buffered solutions of plasma proteins caused a decrease in the quantity of protein adsorbed from these solutions to a polyethylene surface. The present work extends these observations to the glass–fibrinogen system, and provides new information relevant to the mechanism of adsorption inhibition. In particular, we wanted to establish whether the red cell effect has intracellular or membrane origins. Therefore, separate experiments were carried out in the presence of hemolysate from red cells and red cell ghosts.

Experimental

Materials. Fibrinogen (human, Grade L) was obtained from Kabi (Stockholm, Sweden). The lyophilized product was dissolved in distilled water (concentration: 1 g/100 mL) and dialyzed against an appropriate buffer, usually isotonic phosphate-buffered saline (PBS), pH 7.35 (see below). The solution was frozen in 5-mL portions until required. Hemoglobin (human, Type IV, twice crystallized) was purchased from Sigma Chemical Co. and was used as received. The $Na^{125}I$ was from New England Nuclear. Glass tubing (0.25 cm in diameter) was Corning code 7740, Pyrex glass, and was washed for 1 h with chromic acid cleaning mixture (Chromerge), then rinsed with copious amounts of distilled water. The surface of this glass previously has been shown to be essentially smooth and featureless from a topographical standpoint by electron microscopy (12).

The "normal" adsorption medium was isotonic PBS (0.15M, pH 7.35) containing labeled fibrinogen at a specified concentration. To this medium were added, variously, washed whole red cells, red cell ghosts, or red cell hemolysate in sufficient quantity to give a specified final concentration of hemoglobin. Fibrinogen concentrations for the media containing red cells or ghost cells were based on free fluid volume rather than total volume.

Fibrinogen Labeling. Labeling with ^{125}I was carried out as described previously (12), using a twofold molar excess of iodine monochloride. This procedure gives labeled fibrinogen identical in its adsorption on glass to unlabeled protein (13). Other properties of fibrinogen, including biological properties, also are unaffected by this labeling method (14, 15). In general, the fibrinogen solutions used in the present work contained 30% labeled and 70% unlabeled material.

Preparation of Washed Red Cells. Freshly drawn human blood, collected into acid citrate dextrose (ACD) anticoagulant, was centrifuged for 15 min at 630 × g, and the plasma and buffy coat were removed. The red cells were washed three times using 3–4 volumes of PBS, centrifuging between each wash at 2000 × g for 10 min. Packed red cells [hematocrit (HCT) about 90%] were added to appropriate volumes of fibrinogen solution (in PBS) to give the required hematocrit.

Preparation of Ghost Cells. The method of Steck (16) was modified for use in the present work. Washed, packed red cells prepared as indicated above were lysed in 40 volumes of 5mM sodium phosphate (pH 8.0), then washed three times using 40 volumes of 5mM sodium phosphate. This procedure gives so-called "unsealed" ghost cells (16) from which essentially all the hemoglobin has been removed. At the same time, normal red cell morphology (biconcave disc) and size are maintained as shown by the results of scanning electron microscopy (SEM) (Figure 1). Cells were prepared for SEM by allowing them to settle on Nuclepore polycarbonate membranes. They were then fixed sequentially with glutaraldehyde and osmium tetroxide, and dehydrated with ethanol.

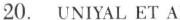

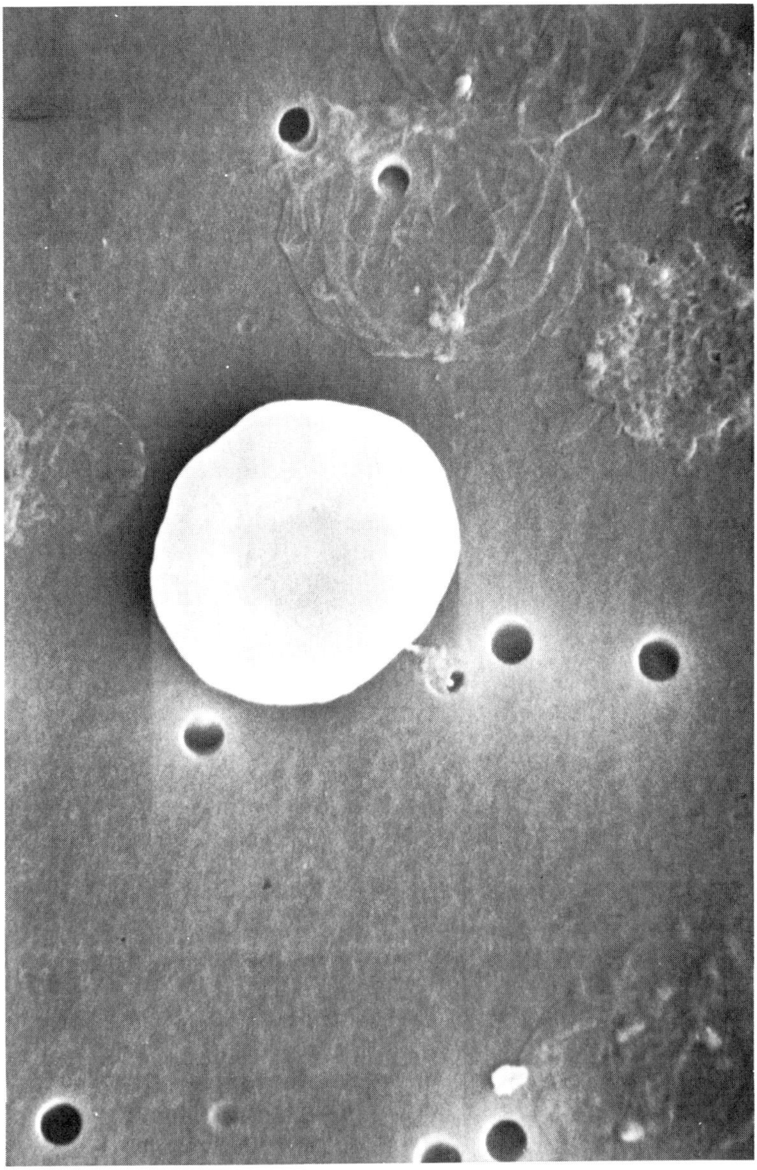

Figure 1. SEM of a typical ghost cell. Cells were deposited on a polycarbonate membrane (Nuclepore) whose pores are visible. The small white marker lines represent 1 μm.

In addition to SEM, size analysis of the ghost cells was performed with a Coulter counter, and as shown in Figure 2, the size distribution is similar to that of the washed red cell preparation.

Sodium dodecyl sulfate polyacrylamide gel electrophoresis (SDS–PAGE) of ghost membrane proteins was performed by a modification of the method of Laemmli (17). Samples were reduced with β-mercaptoethanol and run in 11% gels. Molecular weight (MW) standards were obtained from Pharmacia Canada Ltd.

Media containing ghost cells for adsorption studies were prepared by mixing appropriate volumes of packed ghost cells and labeled fibrinogen in PBS. Ghost hematocrits were determined by cell counting (Coulter counter), assuming an average ghost cell volume of 75 μm^3.

Preparation of Hemolysate. Washed red cells were lysed in distilled water (20% HCT) for 15 min. The stroma was extracted in carbon tetrachloride, and the aqueous layer containing the hemolysate was recovered. This solution was diluted appropriately with PBS to a specified hemoglobin concentration, and labeled fibrinogen was added. The final solution was adjusted to isotonicity and pH 7.35. Hemoglobin concentrations were determined by the cyanmethemoglobin method (18).

Adsorption Experiments. Adsorptions were carried out as described previously (11). A circuit was set up consisting of several glass tubing segments and a roller pump connected in series. The tubes were positioned vertically, and were connected together using Silastic medical-grade tubing (Dow–Corning) and three-way valves. The total length of the Silastic connectors was about one-third that of the glass test segments. The circuit was primed with PBS, which was then displaced by the test medium (a suspension of red blood cells, ghosts, etc.) in a manner (using the three-way valves to eliminate air bubbles) such that no air–solution–solid interface was created. Experiments were run at a flow rate of 50 mL/min (540 s^{-1} surface shear rate) at room temperature. To determine the time course of adsorption, tubing segments were disconnected at various times up to 4 h and were rinsed three times with PBS (20 volumes), and the associated radioactivity was determined (Beckman Biogamma system). An aliquot of the labeled fibrinogen solution (of known concentration) prepared for a given experiment also was counted, and surface concentration Γ (μg/cm^2) was calculated from the relation:

$$\Gamma = \frac{C_p R_f}{A R_s}$$

where C_p is the solution concentration of fibrinogen (μg/mL); R_f, the count rate of surface; R_s, the count rate of solution (per mL); and A, the area of surface (cm^2).

In experiments where the extent of hemolysis was needed, samples of test fluid were withdrawn from the circuit at various times, and the hemoglobin concentration in the supernatant was measured (18).

Results

Effect of Whole Red Cells. As indicated in Figure 3, whole red cells cause a diminution in the quantity of fibrinogen adsorbed to a glass surface. The extent of this "inhibition" increases with increasing hematocrit, and at 40% HCT, the surface concentration after 4 h was reduced to about 50% of its value in the absence of cells. It was shown previously (11), that such an effect was not due to the depletion of fibrinogen from the aqueous phase by adsorption to the cell surfaces. Although this may occur to some extent, it is insufficient to cause any detectable alteration in the concentration of fibrino-

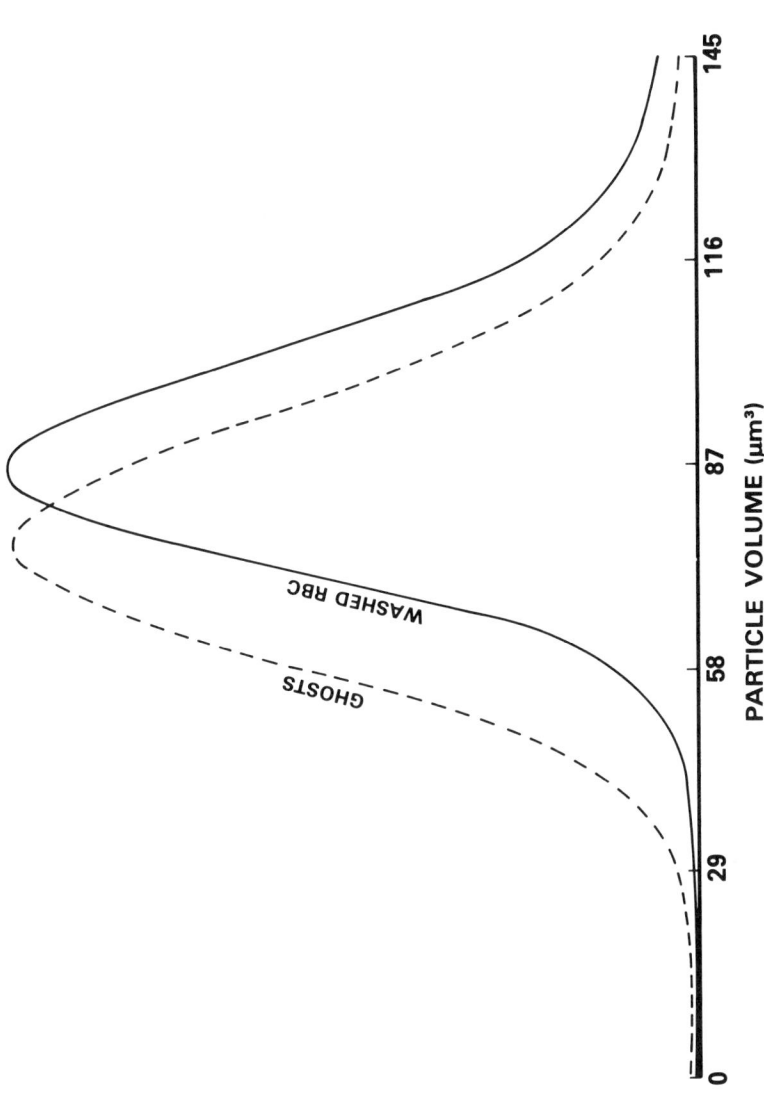

Figure 2. Distributions of cell volumes of typical red cell and ghost cell preparations, obtained by Coulter counter. Key to mean cell volumes: red cells, 87 μm^3; and ghost cells, 76 μm^3.

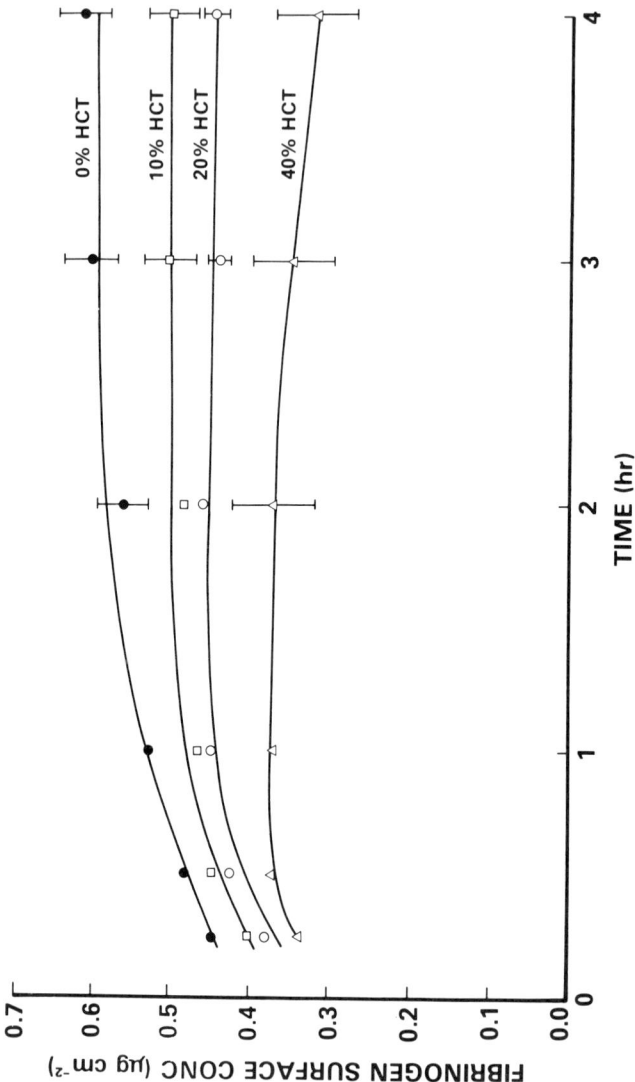

Figure 3. Adsorption of fibrinogen on glass as a function of time at various hematocrits. Conditions: buffer—PBS, pH 7.35; fibrinogen concentration—1.0 mg/mL in free volume; and shear rate at the surface—540 s^{-1}. Values are the average of at least three experiments; error limits are standard deviations. Key: ●, 0% HCT; □, 10% HCT; ○, 20% HCT; and △, 40% HCT.

gen in the liquid phase. In addition, for all suspensions used, the concentration in the cell-free volume was kept constant at 1.0 mg/mL. Unlike the results for polyethylene, published previously (11), the surface concentration does not pass through an early maximum. Instead, it shows "typical" kinetic behavior, approaching a steady-state value in times on the order of 1–2 h. In the case of the 40% HCT suspension, the surface concentration began to decrease from its steady-state value after 2–3 h.

Hemolysis During Experiments with Whole Red Cells. Although it was previously concluded (11) that hemolysis in these experiments is less than 1% and probably of no account, we wanted to ascertain the exact concentration of free hemoglobin and to determine whether this concentration increases with time. Horbett et al. (19) suggested that hemoglobin is a protein of high surface activity, and is preferentially adsorbed from plasma relative to fibrinogen and albumin. Thus, at least a part of the red cell–related inhibition of adsorption possibly could be due to preferential adsorption of hemoglobin. Figure 4 shows that the free hemoglobin concentration does indeed increase with time in typical adsorption experiments, suggesting that some hemolytic damage to cells is occurring. The effect is minimal at the lower hematocrit, but at 40% HCT, the concentration of free hemoglobin reaches a value on the order of 1.0 mg/mL, comparable to that of fibrinogen. The initial concentration of hemoglobin is finite and increases with increasing hematocrit. With the manipulations involved in preparing the red cells, this "residual" free hemoglobin could not be eliminated. Even at 20% HCT, the initial hemoglobin concentration was about 0.04 mg/mL.

Effects of Hemoglobin and Hemolysate. Because substantial concentrations of hemoglobin exist in the adsorption media, we wanted to know whether hemoglobin per se would exert an inhibitory effect on fibrinogen adsorption. Experiments using hemoglobin from a commercial source were thus carried out, using concentrations at the low and high ends of the range actually encountered in the red cell suspensions. Figure 5 shows the kinetics of adsorption at hemoglobin concentrations of 0.09 and 0.8 mg/mL, and indicates a strongly inhibitory effect such that adsorption of fibrinogen is all but eliminated at the higher concentration. The shape of the curves suggests that a certain amount of the fibrinogen adsorbed at short times is removed later. The spectacular effect of hemoglobin shown in Figure 5 is, in fact, greater than the red cell effect itself, suggesting that if the latter is due entirely to leakage of cell contents, then hemolysate is relatively less inhibitory than pure hemoblogin. To investigate further the role of cell contents, adsorption experiments were performed in the presence of controlled amounts of hemolysate, such that free hemoglobin concentrations were again in the range encountered in the red cell experiments. The results of these experiments are shown in Figure 6; the hemolysate effect was very small, and effectively negligible up to a hemoglobin concentration of 1.0 mg/mL. A slight decrease in the steady-state level of adsorption occurred at the higher

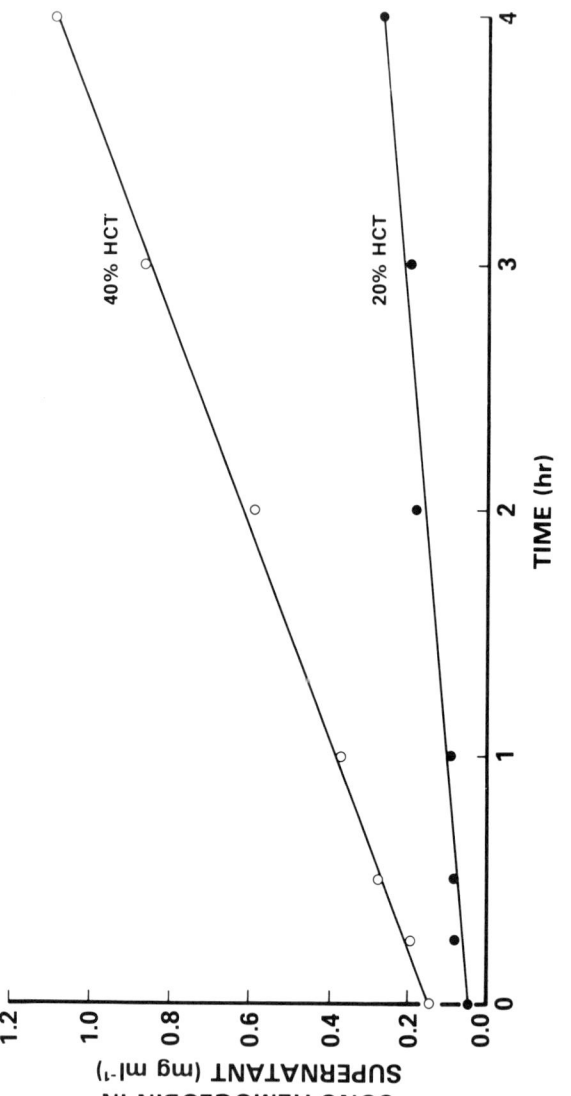

Figure 4. Development of hemoglobin in supernatant as a function of time during red cell experiments at two hematocrits. Values are the average of at least three experiments. Key: ○, *40% HCT and* ●, *20% HCT.*

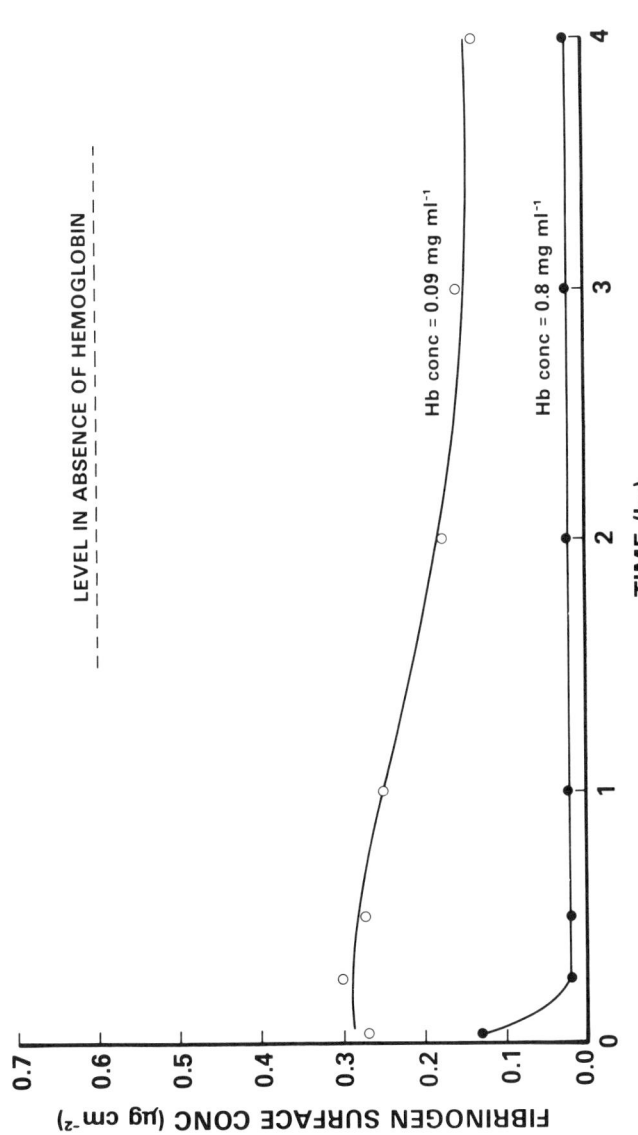

Figure 5. *Adsorption of fibrinogen on glass in the presence of Sigma hemoglobin. Conditions: buffer—PBS, pH 7.35; fibrinogen concentration—1.0 mg/mL; and shear rate at the surface—540 s⁻¹. Values are the average of three experiments. Key to hemoglobin concentration:* ○, *0.09 mg/mL and* ●, *0.8 mg/mL;* ---, *level in absence of hemoglobin.*

hemoglobin concentrations. The difference between the effects of the commercial hemoglobin and hemolysate is very pronounced. Among possible explanations is that other constituents of hemolysate act in opposition to hemoglobin. However, Figure 7 suggests another, perhaps more plausible, explanation. From this figure, showing visible spectra of the hemolysate and Sigma hemoglobin, the hemolysate hemoglobin is in the form of oxyhemoglobin, whereas the Sigma hemoglobin is in the form of methemoglobin (20). Consequently, methemoglobin appears to be adsorbed strongly in preference to fibrinogen, whereas oxyhemoglobin is not.

Effect of Ghost Cells. The results of the experiments in the presence of hemolysate suggest that cell contents, per se, do not influence fibrinogen adsorption, thus implicating the cell membranes directly, or alternatively, the particulate character of the cells, as being responsible for the effect. To investigate this possibility, experiments with ghost cells were conducted. The preparative technique resulted in ghost cells of normal shape and size. Thus, SEM results such as those presented in Figure 1 show retention of bioconcave shape and a cell diameter between 6 and 7 μm. Coulter counter analysis (Figure 2) showed the distribution of cell volumes to be substantially maintained, although the mean cell volume was somewhat less than for the normal cells. Two concentrations of ghost cells, namely, 15% and 45% by volume, were used in these experiments. The results, presented in Figure 8, show a marked diminution in quantity adsorbed (on the order of 50% and 80% at 15% and 45% by volume of ghost cells, respectively). Again, as with

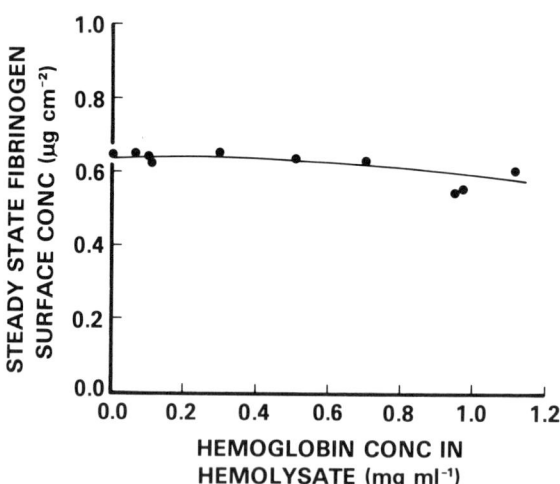

Figure 6. Adsorption of fibrinogen on glass in the presence of red cell hemolysate. Conditions: buffer—PBS, pH 7.35; fibrinogen concentration—1.0 mg/mL; and surface shear rate—540 s^{-1}. Values are the average of three experiments.

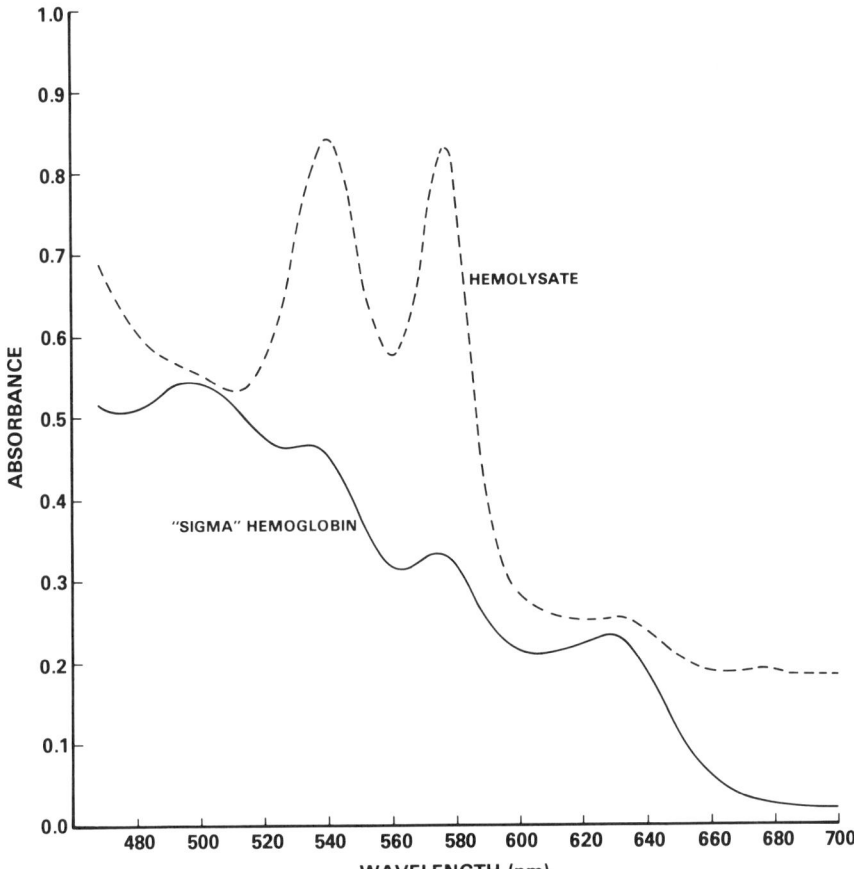

Figure 7. Visible spectra of hemolysate preparation and Sigma hemoglobin in the wavelength range 460–700 nm. Key: ---, hemolysate and —, Sigma hemoglobin.

the kinetics in the presence of methemoglobin, the ghost cells appear to be able to remove initially adsorbed fibrinogen.

SDS–PAGE of Adsorption Media. SDS–PAGE of various media used in this study was undertaken to obtain additional information on their protein compositions. Typical gels are presented in Figure 9. Gel 3 corresponds to the proteins from ghost cell membranes and shows a complex pattern of bands that agrees well with previously published results, for example, those of Fairbanks et al. (21).

Comparison of Gels 2 and 4, corresponding to Kabi fibrinogen and fibrinogen plus supernatant from a ghost cell suspension, respectively, shows the presence of an additional band in Gel 4 at a molecular weight of about 37,000. This protein presumably originated in the ghost membranes, and

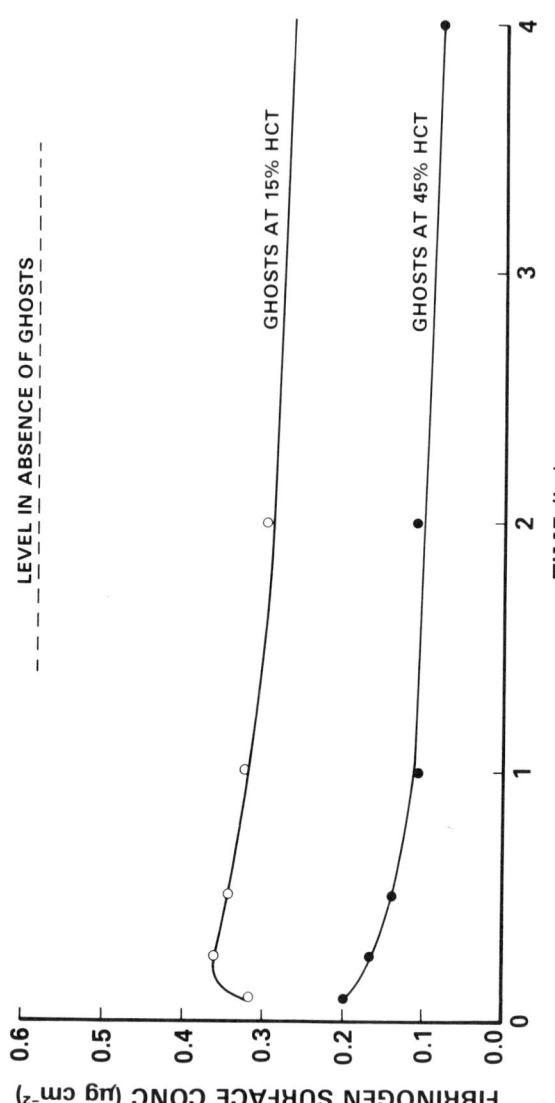

Figure 8. Adsorption of fibrinogen on glass in the presence of ghost cells. Conditions: buffer—PBS, pH 7.35; and fibrinogen concentration—1.0 mg/mL in free volume. Values are the average of three experiments. Key: ○, ghosts at 15% HCT; ●, ghosts at 45% HCT; and ---, level in absence of ghosts.

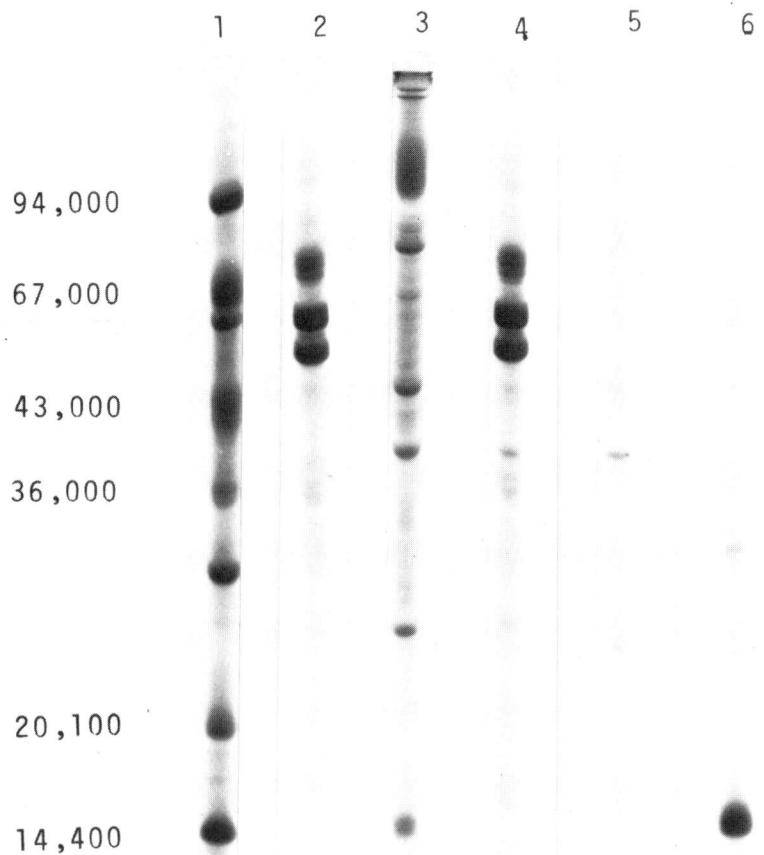

Figure 9. SDS–PAGE of various materials.
Numbers on left are molecular weights of standards shown in Gel 1. Key to gels: 1, molecular weight standards; 2, human fibrinogen (Kabi); 3, ghost cell membrane polypeptides; 4, fibrinogen with supernatant from ghost cell preparation; 5, ghost cell supernatant alone; and 6, hemolysate from red cells.

appears to correspond to "Band 6" in the nomenclature of Fairbanks et al. (21). Band 6 has been identified with the monomeric form of glyceraldehyde-3-phosphate dehydrogenase (22), which is believed to be an "extrinsic" protein, loosely bound to the cytoplasmic surface of the membrane. Gel 5 represents a sample of hemolysate, and shows essentially a single band corresponding to the hemoglobin subunit, thus confirming that the hemolysate does not contain any membrane or plasma protein contaminants.

Discussion

The three principal conclusions emerging from this study are that: (1) the "red cell effect" can now be further generalized to include glass surface; (2) a considerable difference in competitive adsorption exists between oxyhemoglobin and methemoglobin; and (3) inhibition of adsorption by red cells appears to be a cell membrane–related effect.

With regard to the first point, initial work with polyethylene (11) postulated that the mechanism of adsorption inhibition involved collision of red cells with the surface, and transfer of some material from the cell surface to the tube wall. Such an effect might be considered to be more probable if it involved hydrophobic interactions, which would be more likely for polyethylene than for glass. However, as is shown by the present study, the extent of inhibition is about the same for both surfaces, so that whatever the mechanism or mechanisms, the inhibition appears equally likely for hydrophobic and hydrophilic surfaces. The effect may be a general one that would occur for any surface.

Vroman et al. (9) observed transient adsorption (i.e., adsorption followed by rapid desorption) of fibrinogen on glass in the presence of plasma, and attributed this result to replacement of fibrinogen with high molecular weight kininogen. The present results could possibly be explained by this plasma effect resulting from carry over of plasma with the red cells. Since the cells are washed very extensively, we do not believe such an effect would be important. In addition, we have observed a red cell effect for other proteins including albumin (11) and IgG (23).

The dramatic difference between the effects of hemolysate and Sigma hemoglobin is perhaps somewhat surprising, and must remain, for the moment, without explanation. Certainly, however, only the oxyhemoglobin situation is relevant to blood, since methemoglobin constitutes only 0.5–3% of total hemoglobin (24). The observations of Horbett et al. (19), suggesting that hemoglobin adsorption might be important in extracorporeal circulations where hemolysis is more likely to occur, were based on work with methemoglobin (25). Therefore, the question of the possible role of hemoglobin in blood–surface phenomena needs to be re-examined. From a more fundamental standpoint, how such differences in adsorption behavior might arise should be considered based on subtle structural differences between the various hemoglobin types. Apparently, the oxidation state of the iron affects adsorption properties, thus suggesting that the heme groups may be involved. Clearly, more systematic studies relevant to this question are required to resolve the various issues.

The results with ghost cells suggest that the membranes play a key role in the "red cell effect." This point of view is in accord with conclusions from our earlier work (11) that the red cell–surface collision results in transfer of material from the cell to the surface. Keller and Yum (26) also provided evidence that such a transfer of material may occur. Two possible mechanisms probably are operative in this connection: (1) the deposition of material from the cell as just noted, providing a new surface that is less adsorptive toward proteins than the original substrate, and (2) the ability of the red cell to "strip" the surface of previously adsorbed protein, as suggested by the shape of the curves in Figures 5 and 8. In the case of polyethylene (11), red cells circulated over a previously adsorbed protein layer did not remove the layer. Such experiments were not performed in the present work, but probably should be carried out to test the possibility that stripping can occur.

The relevance of these results to blood–biomaterial interactions has several facets. If red cell material is deposited on the surface, then this becomes an interaction of potential importance that has not been recognized previously. Previous observations of early events in blood–material interactions (1, 3) have emphasized the rapid deposition of a protein layer, generally assuming it to consist of proteins originating from the plasma. However, red cell interactions also may possibly contribute to this layer. Identification of material deposited from the red cell and the acquisition of knowledge of how its presence on the surface might influence subsequent interactions such as platelet adhesion, are clearly tasks of some significance. In addition, whether the quantity and composition of the deposit depend on the specific biomaterial surface should be investigated.

Red cell–surface interactions may play a role in the dynamics of protein adsorption. We have been investigating the turnover of protein between solution and surface for several years (27–29), and have established that turnover occurs on a variety of surfaces. The rate and extent of turnover depend strongly on the surface character, with hydrophilic materials, for example, showing much more rapid turnover than hydrophobic materials. If red cells have the ability to strip protein off a biomaterial surface, then clearly this effect could influence the characteristics of the turnover process, particularly from a rate point of view. This process, in turn, could affect the development of the protein layer over a period of time.

Finally, based on results from the present work, if studies of protein adsorption are to be meaningful in terms of blood–biomaterial interactions, then they should be carried out in the presence of red blood cells.

Acknowledgments

Financial support of this work by the Medical Research Council of Canada, the Ontario Heart Foundation, and the Canada–Soviet Union scientific exchange program is gratefully acknowledged.

Literature Cited

1. Baier, R. E.; Dutton, R. C. *J. Biomed. Mater. Res.* **1969**, *3*, 191.
2. Baier, R. E. *Ann. N.Y. Acad. Sci.* **1977**, *283*, 17.
3. Brash, J. L.; Lyman, D. J. *J. Biomed. Mater. Res.* **1969**, *3*, 175.
4. Morrissey, B. W.; Stromberg, R. R. *J. Colloid Interface Sci.* **1974**, *46*, 152.
5. Lee, R. G.; Adamson, C; Kim, S. W. *Thromb. Res.* **1974**, *4*, 485.
6. Horbett, T. A.; Hoffman, A. S. *Am. Chem. Soc. Div. Colloid Surface Chem.* **1975**, *145*, 230.
7. Brash, J. L.; Uniyal, S. *J. Polym. Sci.* **1979**, *C66*, 377.
8. Brash, J. L.; Uniyal, S., unpublished data.
9. Vroman, L.; Adams, A. L.; Fischer, G. C.; Munoz, P. C. *Blood* **1980**, *55*, 156.
10. Turitto, V. T.; Weiss, H. J. *Science* **1980**, *207*, 541.
11. Brash, J. L.; Uniyal, S. *Trans. Am. Soc. Artif. Intern. Organs* **1976**, *22*, 253.
12. Brash, J. L.; Davidson, V. J. *Thromb. Res.* **1976**, *9*, 249.
13. Brash, J. L.; Uniyal, S., unpublished data.
14. McFarlane, A. S. *J. Clin. Invest.* **1963**, *42*, 346.
15. Harwig, S. S. L.; Harwig, J. F.; Coleman, R. E.; Welch, M. J. *Thromb. Res.* **1975**, *6*, 375.
16. Steck, T. L. In "Methods in Membrane Biology"; Korn, E. D., Ed.; Plenum: New York, 1974; Vol. 2, p. 245.
17. Laemmli, U. K. *Nature* **1970**, *227*, 680.
18. "Sigma Technical Bulletin No. 525, Total Hemoglobin in Whole Blood at 530–550 nm," Sigma Chemical Co., St. Louis, 1976.
19. Horbett, T. A.; Weathersby, P. K.; Hoffman, A. S. *Thromb. Res.* **1978**, *12*, 319.
20. Bunn, H. F.; Forget, B. G.; Ranney, H. M. "Human Hemoglobins"; W. B. Saunders Co.: Philadelphia, 1977; p. 34.
21. Fairbanks, G.; Steck, T. L.; Wallach, D. F. H. *Biochemistry* **1971**, *10*, 2606.
22. Marchesi, V. T.; Furthmayr, H. *Ann. Rev. Biochem.* **1976**, *45*, 667.
23. Brash, J. L.; McLeod, L., unpublished data.
24. Lehmann, H.; Huntsman, R. G. "Man's Hemoglobins"; Elsevier North Holland: Amsterdam, 1974; p. 205.
25. Horbett, T. A., personal communication.
26. Keller, K. H.; Yum, S. I. *Trans. Am. Soc. Artif. Intern. Organs* **1970**, *16*, 42.
27. Brash, J. L.; Uniyal, S.; Samak, Q. *Trans. Am. Soc. Artif. Intern. Organs* **1974**, *20*, 69.
28. Brash, J. L.; Samak, Q. M. *J. Colloid Interface Sci.* **1978**, *65*, 495.
29. Chan, B. M. C.; Brash, J. L. *J. Colloid Interface Sci.* **1981**, *82*, 217.

RECEIVED for review January 16, 1981. ACCEPTED September 16, 1981.

21

Protein Adsorption on Polymers

Visualization, Study of Fluid Shear and Roughness Effects, and Methods to Enhance Albumin Binding

ROBERT C. EBERHART, MICHAEL E. LYNCH[1], FERTAC H. BILGE, JOHN F. WISSINGER[2], MARK S. MUNRO, STEPHEN R. ELLSWORTH, and ALFRED J. QUATTRONE[3]

University of Texas Health Science Center, Department of Surgery, Dallas TX 75235 and the University of Texas, Biomedical Engineering Program, Austin, TX 78712

We visualized protein adsorbates on Teflon, silicone rubber, and polyurethane by partial gold decoration transmission electron microscopy, and the results were verified by several methods. Critical-point–dried Cohn I fibrinogen adsorbates formed extensive, reticulated networks; γ-globulin adsorbates resembled these networks but appeared to have weaker protein–protein bonds. In contrast, critical-point–dried albumin formed irregular, unconnected adsorbates with lower surface coverage. Fibrinogen preferentially adsorbed in surface cracks but albumin did not, and albumin was desorbed by a wall shear rate greater than $1500\ s^{-1}$ but fibrinogen was not. Polymers treated by covalently binding C_{18} alkyl residues selectively enhanced albumin affinity. Simultaneous albumin–fibrinogen exposure to alkylated surfaces showed that fibrinogen adsorption was reduced in proportion to enhancement of albumin adsorption.

One aspect of the question of blood–polymer compatibility that is receiving much attention is the interaction between plasma proteins and the polymer substrate. An increasing body of evidence suggests that these events, particularly the initial glycoprotein–polymer interaction, set the stage for thrombogenesis, both in terms of platelet adhesion and aggregation (1–3) and in terms of contact-activated coagulation (4). Recent evidence also suggests that a larger class of cell adhesion phenomena is governed by the nature of the protein adsorbate (5). Cell adhesion in this more general view may

[1]Current address: Westinghouse, Round Rock, TX 78664
[2]Current address: U.T. Medical Branch, Galveston, TX 77550
[3]Current address: Lab Procedures West, Woodland Hills, CA 91367

0065–2393/82/0199–0293$06.00/0
© 1982 American Chemical Society

govern the total response of blood and tissue to polymer-based implants in terms of pannus formation (6) and, perhaps, calcification (7).

Under the impetus of critical reviews of the state of knowledge concerning the physicochemical surface properties of implant polymers (8), and the detailed nature of the blood–polymer interaction (9), a number of methods for physicochemical and biological analysis have been applied to the blood compatibility problem. We developed additional methods, visualizing, by partial gold decoration transmission electron microscopy (PGDTEM), the polymer surface and the protein adsorbate. This visualization method may be useful for several tasks in protein–polymer sorption studies: to elucidate the adsorption patterns of plasma proteins (10), to quantify the surface free energy distribution (11), to evaluate the contribution of surface roughness in protein adsorption and desorption, to characterize the protein species interacting with the polymer in competitive adsorption studies (4), and to document the effects of environmental parameters such as fluid shear stress, temperature, etc., on protein adsorption (12). The results of some of these studies are reviewed and extended in this chapter. One of the more significant results of these studies is the ability of spontaneously adsorbed albumin to inhibit adsorption of Cohn I fraction, composed of fibrinogen, γ-globulin, and fibronectin. These proteins are thought by many to play central roles in cell attachment to surfaces and thrombogenesis (2, 3, 5). Unfortunately, spontaneously bound albumin is only weakly bound to the surface, and long-term prospects for inhibition of adsorption of other plasma proteins are not good (12).

We, therefore, developed a new method for enhancing albumin adsorption, a method that may provide indefinite protection against thrombogenesis and cell adhesion. The method takes advantage of the hydrophobic affinity and reversible dynamic binding of albumin from plasma to C_{18} alkyl residues that are, in turn, covalently bound onto various polymer surfaces.

Experimental

Test polymers for visualization studies were polyurethane (Pellethane, 2363–80A, Upjohn), filler-free polydimethylsiloxane (Sil-Med Corporation), two forms of Teflon, sintered (TFE, DuPont) and Fluorofilm (Dilectrix Corporation), and polyurethane–silicone rubber copolymer (AVCOthane 51, AVCO). Samples of 1 cm^2 or, for shear studies, $5 \times 20 \times 0.5$-cm sheets, were washed in ionic detergent solution (Alconox) at 60°C for 1 h, rinsed in deionized water, and refluxed in absolute ethanol for 1 h. Materials were dried and stored in a desiccator until use.

For the visualization studies the proteins were crystalline human albumin, 99% pure (Miles Laboratories and U.S. Biochemical Corporation), bovine γ-globulin, Cohn fraction II (U.S. Biochem.), human fibrinogen, Cohn fraction I, 65% clottable (U.S. Biochem.), and ferritin-conjugated rabbit antibovine albumin (immunoglobulin G, IgG) solution (Cappel Labs). For the albumin enhancement studies the proteins were crystalline (fraction V) fatty acid–free human albumin, and plasminogen-free fibrinogen (Pentex, Miles Laboratories). The major component of the Cohn I fibrinogen fraction is fibrinogen, but other proteins, notably γ-globulins and plasma fibronectin, are included.

Phosphate-buffered saline (PBS) at pH 7.4 was prepared from a stock concentrate. Following dilution, the solution was placed in a vacuum flask and degassed for 1 h. The solution was retained under vacuum and used subsequently for all solution preparations and wash steps. Crystalline protein was weighed and placed in a dry 500-mL flask, and degassed PBS was transferred to the flask to make the following concentrations: 2500 mg/dL albumin and 300 mg/dL Cohn I and II fractions. The flask was swirled gently and allowed to sit until all proteins had dissolved (30–40 min). Other solutions were prepared from the stock solutions by serial dilution under vacuum. The stock was discarded after 48 h.

The static exposure studies were performed in a closed system consisting of roller-pump (Med Science Electronics) vacuum flasks containing the protein, PBS wash solutions, and four chambers to hold the samples. The samples were initially exposed to PBS to remove any adsorbed gases, followed by 1-h static protein solution exposure (sixfold volume replacement). After the protein exposure, the surfaces were rinsed with degassed PBS (sixfold volume replacement) for 1 h, circulating at a flow rate of 100 mL/min. The shear rate at the sample surface was less than 2 s^{-1}. Sequential protein exposures (albumin–fibrinogen) were straightforward extensions of this regimen; however, they did not include an intervening PBS wash step. At the end of the hour-long rinse the coated surfaces were either air dried in a desiccator or critical-point dried. Alcohol dehydration was carried out according to the following schedule: 20% ethanol for 10 min; 50% for 5 min; 95% for 5 min; and 100% for 10 min. The samples were placed in the critical-point drying bomb with an ethanol-liquid CO_2 mixture, pressurized to 1500 psi and decompressed at a pressure bleed-off rate of 100 psi/min.

The shear experiments were carried out with a carefully constructed plane-parallel flow cell. Details of the shear circuit have been reported previously (12). The recirculation and roller pump sections, accounting for much of the circulation duty cycle, had 3–5 times the test section wall shear rate. The shear system loading, exposure, and wash steps were analogous to those for the static exposure studies. Test surfaces were exposed to one of the following calculated wall shear rates: 0, 100, 500, 800, and 1500 s^{-1}, for 1 h. Wash steps were carried out at a calculated wall shear rate at the test section of 25 s^{-1}. The exposed surfaces were critical-point dried, as described for the static exposure studies. The wall shear rate calculation assumed a steady, plane-parallel flow with no edge effects, and a parabolic velocity profile.

Following the drying steps, samples were prepared for PGDTEM as described previously (10, 13). The primary difference between this technique and conventional biological sample preparation for electron microscopy is the development of a partial gold coat, covering 10–25% of the surface, backed with a carbon film for strength and contrast. PGDTEM has been a sensitive tool in metallurgical analysis for many years (14). Samples prepared this way were examined in a Jeolco JEM 150 transmission electron microscope (TEM) at an accelerating potential of 80 kV. Over 300 grids were examined and analyzed by at least two of us. Photographs of typical and noteworthy regions were taken. For three-dimensional representations, stereo pair photographs were taken on a modified Jeolco stage at a total angle of 20°, rather than the customary 12° angle, in order to enhance the depth effect.

Gold nuclei preferentially formed on protein instead of on the polymers used in this study. Thus the image of the protein could be identified, and the area of the substrate covered with protein could be measured. This was done by tracking the outline of protein deposits and calculating the area inside the closed loops by a modified Simpson's Rule algorithm, using a Tracor Northern NS-800 digitizer computer.

Samples for high-angle scanning electron microscopy (SEM) (to verify PGDTEM images) were fastened onto metal stubs with conductive glue, placed in a Denton DV-502 vacuum evaporator, and pumped down to less than 10^{-6} Torr. The surfaces were sputter coated (20 ma, 60 s) with gold–palladium to obtain a complete conductive film. The samples were then placed in a Jeol JSM-35 scanning electron microscope and were studied at tilt angles from 5° to 30°. Photographs of typical areas were taken.

A modified negative-staining technique also was used to verify the PGDTEM images of the protein deposits, following the method of Brash and Lyman (15). The protein-exposed surfaces were coated with a 5% poly(vinyl alcohol) solution and allowed to dry. The dried films were stripped from the surface and carbon coated in the vacuum evaporator. After dissolving the poly(vinyl alcohol) in hot water and capturing the protein–carbon films on copper grids, the protein on the exposed side of the carbon films was stained with 2% phosphotungstic acid solution (pH adjusted to 7.4 with NaOH). These grids were examined in the TEM.

A ferritin labeling technique also was used to verify protein adsorbate images. Bovine serum albumin (BSA)–coated Fluorofilm Teflon surfaces were placed in a 1% ferritin conjugated rabbit anti-BSA solution. The samples were exposed to 10% rabbit serum before the antibody treatment to prevent nonspecific binding. The protein was stripped off the surface and placed on a copper grid with carbon support, using poly(vinyl alcohol) as described for the negative-staining technique. Samples prepared this way were examined by TEM. Because ferritin is electron dense, the absorbed protein deposits could be visualized without metal-atom image enhancement.

The following formulations were used for the chemical derivatization of polyurethane: sheet Pellethane 2363–80A (Upjohn), tubing Biomer (Ethicon), and a sample tube extruded by Cordis from raw material provided by Mobay. Cleaning agents were redistilled toluene (Fisher, 99% estimated purity), ethanol, dried over molecular seives to 99% purity, and redistilled trimethylpentane, spectro grade (Aldrich, 99% estimated purity). Chemicals were 1-bromooctadecane, reagent grade (Aldrich), octadecyl isocyanate, technical grade (Aldrich), and zinc stearate, reagent grade (MCB). Sodium ethoxide was prepared with pure sodium (Aldrich).

In the two-step derivatization (Figure 1), 10-cm^2 samples were soaked in toluene for 3 min to remove surface impurities. Samples were transferred in 25 mL of 0.04M sodium ethoxide in toluene under dry nitrogen, and were agitated at room temperature for 15 min. In the same vessel, 25 mL of 2.0M 1-bromooctadecane in toluene were added under nitrogen with 15 min mixing at room temperature. The chemically derivatized sheet was removed and soaked consecutively for 30 s at room temperature as follows: toluene, ethanol twice, deionized water twice, 0.1N hydrochloric acid, deionized water twice, followed by air drying for 24 h. A polyurethane was obtained that had random surface N-octadecylamine and urethane substitutions.

The one-step derivatization of polyurethane began with soaking the sample in toluene for 10 min and in ethanol for 20 min. After vacuum drying overnight, the sample was placed in 50 mL of 0.25M n-octadecyl isocyanate in trimethylpentane under dry nitrogen, and was incubated, with mixing, for 1 h at 80°C. The sample was removed, soaked twice for 1 min in ethanol, twice in deionized water, and redried to yield n-octadecyl–derivatized polyurethane.

Albumin was radiolabeled in the following manner. Defatted human serum albumin, 10 mg, was dissolved in 1 mL of PBS. From this solution, 100 μL was placed in an Iodogen-coated reaction vessel (prepared by P. Kulkarni). A 25-μL aliquot of 0.25M phosphate buffer solution (pH 7.52) was added, and the vessel was chilled over ice for 10 min. A 5-μl aliquot of Na^{125}I, 1–1.5 mCi, was then added, and the vessel was rotated slowly several times. The vessel was again placed in an ice bath for 2 min and then incubated for an additional 15 min at room temperature. At the end of the incubation period, 100 μL of PBS was added to the reaction vessel, and the solution

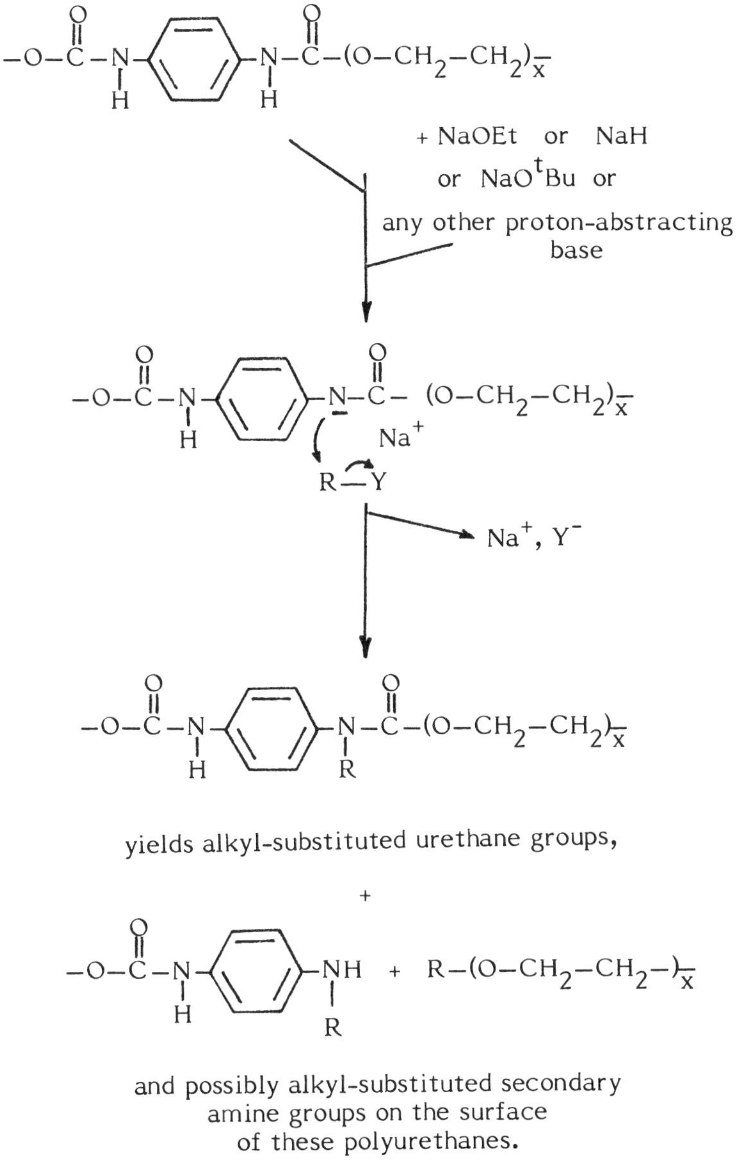

$$-O-\overset{\overset{O}{\|}}{C}-\underset{H}{N}-\underset{}{\underset{}{\bigcirc}}-\underset{H}{N}-\overset{\overset{O}{\|}}{C}-(O-CH_2-CH_2)_{\overline{x}}$$

+ NaOEt or NaH
or NaO^{t}Bu or
any other proton-abstracting base

$$-O-\overset{\overset{O}{\|}}{C}-\underset{H}{N}-\underset{}{\bigcirc}-N-\overset{\overset{O}{\|}}{C}-(O-CH_2-CH_2)_{\overline{x}}$$
$$Na^+$$
$$R-Y$$

→ Na$^+$, Y$^-$

$$-O-\overset{\overset{O}{\|}}{C}-\underset{H}{N}-\underset{}{\bigcirc}-\underset{R}{N}-\overset{\overset{O}{\|}}{C}-(O-CH_2-CH_2)_{\overline{x}}$$

yields alkyl-substituted urethane groups,

+

$$-O-\overset{\overset{O}{\|}}{C}-\underset{H}{N}-\underset{}{\bigcirc}-\underset{R}{N}H + R-(O-CH_2-CH_2-)_{\overline{x}}$$

and possibly alkyl-substituted secondary amine groups on the surface of these polyurethanes.

Figure 1a. Reaction scheme between polyurethanes and alkyl halides. The halide may be a bromide, tosylate, methylsulfonate, etc., and the alkyl residue may vary from C_8 to C_{30}.

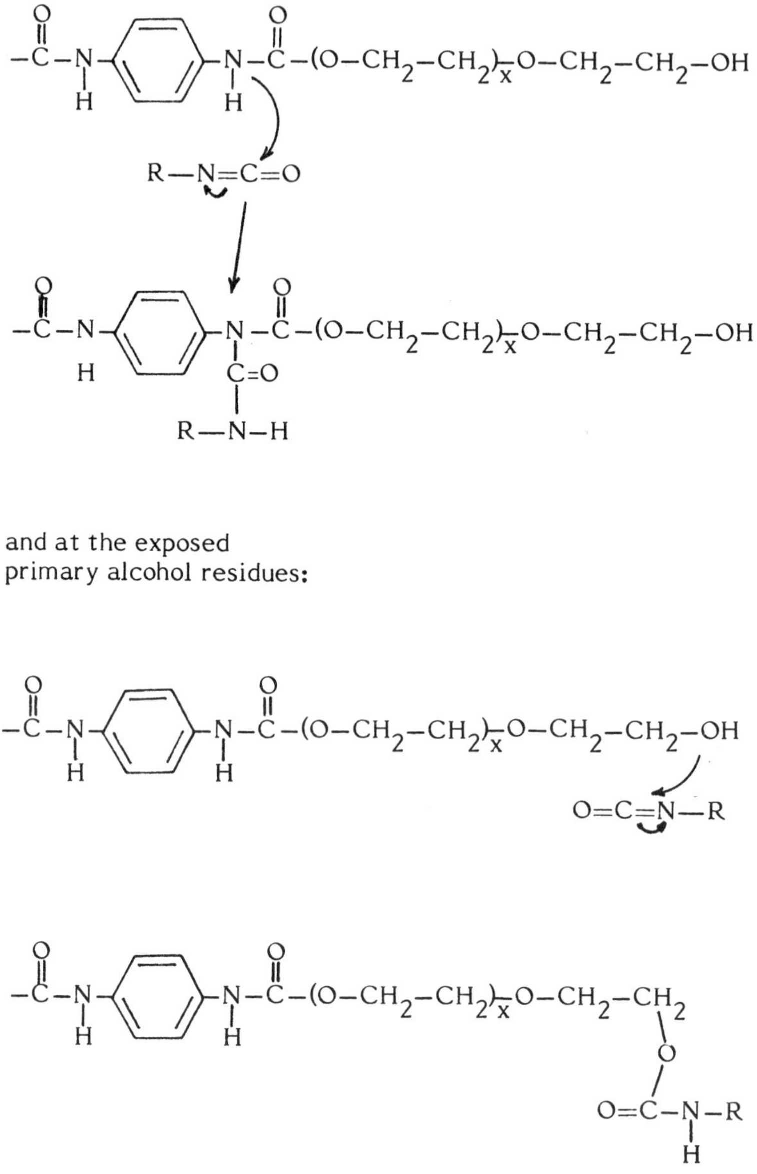

$$-\overset{O}{\underset{H}{\overset{\|}{C}}}-N-\underset{}{\underset{}{\bigcirc}}-\underset{H}{N}-\overset{O}{\overset{\|}{C}}-(O-CH_2-CH_2)_{\overline{x}}O-CH_2-CH_2-OH$$

$$R-N{=}C{=}O$$

$$\downarrow$$

$$-\overset{O}{\underset{H}{\overset{\|}{C}}}-N-\underset{}{\underset{}{\bigcirc}}-N-\overset{O}{\overset{\|}{C}}-(O-CH_2-CH_2)_{\overline{x}}O-CH_2-CH_2-OH$$
$$\underset{}{\underset{R-N-H}{\overset{|}{C}{=}O}}$$

and at the exposed
primary alcohol residues:

$$-\overset{O}{\underset{H}{\overset{\|}{C}}}-N-\underset{}{\underset{}{\bigcirc}}-\underset{H}{N}-\overset{O}{\overset{\|}{C}}-(O-CH_2-CH_2)_{\overline{x}}O-CH_2-CH_2-OH$$

$$O{=}C{=}N-R$$

$$-\overset{O}{\underset{H}{\overset{\|}{C}}}-N-\underset{}{\underset{}{\bigcirc}}-\underset{H}{N}-\overset{O}{\overset{\|}{C}}-(O-CH_2-CH_2)_{\overline{x}}O-CH_2-CH_2$$
$$\underset{O{=}\overset{}{\underset{H}{C}}-N-R}{\overset{|}{O}}$$

Figure 1b. Reaction scheme between polyurethanes and alkyl isocyanates.

was transferred into a Dowex 1 × 8–50 anion-exchange column. PBS, 10 mL, was used to flush the ^{125}I-labeled albumin through the column, giving a final volume of 10 mL with a specific activity of 3.91 µCi/mg. A radio chromatogram was run with 70% methanol, and showed less than 5% free iodide in the solution. Human fibrinogen (Pentex) was radio labeled by a similar technique. The general technique is a modification of a globulin labeling procedure (16).

Exposure of ^{125}I-labeled protein solution to the derivatized and untreated polymer samples was performed by methods different than those described previously. The protein solutions were degassed, but an air–liquid interface existed above the sample in the test chamber. Then, 0.1-mL aliquots of labeled protein were introduced by pipet. Exposures of 30 s to 20 min were carried out with this technique, and a twofold wash with PBS was conducted at the end of the exposure period. In most series, care was taken to ensure that the sample remained well below the air–solution interface. In some series, the sample was introduced through that interface. Either single protein (albumin or fibrinogen) or simultaneous albumin–fibrinogen infusions from separate pipets were performed. Following the wash step, samples with bound radioactivity were transferred to counting vials and were counted for 5 min in a well-type scintillation counter (Tracor Analytic, Model 1191).

Results

Typical gold nucleus distributions on the smooth, and rough Fluorofilm Teflon surfaces are shown in Figures 2a and b, respectively. A range of gold nucleus dimensions were observed, varying from less than 100 Å to 600 Å in size. The larger nuclei, observed for the rough Teflon, possibly resided in grooves of the Teflon surface (Figure 2c). Similar partial coverage gold nuclei were observed for the other polymers, silicone rubber, polyurethane, and AVCOthane 51, with apparently polymer-dependent variations in the nucleus size and spacing distributions.

The gold nucleus density on the γ-globulin adsorbate was considerably higher than that on the polymer substrate (Figure 3a). Comparison of negative-stain technique γ-globulin and ferritin-conjugated IgG adsorbates, obtained in similar experiments shown in Figures 3b and c, respectively, verifies the replication-based gold decoration technique.

The adsorbates in Figure 3 were all air-dried, a process that considerably disrupts the protein film. Results for critical-point–dried γ-globulin at a lower solution concentration are shown in Figure 4 to illustrate the point. The surface film was more extensive with critical-point drying, yet exhibited pores on the order of magnitude of 500 Å in diameter. The pores in these more gently treated films may still be a processing artifact. With this gentler treatment, essentially no variation in surface coverage occurred for 15–100 mg/dL solution concentration.

Figure 5 depicts similar results for Cohn I fibrinogen. Air drying was shown to have a marked disruptive effect on the adsorbate (Figure 5a). The morphology of the adsorbate differed from that of the air-dried γ-globulin; however, the morphology and pore size of the critical-point–dried adsorbate (Figure 5b) were similar to those for γ-globulin. Comparison of the

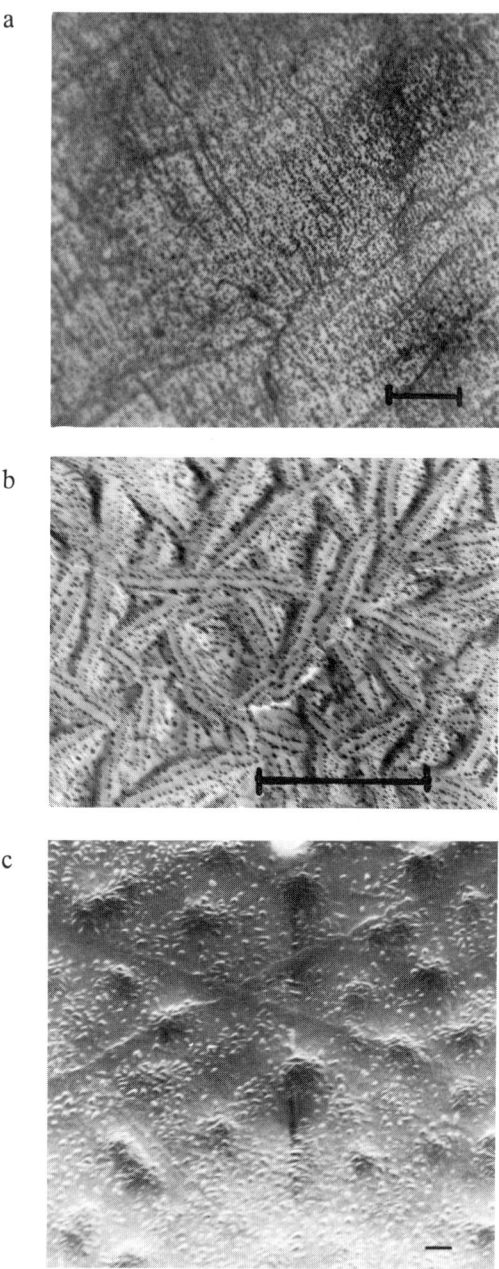

Figure 2. PGDTEM patterns on (a) sintered, 56% crystalline Teflon, (b) Fluorofilm Teflon, and (c) SEM continuous gold–palladium coat on Fluorofilm Teflon. Linear arrays of gold nuclei in (a) are typical, and may reside in surface imperfections. Aggregates of gold nuclei (b) collect at fiber crossovers as shown in (c). Key: bars equal 1 μm.

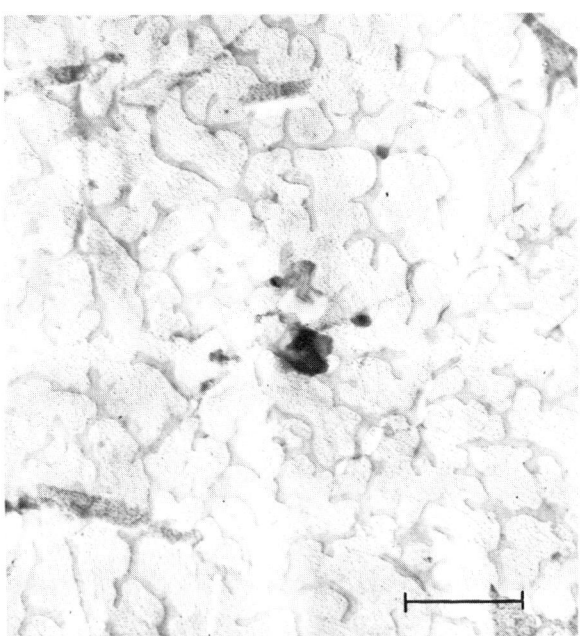

Figure 3a. The γ-globulin adsorbed on the sintered Teflon sample of Figure 2a (air-dry technique). Bovine Cohn II, 100 mg/dL, partial gold decoration. Key: bar equals 1 μm.

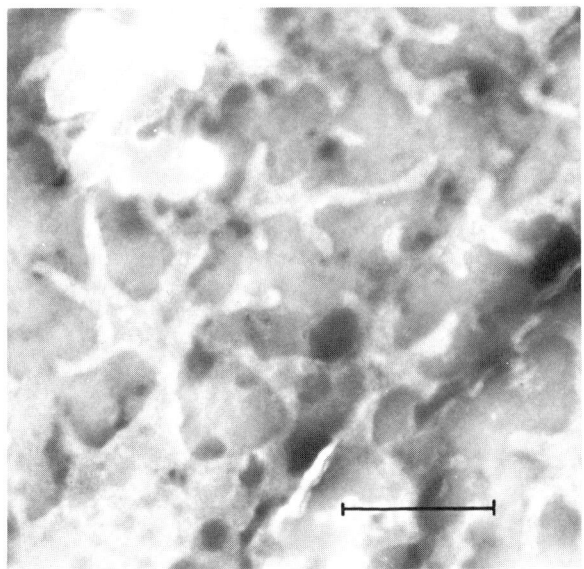

Figure 3b. The γ-globulin adsorbed on the sintered Teflon sample of Figure 2a (air-dry technique). Bovine Cohn II, 100 mg/dL, negative stain. Key: bar equals 1 μm.

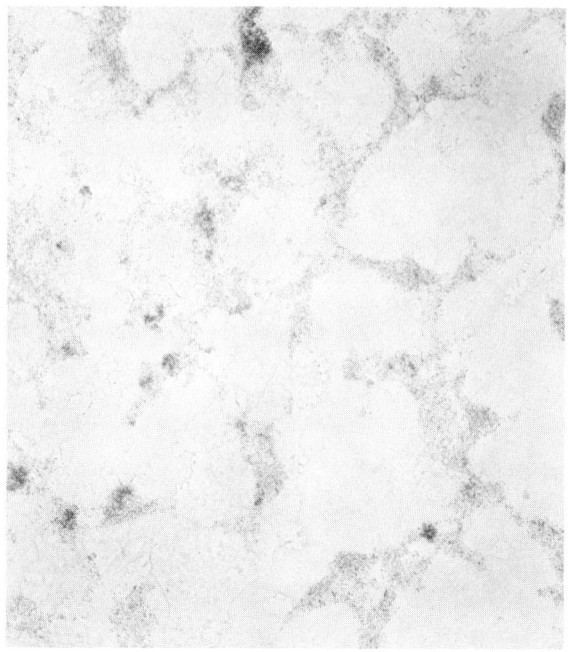

Figure 3c. The γ-globulin adsorbed on the sintered Teflon sample of Figure 2a (dry air technique). Rabbit anti-BSA (IgG), 250 mg/dL, ferritin label, TEM, higher magnification. Key: bar equals 1 μm.

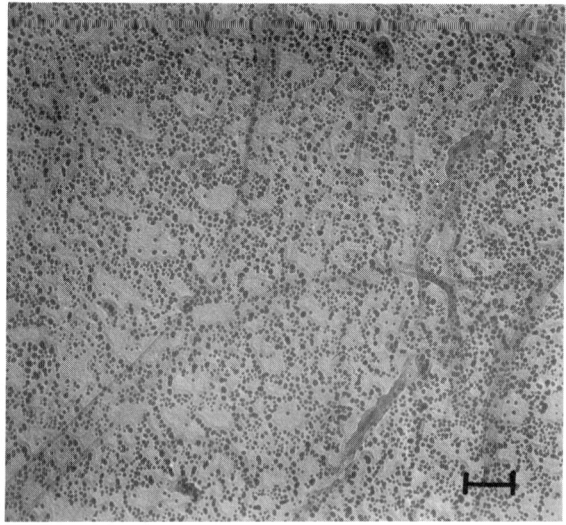

Figure 4. Bovine γ-globulin on sintered Teflon (3 mg/dL solution; critical-point dried, partial gold decoration technique). Key: bar equals 0.1 μm.

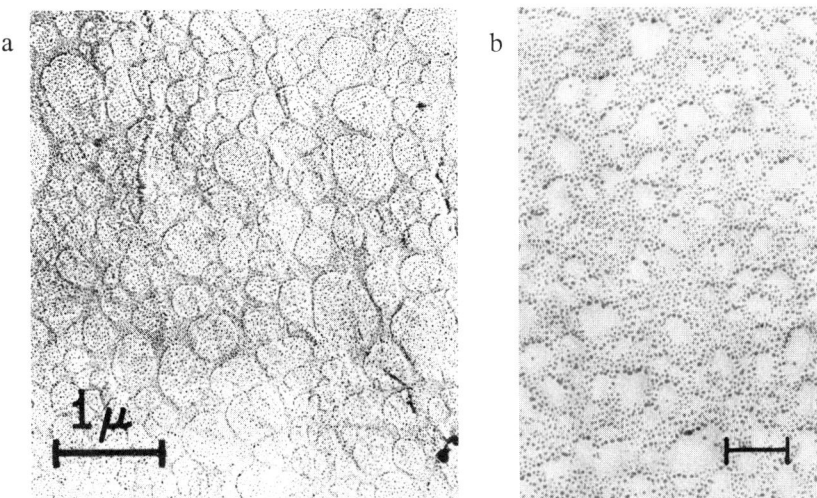
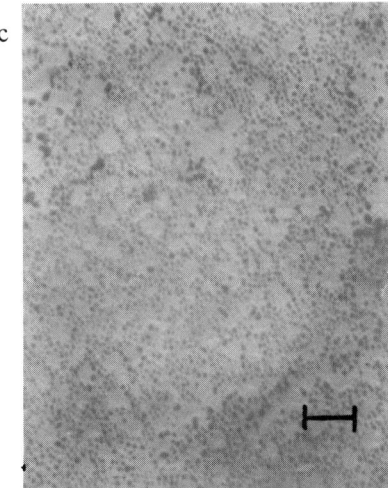

Figure 5. *Cohn I fibrinogen, 3 mg/dL, adsorbed on Teflon (partial gold decoration technique). Key: a, air dried, sintered Teflon; b, critical-point dried, sintered Teflon; and c, critical-point dried, Fluorofilm Teflon. Bar equals 0.1 μm for b and c.*

critical-point–dried protein on the Fluorofilm Teflon (Figure 5c) with that of smoother Teflon (Figure 5b) indicated that no distinguishing surface features discriminated between the adsorbates. This result suggests, in turn, that a protein "blanket" may smooth the rougher surface, utilizing protein–protein bonds to obtain the high surface coverage.

Additional evidence supporting this concept was obtained by stereo pair TEM of critical-point–dried Cohn I fibrinogen. In surface cracks of lengths down to 0.1 μm, Cohn I fibrinogen created a blanket layer, in the crack void, in combination with multiple bifurcating strands of a material that accepts dense gold decoration, and may be fibrin. The strands elaborated from the protein film adjacent to the void also may be derived from the void film. The films existed in several layers in the crack, including a polymer surface–adherent layer. The surface flats exhibited the same reticulated, extensive surface coverage seen in Figures 5b and c.

Air-dried albumin in two-dimensional view exhibited an irregular, partially connected morphology, with blunted ends and an aggregated appearance (Figure 6a), similar to that of air-dried γ-globulin. A nonreplicated sample, high-angle, gold–palladium SEM image from the same surface treatment verified the results (Figure 6b). In contrast to γ-globulin and Cohn I fibrinogen, critical-point–dried albumin exhibited an irregular, unconnected adsorbate, with a characteristic dimension of 200 Å, which appeared to follow the details of surface structure (Figures 7a and b). The albumin adsorbate was characterized by low surface coverage for all polymers studied, in contrast to γ-globulin and Cohn I fibrinogen adsorbates.

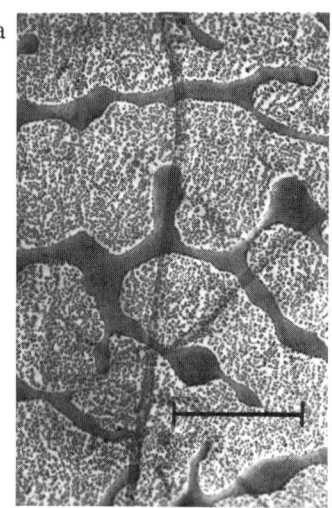 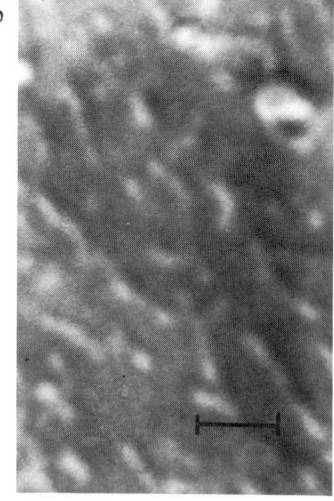

Figure 6. Albumin, 2500 mg/dL solution adsorbed on sintered Teflon (air-dry technique). Key: a, PGDTEM and b, high incidence angle SEM. Bar equals 1 μm.

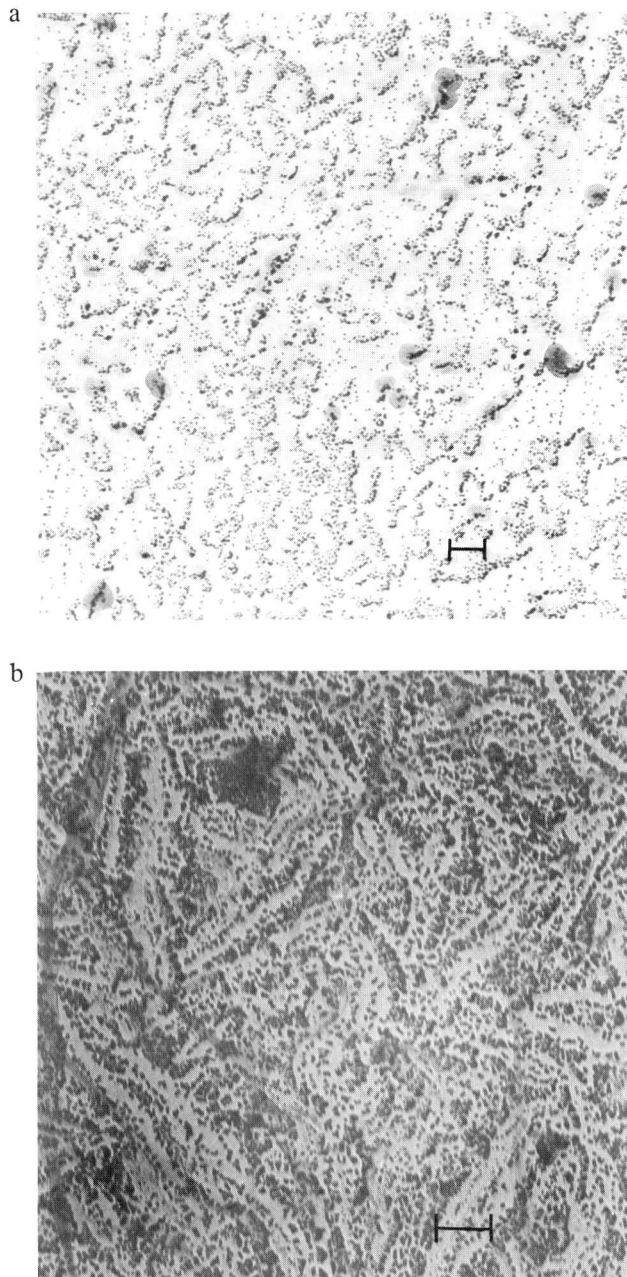

Figure 7. Albumin adsorption by critical-point dry technique. Key: a, sintered Teflon, 250 mg/dL solution and b, Fluorofilm Teflon, 25 mg/dL solution. Bar equals 0.1 μm.

Stereo pair TEM showed that the separation of albumin microadsorbates was preserved in surface holes and cracks, in contrast to the Cohn I fibrinogen results.

Figure 8 summarizes the effects of fluid shear on protein adsorbed to the rough, Fluorofilm Teflon. Cohn I fibrinogen, at 3 and 300 mg/dL, exhibited a weak shear dependence out to a wall shear rate of 1500 s^{-1}. The morphology of the adsorbates did not change; rather, the number of pores in the surface film increased. Albumin was also removed, with a weak dependence on wall shear rate. However, because albumin exposure produced, characteristically, only 20–40% surface coverage, the adsorbate was removed essentially by the 1500-s^{-1} wall shear rate. The gold-decorated adsorbate was difficult to differentiate from the gold nuclei on the substrate for a wall shear rate greater than 800 s^{-1}. Our impression of this result is stronger than can be shown in Figure 8, owing to the artifacts in substrate decoration.

Preexposure of the Flourofilm Teflon surface to albumin, followed by Cohn I fibrinogen (in an air-free, degassed solution environment) and

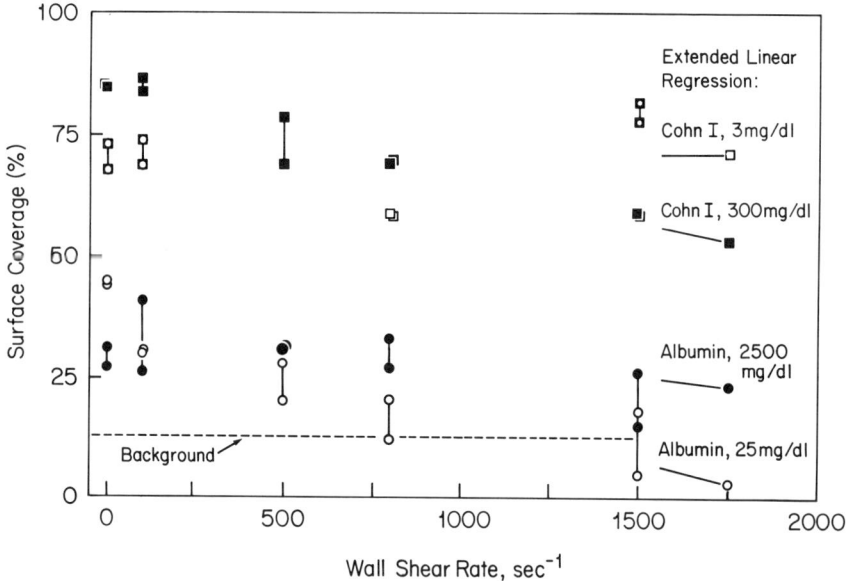

Figure 8. Summary of fluid shear dependence of protein adsorption on Fluorofilm Teflon, using critical-point dry technique for sample preparation and PGDTEM.

Paired data represent high and low area estimates at one set of operating conditions. Lines to the right represent linear regression through all samples at one solution concentration. Key: - - -, average gold nucleus coverage of the Teflon control substrate; □, $r^2 = 0.08$; ■, $r^2 = 0.95$; ●, $r^2 = 0.75$; and ○, $r^2 = 0.79$.

critical-point drying yielded an adsorbate resembling albumin more than Cohn I fibrinogen (Figure 9). Stereo pair TEM of sequential albumin–Cohn I fibrinogen adsorption verified these observations.

These results were supported further in a larger study of several polymers, one in which air drying was used as the final step. The morphologies of the sequential exposure protein adsorbate resembled albumin, not fibrinogen, and the extent of surface coverage was reduced markedly (Figure 10). Thus, the ability of preadsorbed albumin to reduce Cohn I fibrinogen adsorption suggested a potential method for conferring improved thromboresistance on polymers. However, the fragility of the adsorbate, as exemplified by the low extent of surface coverage and weak resistance to shear erosion, suggested that enhancement of polymer affinity for albumin would be necessary to take advantage, in a clinical environment, of albumin's apparent thromboresistive property.

Thus, we turned to alkylation to modify albumin's affinity for polymer surfaces. Chemical derivatization of the polymer surface was evaluated by its ability to adsorb albumin. We verified by optical microscopy that the surfaces

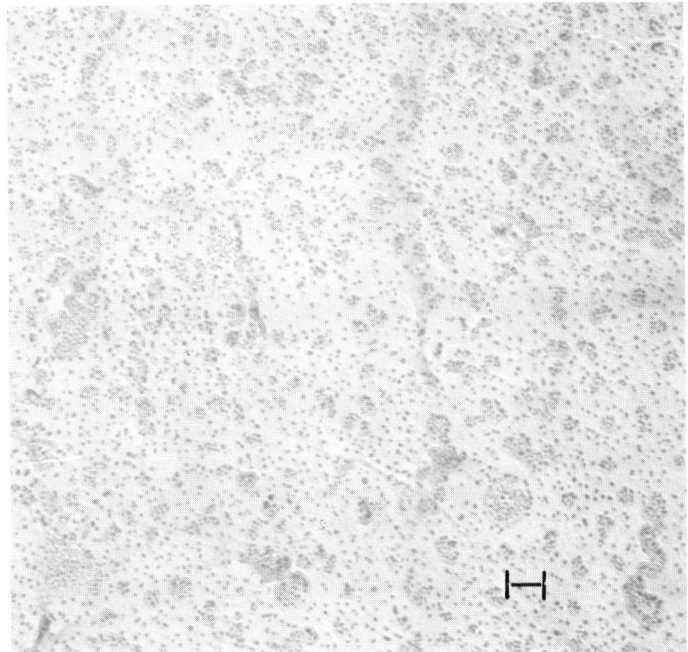

Figure 9. Albumin, 2500 mg/dL solution, preadsorped on sintered Teflon followed by Cohn I fibrinogen, 300 mg/dL, 1h each (critical-point dry and PGDTEM techniques). Key: bar equals 0.1 μm.

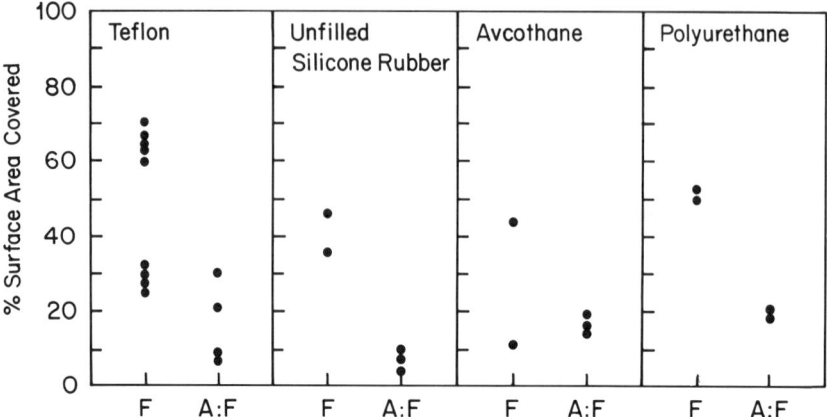

Figure 10. Summary of albumin preadsorption results on a number of polymers. Air drying and PGDTEM were used for all samples. Key: F, 30 mg % fibrinogen (Cohn I) and A:F, 2500 mg % albumin followed by 30 mg % fibrinogen (Cohn I).

were not simply extended by residual solvent swelling or cracking. The effectiveness of the octadecyl residue in binding albumin is shown in Figure 11. Albumin was more rapidly bound to a number of alkylated polyurethanes than to the unmodified surfaces. The extent of normalized but not absolute albumin adsorption was the same after 20–30 min of exposure, insofar as surface concentration is concerned. A series of 5–60-s exposures of the control polyurethane surfaces to ^{125}I albumin solutions of equal concentration showed no change in ^{125}I uptake for 5–15 s, at values equivalent to those obtained by dipping the sample through the air interface film. This result suggests that the ordinate intercept for the control samples represents nonspecific adsorption of air-denatured albumin, and would have occurred for the derivatized samples as well. Thus, we have adopted a conservative interpretation of albumination enhancement by alkylation.

The enhancement of albumin binding, and its potential effectiveness in improving thromboresistance, is further demonstrated in the results of simultaneous fibrinogen–albumin exposure, shown in Figure 12. Reduction of fibrinogen adsorption is proportional to add-on of albumin, presumed to be bound to octadecyl residues. Varying yield may depend on the manufacturer's polymer process variables, the derivatization process variables, and the protein solution exposure technique.

Discussion

Partial gold decoration enhances the protein adsorbate image. Gold vapor atoms condense on the surface to be imaged and migrate until a stable

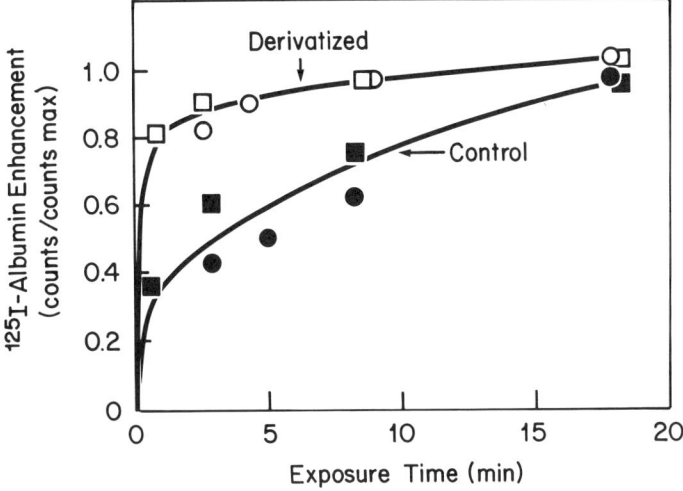

Figure 11. Enhancement of defatted albumin adsorption on Pellethane 2363-80A by binding to octadecyl residues. Symbols represent different derivatization runs.

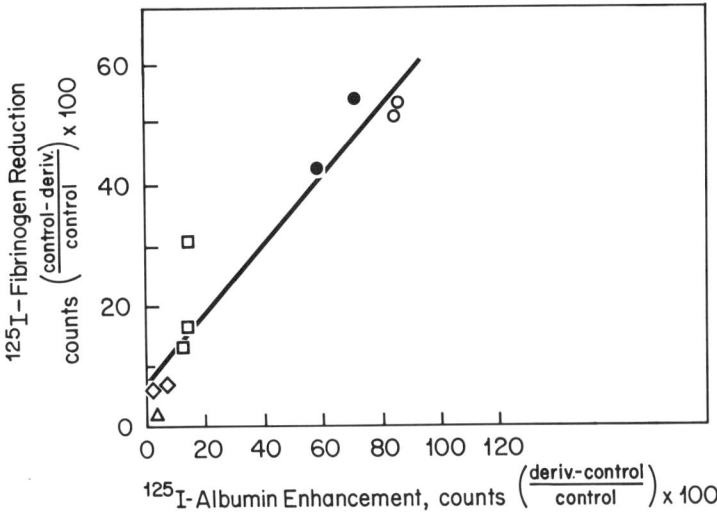

Figure 12. Effect of enhanced binding of defatted albumin to octadecyl residues on reduction of fibrinogen adsorption.

The ordinate gives reduction of fibrinogen adsorption in simultaneous albumin–fibrinogen exposure to the treated samples. The abscissa gives enhancement of albumin adsorption on a duplicate treated sample, using the same albumin solution and identical exposure methodology except for the fibrinogen solution addition. Controls are underivatized samples exposed in the same manner. Both one-step and two-step derivatizations are represented. Distorted Biomer data were corrected by referencing to solvent-treated, but nonderivatized controls. Key: (polyurethanes) ○, Biomer; ●, Biomer (distorted, corrected); □, Pellethane 1; ◇, Pellethane 2; and △, Mobay; $y = 7.6 + 0.57x$; $r^2 = 0.905$; and $S_{y,x} = 6.9$.

gold nucleus is formed. The driving force for the transformation from migrating gold atom to stable nucleus is the free energy difference between the atom and stable nucleus. The gold nucleus density may be described in terms of the impingement rate of gold atoms, their surface residence time, critical nucleus surface density, and rate of growth of nuclei to supercritical dimensions. This value may be expressed by X, the mean distance between stable nuclei, which can be measured experimentally and described analytically (11). The substrate (polymer or protein molecule) modifies the atom–nucleus free energy difference, both in terms of the heat of desorption from the substrate and the heat of diffusion on the substrate surface. Both physical and chemical features of the protein–polymer complex can modify these parameters. The X for all protein adsorbates studied was significantly less than that for the polymer substrates of interest, for partial surface coverage less than 50%. At higher gold coverage fractions, the differences in surface features are obliterated as the gold nuclei grow, coalesce, and form crystals. Empirical observations indicate that a 10–25% coverage of the substrate polymer is best to identify physical and chemical features of the surface.

Comparison of the more gently treated, critical-point–dried γ-globulin and Cohn I fibrinogen adsorbates with air-dried material suggests that protein–protein binding, in combination with protein–polymer binding, creates a tethered network that is in tension during dehydration. This tension is resolved by the circular, reticulated pattern of pores in the film (critical-point drying), which minimizes air–film–surface interfacial tension. Similar patterns have been seen for critical-point dried, purified plasma fibronectin on Teflon (17). Air drying differentiates the γ-globulin and Cohn I fibrinogen films: the γ-globulin film is disrupted and the adsorbate aggregates into extended but unconnected deposits, whereas the Cohn I fibrinogen film always maintains the reticulated pattern. This difference suggests greater strength of the protein–protein bonds for the fibrinogen–γ-globulin–fibronectin complex of Cohn I fraction in the face of dehydration and denaturation forces.

The dramatic stereo pair images of extended fibrinogen films over surface defects provide further and convincing evidence of the strength of the protein–protein bond in this instance. The existence of film pores on surface flats, observed in all cases for Cohn I and II fraction adsorbates, may relate to variations in the conformation of the adsorbed protein, with resultant alteration of binding strength. In the cracks and fissures of the rougher surfaces, the pores were not as prevalent. This result may be due to phenomena that might alter the force balance in the film, for example, concentration of dissolved protein in the defect, protection from shear forces during wash steps, interaction with unremoved microbubbles lodged in cracks, or film support by elaborated fibrin strands.

Observation of strands of fibrin-like material emanating from multiple films of Cohn I fibrinogen in small surface cracks supports the macroscopic, clinical observation of crack-propagated thrombus in extracoporeal circulation and atherosclerotic vascular lesions. This observation also supports findings by Vroman et al. (*18*) based on plasma exposure to a controlled fissure at a sphere–plane–plasma interface. It suggests that surface smoothing techniques must be carried to a high degree of perfection if thromboresistance is to be obtained by this method alone. Identification of the film composition and strand structure may perhaps be carried out by x-ray crystallographic and ferritin-labeled antibody TEM techniques.

Air-exposed albumin aggregates more extensively than the critical-point–dried albumin adsorbate. Yet in both cases, no evidence of the ability (similar to that of fibrinogen, fibronectin, and γ-globulin) to support extensive films in tension during the dehydration process exists.

Identification of the protein adsorbate by the ferritin-conjugated antibody-TEM technique removes one major objection to acceptance of the partial decoration methodology in biomaterials research. However, gold decoration and ferritin-labeled TEM techniques are stop-and-interfere methods, which must be complemented by continuous (*19*) or semicontinuous (*20*) techniques in order to understand the events in blood–material interactions. The partial gold decoration methodology has provided us with superior resolution of all examined protein adsorbates, on surfaces with both physical and chemical inhomogeneity. If, as theory suggests, the metal nucleus decoration method can quantify the chemical inhomogeneity of the polymer surface, it should emerge as a vital tool in biomaterials research.

The weak shear rate dependence of albumin on the Fluorofilm Teflon substrate suggests that the protein–polymer bonds are not strong enough to provide enduring albumin films for this "physiological" range of flow rates. These results are supported by the findings of Brash et al. (*21*). Weak binding also suggests why the surface coverage was incomplete in "static" exposure. Moreover, the apparently complete desorption of albumin above 1500 s^{-1} supports the inferred weak binding from static exposure studies, and casts doubts on the effectiveness of spontaneous albumination as a practical treatment to enhance thromboresistance. Yet preadsorbed albumin, in both air-dried and critical-point–dried settings, gave convincing evidence of inhibition of Cohn I fibrinogen adsorption.

Our protein visualization studies suggest that fibrinogen and globulin fraction proteins rapidly form a tightly bound, extensive coat that is relatively weakly attached to the surface. The coat is weakly, but sufficiently sensitive to fluid shear that shear erosion of the coat will occur at physiological flow rates over extended time periods. Shear erosion would probably increase for smoother surfaces. The "loosely adherent layer" inferred by total internal reflection fluorescence analysis (*19*) may desorb under the influence of flow and/or conformational change to expose the film pores reported above. The film may thicken, elaborate into fibrin-like strands, or adopt other irreversible conformational changes with time. Albumin may modify the conformation of the fibrinogen adsorbate as demonstrated for albumin–fibronectin adsorption (*22*). Preadsorbed albumin apparently occupies the relatively few surface binding sites otherwise available to fibrinogen and γ-globulin, such that a fibrinogen/globulin fraction film may not develop.

Albumin previously has been strongly but irreversibly bound to polymers by a number of methods (*23–25*). The nature of these binding techniques suggests the inability to desorb the material, once the functional biological activity of the surface bound molecule has been lost.

We exploited albumin's high affinity for the hydrophobic function of long-chain fatty acids in the alkyl residue derivatization. We utilized selective high-affinity binding sites on polymer surfaces to bond C_{16-18} carbon aliphatic chains covalently to the surface. Using the 18-carbon chain as the surface substrate provided the advantages of (1) having a near-maximum affinity coefficient (near that of oleate $K_A = 2.6 \times 10^8 M^{-1}$) and (2) being inaccessible to enzymatic degradation (aliphatic chains cannot be degraded via β-oxidation without the presence of a terminal acid function). In the following, we describe two methods of binding aliphatic chains to polymer surfaces. The first consists of a two-step substitution reaction in which polymers with active surface hydrogens (i.e., polyurethane, polyamides, polyesters, etc.) are deprotonated by an aprotonous base (sodium ethoxide) forming an amide ion intermediate. Subsequent treatment with an aliphatic halide which attracts the intermediate in an $S_N 2$ type reaction gives a substituted tertiary amine. The second method of surface substitution is the reaction between an aliphatic isocyanate and active sites of the polymer surface in the presence of a zinc catalyst. In addition to successful and promising results for both methods with polyurethane, these and other reactions also have been carried out successfully on Nylon, polyacrylamide, and other polymers. Dacron has been substituted via transamination and Friedel–Crafts reactions.

By establishing an endogenous albumin adsorbate through selectively increasing the affinity of the surface for albumin, the inherent problems of covalently binding albumin might be eliminated. Denatured and desorbed endogenous albumin might be replaced by additional endogenous albumin which could favorably compete for the open alkyl residues, continuing to maintain the unavailability of the surface to those glycoproteins implicated in cell adhesion and coagulation. Thus, the high albumin affinity substrate, with its biologically functional, renewable endogenous albumin coat may maintain the thromboresistance of a prosthetic device indefinitely.

We produced two types of preliminary evidence to support this hypothesis. First, in radiolabeled albumin studies, alkyl-derivatized polyurethane samples had consistently greater albumin coverage than control samples, with maximal enhancement at short exposure times (Figure 11). Similar results were obtained for other polymers (Nylon, Dacron, polyacrylamide). In addition, modified polyurethane samples exhibited a distinctive two-rate kinetic curve. Based on the similarity between kinetic curves normally seen for high-affinity protein–substrate competitive systems and those of the modified polymer surface, we hypothesize that the initial fast rate represents binding of protein to the available alkyl residues, which is essentially complete within 60 s of exposure. Furthermore, since the second, slower adsorption rate of the modified sample kinetic curve does not reassume that of the unmodified sample, we hypothesize that nonspecific binding sites of the original surface have either been replaced by specific sites through the modification procedure, or have become masked by the specifically bound albumin. Neither hypothesis has been substantiated at this time. Second, in simultaneous albumin–fibrinogen adsorption studies (Figure 12), inhibition of fibrinogen adsorption was proportional to enhancement of albumin adsorption, referenced to underivatized controls. The effect was observed for a number of polyurethane formulations. Furthermore, this effect represents substantial improvement for some of the most blood-compatible polymers currently under investigation (26). Work remains to be done to verify the postulated desorption of albumin at the hydrophobic binding site (27). The results, favorable in the short term, must be validated in the long term, and also in the blood environment. Nevertheless, a method of promise apparently has been developed in the search for materials of improved blood compatibility.

Conclusions

The PGDTEM technique produced superior protein adsorbate images, which have been verified by independent methods. Gold decoration images may not discriminate between protein species adsorbates, however, ferritin-conjugated antibodies may be used for this purpose. Visualization is difficult for protein deposits at low surface concentration. Cohn I fibrinogen adsorbates following a gentle wash (critical-point–dried), are reticulated and connected, with a pore dimension of 400 Å and high surface coverage. Cohn I fibrinogen adsorbates on a Fluorofilm Teflon surface have a weak negative shear dependence at wall shear rates less than 1500 s^{-1}. Adsorption and conversion of the Cohn I fibrinogen may be enhanced in surface defects, and adsorption of Cohn I fibrinogen is inhibited by albumin preadsorption. The results suggest that protein–protein binding is involved in the extension of surface coverage by Cohn I fibrinogen and by γ-globulin. Albumin adsorbates (critical-point–dried) are irregular and unconnected, with a characteristic dimension of 200 Å, and a low surface coverage is observed following gentle wash. Adsorbed albumin is essentially removed by a wall shear rate greater than 1500 s^{-1}, and the adsorbate is unchanged by surface structural detail down to 1000 Å.

Polymers of biomedical interest can be treated in order to covalently bind C_{18} analogs of aliphatic chains. The treatment enhances binding of defatted albumin in short-term exposure, and reduces fibrinogen adsorption, in proportion to enhancement of albumin adsorption. The treatment appears promising for general improvement of blood compatibility of a number of polymers.

Acknowledgments

We gratefully acknowledge the contributions of many skilled colleagues: in protein radiolabeling, P. Kulkarni; in electron microscopy techniques, H. Hagler and W. Schulz; and in fluoroescence technique, F. Grinnell. In addition, the helpful discussions with M. Prager, B. Brink, J. LoSpalluto, M. A. Wilkov, J. Wilson, and F. Grinnell, and the efficient manuscript typing by Katherine Rhodes, are also gratefully acknowledged.

Literature Cited

1. Packham, M. A.; Evans, G.; Glynn, M. F.; Mustard, J. F. *J. Lab. Clin. Med.* **1969**, *73*, 686.
2. Lee, E. S.; Kim, S. W. *ASAIO J.* **1980**, *3*, 50.
3. Jamieson, G. A.; Urban, C. L.; Barber, A. J. *Nature (London), New Biol.* **1971**, *234*, 5.
4. Eberhart, R. C.; Wissinger, J. F.; Wilkov, M. A. *Trans. Soc. Biomaterials* **1978**, *11*, 136.
5. Grinnell, F. *Int. Rev. Cytol.* **1978**, *53*, 65.
6. Harasaki, H.; Kambic, H.; Whalen, R.; Murray, J.; Snow, J.; Murabayashi, S.; Hillegrass, D.; Ozawa, K.; Kiraly, R.; Nose, Y. *Trans. Am. Soc. Artif. Intern. Organs* **1980**, *26*, 470.
7. Pierce, W. J.; Donachy, J. H., Rosenberg, G., Baier, R. E. *Science* **1980**, *209*, 601.
8. Keller, K. H., Ed. "Guidelines for Physicochemical Characterization of Biomaterials," NIH Publication 80–2186, U. S. Dept. Health and Human Services, September 1980.
9. Mason, R. G., Ed. "Guidelines for Blood-Material Interactions," NIH Publication 80–2185, U. S. Dept. Health and Human Services, September 1980.
10. Eberhart, R. C.; Prokop, L. D.; Wissinger, J. F.; Wilkov, M. A. *Trans. Am. Soc. Artif. Intern. Organs* **1977**, *23*, 134.
11. Bilge, F. H., unpublished data.
12. Eberhart, R. C.; Lynch, M. E.; Bilge, F. H.; Arts, H. A. *Trans. Am. Soc. Artif. Intern. Organs* **1980**, *26*, 185.
13. Wissinger, J., M. S. Thesis, Univ. of Texas, Austin, 1977.
14. Neugebauer, C. A. In "Handbook of Thin Film Technology"; Maissel, L. I.; Glang, R.; Eds.; McGraw Hill: New York, 1970; Chap. 8.
15. Brash, L. L.; Lyman, D. J. In "The Chemistry of Biosurfaces"; Hair, M. L., Ed.; Marcel Dekker: New York, 1971, Vol. 1.
16. Fraker, P. J.; Speck, J. C., Jr. *Biochem. Biophys. Res. Commun.* **1978**, *80*, 849.
17. Eberhart, R. C., unpublished data.
18. Vroman, L. et al. Chap. 19 in this book.
19. Watkins, R. W.; Robertson, C. R. *J. Biomed. Mater. Res.* **1977**, *11*, 915.
20. Ihlenfeld, J. V.; Mathis, T. R.; Barber, T. A.; Mosher, D. F.; Updike, S. J.; Cooper, S. L. *Trans. Am. Soc. Artif. Intern. Organs.* **1978**, *24*, 727.
21. Brash, J. L.; Uniyal, S.; Samak, Q. *Trans. Am. Soc. Artif. Intern. Organs* **1974**, *20*, 69.

22. Grinnell, F.; Feld, M. K. *J. Biomed. Mater. Res.*, in press.
23. Hoffman, A. S.; Schmer, G.; Harris, C.; Kraft, W. G. *Trans. Am. Soc. Artif. Intern. Organs* **1972**, *18*, 10.
24. Platé, P. A., Matrosovich, M. N. *Doklady Akad. Nauk SSSR* **1976**, *229*, 496.
25. Imai, Y.; von Bally, K. Nose, Y. *Trans. Am. Soc. Artif. Intern. Organs* **1970**, *26*, 17.
26. Schultz, J. S.; Barenburg, S.; Ciarkowski, A. A.; Lindenauer, S. M.; Penner, J. A. "Evaluation of Compatibility of Biomaterials, Devices and Technology Branch Contractors Meeting," NHLBI, U. S. Dept. H.E.W. **1979**, 121.
27. Tanford, C. *Science* **1978**, *200*, 1012

RECEIVED for review January 16, 1981. ACCEPTED March 23, 1981.

Plasma Proteins: Their Role in Initiating Platelet and Fibrin Deposition on Biomaterials

BRIAN R. YOUNG, LINDA K. LAMBRECHT, and STUART L. COOPER

University of Wisconsin, Department of Chemical Engineering, Madison, WI 53706

DEANE F. MOSHER

University of Wisconsin, Department of Medicine, Madison, WI 53706

Purified plasma proteins adsorbed onto polyvinyl chloride and Silastic arteriovenous shunts prior to ex vivo implantation in mongrel dogs altered the time course and amount of thrombus deposition on these surfaces and also the extent of thrombus dissolution. This behavior was observed in in vivo experiments measuring fibrin and platelet deposition profiles from unheparinized blood at shear rates of 600–1900 s^{-1}. Preadsorbed fibrinogen, γ-globulin, fibronectin, von Willebrand factor, and, to a lesser extent, α_2-macroglobulin enhanced thrombosis whereas preadsorbed albumin diminished thrombosis. In similar experiments, heparinized dogs were used to determine specific protein adsorption profiles. Adsorption of fibrinogen, γ-globulin, albumin, and fibronectin was found to be surface dependent.

The first event that generally occurs after blood contacts a polymer surface is the formation of a protein layer at the blood–polymer interface (1). The formation of this protein layer is followed by the adherence of platelets, fibrin, and possibly leukocytes (2). Further deposition with entrapment of erythrocytes and other formed elements in a fibrin network constitutes thrombus formation. The growth of the thrombus eventually results in partial or total blockage of the lumen unless the thrombus is sheared off or otherwise released from the surface as an embolus (3). Emboli can travel downstream, lodge in vital organs, and cause infarction of tissues. The degree to which the polymer surface promotes thrombus formation and embolization, hemolysis, and protein denaturation determines its usefulness as a biomaterial (4).

Vroman and Adams (5, 6, 7) found that fibrinogen is adsorbed rapidly and preferentially out of plasma onto glass and other surfaces. Vroman and Zucker (8) found that fibrinogen apparently mediates adhesion of blood platelets to surfaces. Chiu et al. (9) suggested that the conformation of fibrinogen adsorbing to low-temperature isotropic carbon and to glass is substantially different, and that surface-induced activation through conformational changes may determine the thrombogenicity of adsorbed fibrinogen. Morrissey and Stromberg previously had obtained data supporting the concept of adsorption-induced conformational changes. However, the observed data also may be explained by other mechanisms (10).

In addition to fibrinogen, γ-globulin preadsorbed to artificial surfaces enhanced the platelet release reaction in vitro (11). In contrast, serum albumin passivated the surface towards platelet adhesion (11). Kim and Lee (12) proposed mechanisms whereby the platelet–protein interactions were mediated via glycosyl transferase reactions involving incomplete terminal oligosaccharide units. These groups are present in fibrinogen, γ-globulin, and many other glycoproteins in plasma, but are absent in albumin.

We evaluated the possible role of various plasma proteins in platelet adherence to and fibrin formation on polymer surfaces in vivo. The proteins preadsorbed to polyvinyl chloride (PVC) tubing were purified fibrinogen, unpurified fibrinogen (containing fibronectin and von Willebrand factor, albumin, γ-globulin, fibronectin, von Willebrand factor, and α_2-macroglobulin. The unpurified fibrinogen was probably similar to the fibrinogen preparations used in static systems of platelet adhesion (8, 11). The magnitude of the deposition and time response of thrombus formation and embolization on the different protein-coated surfaces may suggest possible mechanisms of protein–surface, protein–thrombus, and/or protein–platelet interactions. Several of the proteins preadsorbed onto the PVC tubing were studied additionally on medical grade Silastic tubing so that comparison of the effects of the tubing substrate on the protein–thrombus and protein–surface interactions could be made. Finally, the time sequences of protein adsorption from plasma in vivo to both uncoated PVC and Silastic were determined for fibrinogen, γ-globulin, albumin, and fibronectin in heparinized dogs.

Experimental

Preparation of Blood Plasma Proteins. Canine fibrinogen, canine serum albumin, human fibrinogen, and human fibronectin were purified as described previously (13, 14). Purified human fibrinogen was free of plasminogen, fibronectin, and von Willebrand factor, and had a clottability greater than 98%. Purified fibronectin at its physiological concentration contained less than 1% of the plasma concentration of von Willebrand factor and less than 0.5% of the plasma concentration of human fibrinogen. Unpurified human fibrinogen at its physiological concentration contained approximately 50% of the plasma concentration of von Willebrand factor and fibronectin.

Canine γ-globulin (Pentax, Miles Laboratories) was used as received, its purity verified by SDS gel electrophoresis. The method of Sodetz et al. (15) was used to purify von Willebrand factor, and α_2-macroglobulin was purified according to Harpel (16) or Kurecki et al. (17).

Preparation of Surfaces and Preadsorption of Proteins. Plasticized PVC (Tygon R3603, Norton Plastics; 0.125 in. i.d.) and Silastic (Dow Corning, Medical Grade; 0.132 in. i.d.) were cut and used in 140-cm sections as shunts for implantation. When tubing samples for electron microscopy were to be removed, 178-cm sections were used. Each tubing section was washed at room temperature with 200 mL of dilute Ivory detergent (0.125% solution) and rinsed with 600 mL of distilled water. The tubing was then filled with Tyrode's solution (pH 7.35) and left at 4°C overnight. Surface tension measurements of the Tyrode's solution and of the Tyrode's solution that was in contact with the tubing overnight were compared to insure that no soap remained in the tubing after rinsing. Contact angle measurements on the tubing after equilibration overnight with Tyrode's solution were performed to ensure that the surface properties were characteristic of previously used materials.

Shunts were filled with the protein solution of interest by displacing the Tyrode's solution from the shunt, thus preventing any protein-air interfacial contact. The protein solution remained in the tubing at room temperature for 2 h before being rinsed from the tubing with 60 mL of Tyrode's solution. The tubing was then implanted immediately in the test animal.

Bulk protein concentrations used for preadsorption were 0.9 mg/mL for purified fibrinogen and albumin, 0.5 mg/mL for unpurified fibrinogen, 0.12 mg/mL for von Willebrand factor, and 0.33 mg/mL for γ-globulin, α_2-macroglobulin, and fibronectin. Proteins at these bulk concentrations adsorbed to the surface after 2 h of contact with Silastic and PVC (respectively) to yield surface concentrations (of approximately) 3.6 and 2.2 $\mu g/cm^2$ for fibrinogen, 1.4 and 0.5 $\mu g/cm^2$ for albumin, 1.6 and 1.4 $\mu g/cm^2$ for γ-globulin, and greater than 1.0 and 0.6 $\mu g/cm^2$ for fibronectin (18). The surface concentration of adsorbed α^2-macroglobulin and von Willebrand factor has not been measured yet. Surface concentrations were determined by incubating radiolabeled protein of known specific activity ($\mu Ci/\mu g$) with the tubing of interest under the same conditions used for precoating the surface with unlabeled protein. The bulk protein was then flushed from the tubing with Tyrode's solution until constant radioactivity was achieved. The surface was counted in a well γ-detector. With the proper corrections for background, and knowing the specific radioactivity of the bulk protein and the concentration of the bulk protein, the surface concentration was calculable.

Protein Radiolabeling. Two methods for iodine labeling of the proteins were utilized. Early in our study, a method involving free lactoperoxidase (19) was employed; in the latter part of the study, lactoperoxidase bound to solid-phase Enzymobeads (20) (Bio Rad Laboratories) was used for convenience and for gentler treatment of the protein, since high concentrations of harsh reagents were avoided. Iodine-125 (New England Nuclear) was used to label fibrinogen, fibronectin, and albumin, and ^{131}I was used to label γ-globulin. The ^{125}I-albumin and ^{131}I-γ-globulin in vivo protein adsorption were measured simultaneously in the same experiment.

The viability of ^{51}Cr-labeled platelets was demonstrated for our experiment (21). The ^{125}I-labeled fibrinogen retained its clottability, and all radiolabeled proteins retained their native electrophoretic mobilities. Preliminary data for fibrinogen, γ-globulin, albumin, and fibronectin showed that the affinity of the protein for a surface was unchanged upon labeling. This result was demonstrated in vitro. Identical surface coverages for adsorption from solutions of various molar ratios of labeled and unlabeled protein were determined.

All procedures for treatment of the labeled protein and ^{51}Cr-labeled canine platelets are discussed in more detail by Ihlenfeld et al. (13).

Platelet and Fibrin Deposition Measurements. Adsorption of ^{51}Cr-labeled platelets and ^{125}I-labeled fibrinogen was monitored during the first 2 h of blood contact with PVC or silicone rubber tubing in an ex vivo arteriovenous (AV) shunt configuration using anesthetized mongrel dogs. Shear rates in the shunts (600–1900 s^{-1}) were similar to those found in large arteries in vivo (22). Figure 1 illustrates the experimental arrangement used to measure fibrin(ogen) and platelet deposition on ex vivo AV polymer shunts. (The distinction between formed fibrin and adsorbed fibrinogen was not made in this study, and fibrin(ogen) is used to designate this uncertainty.) The sodium iodide crystal within the lead shield was wrapped with 61 cm of tubing and the lead shield was held at 39°C. Prior to implantation of the ends of the tubing into the femoral artery and vein, the animal was injected with ^{125}I-labeled fibrinogen and ^{51}Cr-labeled platelets. The labeled canine fibrinogen and platelets were injected 30 min and 18 h, respectively, before the surgery. The amounts of fibrin(ogen) and platelets adhering to the tubing surface were calculated by measuring the radioactivity of ^{125}I-labeled canine fibrin(ogen) and ^{51}Cr-labeled platelets adhering to the surface (μCi/cm^2 and μCi/1000 μm^2, respectively). This procedure was done after blood was flushed from the shunt by clamping the artery shut and flushing with 60 mL of Tyrode's solution through the flush line (see Figure 1). These values were converted to the proper units by first measuring the ^{125}I-radioactivity/unit weight of fibrinogen (μCi/μg) and the ^{51}Cr-radioactivity/platelet (μCi/platelet) in the circulating blood and then dividing these values into the measured adherent fibrin(ogen) (μCi/cm^2) and platelets (μCi/1000 μm^2). With the proper manipulations and corrections for decay and background, the results are reported in μg/cm^2 or platelets/1000 μm^2 ± standard error from the mean (sem).

Blood flow rate was measured continuously throughout the experiment using an electromagnetic flow probe and physiograph recorder (Gould, SP2202, and Narco Bio-System, MK III, respectively). The probe was placed proximal to the test section around the femoral artery.

Platelet and fibrin(ogen) sampling periods were 2, 5, 10, 15, 30, 45, 60, 90, and 120 min of blood contact.

The influence of flushing the blood from the tubing with Tyrode's solution to enable counting of the adhering fibrin and platelets on subsequent platelet and fibrin deposition, and the apparent time for embolization have been addressed previously. Ihlenfeld et al. (3) showed that the thrombotic response on PVC determined using the flushing technique was similar to the response on shunts implanted sequentially for various lengths of time.

Details of the tests performed on screen animals prior to surgery, hematological tests performed during surgery, surgical procedure, and method of data analysis have been published previously (3).

Protein Deposition Measurements. The procedures for measuring protein adsorption in vivo were identical to those for platelet and fibrin deposition studies with the exception of: (1) the test animal was given an initial dose of 125 units/kg of sodium heparin (Porcine Mucosal, Lypho-Med., Inc.) followed by 40 units/kg given once every hour to prevent thrombus formation (this regimen prolongs blood clotting time more than 1 h); (2) the test animal was injected with either ^{125}I-labeled canine fibrinogen, ^{125}I-labeled fibronectin, or both ^{125}I-labeled serum albumin and ^{131}I-labeled γ-globulin; and (3) hematological tests were omitted during the experiment. Experimental data were converted to units of (cpm/cm^2 tubing)/(cpm/cm^3 blood). Additional information about the calculations and experimental details have been published previously by Ihlenfeld and Cooper (23).

To present the data in a more useful form, the results tabulated as (cpm/cm^2 tubing)/(cpm/cm^3 blood) were converted to (ng adsorbed protein)/(cm^2 of tubing

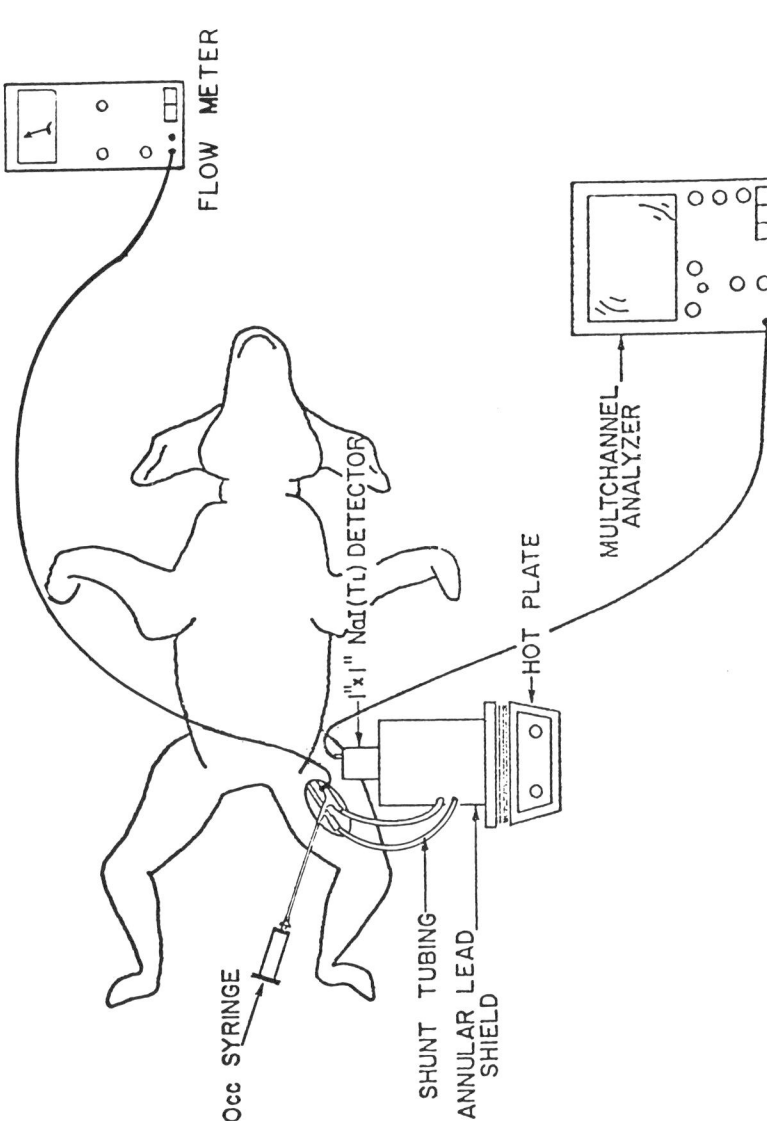

Figure 1. *Experimental arrangement for transient thrombus deposition measurements. Twenty-four inches of shunt tubing are in contact with the shielded detector.*

surface). This conversion was accomplished by multiplying (cpm/cm^2 tubing)/(cpm^3 blood) ± sem by the average physiological blood protein concentration of the protein being studied. These concentrations were determined from blood samples taken from randomly chosen dogs used in our experiments. The average hematocrit value used in these calculations was 41.9 ± 6.57 ($N = 40$). The calculated γ-globulin concentration in blood was 3.14 ± 0.83 mg/cm^3 ($N = 10$). This result was determined from a total globulin measurement based on the Hopkins–Cole reaction (24) according to the procedure in Sigma's Technical Bulletin No. 560; 19.5% of the total globulin was assumed to be γ-globulin (25). The calculated concentration of albumin in blood was 20.3 ± 3.58 mg/cm^3 ($N = 10$). This measurement was based on a measurement described by Doumas et al. (26), and was modified according to the procedure given in Sigma's Technical Bulletin No. 630. A concentration of 1.14 ± 0.18 mg/cm^3 ($N = 40$) in blood was determined for fibrinogen, and a value of 0.18 mg/cm^3 in blood was used for fibronectin based on the observed value of 0.33 mg/cm^3 in human plasma (27) and assuming a hematocrit of 44 (25).

For the data reported in Figures 4 and 7, the magnitude of the ordinate values should be interpreted with the understanding that the adsorbed protein magnitudes were calculated on average concentrations in canine blood and, in the case of fibronectin, extrapolated from human plasma concentration values.

Electron Microscopy Samples. Approximately 2-cm lengths of tubing were excised distal to the counted tubing section at blood contact times of 0, 2, 5, 10, 15, 30, 45, 60, 90, and 120 min for analysis by scanning electron microscopy. These samples were fixed in 1.5% glutaraldehyde and 1% osmium tetroxide, and were dehydrated using increasing concentrations of ethanol. The dehydrated sample specimens were then critical-point dried and coated with carbon and gold palladium for scanning electron microscopy.

Results

Protein and Thrombus Response to Uncoated PVC and Silastic. The animal model presented in this chapter yielded platelet and fibrin(ogen) deposition data during the first 120 min of blood exposure. Because growth of thrombus on the surface is an indication of thrombogenicity, the magnitude of the maximum deposition is important when comparing thrombus deposition patterns on two different surfaces. In addition, a thrombus can be sheared from the surface as an embolus, and the degree to which thrombus is released from the surface after maximum deposition is also important in determining biocompatibility. The parameters of maximum thrombus deposition and percent embolization (which will be defined later) were based on the initial 120 min of blood exposure. Caution should be exercised in extrapolating these results to blood exposure situations involving different flow conditions or longer blood contact times.

Upon contact with blood, uncoated PVC (shown in Figures 2 and 3) initiated rapid thrombus deposition which was followed by substantial embolization. The time course of the platelet and fibrin(ogen) deposition curves showed that increases in platelet coverage were directly related to increases in the amount of fibrin(ogen) on the surface. This result suggests that the fibrin(ogen) and platelets are interwoven in a network. Although other interpretations are conceivable, previous studies utilizing scanning and transmission electron microscopy support this contention (28).

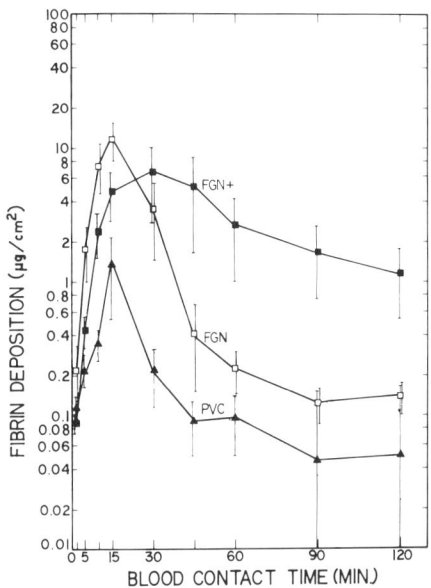

Figure 2. Transient fibrin deposition (±sem) on adsorbed protein substrates. Key: ▲ *(PVC), uncoated PVC (N = 8);* □ *(FGN), fibrinogen free of fibronectin and vWf on PVC (N = 4); and* ■ *(FGN+), fibrinogen containing fibronectin and vWf on PVC (N = 7).*

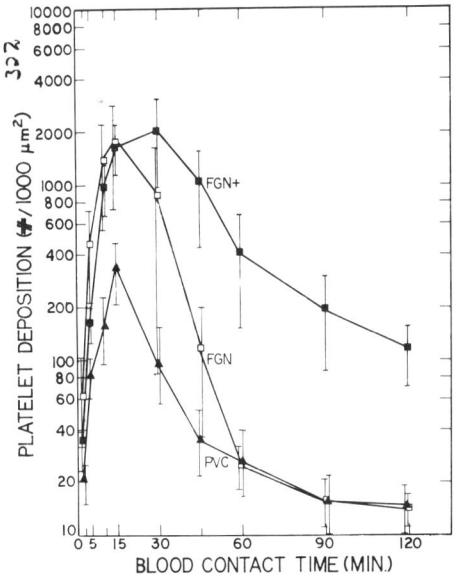

Figure 3. Transient platelet deposition (±sem) on adsorbed protein substrates. Key: ▲ *(PVC), uncoated PVC (N = 10);* □ *(FGN), fibrinogen free of fibronectin and vWf on PVC (N = 4); and* ■ *(FGN+), fibrinogen containing fibronectin and vWf on PVC (N = 7).*

Data obtained using heparinized dogs (29) (Figure 4) showed that at 2 min of blood contact, serum albumin, γ-globulin, fibrinogen, and fibronectin adsorbed to the surface in the relative ratios of 100 : 100 : 75 : 3, respectively, where the surface concentration of serum albumin was 200 ng/cm^2.

The thrombotic response (the time vs. platelet and fibrin deposition pattern) for uncoated PVC (shown in Figures 2 and 3) is a response to PVC that is coated with a complex mixture of proteins in the initial seconds of blood contact. Therefore, at least part of the thrombotic response on PVC is generated by a complex protein-coated surface composed of many proteins adsorbed in various conformations, including serum albumin, γ-globulin, fibrinogen, and fibronectin. However, these four proteins account for only 75% of the total protein in plasma and, therefore, significant amounts of other proteins not accounted for by our measurements may be adsorbed to the test surface.

The thrombotic response to uncoated PVC and to uncoated Silastic would be expected to be identical if thrombosis is surface nonspecific or if the surfaces initially adsorb the same proportion of the various plasma proteins that influence thrombosis. Comparisons of the responses of the uncoated surfaces (Figure 2 with 5 and 3 with 6) reveal that both the fibrin(ogen) and platelet deposition profiles on uncoated Silastic were significantly different than those on PVC. Fibrin(ogen) deposition proceeded at a slower rate on uncoated Silastic than on uncoated PVC, and peaked after 30 min of blood

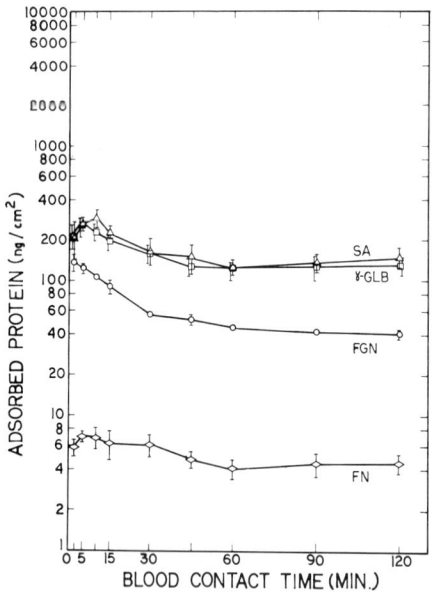

Figure 4. Transient in vivo protein adsorption (±sem) in heparinized dogs on PVC (29). Key: □ (γ-GLB), γ-globulin (N = 4); △ (SA), albumin (N = 3); ○ (FGN), fibrinogen (N = 3); and ◇ (FN), fibronectin (N = 4).

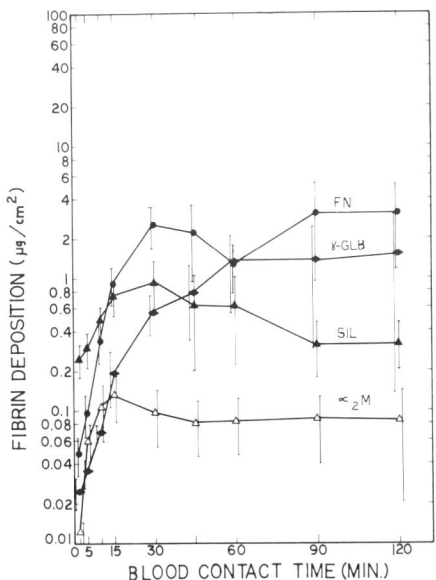

Figure 5. Transient fibrin deposition (±sem) on adsorbed protein substrates. Key: ▲ *(SIL), uncoated Silastic (N = 5);* ♦ *(γ-GLB), γ-globulin on Silastic (N = 3);* ● *(FN), fibronectin on Silastic (N = 6); and* △ *(α_2M), α_2-macroglobulin on Silastic (N = 4).*

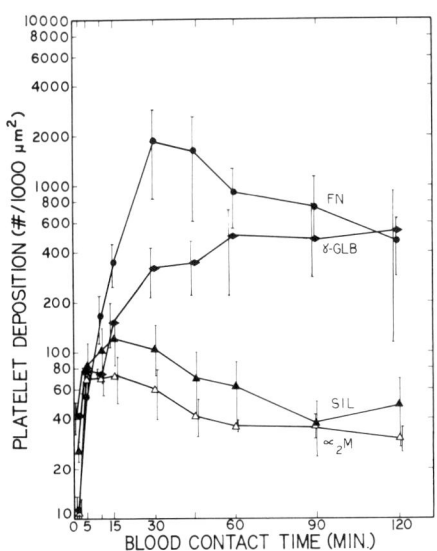

Figure 6. Transient platelet deposition (±sem) on adsorbed protein substrates. Key: ▲ *(SIL), uncoated Silastic (N = 5);* ♦ *(γ-GLB), γ-globulin on Silastic (N = 3);* ● *(FN), fibronectin on Silastic (N = 6), and* △ *(α_2M), α_2-macroglobulin on Silastic (N = 5).*

contact time. Platelet deposition on Silastic proceeded very rapidly from 2 to 5 min of blood contact time, gradually increased to a maximum at 15 min, and then gradually decreased. This observation is in sharp contrast to the response on uncoated PVC where a sharp peak in platelet and fibrin(ogen) thrombus deposition centered at 15 min was observed. The degree of platelet and fibrin(ogen) dissolution on uncoated Silastic also was much less than that on uncoated PVC.

Comparison of fibrin(ogen) and platelet deposition on uncoated Silastic makes it apparent that fibrin(ogen) deposition and embolization were not proportional to platelet adherence and embolization. In work published previously, scanning electron micrographs showed isolated platelet clumps on Silastic that were slightly smaller than those on PVC. Small patches of basal fibrin also were observed on Silastic (28). Together with the electron microscopy work, the rapid platelet accumulation suggests that the platelets are both adhering uniformly on the surface in monolayer fashion and forming platelet clumps. At the same time, apparently, fibrin strands are gradually forming a network independent of the deposited platelets.

Figure 7 shows that Silastic initially (2 min of blood contact) adsorbed albumin, γ-globulin, fibrinogen, and fibronectin in the relative ratios of 100 : 52 : 33 : 3, where the surface concentration of serum albumin was 300

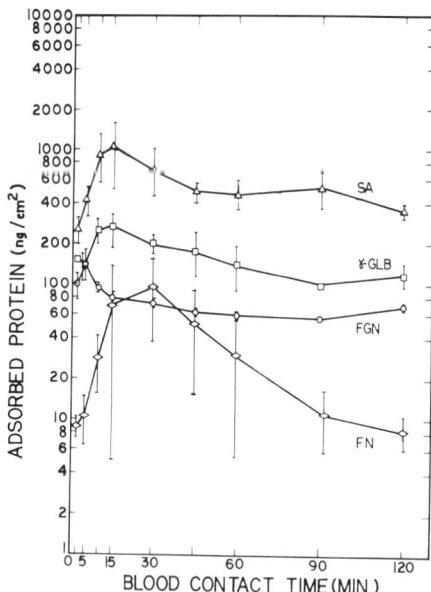

Figure 7. Transient in vivo protein adsorption (±sem) in heparinized dogs on Silastic (29). Key: □ *(γ-GLB), γ-globulin (N = 3);* △ *(SA), albumin (N = 3);* ○ *(FGN), fibrinogen (N = 3); and* ◇ *(FN), fibronectin (N = 5).*

ng/cm^2. These data compare to 100:100:75:3 for protein adsorption onto PVC (where the surface concentration of albumin was 200 ng/cm^2). Based on the thrombotic responses discussed so far, PVC might be classified as more thrombogenic than Silastic because smaller thrombi and less embolization occurred on the Silastic surface. In addition, albumin, which is less thrombogenic in preadsorption studies (see below), had a higher initial surface concentration on Silastic than on PVC. Consequently, the differences between the thrombotic responses on PVC and Silastic may be due to surface and physical property differences of the polymers which control the relative amounts of proteins adsorbed initially.

The marked difference between fibronectin adsorption on Silastic and PVC (Figure 7 vs. Figure 4) is interesting. The greater fibronectin adsorption on Silastic might explain why the thrombi formed on the Silastic surface embolize to a lesser extent than those formed on PVC because fibronectin appears to play a role in both cell-to-cell and cell-to-substratum adhesion (30, 31). However, fibronectin adsorption on Silastic varied widely among test animals.

Thrombotic Response to Protein-Coated Surfaces. OVERVIEW. Although Figures 2, 3, 5, 6, and 8–11 show fibrin(ogen) and platelet responses to many different surfaces, all of the curves have a similar appearance. At the first datum of 2 min, an initial amount of deposition was gener-

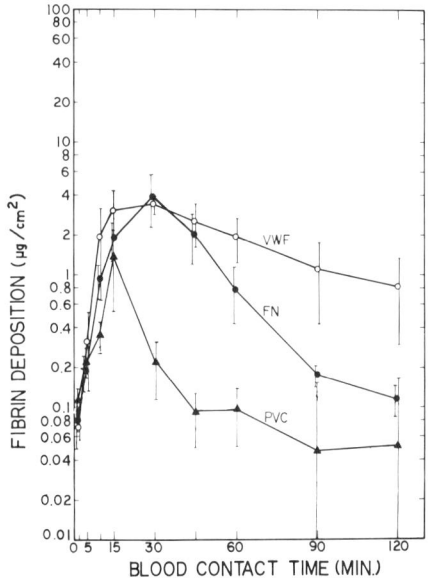

Figure 8. Transient fibrin deposition ($\pm$sem) on adsorbed protein substrates. Key: ▲ *(PVC), uncoated PVC (N = 8);* ● *(FN), fibronectin on PVC (N = 4); and* ○ *(vWf) vWf on PVC (N = 5).*

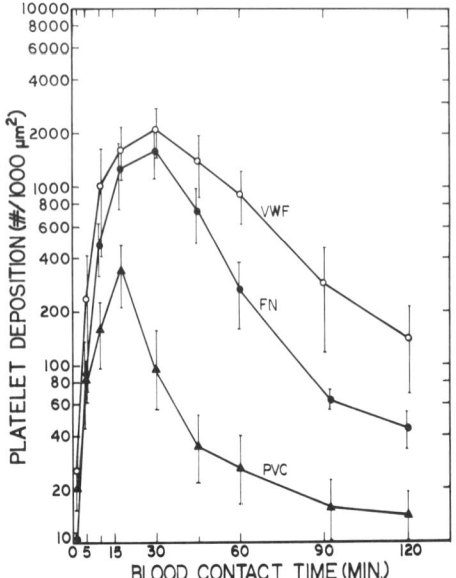

Figure 9. Transient platelet deposition (±sem) on adsorbed protein substrates. Key: ▲ *(PVC), uncoated PVC (N = 9);* ● *(FN), fibronectin on PVC (N = 5); and* ○ *(vWf), vWf on PVC (N = 5).*

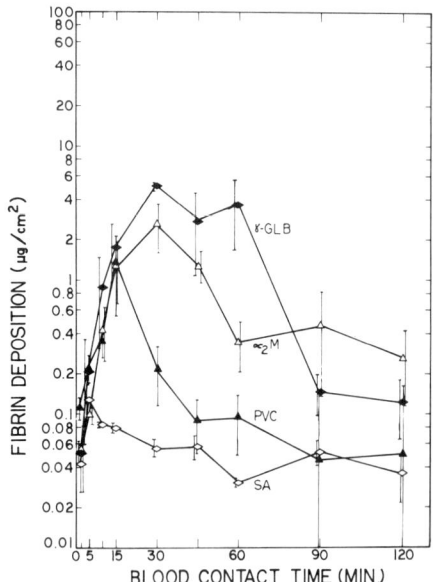

Figure 10. Transient fibrin deposition (±sem) on adsorbed protein substrates. Key: ▲ *(PVC), uncoated PVC (N = 8);* ♦ *(γ-GLB), γ-globulin on PVC (N = 3);* △ *($α_2$M), $α_2$-macroglobulin on PVC (N = 4); and* ◇ *(SA), albumin on PVC (N = 3).*

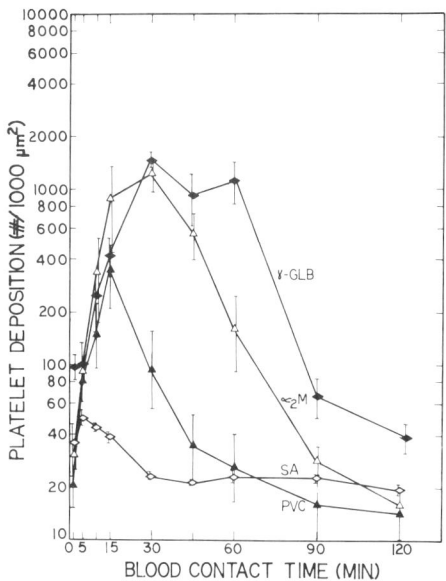

Figure 11. Transient platelet deposition (±sem) on adsorbed protein substrates. Key: ▲ *(PVC), uncoated PVC (N = 9);* ◆ *(γ-GLB), γ-globulin on PVC (N = 3);* △ *(α_2M), α_2-macroglobulin on PVC (N = 4); and* ◇ *(SA), albumin on PVC (N = 3).*

ally lower than or equal to other values occurring during the subsequent 118 min of blood contact. With increasing time the amount of fibrin(ogen) or platelets adhering to the surface increased to a maximum value. The maximum was followed by the release of the thrombi, presumably as emboli.

The thrombotic responses to the various surfaces can be characterized by specifying the initial rate of thrombus deposition for the period from 0 to 2 min of blood contact, the time (or time range) and magnitude of maximum thrombus deposition, and the extent of embolization after 120 min of blood exposure. This characterization is presented in Table I for the fibrin(ogen) and platelet deposition profiles on the protein-coated surfaces. To obtain the entries in Columns 2–4 of Table I, the numerical values of the fibrin(ogen) and platelet data from the protein-coated surface (Figures 2, 3, 5, 6, and 8–11) were divided by the corresponding numerical value of the fibrin(ogen) or platelet data from the uncoated surface.

In addition, the ratio of the amount of the protein preadsorbed onto the surface (μg/cm^2) to the amount of the protein adsorbed initially onto the uncoated surface in vivo (from Figures 4 and 7 at 2 min of blood contact time) is presented in Column 1 of Table I (Amount Preadsorbed).

Presumably, a surface precoated with protein would initially adsorb less protein from the blood than an uncoated surface. Data on the uncoated surfaces are shown in Figures 4 and 7. From in vitro adsorption studies of

Table I. Reduced Data

Surface	Protein Preadsorbed	Protein Preadsorbed[a]	Initial Rate of Deposition[b]		Time of Maxima[c]		Amount Adhering at Maxima[d]		Extent of Embolization at 120 Min. (%)[e]	
			Fibrin	Platelets	Fibrin	Platelets	Fibrin	Platelets	Fibrin	Platelets
PVC	Fibrinogen	17	1.9	2.9	1	1	8.7	5.4	99	98
	Fibrinogen+ von Willebrand factor	17	0.77	1.6	1–3	1–3	4.9	6.3	82	94
		—	0.62	1.2	1–4	1–4	2.5	6.3	76	93
	Fibronectin	>86	0.70	0.42	1–3	1–3	3.0	4.8	97	97
	γ-Globulin	5	0.44	4.5	2–4	2–4	1.3	4.5	98	97
	$α_2$-Macroglobulin	—	0.47	1.4	1–3	1–3	2.0	3.7	90	99
	Albumin	1.7	0.37	1.6	0.33	0.33	0.10	0.15	72	61
	Uncoated	1.0	1.0	1.0	1	1	1.0	1.0	96	96
Silastic	Fibronectin	>91	0.19	0.44	1.5	2	2.8	15	0	75
	γ-Globulin	11	0.10	1.6	4	8	1.7	4.3	0	0
	$α_2$-Macroglobulin	—	0.049	0.42	0.5	1	0.14	0.60	36	57
	Uncoated	1.0	1.0	1.0	1	1	1.0	1.0	64	60

[a] Amount of protein preadsorbed/amount of that protein adsorbed in vivo after 2 min of blood contact on uncoated surface.
[b] Amount adhering at 2 min of blood contact/amount adhering at 2 min on the uncoated surface.
[c] Time of maxima/time of maxima on uncoated surface.
[d] Amount adhering at maxima/amount adhering at maxima on uncoated surface.
[e] $100 × (1 − $[amount adhering at 120 min]/[amount adhering at maxima]$)$.

several of the proteins used in this work, we calculated that nearly monolayer coverage on the surface occurs under the preadsorption conditions used in our experiments. (*See* section on Preparation of Surfaces and Preadsorption of Proteins). If exchange of these preadsorbed proteins with fibrinogen from blood is not substantial and if adherence of fibrinogen to the surface is low during the first 2 min of blood contact time, then the normalized initial rate of deposition of fibrin(ogen) shown in Column 2 of Table I should be less than unity. This is the case for all of the preadsorbed proteins tested except for purified fibrinogen on PVC. As discussed below, the value of 1.9 for preadsorbed fibrinogen on PVC probably was due to binding of fibrin(ogen) in the blood with fibrinogen preadsorbed to the surface. Apparently, the initial rate (within 2 min of blood contact) of fibrin formation or fibrinogen adsorption on the PVC surface precoated with fibrinogen is at least 3 times greater than on any of the other protein-coated surfaces.

γ-GLOBULIN. From Table I, apparently 5 times more γ-globulin was preadsorbed onto PVC than would be adsorbed in vivo onto uncoated PVC after 2 min of blood exposure. On this surface, initial fibrin formation decreased significantly while the initial platelet adhesion increased 4.5 times. This initial rate of adsorption of platelets on γ-globulin–coated PVC was much larger than that on any other protein-coated surface. In addition, the thrombi appeared to be anchored to the surface more securely, allowing growth of the thrombi to proceed 2 to 4 times longer than on uncoated PVC. The thrombus at the maximum in deposition contained 4.5 times the number of platelets but only 1.3 times the amount of fibrin(ogen) when compared to the thrombus formed on the uncoated PVC surface. Because less fibrin(ogen) was adsorbed on the γ-globulin layer initially, the thrombus formed subsequently also contained less fibrin(ogen). At 120 min, the thrombus had embolized almost completely, removing platelets and fibrin(ogen) together in equal proportions.

Figures 12 and 13 are scanning electron micrographs showing the surface of γ-globulin–coated PVC after 5 min of blood contact time. Platelets appear to cover the surface uniformly with little evidence of basal fibrin. The large spherical platelet thrombus in Figure 12 also contained no visible fibrin basal to the platelet thrombus.

The fibrin(ogen) and platelet response to γ-globulin–coated Silastic was similar to that on γ-globulin–coated PVC. On both surfaces the relative rate of deposition of fibrin(ogen) initially (Table I) was much less than that of the platelets. On Silastic, the preadsorbed γ-globulin was 11 times more concentrated than the amount that would be adsorbed onto the uncoated surface. Not much embolization occurred during an experimental blood exposure time of 120 min.

Thus, γ-globulin appears to promote a faster rate of platelet adhesion to the surface while limiting fibrinogen adsorption and subsequent fibrin formation. In addition, embolization either was reduced or the time of emboli-

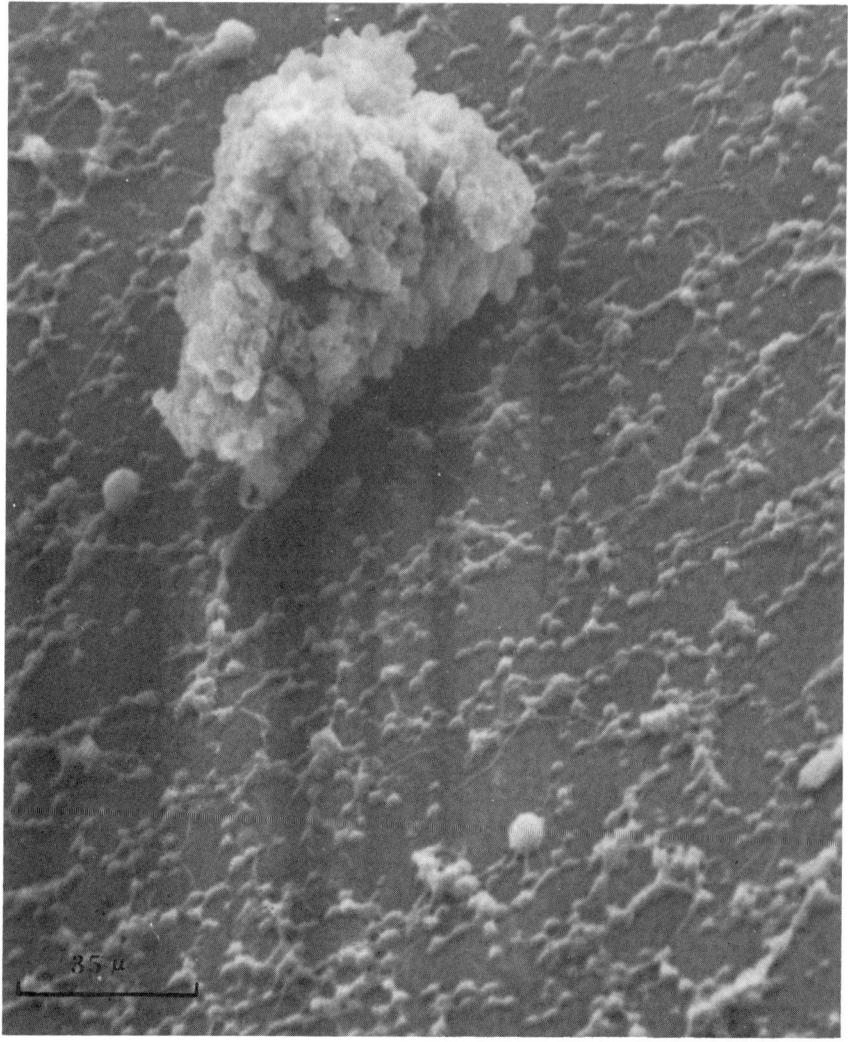

Figure 12. The γ-globulin coated–PVC after 5 min of blood exposure showing randomly scattered platelets, occasional leukocytes, and a large spherical platelet thrombus.

zation was prolonged excessively on the γ-globulin–coated surface vs. the uncoated surface. Apparently, the adhesion between the surface and the protein layer and between the protein layer and platelet clumps is stronger for a γ-globulin–coated surface than the adhesion between a thrombus and the mixed protein layer initially laid down on the uncoated surface.

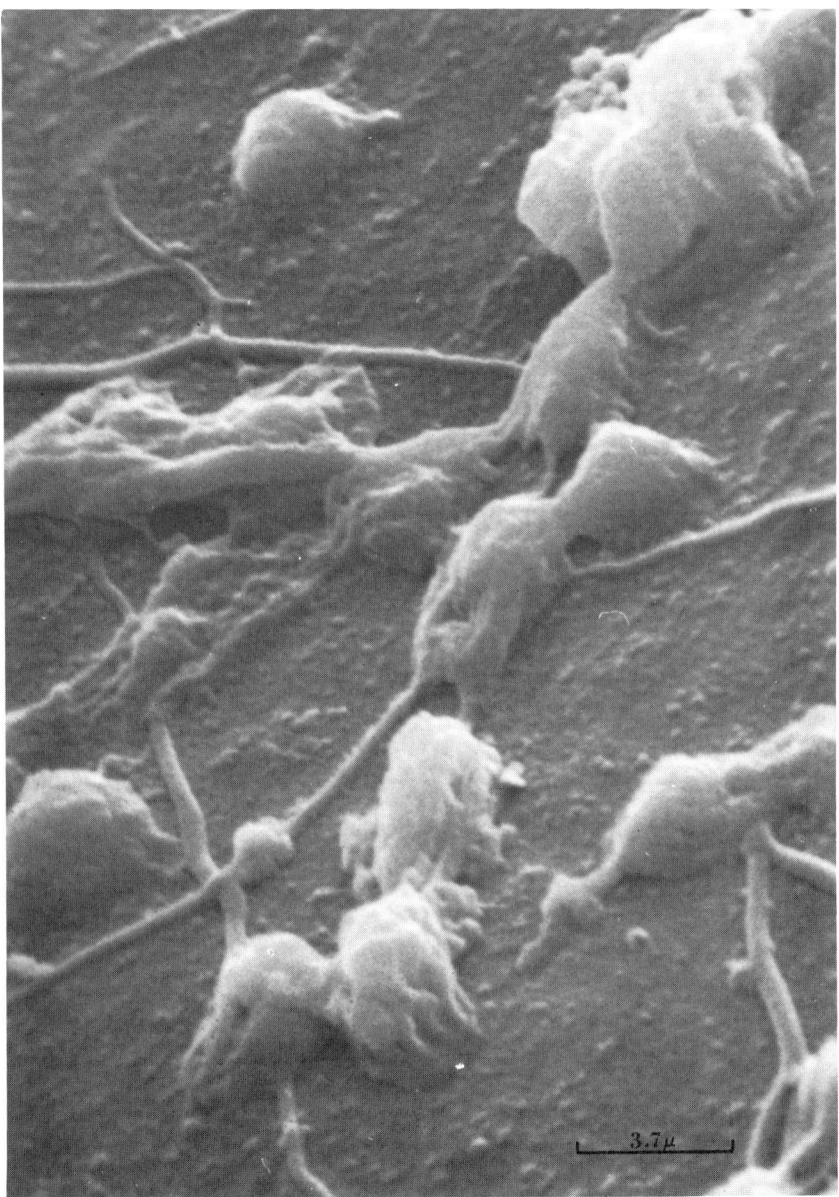

Figure 13. A higher magnification of a section of Figure 12 showing platelets randomly attached to the surface.

α_2-MACROGLOBULIN. Of the three proteins preadsorbed onto both Silastic and PVC, only α_2-macroglobulin appeared to increase thrombosis on one surface while reducing thrombosis on the other. The data of Table I show that when α_2-macroglobulin was preadsorbed onto PVC, fibrin(ogen) and platelet deposition greater two to three times than that observed on uncoated PVC. On Silastic at maximum deposition, α_2-macroglobulin decreased platelet deposition roughly by a factor of 2, and fibrin deposition by a factor of 7 over the deposition on the uncoated surface. On PVC, α_2-macroglobulin lengthened the time period before maximum deposition was reached, while on Silastic, α_2-macroglobulin decreased the time prior to the peak thrombus deposition. Several explanations could account for this behavior. On Silastic, the cell binding portion of α_2-macroglobulin may not have been available to the platelets for binding, or, if the platelet did bind to the protein, the protein may have been unable to secure itself effectively to the Silastic surface. The micrograph of Figure 14 shows a uniform layer of platelets on α_2-macroglobulin adsorbed to PVC after 5 min of blood exposure with thrombi composed of both platelets and fibrin. Figure 15 shows a uniform layer of thrombus adhering to α_2-macroglobulin–coated Silastic after 2 min of blood contact. The micrograph also shows a large patch (upper center) that appears void of platelets and other formed elements. If this area were exposed by the "peeling off" of the uniform layer in this region, then the second hypothesis which states that the protein is unable to secure itself effectively to the Silastic surface would probably be more correct. Even without reference to the large patch, which may be due to an artifact caused by the sample preparation, the loose coupling to the surface of the large thrombi as shown in Figure 15 (α_2 macroglobulin–coated Silastic after 5 min of blood contact) can be contrasted with the apparent firmness of the attachment of the thrombi to PVC (Figure 14).

FIBRONECTIN. When fibronectin was preadsorbed onto Silastic or PVC at roughly 100 times the concentration initially adsorbed in vivo to the uncoated surface, the initial rate of both platelet and fibrin(ogen) deposition decreased. However, the fibrin(ogen) deposition on fibronectin-precoated PVC and Silastic did not decrease as much as on the γ-globulin precoated surfaces. This result is consistent with findings that indicate that fibronectin binds and cross-links to fibrin (through the α-chain of fibrin) (32). Because platelet deposition is inhibited initially, there should be a fibrin layer basal to the platelets and thrombi. In Figure 16, which shows the surface of fibronectin-coated PVC after 5 min of blood contact, fibrin strands are between single platelets and basal to the thrombus (upper right). More fibrin is seen in Figure 16 than in Figure 12, which shows γ-globulin–precoated PVC at 5 min of blood contact.

The thrombotic response at longer blood contact times on fibronectin-coated PVC followed the pattern of the response on γ-globulin–coated PVC except that more fibrin(ogen) was found on the fibronectin-coated surface.

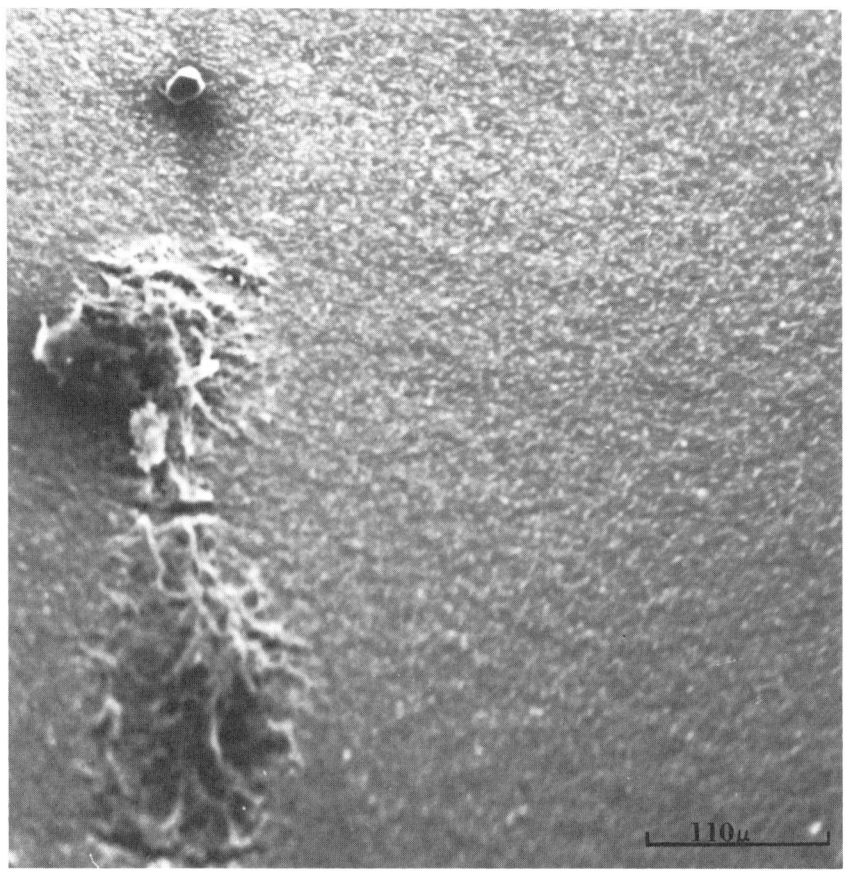

Figure 14. Uniform layer of platelets and fibrin on α_2-macroglobulin-coated PVC after 5 min of blood contact. Securely anchored thrombi composed of fibrin and platelets are present (center).

Although affinity of preadsorbed fibronectin for platelets may be less than that of preadsorbed γ-globulin for platelets, the increased fibrin formation on the fibronectin-coated surface is sufficient to generate similarly sized thrombi. The interaction of fibronectin with PVC is probably similar in magnitude to that of γ-globulin with PVC because the time and magnitude of maximum deposition were similar.

On Silastic, however, the thrombotic response to the fibronectin-coated surface was quite different than the response to the γ-globulin–coated surface. Initially, more fibrin(ogen) was deposited on the fibronectin-coated surface, whereas platelet adhesion was greatly diminished. At later times of blood contact, platelet adhesion to the fibronectin-coated surface increased

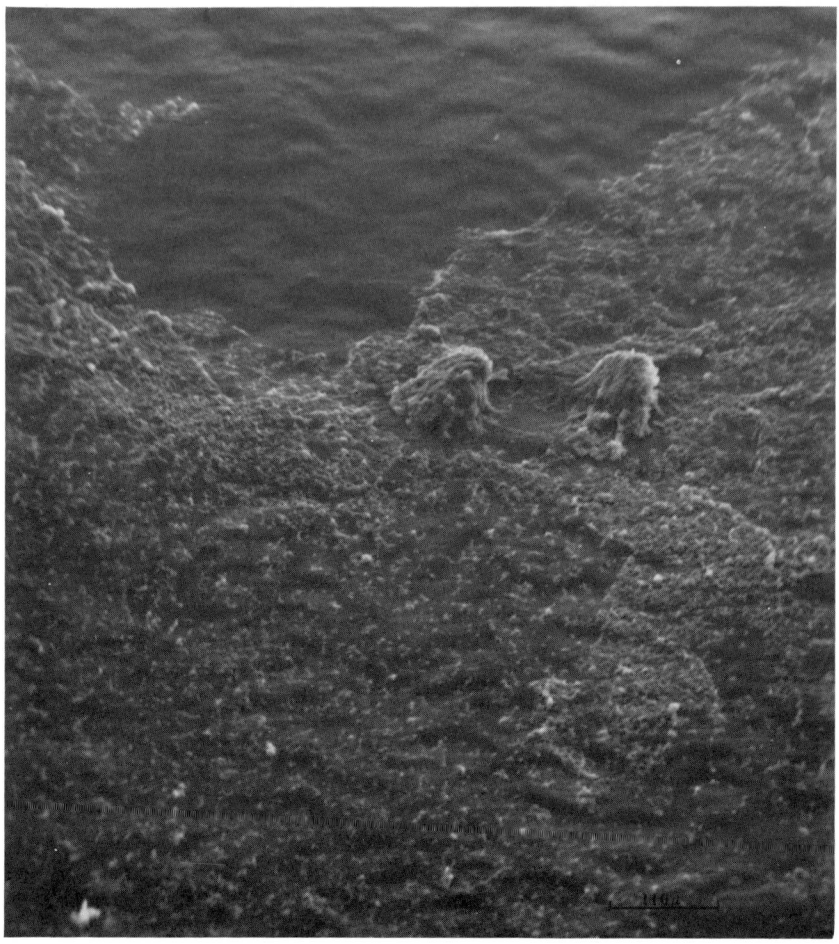

Figure 15. Uniform layer of platelets and fibrin (lower half of picture) on α_2-macroglobulin-coated Silastic after 5 min of blood contact. Thrombi (upper center) are in the process of embolization. Embolization probably has occurred in upper center of the micrograph.

far more than adhesion to the γ-globulin–coated surface, while fibrin(ogen) deposition was only moderately higher.

The embolization process on the fibronectin-coated PVC surface was quite different than the embolization process on fibronectin-coated Silastic. On fibronectin-coated PVC, 97% of the deposited thrombus [both platelets and fibrin(ogen)] were shed after 120 min of blood contact, while on fibronectin-coated Silastic only 75% of the deposited platelets and none of the fibrin(ogen) was released. This behavior is consistent with the observations shown in Figures 17 and 18 (fibronectin-coated PVC at 30 min and

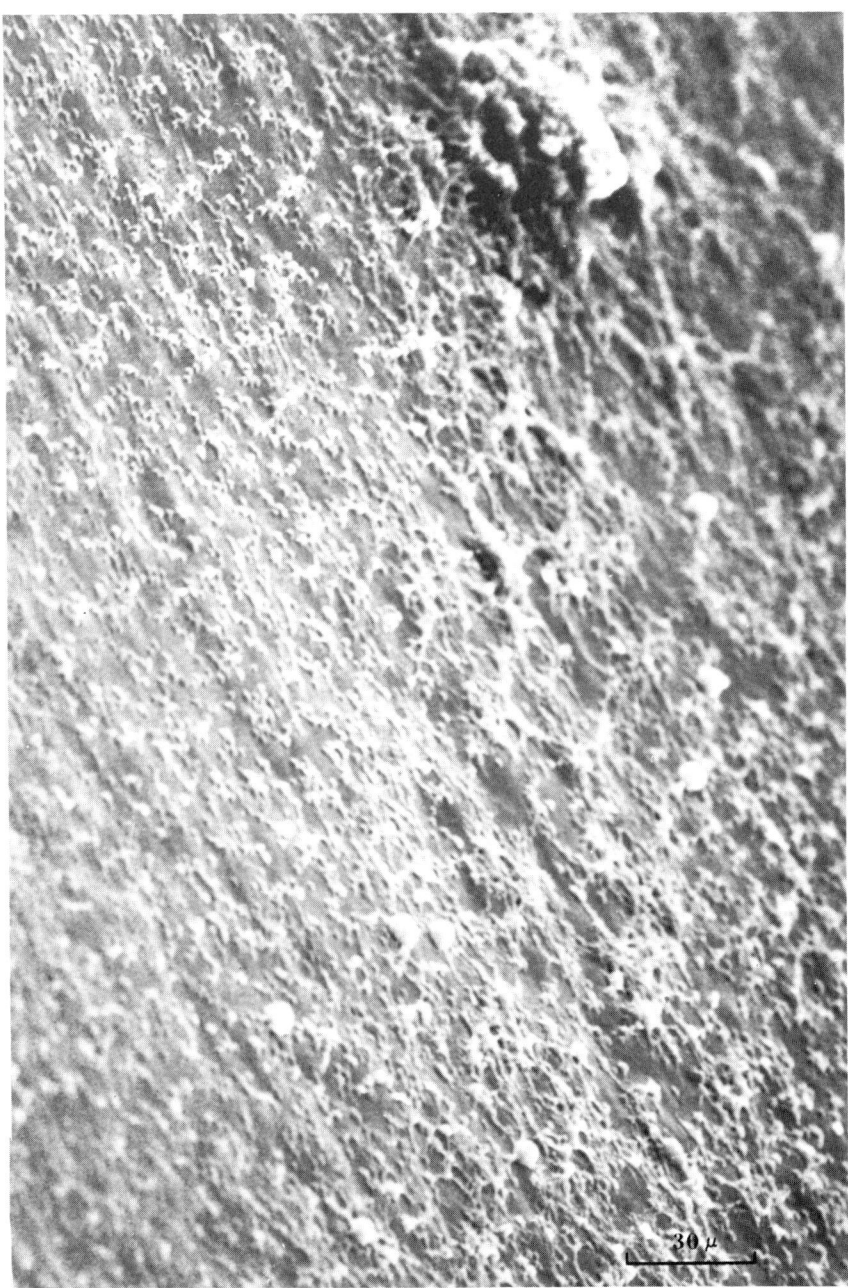

Figure 16. Fibronectin-coated PVC after 5 min of blood contact. Uniform layer of fibrin and scattered platelets with occasional leukocytes are present. Fibrin appears basal and throughout formed thrombus (upper right).

fibronectin-coated Silastic at 30 min, respectively). On PVC, the fibrin and platelets were concentrated primarily in large thrombi surrounded by a very thin, uniform layer of fibrin and platelets. On Silastic, the platelets were associated primarily with large thrombi, and fibrin surrounded these thrombi in a uniformly thick layer. During embolization, both fibrin and platelets were released from the PVC surface, while on Silastic, a large majority of the platelets were shed while the fibrin remained fixed to the surface in the thicker, uniform layer.

From these data, fibronectin apparently associated primarily with fibrinogen or fibrin, which then bound platelets.

SERUM ALBUMIN. The preadsorption of albumin on PVC resulted in a surface concentration of albumin that was 1.7 times (Table I) larger than the surface concentration that would adsorb in vivo to the uncoated PVC surface within 2 min of blood contact. However, this relatively small increase in surface coverage with the exclusion of other serum proteins resulted in a drastic decrease in the number of platelets and amount of fibrin(ogen) adhering to the surface at maximum deposition.

At early blood contact times, the number of adhering platelets on the albumin-coated PVC surface was similar to the other protein-coated surfaces investigated. Figures 19 and 20 show that the albumin-coated surface after 5 min of blood contact time (corresponding to the maximum thrombus deposition on albumin-coated PVC) was covered by a uniform yet sparse layer of platelets with some fibrin. This layer is similar to the other protein-coated surfaces shown in Figures 12–16. From the data shown in Figures 6 and 7, and Table I, albumin apparently prevented the formation of large thrombi over the entire 120 min of blood contact time studied. Yet, albumin allowed platelets and fibrin(ogen) to form on its surface at early blood contact times. One explanation is that the platelets or fibrinogen are not activated towards thrombosis upon surface contact. Another, simpler explanation is that the interaction between the surface and albumin is much stronger than the interaction between albumin and platelets or fibrin(ogen). Only single platelets or small fibrin strands would be able to adhere to the albumin. The aggregation of several platelets into a clump would increase the torque applied by the shear forces from the flowing blood to the basal portion of the platelet clump. Consequently, the aggregate would be sheared from the surface before a substantial thrombus could form. This mode is consistent with the very early contact time for maximum deposition (5 min). The amount of platelets and fibrin(ogen) adsorbed onto the surface after this shallow maximum reached a low asymptotic value at longer blood contact times. This behavior supports the idea that albumin is not torn from the surface upon embolization of the fibrin(ogen) and platelets. If the albumin were removed from the surface after 5 min of blood contact together with the fibrin(ogen) and platelets, other proteins and subsequently platelets and fibrin(ogen) would be expected to anchor to the surface in their place, ini-

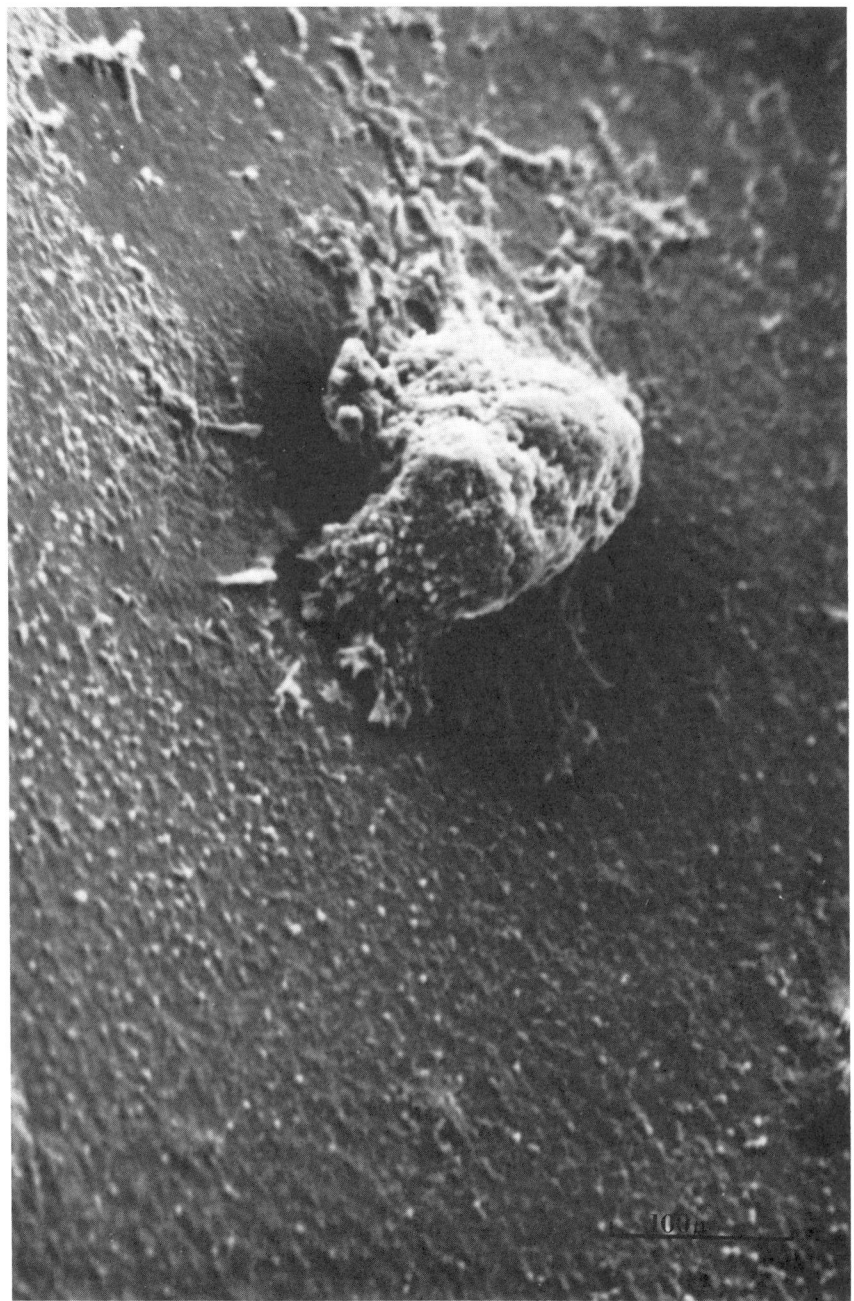

Figure 17. Fibronectin-coated PVC after 30 min of blood contact. Large thrombi consisting of both fibrin and platelets are beginning to embolize. Surrounding surface coverage is uniform but very thin.

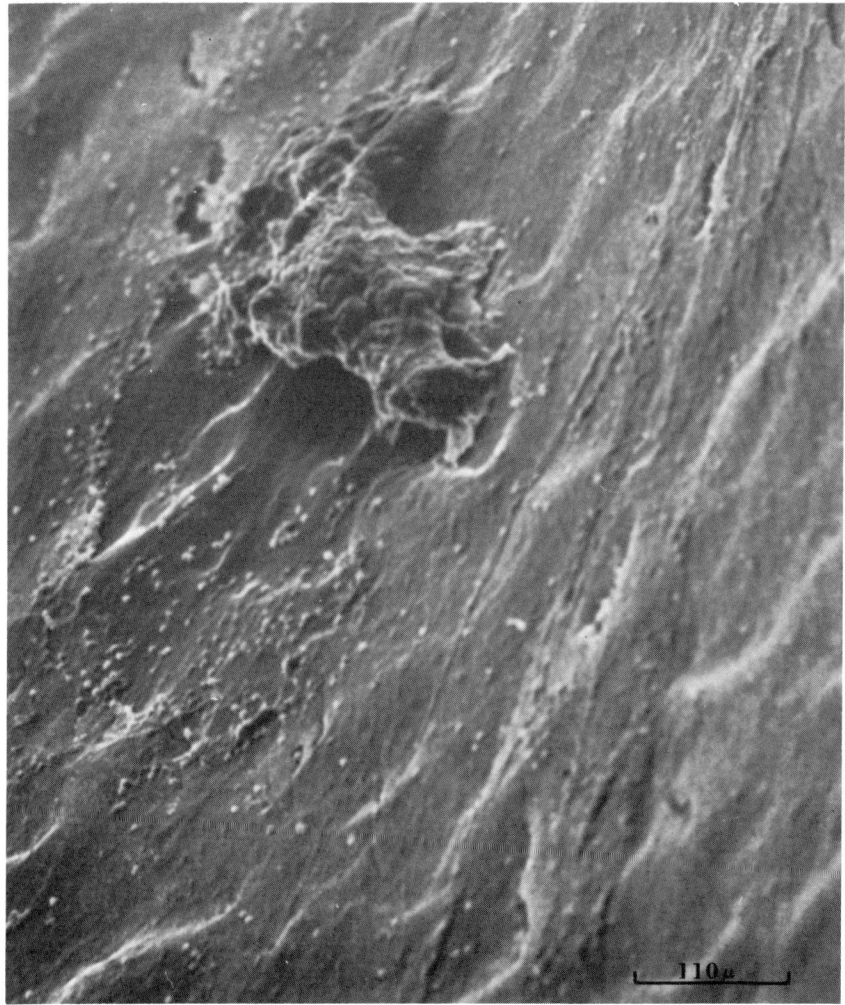

Figure 18. Fibronectin-coated Silastic after 30 min of blood contact. Large adherent thrombus (center) is beginning to embolize. Surrounding surface coverage appears to be mostly fibrin with a few adherent platelets.

tiating another increase in deposition at longer blood contact times. Such a complex deposition pattern is not observed on albumin-coated PVC.

FIBRINOGEN AND VON WILLEBRAND FACTOR. The thrombotic response on PVC coated with fibrinogen containing both fibronectin and von Willebrand factor, purified fibrinogen, and von Willebrand factor are discussed together because the responses appear to be interrelated.

When purified fibrinogen was preadsorbed to PVC (fibrinogen, Table I), the initial rate of fibrin(ogen) deposition was much larger than that on the

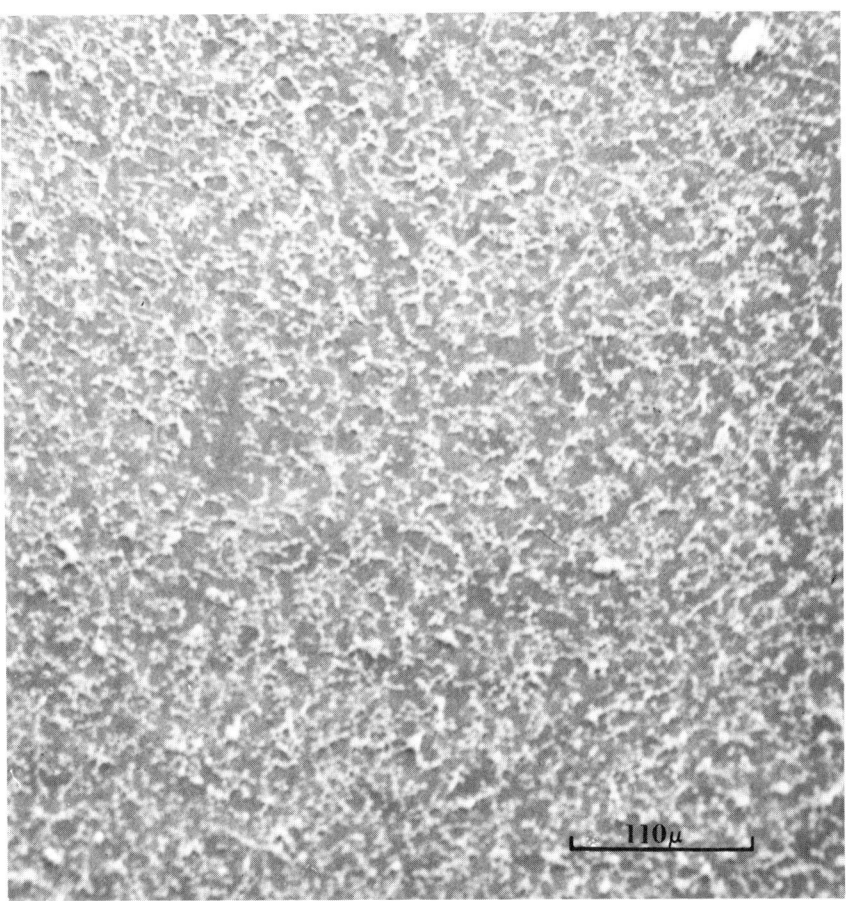

Figure 19. Albumin-coated PVC after 5 min of blood contact. This blood contact time represents the maximum thrombus deposition as measured by radioisotope-labeled fibrinogen and platelets. No large adherent thrombi are present.

uncoated surface. Platelet attachment was greater than on uncoated PVC but not as large as on γ-globulin–coated PVC. The preadsorption of fibrinogen thus appears to encourage fibrin polymerization and the adherence of platelets. Figure 21 shows a fibrin network adhering to the fibrinogen-coated surface. Single platelets and small platelet clumps appear randomly attached to this surface. The deposition maximum on fibrinogen-coated PVC occurred at the same time as that on uncoated PVC, although the amount of adhering fibrin(ogen) at this maximum was 9 times larger and the number of adhering platelets was 5 times larger than on uncoated PVC. Figure 22 shows that at 15 min of blood contact time an extensive fibrin network was present both

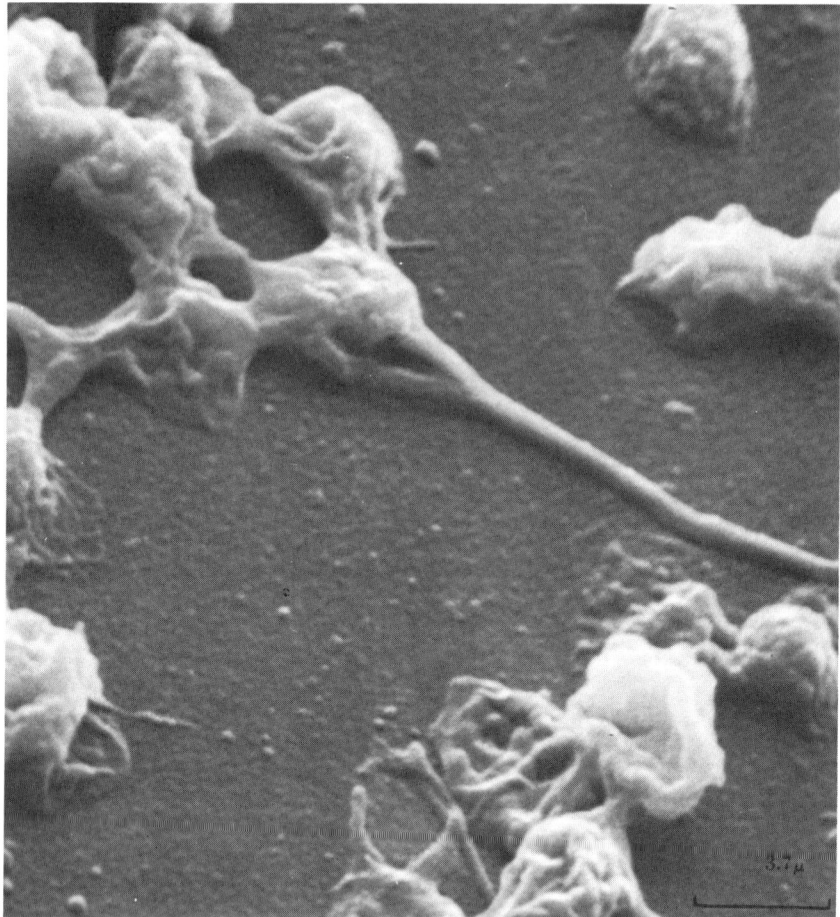

Figure 20. Higher magnification of a section of Figure 19 showing primarily platelets with extended pseudopodia. No platelet clumps are present.

basal to and within the platelet masses. At times greater than 15 min, embolization of fibrin(ogen) and platelets proceeded rapidly and extensively.

When partially purified fibrinogen containing both fibronectin and von Willebrand factor was preadsorbed to PVC, the thrombotic response was quite different than the response on the surface coated with purified fibrinogen. Compared to fibrinogen-coated PVC, the initial rate of platelet and fibrin(ogen) deposition to PVC precoated with partially purified fibrinogen decreased, while the time of maximum thrombus formation increased. In addition, the maximum level of fibrin deposition decreased whereas platelet adhesion increased, and the extents of embolization of both fibrin(ogen) and platelets decreased. The differences in these responses are remarkable because the amount of fibrinogen in the mixture of preadsorbed proteins was much larger than the amount of von Willebrand factor and fibronectin. To explain this phenomenon, the results with von Willebrand factor preadsorption must be considered alone.

Table I summarizes thrombotic response data on fibrinogen–, partially purified fibrinogen–, and von Willebrand factor–coated PVC. As one proceeds down any fibrin or platelet column (Columns 2–5), the values go either from high to low or low to high. These trends suggest that von Willebrand factor is controlling much of the response on the surface coated with partially purified fibrinogen. In comparing Figures 2 with 8 and 3 with 9, the fibrin(ogen) and platelet deposition curves for PVC preadsorbed with von Willebrand factor and partially purified fibrinogen are nearly identical and much different than the curves for fibrinogen-coated PVC. von Willebrand factor retarded the initial formation of fibrin(ogen) and, to a lesser extent, the adherence of platelets. At later blood contact times, platelet adhesion was

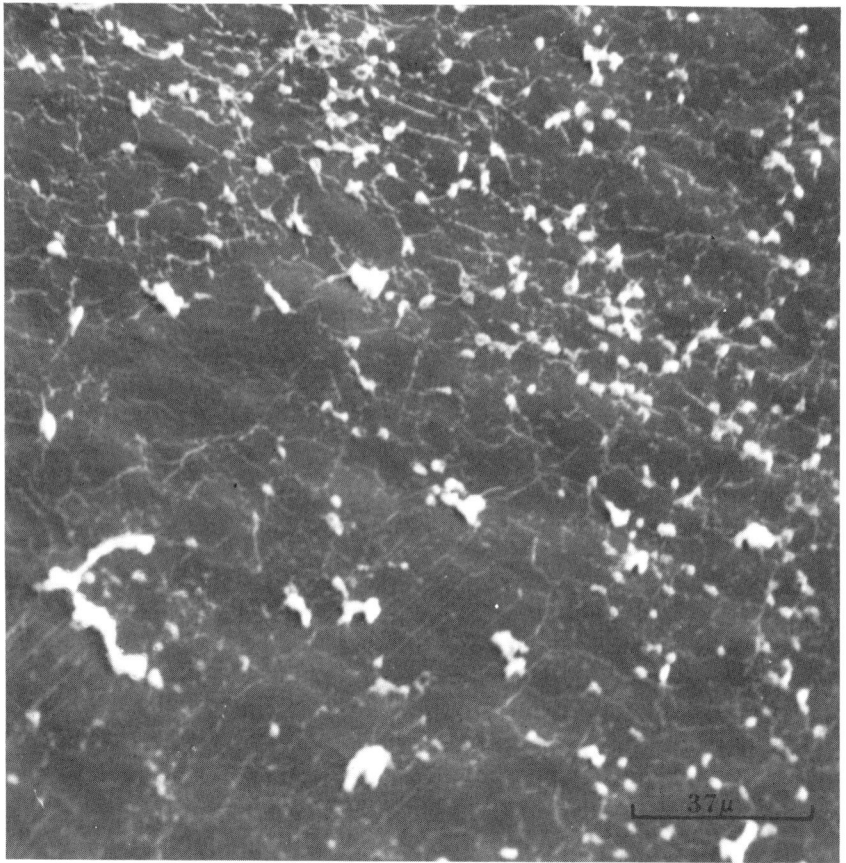

Figure 21. Fibrinogen-coated PVC after 2 min of blood contact. Uniform fibrin networks appear to cover the surface. Small platelet clumps and single platelets are attached.

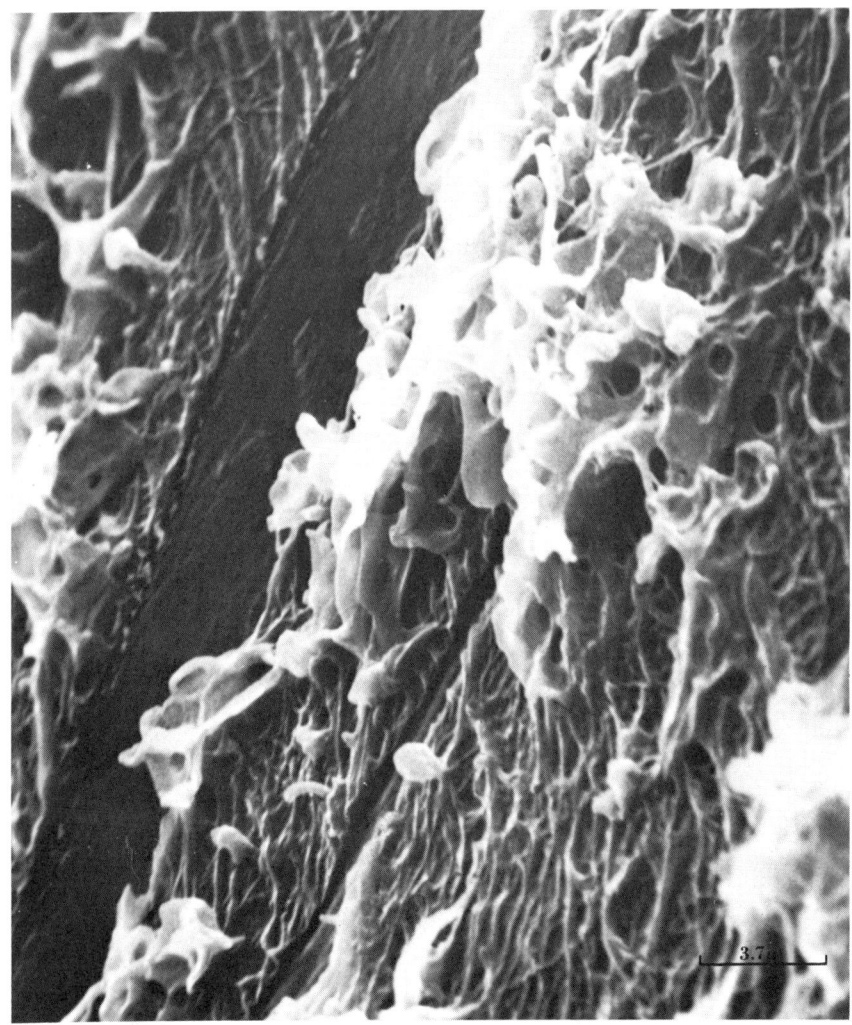

Figure 22. Fibrinogen-coated PVC after 15 min of blood contact (representing time of maximum deposition). Extensive fibrin network basal to attached platelets and platelet clumps is shown. Fibrin is the predominant species present.

enhanced greatly, while fibrin(ogen) deposition was only moderately enhanced. Figure 23 shows platelets attached to von Willebrand factor at 2 min of blood contact time. Little fibrin is seen on this surface compared to the fibrin observed on fibrinogen-coated PVC after 2 min of blood contact (Figure 21).

The von Willebrand factor, which is a multimer of a subunit of molecular weight 200,000, can range in molecular weight from 1×10^6 to 2×10^7. It is the portion of factor VIII complex proteins that is necessary for platelet function. Qualitative or quantitative abnormalities of von Willebrand factor cause the bleeding symptoms of von Willebrand's disease *(33)*. Given the importance of this factor in hemostasis, especially at high shear rates *(34)*, it is not surprising that von Willebrand factor has a dominant effect on thrombus formation in our model.

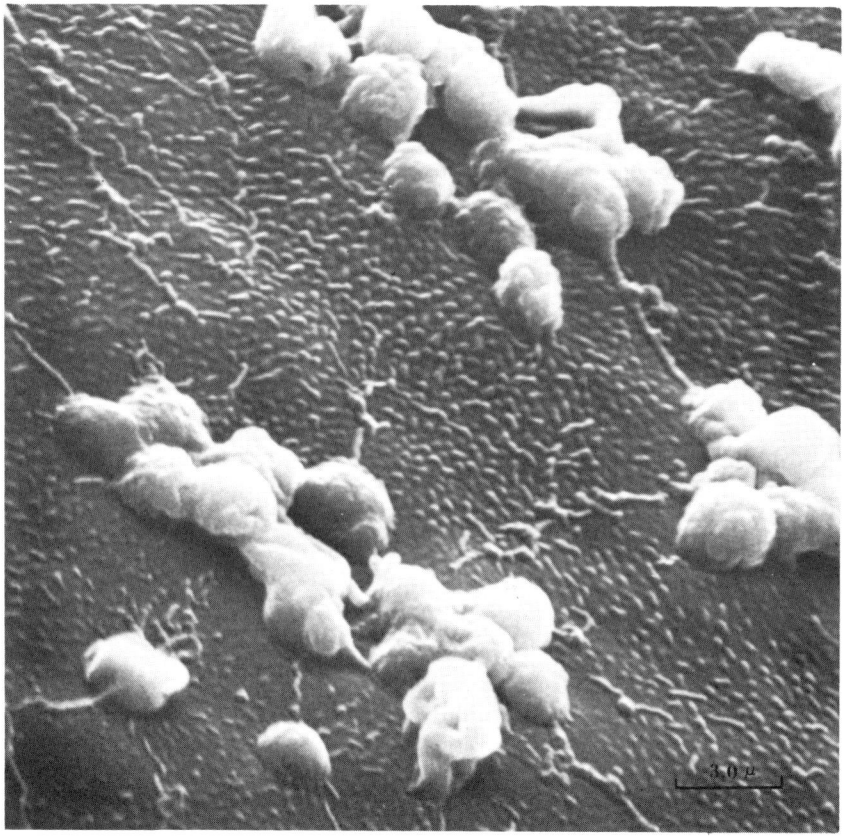

Figure 23. von Willebrand factor–coated PVC after 2 min of blood exposure. Platelets appear in groups and are attached to the surface, and the presence of fibrin is minimal.

Discussion

Protein Surface Interactions. The potential linking of specific proteins to platelets via nucleotide diphosphate monosaccharide residues in the protein has been suggested by Kim *(12)*. The experimental results show greater maximum platelet and fibrin(ogen) deposition on all of the protein-coated surfaces except albumin-coated PVC and Silastic and α_2-macroglobulin–coated Silastic. Because all of the proteins except albumin contain carbohydrate groups, the hypothesis presented by Kim *(12)* may be generally correct. However, significantly different thrombotic responses were observed on the carbohydrate containing protein-coated surfaces studied. Thus, although one determinant of thrombogenicity may be the carbohydrate moiety (e.g., the type of saccharide at the terminal end of the carbohydrate), another and more important factor may be the structure of the protein itself and the protein's interaction with platelets, fibrin(ogen), and the surface.

The influence of the surface on the thrombotic response was most apparent in the case of α_2-macroglobulin. On PVC, α_2-macroglobulin promoted greater thrombus formation whereas on Silastic it prevented extensive thrombus buildup. This behavior indicates that different molecular interactions are taking place between the surface and the protein and between the protein and blood.

In addition to influencing the extent to which various proteins adsorb upon initial blood contact, the surface also affects the thrombotic response once a protein has adsorbed. However, this behavior depends on the concentrations of the various formed elements in the blood and the hemodynamic environment at the interface.

The presence of low concentrations of proteins such as fibronectin and/or von Willebrand factor can drastically alter the thrombotic response on a fibrinogen-coated surface, indicating that proteins that have yet to be characterized may contribute greatly to thrombosis.

Leukocyte Involvement. A topic not previously discussed in this chapter concerns the question of why the large thrombi, as observed in several of the electron micrographs (Figures 12 and 14–18), were scattered over the surface in what appears to be a random fashion rather than uniform coverage. In an earlier paper by Barber et al. *(35)*, an attempt was made to correlate the adhesion of leukocytes to protein covered surfaces with the presence of large thrombi. Because the procoagulant and thrombogenic powers of leukocytes have been accepted for some time *(36, 37)*, and leukocyte adsorption onto polymers has been noted by other researchers *(38, 39)*, leukocyte–surface interactions should be considered when developing a mechanism describing thrombosis induced by artificial surfaces. Several transmission electron micrographs presented by Barber et al. *(35)* show that monocytes or polymorphonuclear neutropils are found basal to the thrombus. Large thrombi may form over those leukocytes that adhere randomly over the surface. However, how and why fibrin, platelets, and leukocytes adhere to a given surface initially is still unclear.

The Canine Model. While ex vivo models often are considered to be an improvement over in vitro biocompatibility test systems, the problem of describing extremely complex blood–polymer interactions still remains. In this study, we used radioisotope-labeled proteins and platelets and scanning electron microscopy. In other studies, we applied immunolabeling techniques and transmission electron microscopy. The application of these tools to an in vivo or ex vivo system provides more pertinent data than that often obtained in an in vitro system. Through this approach we hope to gain some insights into the complicated interactions of blood with biomaterials.

To lessen the influence of system variability on our results, we chose acceptable range limits for various parameters. Turitto et al. (40) found that thrombus formation increased with a shear rate over a range of 1000–10,000 s^{-1}, which emphasizes the need for controlled flow rate. In our system, the maximum blood flow rate was determined by the dog's cardiac output and shunt diameter. Since we continuously monitored blood flow rate through the shunt by an electromagnetic flow probe, we were able to adjust the degree of constriction of the tubing at the venous return in order to limit the shear rates to a range of 600–1900 s^{-1}. If the shear rate fell below 600 s^{-1}, the data were discarded. Prior to and during animal surgery, we required that fibrinogen levels remained in the range from 100 to 300 mg/dL, platelet count from 150×10^3 to 400×10^3/mL, and hematocrit from 35 to 50. In addition, we required that the white blood count be less than 20×10^3/mL, euglobulin lysis time be greater than 1.5 h, spontaneous platelet aggregation and ADP-induced platelet aggregation be normal (for canines), and plasma protamine paracoagulation be negative prior to surgery. The activated partial thromboplastin time was monitored before and during experiments; no evidence of gross depletion of procoagulant factors or generation of anticoagulants was noted. The allowed variations in these parameters apparently were small enough to prevent extreme variations in the specific thrombotic responses, because relatively small standard errors from the mean were observed and the responses were unique to the surface tested.

Human fibrinogen containing fibronectin and von Willebrand factor, purified human fibrinogen, von Willebrand factor α_2-macroglobulin, and fibronectin used for preadsorption to the surfaces in this study were chosen primarily because of their increased accessibility over the canine analogs. Fibronectin is very similar in structure in all mammalian species tested so far, and all types of fibronectin have similar effects on cultured cells and cross-react with antibodies elicited in rabbits to one species of fibronectin. Thus, the use of human fibronectin is probably justified. Recent unpublished data of W. J. Dodds and G. S. Johnson suggest that washed canine platelets will not respond to human factor VIII concentrates in the ristocetin-induced platelet aggregation test. From these results, the conclusions for the von Willebrand factor work in our study may be questioned. However, preliminary studies using canine fibrinogen and canine von Willebrand factor–coated PVC showed similar response to those on the human protein-coated PVC. The primary difference was that the magnitude of the thrombotic response was somewhat greater on the canine protein-coated PVC. Consequently, the conclusions made in this study using human proteins in canine subjects should be substantiated upon completion of our studies using canine proteins. Work on canine α_2-macroglobulin has not begun; however, a human albumin run was completed, and showed results nearly identical to the results with canine albumin presented in this chapter.

The use of an appropriate mammalian species for biocompatibility studies often has been a topic of heavy debate. The rationale for use of the dog in our system was based primarily on availability of subjects and cost. In addition, the adherence of dog platelets to cuprophane membranes was reported to be three orders of magnitude greater than the adherence of human platelets *(41)*. The dog is also thought to have a highly potent fibrinolytic system *(42)*. Thus, the dog should be a very sensitive animal for studying clot formation and dissolution. A clearer visualization of the mechanisms involved should therefore be possible. We believe that fundamental mechanisms underlie artificial surface-induced thrombosis and embolization in dogs, humans, and other mammalian species.

Conclusions

The findings of this work are (1) the properties of the polymer surface influence the composition of the protein film adsorbed upon blood contact and (2) the composition of adsorbed protein influences the subsequent thrombotic response.

Silastic adsorbed a higher percentage of serum albumin initially than PVC. The albumin may have prevented the formation of large thrombi by allowing embolization of smaller platelet clumps before large thrombi could be produced. Preadsorbed albumin lessened thrombus generation on both surfaces probably by forming weak protein–platelet and protein–fibrin(ogen) bonds, possibly due to its lack of carbohydrate residues. Preadsorbed γ-globulin promoted platelet adhesion. The platelet layer formed facilitated fibrin(ogen) and platelet adhesion since surface–γ-globulin–thrombus interactions were relatively strong. Preadsorbed fibronectin increased fibrin(ogen) deposition, most likely through cross-linking with the fibrin. In addition, the fibrin network probably mediated increased platelet adhesion and more fibrin formation through a strong surface–protein–thrombus interaction. Preadsorbed α_2-macroglobulin increased thrombus deposition on PVC, but to a lesser degree than the other globulins. The α_2-macroglobulin appeared to bind platelets on Silastic but did not produce significant thrombus formation. The α_2-macroglobulin effect could result from weak protein–

thrombus or protein–surface interactions, thereby allowing embolization prior to substantial platelet and fibrin(ogen) deposition. Preadsorbed fibrinogen promoted fibrin(ogen) formation with concurrent adhesion of platelets in a fibrin network. Preadsorbed von Willebrand factor promoted platelet adhesion and appeared to dominate the response when adsorbed as a portion of impure fibrinogen. This result may be due to von Willebrand factor's large size and ability to aggregate platelets. von Willebrand factor also appeared to function as a strong anchor for the thrombus on the surface.

Acknowledgments

This work was supported in part by the National Heart, Lung, and Blood Institute of the National Institutes of Health through grants HL-21001, HL-24046, and HL-21644, and by a fellowship award from Phillips Petroleum Company. Deane F. Mosher is an Established Investigator of the American Heart Association and its Wisconsin Affiliate.

The authors thank Arlene P. Hart for the hematological services she performed, James M. Vann for obtaining electron micrographs, Randy J. Stafford and Richard E. Stafford for their laboratory and surgical assistance, Ruth B. Johnson for purifying proteins, and Mark G. Goode for assistance in surgery.

Literature Cited

1. Baier, R.E.; Dutton, R.C. *J. Biomed. Mater. Res.* **1969**, *3*, 191.
2. Mason, R.G.; Zucker, W.H.; Shinoda, B.A.; Chuang, H.Y.; Kingdon, H.S.; Clark, H.G. *Lab. Invest.* **1974**, *31:2*, 143.
3. Ihlenfeld, J.V.; Mathis, T.R.; Riddle, L.M.; Cooper, S.L. *Thromb. Res.* **1979**, *14*, 953.
4. Falb, R.D.; Grode, G.A.; Leininger, R.I. *Rubber Chem. Technol.* **1966**, *39*, 1288.
5. Vroman, L.; Adams, A.L. *J. Polym. Sci. Part C.* **1971**, *34*, 159.
6. Vroman, L.; Adams, A.L. *Thromb. Diath. Hemorrhag.* **1967**, *18*, 510.
7. Vroman, L.; Adams, A.L. *J. Biomed. Mater. Res.* **1969**, *3*, 43.
8. Zucker, M.B.; Vroman, L. *Proc. Soc. Exp. Biol. Med.* **1969**, *131*, 318.
9. Chiu, T.-H.; Nyilas, E.; Lederman, D.M. *Trans. Am. Soc. Artif. Intern. Organs* **1976**, *12*, 498.
10. Morrissey, B.W.; Stromberg, R.R. *Am. Chem. Soc., Div. Org. Coat. and Plast. Chem. Prepr.* **1973**, *33*, 333.
11. Packham, M.A.; Evans, G.; Glynn, M.F.; Mustard, J.F. *J. Lab. Clin. Med.* **1969**, *73*, 686.
12. Kim, S.W.; Lee, E.S. *J. Polym. Sci., Polym. Symp.* **1979**, *66*, 429.
13. Ihlenfeld, J.V.; Mathis, T.R.; Barber, T.A.; Mosher, D.F.; Riddle, L.M.; Hart, A.P.; Updike, S.J.; Cooper, S.L. *Trans. Am. Soc. Artif. Intern. Organs* **1978**, *24*, 727.
14. Jakobsen, R.; Kierulk, P. *Thromb. Res.* **1973**, *3*, 145.
15. Sodetz, J.M.; Pizzo, S.V.; McKee, P.A. *J. Biol. Chem.* **1977**, *252*, 5538.
16. Harpel, P.C. "Methods in Enzymology"; Academic: New York, 1976; p. 639.
17. Kurecki, T.; Kress, L.M.; Laskowski, M., Sr. *Anal. Biochem.* **1979**, *99*, 415.
18. Young, B.R., unpublished data.

19. Marchalonis, J.J. *Biochem. J.* **1969**, *113*, 299.
20. "Bio Radiations," Chemical Division of Bio-Rad Laboratories, Richmond, Georgia, Oct. 32, 1979, p. 3.
21. Mathis, T.R., M.S. Thesis, Univ. of Wisconsin, 1978.
22. Mosher, D.F. In "Interaction of Blood with Natural and Artificial Surfaces"; Salzman, E., Ed.; Dekker: New York, 1981; p. 85.
23. Ihlenfeld, J.V.; Cooper, S.L. *J. Biomed. Mater. Res.* **1979**, *13*, 577.
24. Hopkins, F.G.; Cole, S.W. *Proc. Roy. Soc., London, Ser. B.* **1901**, *68*, 21.
25. Mitruka, B.M.; Rawnsley, H.M. "Clinical Biochemical and Hematological Reference Values in Normal Experimental Animals"; Masson: New York, 1977.
26. Doumas, B.T.; Biggs, H.G. "Standard Methods of Clinical Chemistry"; Academic: New York, 1972; Vol. 7, p. 175.
27. Mosesson, M.W.; Umfleet, R.A. *J. Biol. Chem.* **1970**, *245*, 5728.
28. Barber, T.A.; Mathis, T.R.; Ihlenfeld, J.V.; Cooper, S.L.; Mosher, D.F. *Scanning Electron Microsc.* **1978**, *2*, 431.
29. Cooper, S.L.; Young, B.R.; Lelah, M.D. In "Interaction of Blood with Natural and Artificial Surfaces"; Salzman, E., Ed.; Dekker: New York, 1981; p.1.
30. Grinnell, F.; Hays, D.A. *Exp. Cell Res.* **1976**, *102*, 51.
31. Hook, M.; Rubin, K.; Oldberg, B. *Biochem. Biophys. Res. Commun.* **1977**, *145*, 230.
32. Mosher, D.F. *J. Biol. Chem.* **1976**, *251*, 1639.
33. Fass, D.N.; Knutson, G.J.; Bowie, E.J.W. *J. Lab. Clin. Med.* **1978**, *91:2*, 307.
34. Weiss, H.J.; Turitto, V.T.; Baumgartner, H.R. *J. Lab. Clin. Med.* **1978**, *92*, 750.
35. Barber, T.A.; Lambrecht, L.K.; Mosher, D.F.; Young, B.R.; Ihlenfeld, J.V.; Cooper, S.L. *Scanning Electron Microsc.* **1979**, 3, 881.
36. Niemetz, J.; Fani, K. *Blood* **1973**, *42*, 47.
37. Niemetz, J.; Muhlfelder, T.; Churego, M.E., Troy, B. *Ann. N.Y. Acad. Sci.* **1977**, *283*, 208.
38. Kurusz, M.; Stooer, L.R.; Rosenberg, G.; Donachy, J.H.; Pierce, W.S. *Scanning Electron Microsc. 2*, **1978**, 2221.
39. Stewart, G.J.; Finch, P.R.; Rechle, F.A.; Richies, W.G.; Smith, A.; Schaub, R.G. *Ann. N.Y. Acad. Sci.* **1977**, *283*, 179.
40. Turitto, V.T.; Muggli, R.; Baumgartner, H.R. *Ann. N.Y. Acad. Sci.* **1977**, *283*, 284.
41. Grabowski, E.F.; Herther, K.K.; Didisheim, P. *J. Lab. Clin. Med* **1976**, *88*, 368.
42. Mason, R.G.; Read, M.S. *J. Biomed. Mater. Res.* **1971**, 5, 121.

RECEIVED for review January 16, 1981. ACCEPTED March 30, 1981.

23

Probing Protein Adsorption: Total Internal Reflection Intrinsic Fluorescence

R. A. VAN WAGENEN, S. ROCKHOLD, and J. D. ANDRADE

University of Utah, Department of Bioengineering, College of Engineering, Salt Lake City, UT 84112

> *Interfacial intrinsic fluorescence induced by evanescent wave total internal reflection was developed to study protein adsorption at solid–aqueous buffer solution interfaces. The technique has a number of advantages over conventional methodologies for the study of adsorption including (1) continuous, real-time sampling with 0.1-s resolution; (2) in situ sensing; (3) application to biomedically relevant, flat, low surface area samples; (4) quantitation of the amount adsorbed calculated on the basis of an internal standard; and (5) ability to obtain fluorescence emission spectra of intrinsic tryptophan moieties that are sensitive to local microenvironmental changes produced during the protein adsorption process. These advantages are illustrated for bovine serum albumin and γ-globulins adsorbed on hydrophilic quartz.*

An understanding of protein adsorption behavior is applicable in numerous fields including blood–synthetic materials interfaces, macromolecular-membrane interactions, receptor interactions, enzyme engineering, adhesion, and protein separation on chromatographic supports. Many methods have evolved to study interfacial adsorption, but no single independent method seems adequate. The ideal technique should produce quantitative, real-time, in situ data concerning the amount, activity, and conformation of proteins adsorbed on well-characterized surfaces. All adsorption techniques are approximations to this optimum.

Protein solution depletion via adsorption on finely divided substrates is quantitative, but applicability to low surface area materials of biomedical relevance is often minimal. Adsorption of radiolabeled macromolecules is quantitative on low surface area substrates; however, the presence of an extrinsic label may alter protein physical properties and subsequent adsorption behavior. Automated ellipsometry can, in principle, provide in situ, real-time information on film thickness and refractive index, but the minute differences in substrate, film, and buffer refractive indices often preclude this approach. Multiple internal reflection infrared spectroscopy is complicated by strong water signals that obscure protein amide bands and, while Fourier transform analysis seems promising, the interpretation remains difficult and the equipment is expensive.

Interfacial protein fluorescence induced by internal reflection evanescent wave excitation offers a number of advantages over conventional adsorption techniques. The total internal reflection fluorescence (TIRF) concept was originally patented by Hirschfeld (1) and applied to protein adsorption by Harrick and Loeb (2). Since then TIRF has been utilized in a limited number of investigations to study the adsorption of extrinsic fluor-labeled plasma proteins on quartz (3, 4), hapten-protein conjugates (5), and polydimethylsiloxane films (6). Our preliminary development of TIRF also employed covalently bound fluorescein isothiocyanate (FITC) as an extrinsic fluor (7, 8); however, research has indicated that FITC labeling of albumin is labile and also alters the proteins chromatographic and electrophoretic properties (9). Extrinsic labels per se are not objectionable as long as the presence of the label can be shown not to alter the biochemical and physicochemical properties of the molecule being studied. However, the attractiveness of intrinsic TIRF is that the difficulties in labeling and confirming the inertness of the label are completely obviated. We report here the successful development of intrinsic, interfacial protein fluorescence based on tryptophan excitation. The advantages offered by intrinsic TIRF are illustrated with data for albumin and γ-globulin adsorption on quartz.

Principles of Internal Reflection Fluorescence

When light of wavelength λ, traveling in a medium of refractive index n_1, encounters a second medium of refractive index n_2 ($n_2 < n_1$), it undergoes total internal reflection if the angle of incidence, θ, exceeds the critical angle θ_c, where $\theta_c = \sin^{-1}(n_2/n_1)$. The rectangular coordinate system of Figure 1 illustrates this phenomenon. The electric field vectors may be resolved into components parallel, $E_\parallel$, and perpendicular, $E_\perp$, to an optical plane delineated by the incident and reflected beams. The superposition of incident and reflected radiation establishes a standing wave normal to the reflecting interface as illustrated in Figure 1. The electric field amplitude has a nonzero value E° at the surface, which then decays exponentially into the less dense medium. The perpendicular polarization-mode electric field amplitude at

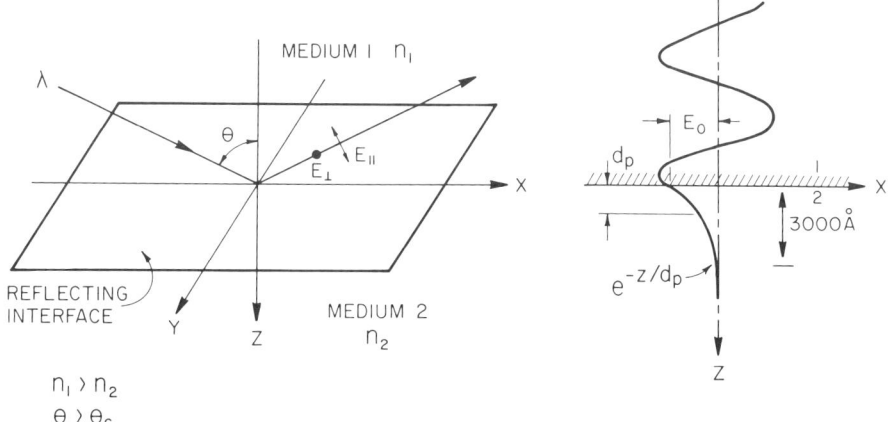

Figure 1. Left: Schematic of the coordinate system at a totally reflecting interface separating two media of refractive index n_1 and n_2. Right: Standing wave pattern and exponential decay of the electric field vector into the less dense medium, 2.

the interface (10), $E_\perp{}^\circ$, can be represented as

$$E_\perp{}^\circ = E_y{}^\circ = \frac{2 \cos \theta}{[1 - (n_{21})^2]^{1/2}} \qquad (1)$$

where $n_{21} = (n_2/n_1)$.

An electromagnetic disturbance termed the evanescent wave penetrates the rarer medium to a finite depth. It has a wavelength λ and is continuous with the sinusoidal field of the standing wave, but the electric field amplitude E decreases exponentially with distance from the surface z as

$$E = E^\circ \exp[-z/d_p] \qquad (2)$$

The effective wave penetration depth d_p is the distance z, where the electric field amplitude E has decayed to e^{-1} of its surface value E°, as given by Equation 3.

$$d_p = \frac{\lambda}{2\pi n_1 [\sin^2\theta - (n_{21})^2]^{1/2}} \qquad (3)$$

The value of d_p decreases at shorter wavelengths, greater index mismatching ($n_1 \gg n_2$), and incident angles approaching the critical angle ($\theta \to \theta_c$).

Interfacial fluorescence provides an excellent means of studying protein adsorption. The maximum energy available for excitation is localized within a few hundred angstroms of the surface where most of the protein is concentrated. Consequently, the vast majority of the fluorescence signal arises from adsorbed protein molecules. An adsorbed interfacial film of refractive index n_3 complicates the analysis of interfacial electric field distribution. Generally, the film is assumed to be much thinner than d_p and the film electric field distribution is assumed to be uniform. The field distribution for the parallel component depends strongly on n_3, but the perpendicular field component $E_\perp$, is not affected by the thin film and remains defined by Equation 1. Macromolecular properties may alter the film refractive index n_3, which in turn could affect the available excitation energy distribution and resulting flourescence signal levels. Consequently, the perpendicular component $E_\perp$ was used in this research. (*See* Refs. *8*, *10*, *11*, and *12* for more details on TIRF principles.)

The study of macromolecular adsorption on thin polymer films should also be feasible. Adsorption isotherms can be obtained on any nonfluorescing polymer that can be deposited in thin-film form on quartz. The only limitation is that the film be nonabsorbing at the excitation wavelength and exhibit minimal fluorescence. Thin films of depth d can be studied if $[2\pi d/\lambda] < 0.1$ and if the film attenuation index κ is less than 0.1 (*10*). Thin films on quartz substrates can then be characterized by other surface analytical techniques.

Molecular interaction with radiation is proportional to the radiation intensity, and thus to the square of the electric field vector, $E_\perp^2$. Equations 1–3 were used to generate Figure 2 which illustrates the variation of $E_\perp^2$ with z for both intrinsic and extrinsic TIRF at the quartz–aqueous electrolyte interface. Intrinsic fluorescence is more localized in the interfacial region ($d_p = 1040$ Å) than is extrinsic fluorescence using FITC ($d_p = 2235$ Å).

Experimental

Figure 3 illustrates the experimental configuration. The light source (A) was a 200-W mercury–xenon high-pressure lamp, and the monochromator (B) selected the fluorescence excitation wavelength. A 10-cm focal length quartz lens (L) reduced the beam diameter and, in conjunction with a front-surface, silvered mirror (M), redirected the light through a UV-polarizing filter (Oriel 2732) (0) oriented to pass the perpendicular component of radiation. Light entered one face of the quartz dove tail prism (Q), and illuminated approximately 1/cm^2 of the central prism face contacting the aqueous buffer in the flow cell (F). The prism was UV-grade quartz (Markson Science Inc.)—3-cm wide, 9-cm long, and 2.9-cm thick with face angles of 70° to the base. The flow cell base was a 3-cm wide, 9-cm long, and 1.3-cm thick block of marine-grade aluminum alloy (5086-Hll) anodized flat black after machining rectangular slit-flow ports at the surface of each end. Aluminum was chosen because of its ease of machining, passivity to cleaning solvents, and good thermal conductivity. The anodized film endowed the cell base with excellent inertness to aqueous saline solutions. The flow cell base and prism were separated by a Silastic rubber medical-grade polydimethylsiloxane gasket 0.05 cm thick. The effective cell flow field was $7.9 \times 2.1 \times 0.05$ cm. Flow rates during sample injection and flush ranged from 1.5 to 2.0 mL/s. Flow at the sampling area was laminar (Reynolds numbers 140–190) and well established (flow development length 0.12 cm). Flow cell surface area and

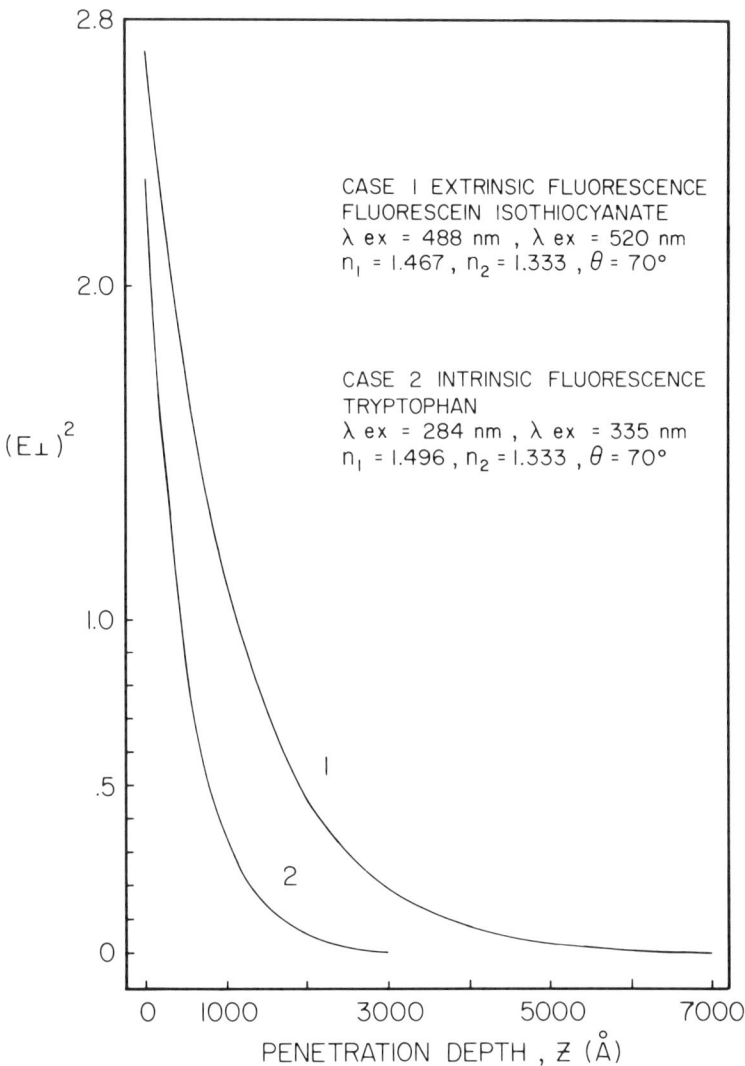

Figure 2. Exponential decay in $(E_\perp)^2$ with distance z from the reflecting interface.

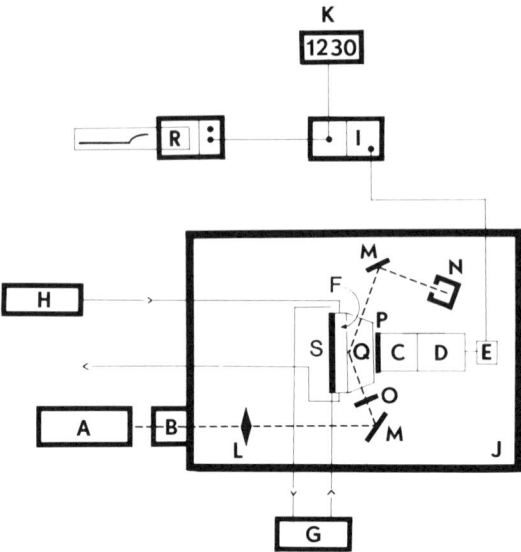

Figure 3. Schematic of experimental system.

Light source (A), excitation and emission monochromators (B and C, respectively), PMT (D), preamplifier (E), flow cell (F), constant temperature recirculator (G), syringe pump (H), photon counter (I), light tight enclosure (J), digital disc storage (K), quartz lens (L), mirrors (M), beam stop (N), excitation and emission polarizing filters (O and P, respectively), trapezoidal quartz prism (Q), chart recorder (R), and copper heat exchanger base plate (S).

volume were 34.1 cm^2 and 0.83 cm^3, respectively. The amount of bulk solution depletion due to protein adsorption on the cell walls was not measured, but order of magnitude calculations suggest that it could be significant for C_B less than 0.1 mg/mL. However, this result depends on how much protein is assumed to adsorb to the flow cell walls. Flow cell base temperature and all solutions entering the cell were maintained at 37° ± 1°C by an attached copper base plate (S) thermally linked to a constant-temperature bath (G).

A fraction of the interfacial fluorescence penetrated the prism and entered an emission monochromator (C). Both monochromators (B) and (C) (Jobin Yvon, H-10) were used with 16-nm bandpass resolution, the only exception being for spectra scans where the emission monochromator bandpass was 4 nm for optimal resolution. Fluorescence quantitation was accomplished by using an RCA 8850 photomultiplier tube (D) linked to an Ortec photon counting system with the following components: preamplifier 9301 (E), amplifier-discriminator 9302, photon counter 9315 (I), sampling control module 9320, and digital data storage using a 5¼-in. floppy disk on an Apple II Plus Computer (K). Digital signals were converted to analog (Ortec 9325) and displayed on a Pharmacia 481 strip chart recorder (P). Well-defined flow parameters were maintained by a Sage Instruments 341 syringe pump (H). An acrylic, light tight housing (J) and beam stop (N) helped keep extraneous light signals at low levels.

All solutions were made with analytical-grade reagents and low-conductivity (6 megohm) water purified by a combination of reverse osmosis, ion exchange, activated-carbon adsorption, and microfiltration. Phosphate-buffered saline (PBS) (0.145M NaCl, $2 \times 10^{-4}M$ KH$_2$PO$_4$, $8 \times 10^{-4}M$ Na$_2$HPO$_4$) had a pH of 7.3 and osmolarity of 310 mosmol. All solutions were deaerated initially, but because this procedure had no effect on fluorescence intensity, deaerating was not a routine procedure.

Proteins were obtained from Miles Laboratories as bovine serum albumin (BSA) monomer standard Fraction V (81-028-1-P338) and bovine γ-globulins Fraction II (82-041-2-1086). L-Tryptophan (Matheson Coleman & Bell), 0.3 mg/mL in PBS, was used as an intrinsic fluorescence experimental reproducibility standard.

The quartz prism surface was cleaned prior to each experiment in the following sequence: (1) 5 min soak in 2% (v/v) Microclean, (2) 15-min soak in dichromate–sulfuric acid (25/mL Manostat Chromerge chromic acid in 4.1 kg of concentrated sulfuric acid), (3) thorough rinse in low-conductivity, filtered water, (4) rinse in filtered, absolute ethanol, (5) 5-min vapor degreasing in Freon TES-ethanol azeotrope vapor, (6) 2-min radiofrequency (RF) glow discharge at 30 W tuned RF power (Tegal, Plasmod), 200 μm mercury pressure oxygen plasma, and (7) 10-min purge in ultrapure (99.999%) oxygen. All surface cleaning and assembly were carried out under Class 10,000 clean room conditions to minimize particulates and enhance experimental reproducibility.

Figure 4 illustrates schematically the time course of a TIRF experiment. The PBS background is due to scatter in the primed flow cell and stray light passed by the wide monochromator slits. The fluorescence signal intensity is expressed as counts per unit time above the PBS background. Injection of a tryptophan standard was used as an internal reference point for comparing the reproducibility of each experiment. With high recording speeds (10 cm/s), short count times (0.1 s), and rapid solution injection (1.5–2.0 mL/s), the speed with which the tryptophan bulk signal reached its equilibrium count level was determined. This procedure typically required 1–2 s after the first hint of signal increase. Similarly, the time required to remove all of the tryptophan from the cell at 2.0 mL/s was about 2 s. The cell priming volume, including flow ports, was 1.5 cm^3. No indication that tryptophan adsorbed irreversibly was observed, since count rates before and after the standard were identical.

Protein was introduced under the same sampling and flow conditions. At bulk concentrations greater than 0.5 mg/mL, a small signal step of 1–2 s, N_B, was immediately evident on the recorder at high speed and short sampling times (see Figure 5). The adsorption signal then rapidly developed on top of N_B. With the exception of injecting and flushing out protein solutions, all adsorption and desorption occurred under nonflow conditions. After reaching equilibrium signal level for any particular bulk protein concentration, the bulk protein was removed via a 50-mL flush of PBS at 2 mL/s. A rapid incremental signal drop N_B occurred due to removal of the bulk solution contribution followed by a slower decrease in signal as the protein molecules desorbed from the surface (see Figure 4). Protein adsorption dynamics could then be monitored. Alternatively, additional protein at a greater bulk concentration could be added in a stepwise manner to determine the adsorption isotherm. Solutions of higher bulk protein concentration were added when the equilibrium plateau signal had remained stable for 10–15 min. Since the time required to reach the plateau was generally about 20 min, the total elapsed time between different concentrations was typically 40 min. This entire step isotherm was determined on a single surface rather than the more classical and lengthy approach of obtaining one datum point at a particular C_B on a single fresh surface. Emission spectra of adsorbed protein were taken following the PBS flush. In this way only the spectra of adsorbed protein were determined. These spectra were then compared to bulk solution spectra of non-adsorbed protein obtained with the same equipment, but with the TIRF prism and cell replaced by a conventional transmission fluorescence bulk cell. Tryptophan amino acid emission spectra were recorded both in a conventional spectrofluorometer bulk cell and with the standard in the TIRF flow cell.

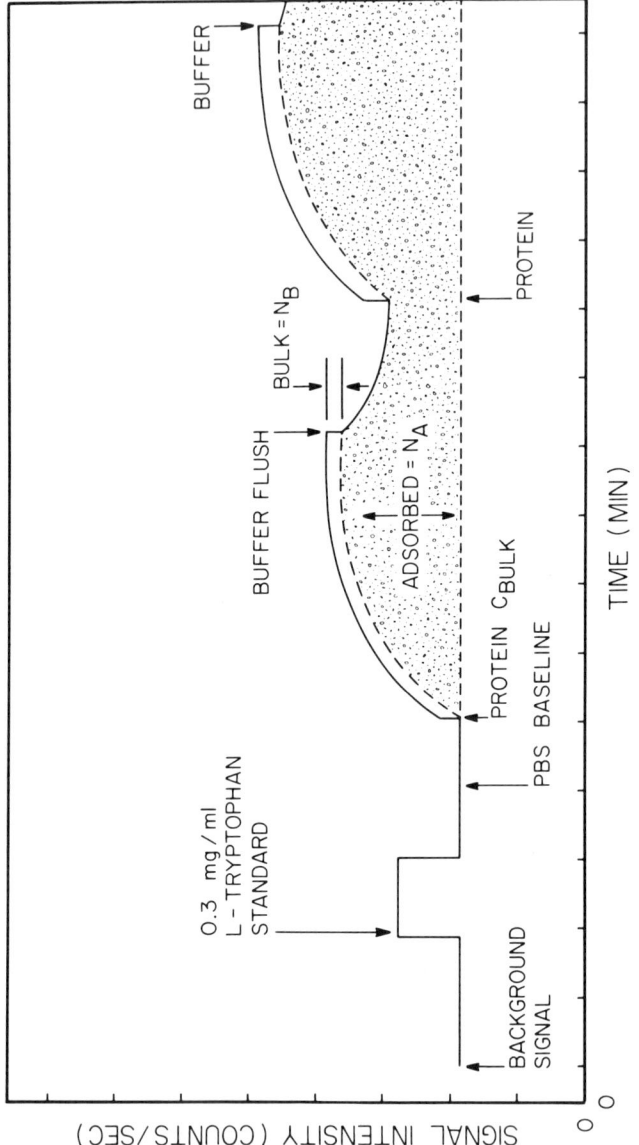

Figure 4. Schematic of TIRF data during a typical experiment. A tryptophan standard initiates each experiment. The stippled area represents adsorbed protein producing N_A counts per unit time.

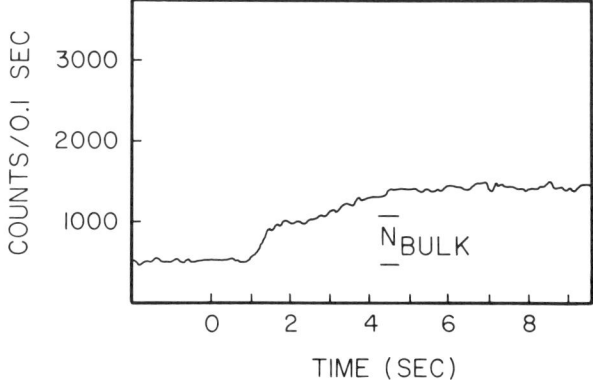

Figure 5. Fluorescence data for γ-globulin on quartz. The bulk signal N_B arises during the first 1–2 s of flow.

Results and Discussion

Interfacial fluorescence signals did not yield direct information on the amount of adsorbed protein. This lack of quantitation appears to be the major weakness of the method. Calibration studies have been attempted (6), but the ideal solution would be a second, independent quantitative technique such as FTIR or use of unaltered radiolabeled protein. An independent calibration method is now being developed.

Our approach was to use the fluorescence background signal N_B emanating from evanescent wave–excited protein in the bulk solution as an internal calibration signal. Consider the 3000-Å decay depth of $E_\perp^2$ for the intrinsic fluorescence case of Figure 2. The evanescent wave penetration depth was divided into 30 lamellae, each 100 Å thick and 1/cm². Adsorption was defined as those molecules occupying the first lamella adjacent to the surface. Molecules in Lamellae 2–30 were considered to have bulk properties and to constitute the bulk signal. The total fluorescence signal was proportional to the area under Curve 2 of Figure 2, but it was unequally weighted to the first few lamellae, where most of the energy was available to excite the majority of the molecules. The area of each lamella was integrated and expressed as field intensity units squared (FIU^2). The first lamella had 2.11 FIU^2 while the sum of Lamellae 2–30 was 9.9 FIU^2. At a bulk protein concentration C_B of 1.0 mg/mL, each bulk lamella contained 1×10^{-9} g of protein. Protein in the bulk lamellae (29×0.001 μg/cm²) was excited by 9.90 FIU^2 and produced N_B counts, while adsorbed protein Γ (μg/cm²) was excited by 2.11 FIU^2 and produced N_A counts. Bulk signal N_B was resolved from adsorbed protein signal N_A during the first 1–2 s of protein injection and flush (*See* Figures 4 and 5). N_B was accurately determined for $C_B \geq 0.5$ mg/mL. Consequently, for the quantitation of N_B at lower bulk concentrations, a linear plot of N_B as a function of $(0.5 \leq C_B \leq 4.0)$ mg/mL was extrapolated to a C_B of 0 mg/mL between $(0.0 \leq C_B < 0.5)$ mg/mL. The equality of Equation 4 results assuming that in both bulk and adsorbed states, a certain quantity of protein excited by a given amount of energy (FIU^2) produced an equal amount of fluorescence signal per unit time, that is, the quantum yields of bulk and adsorbed protein were equal.

$$\frac{(C_B)\ (0.001\ \mu g/cm^2\ \text{lamella})\ (29\ \text{lamellae})\ (9.90\ FIU^2)}{N_B\ \text{counts/unit time}} =$$

$$\frac{(\Gamma)\ (2.11\ FIU^2)}{N_A\ \text{counts/unit time}} \quad (4)$$

The correction for bulk protein concentrations other than 1.0 mg/mL is represented by C_B. Surface concentrations Γ ($\mu g/cm^2$) were calculated on the basis of Equation 4 and presented as a function of time or bulk concentration C_B for adsorption–desorption dynamics or adsorption isotherms, respectively.

This research and its associated quantitation rests on several assumptions. First, lamp power output was assumed to be invariant with times comparable to the course of an experiment. This assumption was reasonable since source intensity monitoring via background counts N for 6–8 h showed no significant drift if the lamp and photon counting system were equilibrated for 1 h prior to an experiment. Count rates N were typically 500 counts and the counting statistics error rarely exceeded $\sqrt{N}$ by more than several (0.1/s) percent. Second, the excited bulk concentration and thus N_B are time invariant. This assumption is probably correct if C_B is not reduced by adsorption within the flow cell and if no photobleaching occurs. Also, our fast sampling data indicated that for both tryptophan standard and protein solution, a bulk signal component could be resolved during the first 1–2 s following sample injection. The protein adsorption signal intensity then builds on top of this. Assuming that C_B is established more slowly by diffusional processes alone, some interfacial time-variant distribution function would have to be incorporated into Equation 4. Such a function would initially lower the interfacial concentration and reduce Γ. Third, quantum yields of adsorbed- and bulk-fluorescing species are identical. This is probably the most questionable assumption, particularly if conformational changes occur following adsorption. Quantum yield determinations of adsorbed species are planned in the future. Fourth, light scattered from both adsorbed molecules and bulk molecules within the evanescent zone does not generate significant bulk protein solution fluorescence. This assumption would have the effect of reducing N_A, increasing N_B, and consequently lowering Γ. Fifth, the adsorbed film is 100 Å thick, that is, it is the first lamella. Assuming that the adsorbed film and thus the first lamella was 50 or 150 Å thick, the calculated value of Γ would be altered by less than ±5%. Sixth, N_B could not be determined accurately below a C_B of 0.5 mg/mL. Consequently, a plot of N_B as a function of $(0.5 \leq C_B \leq 4.0)$ mg/mL was linearly extrapolated to zero in the range $(0 \leq C_B < 0.5)$ mg/mL to yield values of N_B.

Finally, we assume no occurence of interfacial photochemistry. This was generally true for the light intensities and times utilized in our research as illustrated in Case 1 of Figure 6 for adsorbed bovine γ-globulin. Following protein introduction, the surface concentration Γ rose to an equilibrium value, and remained time invariant even when additional protein of the same bulk concentration was injected into the cell. However, when the light source intensity was increased beyond a critical level by either increasing lamp power or replacement with a fresh mercury–xenon lamp bulb, the equilibrium fluorescence signal was not attained. Signal intensity peaked quickly and then decayed continuously. This phenomenon is referred to as Case II behavior and is illustrated in Figure 6.

This behavior is not surprising in that many investigators have detected photoeffects under conventional spectrofluorometric conditions. Studies conducted on the UV-irradiation of lysozyme (13) and L-glutamate dehydrogenase (14) revealed a concomitant loss in enzyme activity and fluorescence emission with irradiation time. The primary photoeffects were destruc-

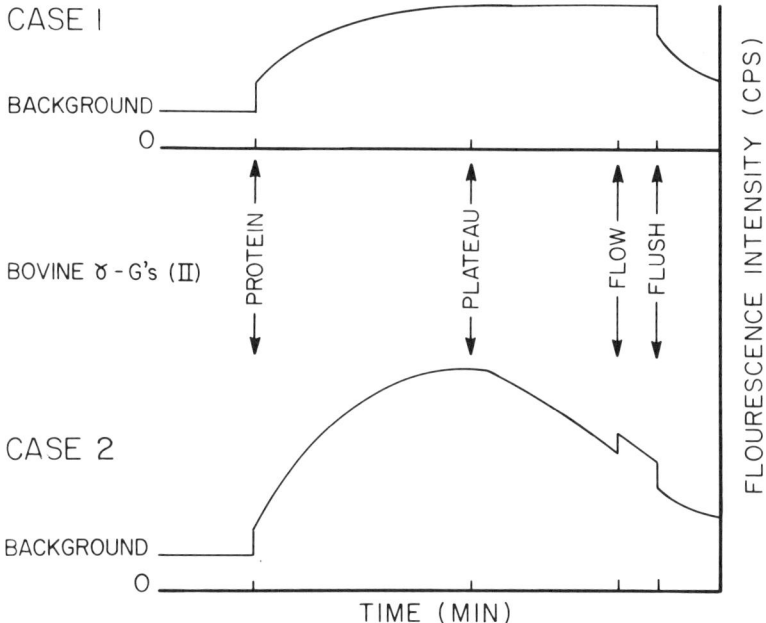

Figure 6. Schematic of typical TIRF data with no photoeffects (Case 1) and with photoeffects causing a time variable signal (Case 2) for bovine γ-globulin adsorbed on hydrophilic quartz.

tion of tryptophan residues and the appearance of SH groups (13) as disulfide bonds were disrupted. Enzymatic inactivation may have resulted from tertiary structure loss due to scission of the four disulfide bonds cross-linking the single polypeptide chain of lysozyme.

The destruction of aromatic and sulfur-containing amino acid residues and resulting loss of helical structure following 68 mW UV-irradiation also have been reported for albumin (15). However, in our research, signal instabilities postulated to result from photochemical effects were always associated with γ-globulin, but not albumin adsorption. Also, our calculated maximum UV light power was typically much less, that is, several megawatts at most. On the basis of tryptophan content alone, 25 residues in γ-globulin and two in BSA, the likelihood of photochemical susceptibility in γ-globulins is great. Both proteins have at least 16 disulfide bridges that maintain structural integrity, but both molecules appear to have substantial chain flexibility. At wavelengths of 270–290 nm or greater, aromatic residues and disulfide bonds of proteins adsorb well, and because tryptophan has the lowest triplet state energy of all the amino acids, light adsorption by other residues results in excited states that may migrate to specific tryptophan moieties via a nonradiative transfer mechanism. One primary oxidation reaction of photoexcited tryptophan is electron transfer to an acceptor molecule and C2–C3 bond cleavage of the indole ring yielding N-formylkynurenine (16).

The adsorption isotherm for bovine γ-globulin on hydrophilic quartz is illustrated in Figure 7. The equilibrium plateau concentration of 3.60 $\mu g/cm^2$ is substantially higher than most other γ-globulin adsorption data on silica and glass substrates, that is, several tenths of a microgram per square centimeter (17, 18). This result probably occurs because TIRF is an in situ technique yielding values of Γ obtained immediately after removal of the bulk signal. This is in contrast to most adsorption methods employing an extensive prequantitation buffer rinse that may cause desorption of a loosely bound, rapidly desorbing layer(s) (6), the presence of which would not be generally discernible.

Quantitation of Γ was made on the basis of bulk background counts N_B determined by a discrete step change in fluorescence intensity occurring either as protein was initially introduced or during the first few seconds of the buffer flush. Alternatively, N_B, and thus Γ, could be determined later during the flush sequence, for example, at 50 mL total flush volume rather than at 4 mL. This would be a closer approximation to sample washing conditions described for the more conventional approaches. The result would be a higher value of N_B, a lower value of N_A, and a value of Γ more than 50 percent lower than our data. In situ fluorescence appears to give larger values of Γ because conventional methods require longer rinse times which in turn remove substantial amounts of loosely adherent molecules.

Preliminary data determined for reproducibility studies at a C_B of 1.0 mg/mL on clean, hydrophilic quartz gave an equilibrium plateau adsorbed

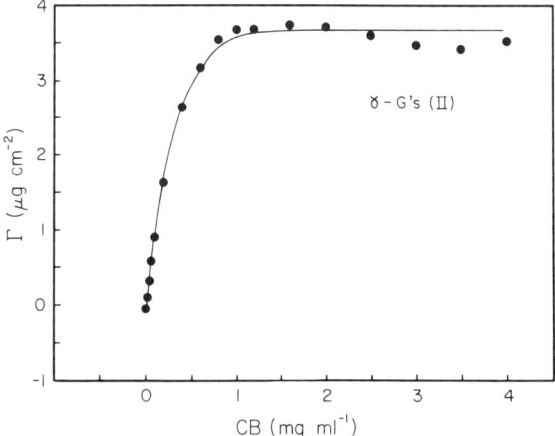

Figure 7. Adsorption isotherm for bovine γ-globulin on hydrophilic quartz at 37°C.

value of 1.69 ± 0.16 μg/cm^2 ($n = 4$). Not surprisingly, step isotherm and discrete adsorption isotherm maxima were substantially different. The conformational state of an adsorbed protein may be a function of surface residence time, solution activity, and number of adsorbed neighbors. Because adsorption is only partially reversible, C_B cannot be increased or decreased to obtain a particular value of Γ, that is, hysteresis effects do occur. Such hysteresis behavior has been well documented in adsorption experiments on well-defined chromatographic substrates (19). The application of TIRF to both desorption and adsorption dynamics as well as both approaches to isotherm determination should make the study of hysteresis effects more productive in the future.

A significant decrease occurred in adsorbed protein signal as reflected in Γ at bulk concentrations exceeding 2 mg/mL. This decrease was also evident in our earlier extrinsic TIRF adsorption studies with γ-globulin-FITC and fibrinogen-FITC (8), and also has been observed by others studying γ-globulin adsorption (3). The actual cause is as yet unresolved. However, this significant drop in fluorescence and thus in apparent Γ may be due to fluorescence quenching at high surface concentrations or protein conformational changes and subsequent lowering of quantum yield that may occur with increased surface packing density. Morrissey et al. (18, 20) have shown that γ-globulin does undergo substrate-induced conformational changes during adsorption on silica, and the degree of conformational alteration appeared to depend on surface concentration.

Since our isotherms are derived in a bulk concentration step-increase fashion, higher bulk concentrations (>2 mg/mL) were not evaluated for several hours after protein first contacted the quartz surface. This delay may provide sufficient time for γ-globulin molecules to change conformationally in such a manner tha quantum yields fall and the corresponding fluorescence signal drops or desorption of altered protein occurs. Transmission circular dichroism (CD) studies have shown major conformational changes during the adsorption and subsequent activation of Hageman factor on quartz (21). Recently, conformational changes associated with the adsorption of albumin, γ-globulin, and fibrinogen on to copolypeptide and silicone substrates were reported (22). Three stages characterized by reversible adsorption, irreversible adsorption, and slow structural alteration and desorption of denatured protein molecules were reported. However, the time course of these events was many hours to several days. Morrissey et al. saw no significant effect of time on the conformation of adsorbed γ-globulin (21).

Alternatively, an ordered, stable array of macromolecules may evolve at the surface with increasing time and/or bulk concentration. Since the excitation light is plane-polarized, the decay in emission signal may be a reflection of preferential orientation of γ-globulin molecules with time or enhanced surface packing densities. Fluorescence emission polarization studies should tell us more about this in the future.

Figure 8 illustrates the adsorption isotherm for BSA on hydrophilic quartz. The value of Γ is now on the order of 0.1 µg/cm^2, and the amount adsorbed is directly proportional to bulk concentration C_B with no hint of plateau saturation below 5.0 mg/mL. These surface concentrations are comparable to data reported by others (23–27) for BSA adsorption on silica and glasses. At a C_B of 1 mg/mL, reported values range from 0.02–0.2 µg/cm^2, depending on pH, temperature, ionic strength, and substrate. Our value of 0.08 µg/cm^2 at the same C_B is intermediate in this range. These results parallel our qualitative findings for BSA-FITC adsorption on quartz (8). Albumin adsorption continues to occur at concentrations exceeding those required for monolayer coverage. This result is at odds with most research, which indicates an equilibrium coverage of several tenths of a microgram per square centimeter at a C_B greater than several milligrams per milliliter. However, the means of obtaining these isotherms are not directly comparable with our TIRF data, where reversible desorption is more accurately based on rapidly removing only the bulk signal prior to reversible desorption of "peripheral protein." The continual buildup of BSA with increasing C_B may result from hydrophobic bonding between molecules comprising different layers. The surface of the BSA molecule may have hydrophobic patches (28), which may in turn facilitate multilayer binding at increasing concentrations via hydrophobic bonding.

Interfacial protein fluorescence is an in situ method that can provide real time data with a resolution of 0.1 s. This technique is a major advantage in that the protein adsorption–desorption dynamics may be determined without resorting to sample manipulation prior to analysis. Figure 9 illustrates adsorption–desorption dynamics for both BSA and γ-globulin at bulk equimolar concentrations of 6.67 µM/L. The γ-globulin required 40 min to reach

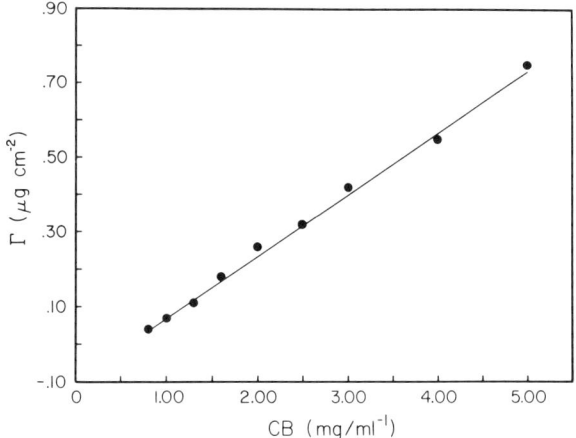

Figure 8. Adsorption isotherm for BSA on hydrophilic quartz at 37°C.

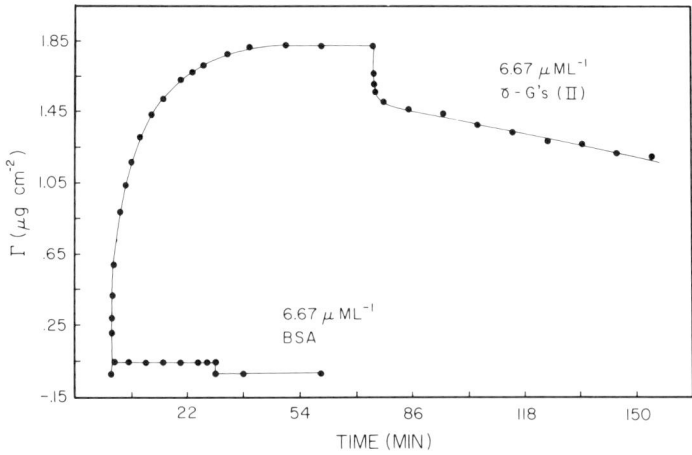

Figure 9. Adsorption–desorption dynamics for equimolar concentrations of BSA and γ-globulin on hydrophilic quartz at 37°C.

an equilibrium of 1.80 μg/cm^2, while the BSA adsorbed to an equilibrium value of 0.06 μg/cm^2 in approximately 8 s, as illustrated in Figure 10. The initial desorption dynamics were extremely rapid for both proteins (see Figure 11). During the first 3 s, BSA desorbed at a rate of 24 ng/cm^2/s, and within 6 s, most of the protein had desorbed. However, a small amount of BSA always seemed to remain irreversibly adsorbed (7), that is, about 0.01 μg/cm^2. Such rapid rates might simply have been the result of bulk solution fluorescence. However, if this were true, the same TIRF behavior would occur on all surfaces, which clearly was not the case, as illustrated already for γ-globulin on hydrophilic quartz. Virtually no data exist in the literature with which we may compare this adsorptive behavior occurring in the first few seconds of surface contact. Dynamic ellipsometry is too slow, and radiolabled protein experiments are inappropriate due to required washing steps.

The initial desorption rate for γ-globulin was linear for the first 30 s at 6.7 ng/cm^2/s. This rapid desorption may be due to the presence of a reversibly adsorbed peripheral layer of γ-globulin. The existence of this adsorbed γ-globulin layer has been reported in other TIRF research as well (3, 6). A transition time of several minutes separates two essentially linear regions of γ-globulin desorption. The second linear desorption phase has a rate of 0.067 ng/cm/s over a 60-min period, that is, a factor one hundred times slower than the initial desorption rate. After more than 1 h of desorption, a substantial amount of γ-globulin remains "irreversibly" adsorbed on the quartz surface. Based on the second phase rate, at least 13 days would be required for all of the γ-globulin to desorb under these conditions. However, over periods exceeding 2 h, the desorption rate was not completely linear, but was weakly exponential. Consequently, irreversibly adsorbed layers of

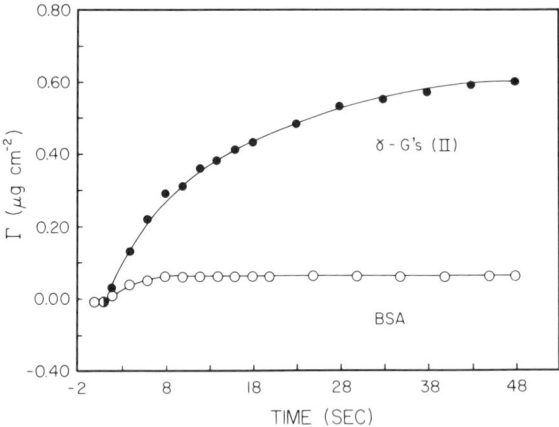

Figure 10. *Adsorption dynamics for 6.67 μM/L BSA (0) and γ-globulin (●) on hydrophilic quartz at 37°C.*

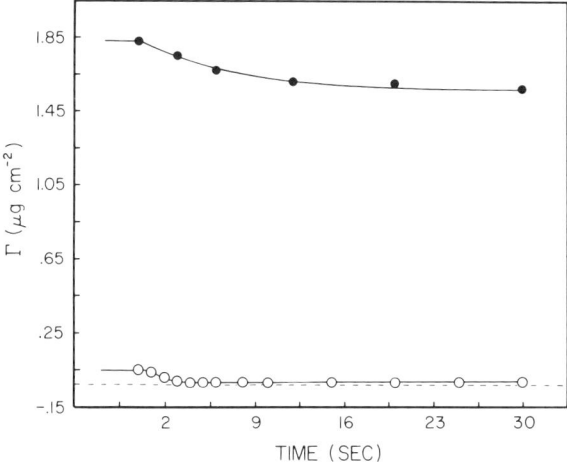

Figure 11. Desorption dynamics for 6.67 μM/L BSA (○) and γ-globulin (●) on hydrophilic quartz at 37°C.

BSA and γ-globulin appear to exist on hydrophilic quartz, and the surface molar ratio of BSA: γ-globulin is 0.02 picomol/cm^2: 8.0 picomol/cm^2 after 1 h of desorption. Since desorption was performed statically, such proteins might contribute to an excess in bulk solution, and "irreversible" protein then would not be in equilibrium with a true zero bulk concentration, but this does not seem to be a significant effect. Preliminary experiments indicate that if additional rinsing occurs during the desorption phase, that is, reestablishing zero for C_B, the desorption rate does not change appreciably.

Perhaps the single greatest advantage of TIRF is its ability to determine an adsorbed protein emission spectrum, which is illustrated in Figure 12 for bulk tryptophan and adsorbed γ-globulin and BSA. In all three cases, the emission spectra are broad (300–460 nm), and several have shoulders at wavelengths exceeding 350 nm, which is understandable for both proteins, particularly γ-globulin. The heterogeneity of the proteins as well as the local microenvironment of particular tryptophan moieties contribute to a wide range of fluorescence emissions. Cellulose acetate electrophoresis indicated that BSA and bovine γ-globulin were 99% pure. However, bovine serum Fraction II γ-globulins comprise a variety of different immunoglobulin types, and each of these may be further subdivided into variations in the F_{ab} section. The local tryptophan microenvironment probably contributes the most diversity to the emission spectra. At least three distinct spectral classes of tryptophan exist, one buried deep in nonpolar regions of the protein and two at the surface, one completely and one only partially exposed to the aqueous environment (29). Such spectral classification for the 26 tryptophans in γ-globulin and the two tryptophans in BSA can be employed to elucidate the

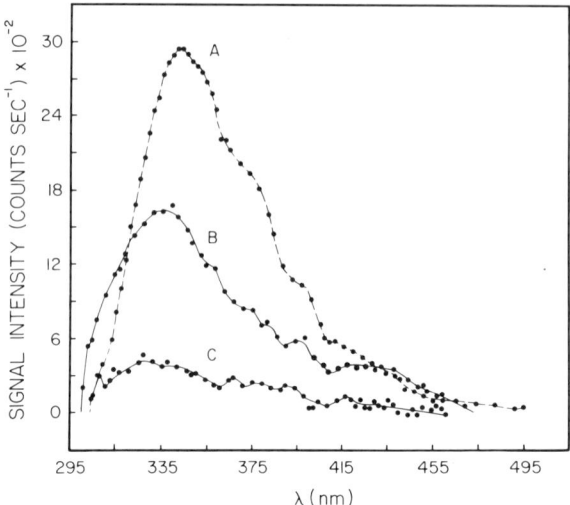

Figure 12. Fluroescence emission spectra for evanescent wave excited "interfacial" L-tryptophan (A), adsorbed bovine γ-globulin (B), and adsorbed BSA (C).

emission spectra of both proteins between 300–360 nm. The amount and kind of fatty acid complexed to BSA molecules affect the λ_{MAX} and intensity of their emission spectrum (30). Note the tyrosine emission peak λ_{MAX} at 305 nm for BSA. Albumin is one of the few proteins that exhibit tyrosine fluorescence primarily because of its low quantum yield and the existence of several quenching mechanisms (31).

The shoulders at wavelengths exceeding 360 nm are difficult to explain, particularly for the tryptophan case. Tryptophan molecules were possibly concentrated at the quartz-buffer interface in some kind of weak, but sufficiently close association to create resonance fluorescence phenomena exhibiting several peaks between 360–460 nm. Similar peaks exist for both BSA and γ-globulin, and since the background spectra were subtracted to leave the corrected spectra of Figure 12, envisioning how an instrumental artifact could cause the phenomena is difficult. Bulk fluorescence spectra taken in a conventional Aminco Bowman spectrofluorometer showed no such shoulder behavior for L-tryptophan, BSA, or γ-globulin; however, the spectral resolution was not as good as that in the TIRF system. Bulk fluorescence emission spectra obtained with a conventional 1-cm quartz cell and the same TIRF optical and electrical equipment produced data comparable to those obtained in the spectrofluorometer. Consequently, the shoulders appear to be independent of the instrumentation, and the strong possibility exists that conformational changes are reflected in altered fluorescence emission spectra that accompany the adsorption of BSA and γ-globulin on quartz.

In summary, TIRF offers a number of advantages over conventional techniques for studying macromolecular adsorption. First, it is an in situ method yielding real time data with resolutions of 0.1 s. Second, the geometry of the prism flow cell system makes possible the study of factors affecting protein adsorption, that is, interfacial shear stress, temperature, buffer properties, etc. Third, fluorescence emission spectra of adsorbed macromolecules are, in principle, capable of providing information on macromolecular conformational changes accompanying adsorption. This fact is particularly true for the intrinsic fluorescence emission of tryptophan residues that are extremely sensitive to local microenvironments within and upon the protein surface. Finally, by selectively labeling one type of protein, studying competitive protein adsorption with all of the previously mentioned advantages should be possible. This theory is, of course, predicated upon the use of a fluor that does not alter the physicochemical and biochemical properties of the macromolecule to which it is attached.

Acknowledgments

We thank Joel M. Harris for constructive advice, and acknowledge NIH Grant HL-18519-05 for financial support of this research.

Literature Cited

1. Hirschfeld, T. U.S. Patent 3, 604, 937, 1971.
2. Harrick, N. J.; Loeb, G. I. *Anal. Chem.* **1973**, *45*, 687.
3. Beissinger, R. L.; Leonard, E. F. *ASAIO J.* **1980**, *3*, 160.
4. Burghardt, T. P.; Axelrod, D. *Biophys. J.*, in press.
5. Kronick, M. N.; Little, W. A. *J. Immunol. Methods* **1975**, *8*, 235.
6. Watkins, R. W.; Robertson, C. R. *J. Biomed. Mater. Res.* **1977**, *11*, 915.
7. Van Wagenen, R. A.; Zdasiuk, B. J.; Andrade, J. D. *Am. Chem. Soc., Div. Org. Coat. Plast. Chem., Prepr.* (Houston, Mar., 1980) *42*, 749.
8. Zdasiuk, B. J., Masters Thesis, Univ. of Utah, 1980.
9. Crandall, R. E.; Janatova, J.; Andrade, J. D. *Prep. Biochem.* **1981**, *11*, 111.
10. Harrick, N. J. "Internal Reflection Spectroscopy"; Interscience: New York, 1967; pp. 25–55.
11. Watkins, R. W., Ph.D. Dissertation, Stanford Univ., 1976.
12. Kronick, M. N., Ph.D., Dissertation, Stanford Univ., 1974.
13. Churchich, J. E. *Biochim. Biophys. Acta* **1966**, *126*, 606.
14. Chen, R. F. *Biochem. Biophys. Res. Commun.* **1964**, *17*, 141.
15. Colson, C.; Frederico, E. *Bull. Cl. Sci. Acad. R. Belg. Ser. 5* **1970**, *56*.
16. Coyle, J. *Chem. Br.* **1980**, *16 Ser. 5*, 460.
17. Bresler, S. E.; Kolikov, V. M.; Katushkina, N. V.; Ponomareva, R. B.; Zhdanov, S. P.; Koromal'di, E. V. *Colloid J. USSR, Engl. Trans.* **1974**, *36*, 682.
18. Morrissey, B. W.; Fenstermaker, C. A. *Trans. Am. Soc. Artif. Intern. Organs* **1976**, *22*, 278.
19. Jennissen, H. P.; Botzet, G. *Int. J. Biol. Macromol.* **1979**, *1*, 171.
20. Morrissey, B. W. *Ann. N. Y. Acad. Sci.* **1977**, *283*, 50.
21. McMillin, C. R.; Walton, A. G. *J. Colloid Interface Sci.* **1974**, *48*, 345.
22. Soderquist, M. E.; Walton, A. G. *J. Colloid Interface Sci.* **1980**, *75*, 386.
23. Bull, H. B. *Biochim. Biophys. Acta* **1956**, *19*, 464.

24. MacRitchie, F. *J. Colloid Interface Sci.* **1972**, *38*, 484.
25. Morrissey, B. W.; Stromberg, R. R. *J. Colloid Interface Sci.* **1974**, *46*, 152.
26. Brash, J. L.; Davidson, V. J. *Thromb. Res.* **1976**, *9*, 249.
27. Tarasevich, Yu.I.; Smirnova, V. A.; Monakhova, L. I. *Colloid J. USSR* **1978**, *40*, 1029.
28. Hofstee, B. H. J.; Otillio, N. F. *J. Chromatogr.* **1978**, *161*, 153.
29. Burnstein, E. A.; Vedenkina, N. S.; Ivkova, M. N. *Photochem. Photobiol.* **1973**, *18*, 263.
30. Spector, A. A.; John, M. K. *Arch. Biochem. Biophys.* **1968**, *127*, 65.
31. Guilbault, G. G. "Practical Fluorescence"; Dekker: New York, 1973, p. 497.

RECEIVED for review January 16, 1981. ACCEPTED June 3, 1981.

24

Fourier Transform Infrared Spectroscopy for Protein–Surface Studies

R. M. GENDREAU, R. I. LEININGER, S. WINTERS, and R. J. JAKOBSEN

Battelle Columbus Laboratories, Columbus, OH 43201

Fourier transform infrared spectroscopy (FTIR) was applied to the study of protein interactions with surfaces. In addition, the various spectroscopic techniques and methods used to interpret adsorbed protein spectra are discussed, including transmission and attenuated total reflection (flowing) experiments using both aqueous solutions of single proteins and aqueous solutions of protein mixtures. Also included are spectral subtraction, spectral derivation, and spectral deconvolution. Use of these techniques showed that in transmission studies of albumin, a conformation change occurred when the protein concentration reached approximately 3% (w/v) in saline. Spectral evidence also indicated the possibility of hydrogen-bonded polymerization of albumin as concentration increased. Studies of albumin–fibrinogen mixtures allowed to adsorb completely onto a surface illustrated that albumin adsorbed initially, followed by fibrinogen adsorption and displacement of albumin. The infrared band at 1400 cm^{-1} of surface-adsorbed γ-globulins correlated quantitatively with the amount of protein adsorbed, as shown by radiolabeling techniques.

The biological spectroscopy program in our laboratory was designed to provide molecular level studies of blood–surface interactions primarily using Fourier transform infrared spectroscopy (FTIR). In addition, the program utilizes flowing blood from a living dog equipped with a shunt to follow molecular level adsorption of blood proteins onto various surfaces in real time. To accomplish these aims, we faced two problems, stated in the following list, together with the studies needed to overcome these problems.

0065–2393/82/0199–0371$07.00/0
© 1982 American Chemical Society

1. Devising methods for obtaining quality FTIR spectra on
   - Aqueous solutions, flowing systems
     Single model proteins and mixtures of model proteins
     Serum, plasma, whole blood (bagged)
   - Ex vivo studies involving live animals
     Dogs
     Sheep
2. Interpreting spectra of adsorbed proteins by
   - Transmission spectra
     Single model proteins
     Mixtures of model proteins
   - Attenuated total reflection (ATR) (flowing)
     Single model proteins
     Mixtures of model proteins

We have completed the first series of shunt studies using live dogs to devise methods for obtaining spectra. The experimental details of this work have been described (1) previously and need not be reported here. Demonstrations of the quality of the spectra obtained on aqueous solutions of model proteins are given in succeeding sections. Thus, this chapter emphasizes the progress made towards overcoming the second problem—that of learning to interpret the FTIR spectra of the adsorbed blood proteins. This progress includes infrared transmission studies of single model proteins and mixtures, and attenuated total reflection (ATR) studies of flowing solutions of single proteins as well as of mixtures of proteins.

Experimental

All spectra were run on a Digilab FTS-10 FTIR system equipped with fast-scan capabilities, a Hycomp 32 data array processor, and a nitrogen-cooled mercury–cadmium–telluride detector. Transmission spectra were obtained using CaF_2 windows with a 6-μm spacer. For each transmission spectrum, 500 scans were co-added at 4-cm^{-1} resolution. Smoothing was not needed on these spectra. All the spectra in this chapter (both transmission and ATR) are subtracted spectra, that is, they are the result of subtracting a saline (H_2O) spectrum from the spectra of the aqueous protein solutions.

ATR techniques were utilized to follow the adsorption of proteins onto various surfaces using 60° germanium crystals mounted in a liquid cell specially designed for flowing liquids by Harrick Scientific Co. The infrared depth of penetration using such crystals is approximately 2000 Å at 1600 cm^{-1}. The scanning sequence during such a flowing protein solution run (flow rate of 15 mL/min) was:

1. The 25-scan, 8-cm^{-1} resolution spectra were collected every 5 s for the first 110 s of flow.
2. The 50-scan, 8-cm^{-1} resolution spectra were collected every 11 s for the next 8 min.
3. The 200-scan, 400-scan, and then 1000-scan, 4-cm^{-1} resolution spectra were collected during the remaining 3 h of the adsorption experiment.

All proteins were used as received from Sigma Chemical (albumin, 97% pure; fibrinogen, 95% clottable; and γ-globulin, 99% pure). All solutions were made in 0.15N NaCl, and in experiments where the pH was regulated, HCl and NaOH were used to hold the pH at 7.4. For experiments where the pH was allowed to vary, it ranged from 6.3 to 7.4.

For the tagging experiments, proteins were labeled with ^{125}I by the lactoperoxidase procedure using the Radio-iodination System Kit produced by New England Nuclear. After termination of the reaction, the sample was chromatographed on a 0.7 × 29–cm column of G-10 Sephadex and eluted with 0.15N NaCl. Fractions of the protein peak were dialyzed overnight against 0.15N NaCl before use. Protein concentration and specific activity were determined from aliquots of the chromatographed, dialyzed protein solution. The labeled protein solution was flowed through the ATR cell with protein adsorption (onto the ATR crystal) monitored by infrared. After a protein film had built up on the ATR crystal, 0.15N saline was substituted for the protein solution, and desorption commenced. Desorption continued until infrared indicated that no further desorption was occurring. The liquid ATR cell was then drained of saline, and the ATR crystal was removed. This crystal was soaked overnight in a 2% Countoff solution (New England Nuclear) to remove the protein. The solution was then counted using a Searle Series 1185 γ-counter adjusted to the blank to determine the number of counts per minute. The amount of protein adsorbed (μg/cm^2) was then calculated from the value of counts per minute, the concentration of the solution, and the area of the ATR crystal.

Transmission Studies—Single Proteins

To interpret the infrared spectra of proteins, transmission studies of aqueous solutions of single proteins were used, because physical parameters such as concentration, pH, heat, etc. can be varied easily, inducing structural changes that are reflected in the infrared spectra. Thus, spectral changes can be related to protein structural changes induced by physical parameter changes. An example is given in Figure 1 which shows transmission spectra of varying concentrations of albumin in saline solution. Of special significance are the changes with concentration occurring in the Amide III spectral region (1200–1350 cm^{-1}). Changes (with concentration) occur in the number, shape, and frequency of the bands near 1300 cm^{-1}, following a definite pattern with concentration as illustrated in Table I. These changes involve only those bands near 1300 cm^{-1} and not those near 1250 cm^{-1}. Thus, they are not likely to be conformational changes of the type involved in changing from (for instance) an α-helix to a β-pleated sheet or a random coil conformation. Conformation changes such as these would be indicated by a change in the ratio of the 1300-cm^{-1} and 1250-cm^{-1} complexes, and frequency shifts in the 1250-cm^{-1} region. Rather, these changes appear to be typical of hydrogen-bond dilution effects, and thus appear to involve changes in the hydrogen bond structure of the proteins. Most likely, these changes involve the formation of hydrogen-bonded dimers or polymers as the concentration increases.

For the solutions shown in Figure 1 and Table I, the concentration was varied, but no attempt was made to hold the pH constant. For these solutions the pH varied from about 6.3 to 7.4. Another series of transmission runs were

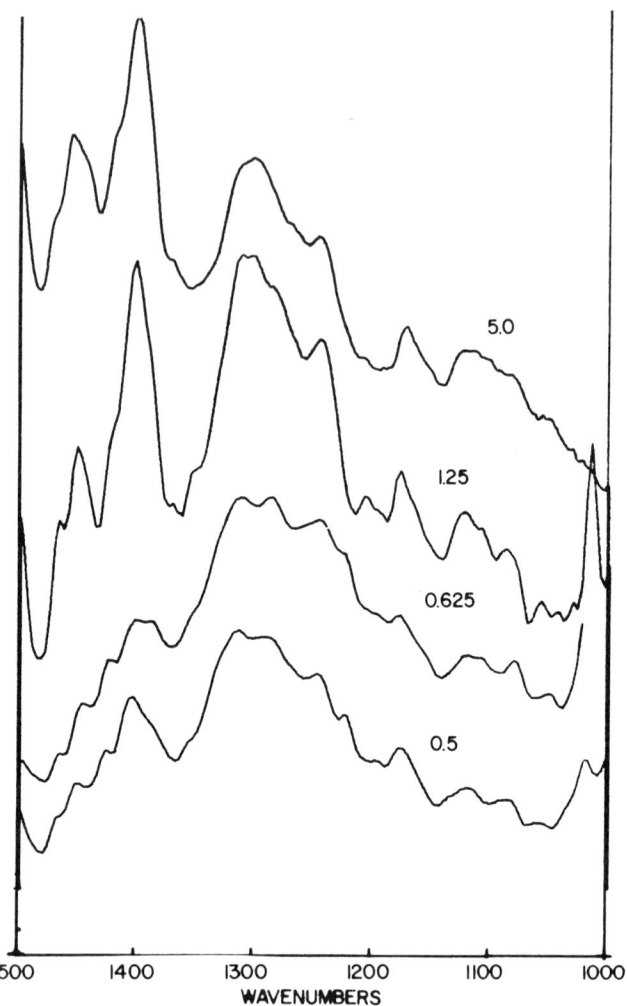

Figure 1. Transmission spectra of albumin in isotonic saline. Concentrations are 0.5, 0.625, 1.25 and 5% (w/v) from bottom to top. Spectra are water-subtracted and plotted at different scale expansions to illustrate differences.

made where the concentration was varied (as before), but the pH was titrated to 7.4 (buffers were avoided to prevent any potential interference with the protein spectra). For both series of solutions, the intensities of various infrared bands were measured.

The intensities of various pairs of adsorption bands were ratioed, and this ratio was plotted against concentration as shown in Figure 2. In both the constant and variable pH solutions, and for both the 1300-cm^{-1}/1250-cm^{-1} ratio and the 1400-cm^{-1}/1300-cm^{-1} ratio, major changes in slope occurred in the interval between 1 and 3% (w/v) concentration. Because infrared bands of the Amide III region are involved in the ratios (just given), and because these Amide III bands have been shown to be sensitive to conformational changes, the change in slope noted indicates that a conformational change occurs with concentration changes in the albumin solution.

The effects of pH are indicated in Figure 3 which shows spectra obtained for solutions of albumin (5% w/v) in which the pH varied from 1.35 to 10.5. In this figure, the ratio of the 1450-cm^{-1} infrared band to the 1400-cm^{-1} band changed as the pH was lowered. At a pH of 1.35, the 1400-cm^{-1} band almost disappeared. Koenig (2) assigned a Raman band at this frequency to the symmetric COO$^-$ stretching vibration of the carboxylate groups of amino acid side chains. This assignment is confirmed by the infrared data shown in Figure 3. For basic solutions (high pH) the carboxylate frequency (1400 cm^{-1}) is strong, but as the pH is lowered the carboxylate band disappears because the protonated form is generated. At low pH distinct changes occur in the Amide III spectral region as compared to the spectra at higher pH values. These changes (Figure 3, pH 1.35) involve a marked intensity increase in the 1250-cm^{-1} band as compared to the 1300-cm^{-1} band, indicating an albumin conformational change at this low pH.

Transmission Studies—Mixtures of Model Proteins

Our previous transmission studies of aqueous solutions of single proteins demonstrated that spectral changes can be related to structural and/or conformational variations in single protein systems. Now we must show that this can be accomplished for mixtures of proteins and most importantly, that

Table I. Transmission Spectra of Aqueous Solutions of Albumin

Concentration (%)	Frequency (cm^{-1})[a]		
0.5	1311		1287
0.625	1312		1290
1.0	1313		1295 Sh[b]
1.25	1314	1300	1286 Sh
2.5	~1315 W, Sh[b]	1301	
3.0	1317 Sh	1306	
5.0	1312 Sh	1302	
10.0	1317 Sh	1305	
15.0	possible 1312–16 Sh	1305	

[a] Computer-generated frequencies. Resolution was 4 cm^{-1}, with data points collected every 1 cm^{-1}.
[b] Sh = Shoulder, W = Weak.

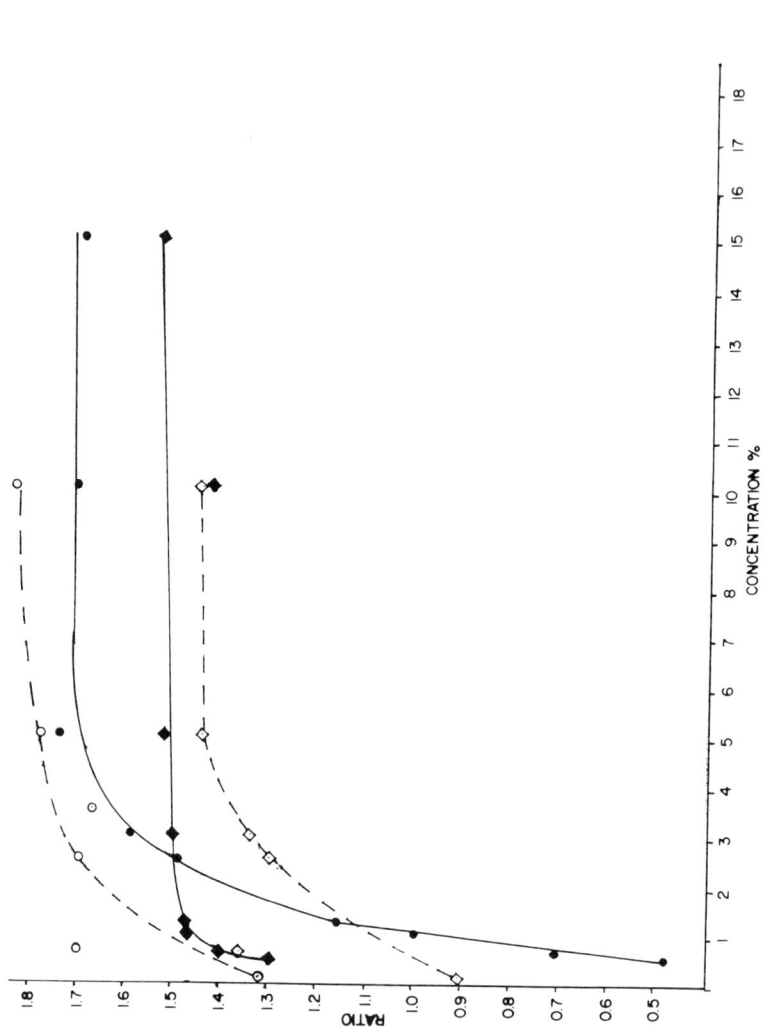

Figure 2. Plots of band intensity ratios for albumin in isotonic saline (water-subtracted transmission spectra). Key: 1300/1250: ◆, no pH control; ◇, pH 7.4; 1400/1300 cm^{-1}: ●, no pH control; ○, pH 7.4.

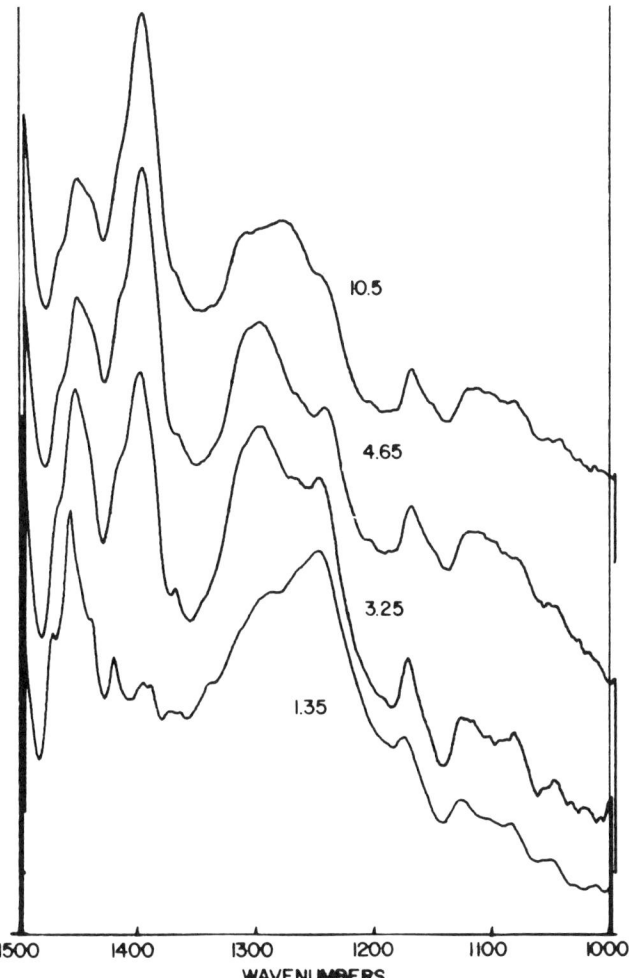

Figure 3. Water-subtracted transmission spectra of albumin in isotonic saline with varying pH. All solutions were 5% (w/v). The pH was adjusted with HCl and NaOH to (from bottom to top) pH 1.35, 3.25, 4.65, and 10.5.

individual proteins can be identified in a mixture. We approached this identification problem in three ways. We worked considerably on the first approach (spectral subtraction), and are just beginning work on the second and third approaches (deconvolution of spectra and second derivative spectra), but all three techniques show great promise for certain applications.

The first approach is illustrated in Figures 4, 5, and 6. Figure 4 shows spectra of γ-globulin (*top*), albumin (*bottom*), and a 1:1 mixture of albumin and γ-globulin (*middle*). The presence of both components could possibly be deduced from the spectra of the mixture by both the bands in the 1400–1450–cm^{-1} region and by the bands in the Amide III region. The ratio

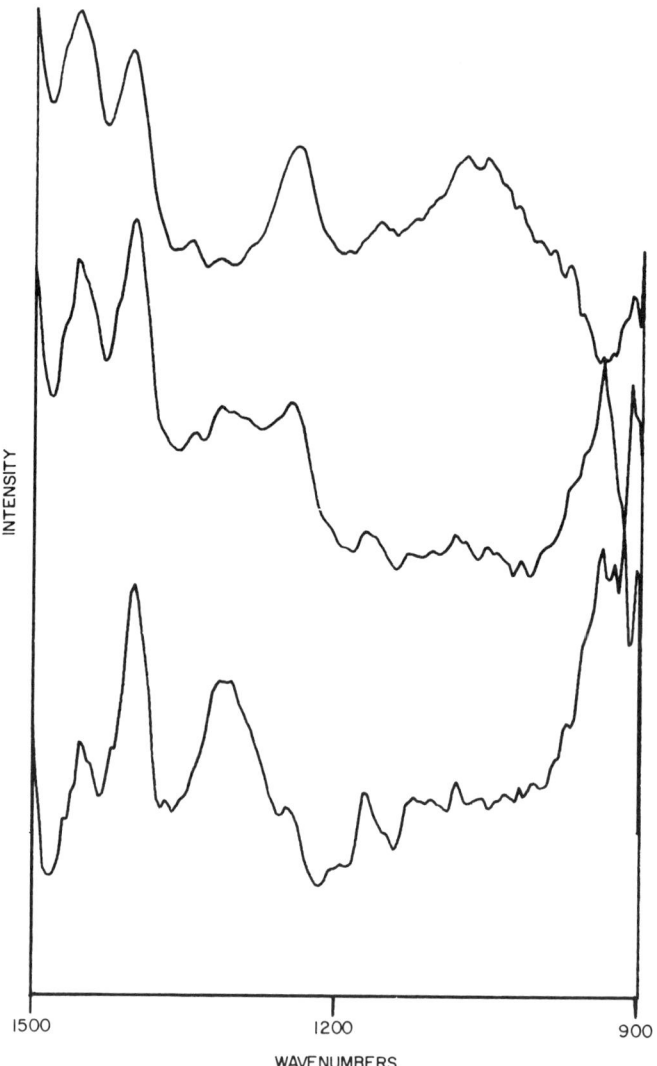

Figure 4. Water-subtracted transmission spectra of 2% (w/v) solutions of albumin (bottom), *γ-globulins* (top), *and a 1:1 mixture of albumin and γ-globulins* (middle).

of the 1400-cm^{-1}/1450-cm^{-1} bands in the spectrum of the mixture is intermediately between that of pure albumin and that of pure γ-globulins. Also, the band near 1320 cm^{-1} in albumin is in the spectrum of the mixture as is the 1250-cm^{-1} band of γ-globulins. However, if this were an unknown mixture, the only real proof of the identity of the components of the mixture

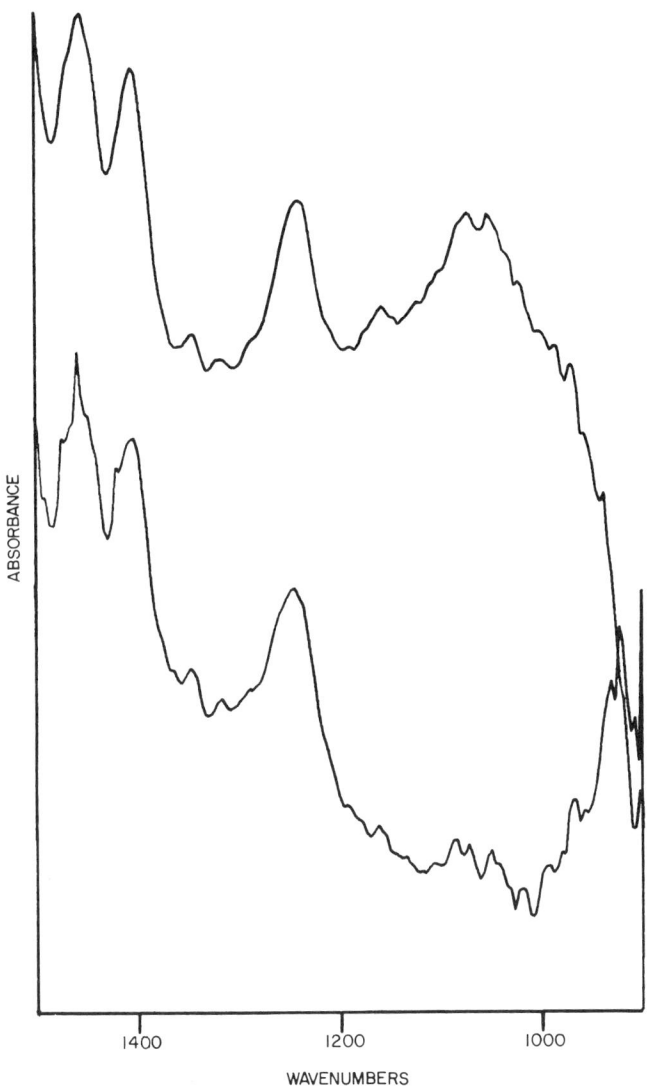

Figure 5. Result of subtracting albumin from albumin–globulins mixture shown in Figure 4 (bottom) and reference spectrum of γ-globulins (top).

would be if the components were separated and the spectrum of a separated component matched a reference spectrum of that component. One method to obtain this result is through spectral subtraction. By subtracting a reference spectrum of one component from the mixture, a spectrum of the other component is generated. This other component then can be identified by comparison to reference spectra. This result is illustrated for the 1:1 albumin–globulins mixture in Figures 5 and 6. Figure 5 shows the result (*bottom*) of subtracting a spectrum of albumin from the spectrum of the mixture. This subtracted spectrum matches the reference spectrum of globulins shown at

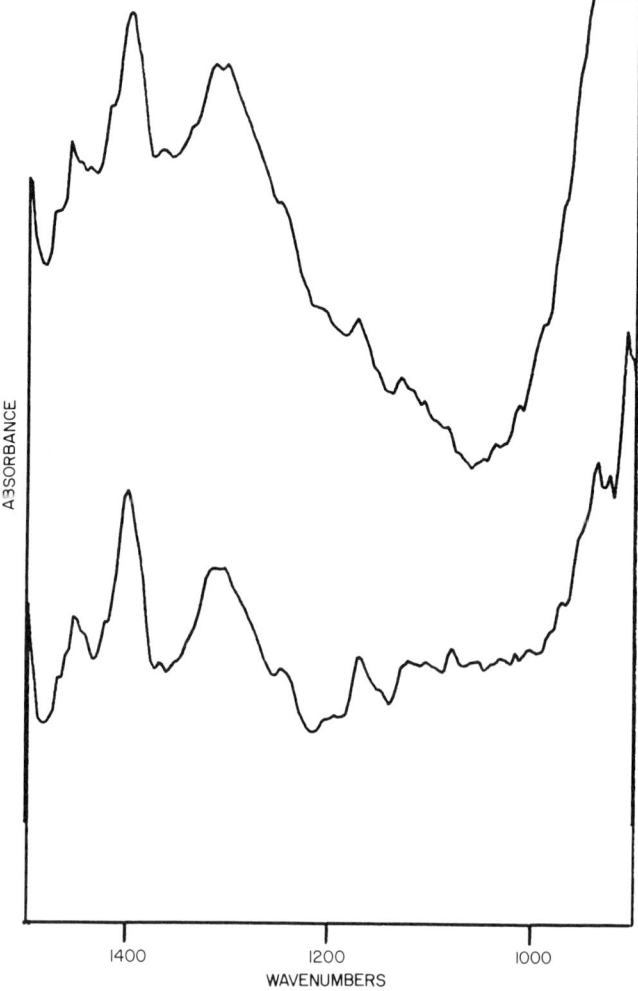

Figure 6. Result of subtracting globulins from albumin–globulins mixture shown in Figure 4 (top) *and reference spectrum of albumin* (bottom).

the top (differences below 1050 cm^{-1} were spectral artifacts, and were not important in this identification). The reverse subtraction is shown in Figure 6 which identifies the other component as albumin.

The second approach to identifying proteins in mixtures is shown in Figure 7. At the top of the figure, a second derivative of the infrared spec-

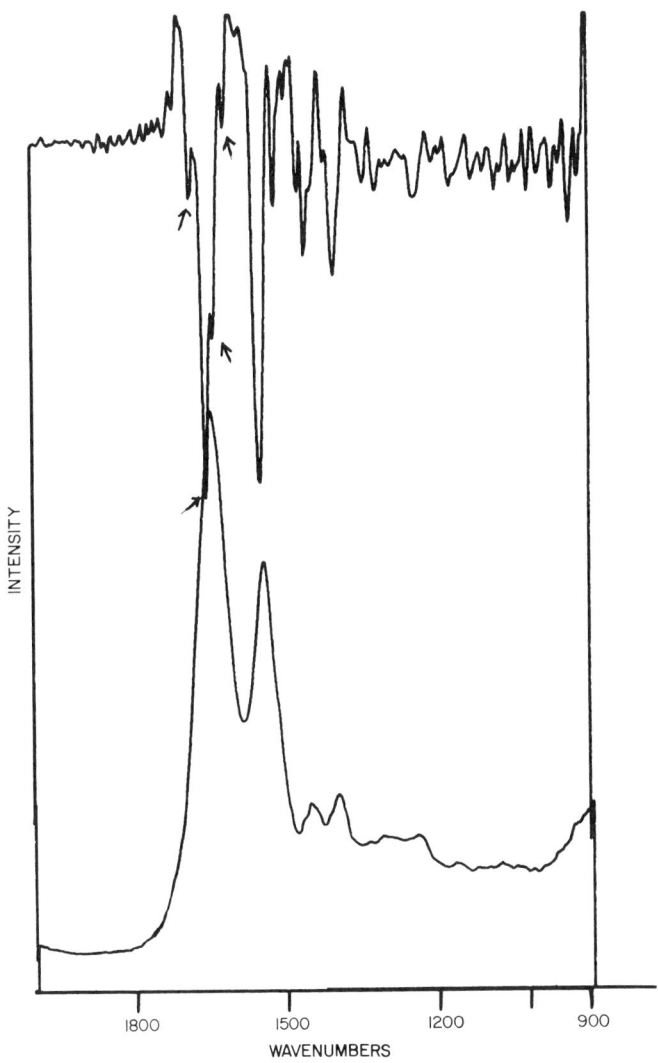

Figure 7. (Top) Spectrum obtained by taking second derivative of spectrum at bottom. Arrows point to second-derivative bands that fall at frequencies where albumin and γ-globulins are known to have second-derivative bands.
(Bottom) Albumin–globulins mixture from Figure 4.

trum of the 1:1 mixture of albumin and γ-globulins is compared to the adsorbance spectrum of this mixture (*bottom*). Although the Amide I band (1650 cm^{-1}) shows a slight low-frequency asymmetry, proving the presence of two components, much less identifying them, would be difficult. However, the second-derivative spectrum of the mixture shows four peaks (marked with arrows) in the Amide I region. The two high-frequency peaks correspond to the frequencies of the two peaks we observed in the second-derivative spectrum of pure albumin, while the two lower-frequency peaks of the mixture correspond to the two peaks seen in the second-derivative spectrum of γ-globulins. Albumin tends to be a mixture of α-helix and β-pleated sheet conformations (*3*). The high-frequency Amide I peaks in the second-derivative spectrum of the mixture agree in frequency with the frequencies assigned (*4*) to α-helix (1655-cm^{-1}) and β-pleated sheet (1685-cm^{-1}) conformations of albumin. In addition, the intensities of the 1685- and 1655-cm^{-1} second-derivative peaks roughly correspond to the reported (*3*) distribution of α-helix conformer (55%) and β-pleated sheet conformer (15%).

Figure 8 illustrates the third approach to identify proteins in mixtures. This figure shows the Amide I and Amide II regions for an absorbance spectrum of the 1:1 albumin–globulins mixture (*top*), and the deconvolution of this spectrum (*bottom*). (The FORTRAN deconvolution program used was generously supplied by David Cameron of the National Research Council of Canada.) The program assumes a band shape and narrows the band width to resolve intrinsically overlapped bands. The authors of the program have published the theory of this approach recently (*5*). The low-frequency asymmetry of the Amide I band (1650 cm^{-1}) is even more apparent in this expanded spectrum, but still would not allow identification of the components. However, in the deconvoluted spectrum (*bottom*), two peaks are clearly discernable at 1656 cm^{-1} and 1643 cm^{-1}, frequencies that correspond to the Amide I frequencies of pure albumin and γ-globulin, respectively. This frequency distinction alone would help in identifying the individual components of the mixtures. Thus, spectral subtraction, deconvolution, and second-derivative spectra all provide information helpful in identifying proteins in mixtures. However, because infrared second-derivative spectra and deconvolution are relatively new and unproven techniques, we are still evaluating their usefulness.

ATR Studies (Flowing Systems)

The transmission FTIR studies of aqueous protein solutions indicate how structural and conformational differences in a protein can be related to spectral changes, and that spectral features can be used to identify proteins in mixtures. However, these studies involve static systems, and our goal was to study flowing systems and the adsorption of proteins onto various surfaces.

To attain this goal, we used ATR techniques which have been described previously (6). A liquid ATR cell can be used to circulate protein solutions (or blood) through the cell while spectrally monitoring the adsorption of proteins onto the surface of the ATR crystal. In addition, the ATR crystal can be coated with a thin layer of polymer, permitting us to follow the adsorption of pro-

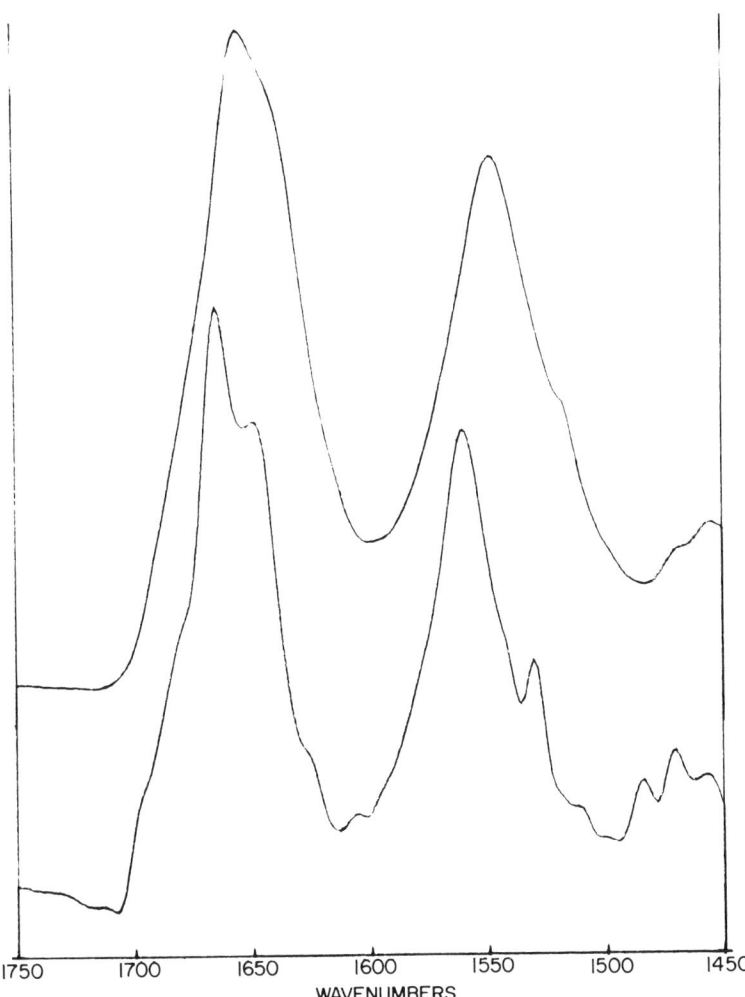

Figure 8. Top: The 1:1 mixture of albumin–γ-globulins shown in Figure 4. Bottom: Result of Fourier transform self-deconvolution. This program operates on the spectral interferogram to cause narrowing of overlapped bands so that they may be resolved. The program provides information about exact peak frequencies while trading off information about exact band shape.

teins onto the polymer surface. All of the work described in the following section is concerned with protein adsorption onto the surface of a germanium ATR crystal.

As indicated earlier, we initially studied the adsorption of proteins from flowing aqueous solutions of single proteins, which allowed us to establish a baseline for the time–adsorption behavior of each of the proteins. The protein buildup was monitored as the adsorbed layer increases in thickness. An example of this is shown in the spectra of Figure 9 which show how the protein layer adsorbed from an albumin solution changes with time. In addition to an increase in the amount of adsorbed protein, changes with time occur in the 1300-cm^{-1} region of the Amide III complex. The adsorbed

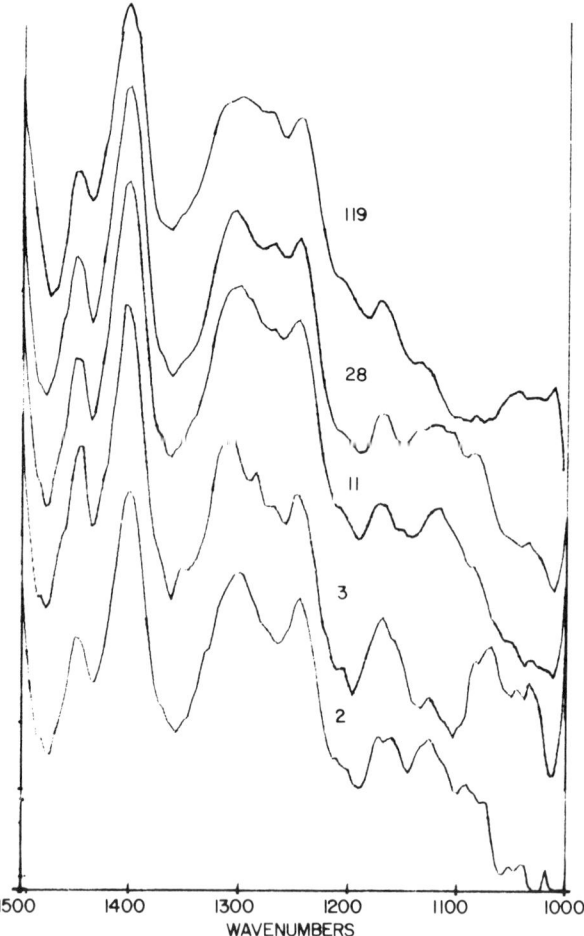

Figure 9. Flowing ATR spectrum of 2% (w/v) albumin, adsorbing onto germanium ATR crystal (flow rate: 3 mL/min). Spectra are taken at (from bottom to top) 2, 3, 11, 28, and 119 min of flow (water-subtracted).

protein layer changes with time of flow, and this behavior can be established for each protein. These changes are discussed in more detail in the section on ATR studies of protein mixtures.

More important is a description of the type of information that can be obtained from the spectra of more complex, flowing mixtures, which can be illustrated by consideration of a 1:1 albumin–fibrinogen mixture in saline. Representative spectra of the protein layer obtained by flowing this mixture past the ATR crystal are shown in Figure 10. In the Amide III (1200–1350-cm^{-1}) spectral region, three types of spectral changes occur with time of flow. Looking only at the series of infrared bands around 1300 cm^{-1}, we find that the number of bands, the frequencies of the bands, and the shape

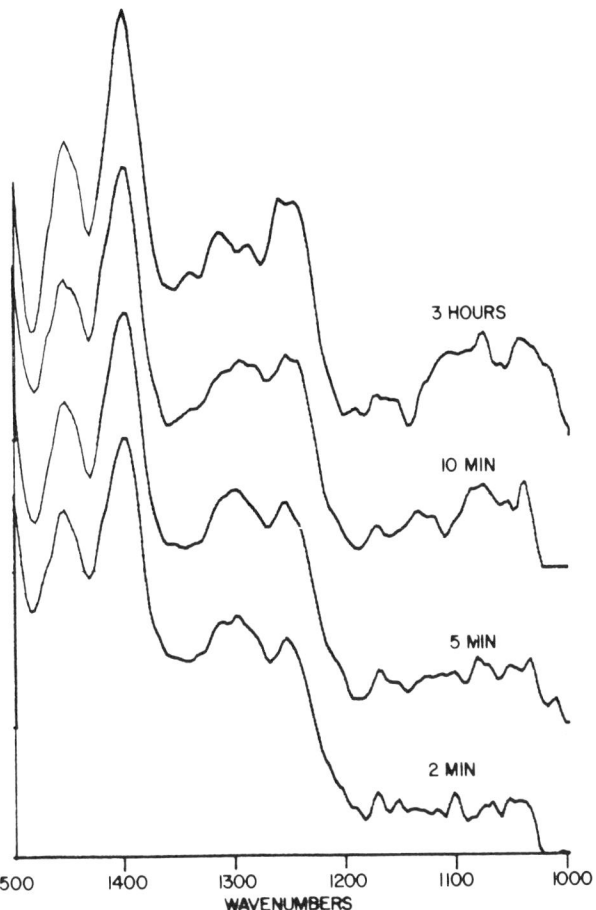

Figure 10. Flowing ATR spectrum of 2% (w/v) 1:1 albumin–fibrinogen adsorbing onto a germanium ATR crystal (flow rate: 15 mL/min). Spectra are taken at (from bottom to top) 2, 5, 10, and 180 min of flow (water-subtracted).

of the bands all change with time. The very same type of behavior is observed for the series of infrared bands near 1250 cm^{-1}. The third spectral change is that the ratio of the intensities of the 1300-cm^{-1}/1250-cm^{-1} bands also changes with time of flow. The significance of these changes is discussed in later sections after other experimental observations are discussed.

If the intensities of various infrared bands are measured and plotted against time of flow, the kinetics or rate of adsorption can be determined. This is only true if infrared bands that are not sensitive to conformation or structural changes are used; the intensity will then be related directly to the total amount of adsorbed material. The two bands that were common to all proteins studied, and that were independent of conformational changes at constant pH are the bands at 1550 cm^{-1} (Amide II) and 1400 cm^{-1}. These bands are shown for the fibrinogen–albumin mixture in Figure 11, where

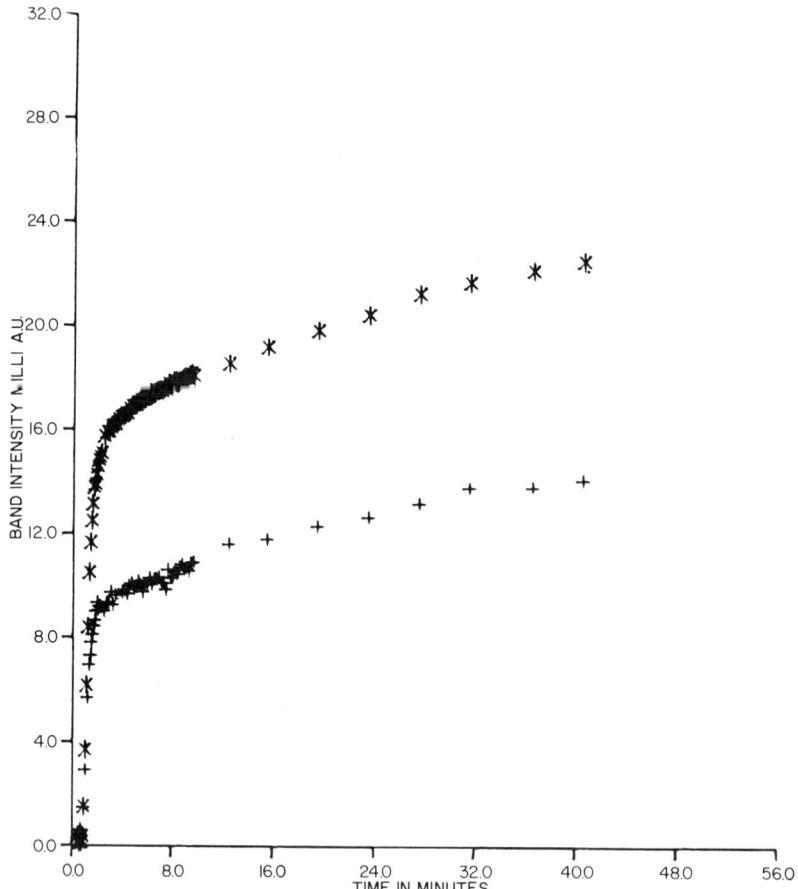

Figure 11. Kinetic plot of intensities (baseline corrected) of (*) Amide II (1550-cm^{-1}) and 1400-cm^{-1} (+, ×3.0) band as a function of time of flow (flow rate: 15 mL/min) for the albumin–fibrinogen mixture shown in Figure 10.

most of the protein adsorbs in the first few minutes of solution flow. At slightly less than 2 min of flow, a marked change in slope occurs, indicating a decrease in the rate of protein adsorption. The possible reasons for this change are discussed with the three types of spectral changes observed in Figure 10. After 2 min the rate of protein adsorption decreased, but adsorption never stopped during the time of this experiment (222 min, although only data up to 42 min is shown in Figure 11). If saline is substituted for the flowing protein solution, then the kinetics of desorption can be studied as shown in Figure 12. Such a plot also can be used to determine the relative amounts of stable adsorbed proteins to unstable or loosely held proteins. Figure 12 shows that roughly 18–20% of the protein was desorbed during the first 2 min of saline flow, but after that time, very little additional protein was desorbed. This stable layer gives an intensity of about 27 milliabsorbance

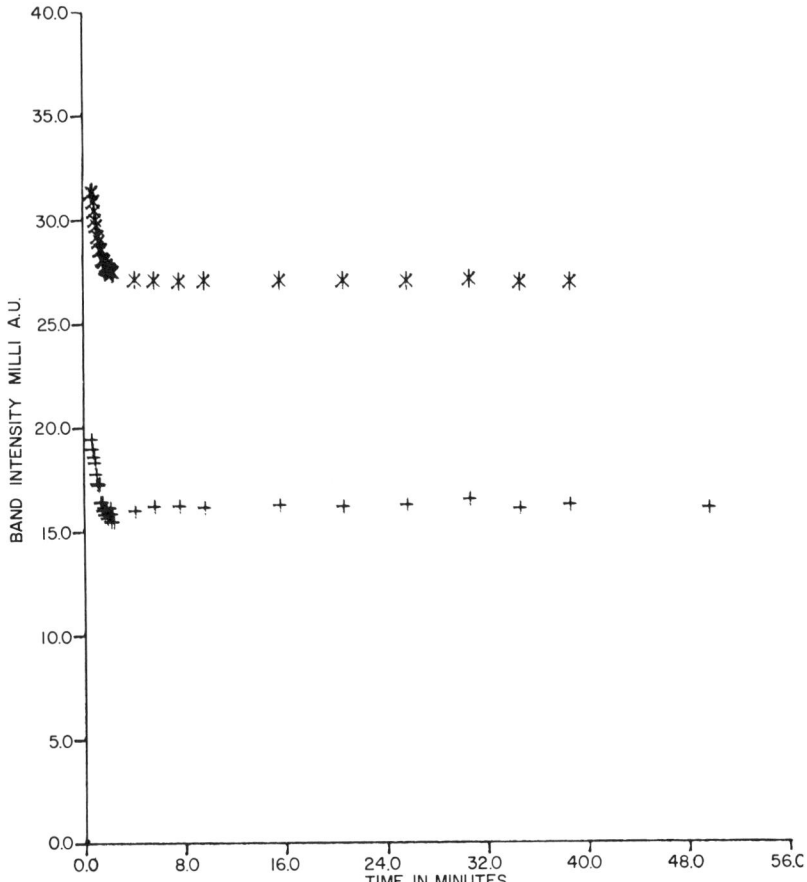

Figure 12. Kinetics of protein desorption from germanium crystal for the mixture shown in Figure 10. Desorption is with isotonic saline flowing at 15 mL/min. Key: *, Amide II band (1550 cm^{-1}) and +, 1400-cm^{-1} band (×3.0).

units for the 1550-cm^{-1} band. Although not shown in Figure 11, the intensity of this band (1550 cm^{-1}) reaches 27 milliabsorbance units at approximately 100 min of flow. Thus, the layer established by 100 min of flow is an amount of protein equal to the amount in the stable layer in the desorption experiment.

Certain bands are insensitive to protein conformational changes and can be used, even in mixtures, to measure the total amount of protein adsorbed. This result was verified using ^{125}I-radiolabeled proteins. Solutions of these tagged proteins (pH 5.3) were adsorbed onto the ATR crystal, and a spectrum of the stable desorbed layer was obtained. The tagged protein was then removed from the crystal and counted. Figure 13 shows such data: a plot of intensity of the 1400-cm^{-1} band against the amount of adsorbed protein (as determined by radioactive counting). This plot shows a reasonably linear relationship with an intercept at zero, indicating that the 1400-cm^{-1} band can be used to measure quantitative rates of protein adsorption and desorption.

Several observations of spectral changes for the fibrinogen–albumin mixture that require further explanation are:

1. The number, frequencies, and shapes of the infrared bands in the 1300-cm^{-1} region change with time.
2. The number, frequencies, and shapes of the infrared bands in the 1250-cm^{-1} region also change with time of flow.
3. The intensity ratio of the 1300 cm^{-1}/1250 cm^{-1} bands changes with time of flow.
4. An amount of protein equal to the amount of protein in the stable layer is adsorbed near 100 min of flow time.

First, we consider the changes that occur in the 1300-cm^{-1} band during the course of the experiment. These changes in frequency of bands around 1300 cm^{-1} are apparent in the spectra of Figure 10, and are listed in tabular form in Table II. Comparing these frequency patterns to those shown in Table I, the frequency changes with time are similar to the frequency changes found with varying concentrations of pure albumin solutions in transmission. This result strongly indicates that the frequency changes in the spectra of the flowing mixture are tracking or following the behavior of albumin as the concentration changes. More albumin is adsorbed in the period from 1.5 to 7.5 min, and thus the frequency changes are similar to those occurring when concentration is increased (Table I). However, after 7.5 min, a reversal occurs, and by comparison to Table I, the albumin is behaving as if it were in an increasingly more dilute environment. To explain this behavior the spectral changes (for the mixture) in the 1250-cm^{-1} region must be considered. These changes are illustrated in Table III, which shows that these bands also give a pattern of change with time of flow. In addition, at the bottom of Table III, the Raman assignments (3) for various conformers of

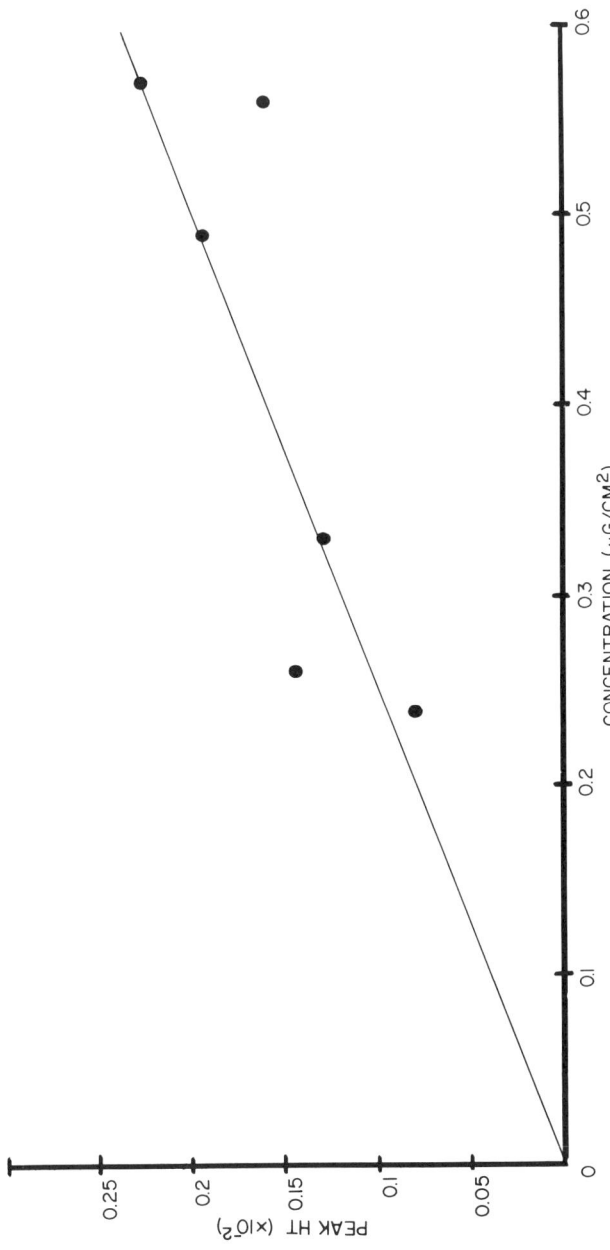

Figure 13. Plot of intensity of 1400-cm^{-1} band of γ-globulins vs. the amount of surface-adsorbed proteins as shown by the radiolabeling experiment. Conditions: slope, 0.00284; slope intercept, 0.000394; and standard deviation, 0.00051.

Table II. Albumin–Fibrinogen 1:1 Mixture (Flowing)

Time (min)	Frequency (cm^{-1})			
1.5–7.5		1300		
7.5–~23	1315 Sh[b]	1300		
~23–~100[a]	1315	1300	1288 Sh[b]	
~100–222	1315		1288	

[a]From 27 to 100 min, the 1315-cm^{-1}/1300-cm^{-1} intensity ratio increases.
[b]Sh = Shoulder.

fibrinogen are listed. These assigned frequencies are reasonably close to those observed in the FTIR spectra of the flowing fibrinogen–albumin mixture, and thus, the changes in the 1250-cm^{-1} region appear to be tracking the conformational behavior of fibrinogen. At 7.5 min, the ratio of the 1300-cm^{-1}/1250-cm^{-1} intensities begins to decrease significantly. Since the 1300-cm^{-1} bands are mainly due to albumin and the 1250-cm^{-1} bands are mainly due to fibrinogen, the 1300-cm^{-1}/1250-cm^{-1} change indicates a change in the ratio of albumin to fibrinogen, that is, at 7.5 min much more fibrinogen begins to be adsorbed. Thus, albumin is behaving (after 7.5 min) as if it were in a more dilute environment, and at this time the amount of fibrinogen is increasing. Therefore, the adsorbed albumin is apparently being diluted with fibrinogen. Because the total amount of protein (as indicated by the 1400-cm^{-1} band) has not increased dramatically at 7 min, fibrinogen is probably replacing adsorbed albumin at the surface, accounting for the large increase in fibrinogen intensity. This result is further emphasized by the spectra of Figures 14 and 15. Figure 14 shows the spectrum of the adsorbed proteins after 2 min of flow. The ratio of the 1300-cm^{-1} to the 1250-cm^{-1} bands indicates a mixture rich in albumin. Yet in Figure 15, after 222 min of flow, the 1300-cm^{-1}/1250-cm^{-1} ratio indicates that the adsorbed proteins are very rich in fibrinogen (probably >90% fibrinogen).

Table III. Albumin–Fibrinogen 1:1 Mixture (Flowing)

Time (min)	Frequency (cm^{-1})		
1.5—19[a]		1254	
19—222	1263		1248
Fibrinogen (Raman)	1264	1254	1242
	30–55%	60%	5–10%
2° Structure	α-helix	random coil	β-sheet

[a]At approximately 7.5 min, the ratio of the 1300-cm^{-1}/1254-cm^{-1} intensities begins to decrease.

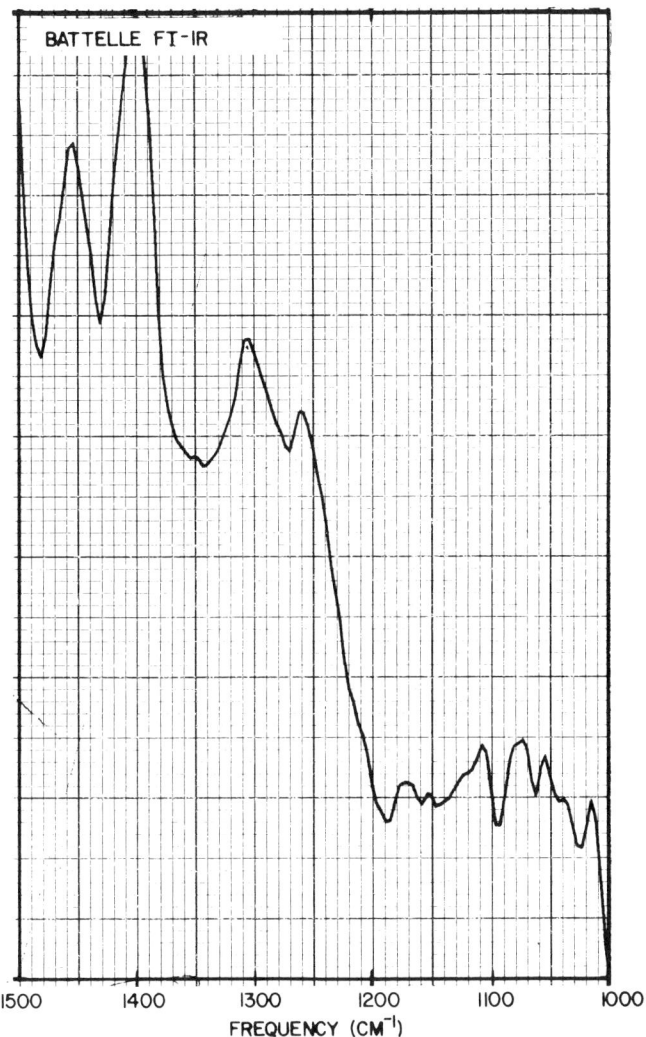

Figure 14. The 1:1 mixture of albumin–fibrinogen adsorbing on germanium (water-subtracted and scale expanded). The spectrum was obtained at 2 min of flow.

Explanations for these spectral observations are summarized below.

1. The spectral changes in the 1300-cm^{-1} region are like the spectral changes that occur when the concentration of pure albumin solutions are varied, that is, the 1300-cm^{-1} spectral changes are tracking the behavior of albumin in the protein layer adsorbed from the albumin–fibrinogen mixture.

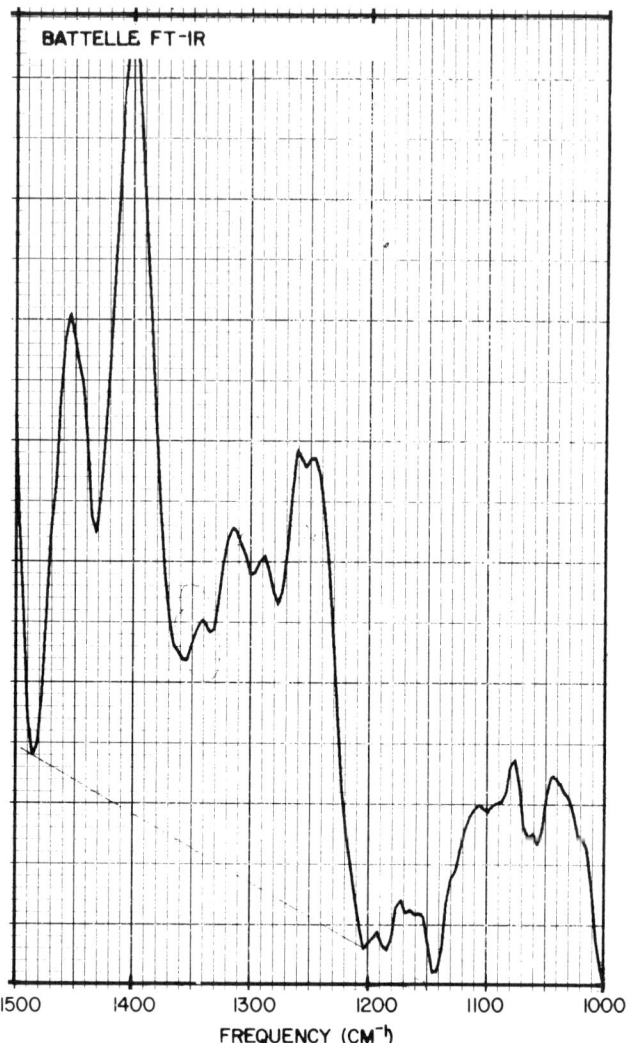

Figure 15. The 1:1 mixture of albumin–fibrinogen adsorbing on germanium (water-subtracted and scale expanded). The spectrum was obtained at 222 min of flow.

2. The spectral changes in the 1250-cm^{-1} region agree with assigned frequencies for conformers of fibrinogen, that is, the 1250-cm^{-1} changes are tracking the conformational behavior of fibrinogen in the adsorbed layer.
3. Since the 1300-cm^{-1} spectral changes track albumin behavior and the 1250-cm^{-1} changes track fibrinogen behavior, then changes in the 1300-cm^{-1}/1250-cm^{-1} intensity ratio indicate

changes in the albumin/fibrinogen ratio, that is, near 7.5 min of flow time, the total adsorbed protein layer becomes appreciably richer in fibrinogen.

4. At 100 min, an amount of protein equal to the amount of protein in the stable layer has adsorbed, and an albumin structural change occurs. At present, the relationship (if any) between these results is unknown.

Point 4 relates to the albumin change after 100 min of flow time and that at this time an amount of protein equal to the stable layer has adsorbed.

Finally, a summary of the flow time behavior of protein adsorption from the 1:1 albumin–fibrinogen solution is listed:

0–1.5 min	• Mixture rich in albumin adsorbs
	• At 1.5 min, fibrinogen conformation changes, as does the rate (slope) of protein adsorbed
1.5–7.5 min	• Amount of albumin increases (behaves as if more concentrated)
	• At 7.5 min, fibrinogen/albumin ratio increases
7.5–~23 min	• Relative amount of albumin decreases (albumin behaves as if more dilute). Since total amount of material only increases slightly, fibrinogen must replace albumin
	• At 19 min, fibrinogen conformation changes
~23–~100 min	• Albumin behaves as if even more dilute
	• At 100 min, amount of material equal to stable layer has adsorbed
~100–~222 min	• Albumin even more dilute—loosely bound?
	• At 222 min, the total adsorbed layer is rich in fibrinogen

In conclusion, the final equilibrium adsorbed layer is rich in fibrinogen. While this result agrees with reports from other investigators, many different events take place before the final equilibrium adsorbed layer is established. Not only can FTIR follow these different events, but the times at which the different events occur can be related to spectral changes, which in turn can be related to the albumin–fibrinogen composition and secondary or tertiary changes in the individual proteins.

While these conclusions are directed towards the fibrinogen–albumin mixture study, this type of FTIR analysis of proteins has general applicability. These results indicate that FTIR can produce usable spectra of flowing aqueous protein solutions, and these spectra can in turn provide useful molecular-level information concerning protein–surface interactions.

Acknowledgment

This work was supported by NIH Grant No. 1 R01 HL24015–2.

Literature Cited

1. Gendreau, R. M.; Winters, S.; Leininger, R. I.; Fink, D.; Hassler, C. R.; Jakobsen, R. J., *Appl. Spectros.* **1981**, *35*(4), 353.
2. Lin, V. J. C.; Koenig, J. L. *Biopolymers* **1976**, *15*, 203.
3. Marx, J.; Hudry-Clergeon, G.; Capet-Antonini, F.; Bernard, L. *Biochim. Biophys. Acta.* **1979**, *578*, 107.
4. Soderguest, M. E.; Walton, A. G. *J. Colloid Interface Sci.* **1980**, *75*, 386.
5. Kauppinen, J. K.; Moffatt, D. J.; Mantsch, H. H.; Cameron, D. G. *Appl. Spectros.* **1981**, *35*(3), 271.
6. Harrick, N. J. "Internal Reflection Spectroscopy"; Interscience: New York, 1967.

RECEIVED for review January 16, 1981. ACCEPTED April 13, 1981.

25

Analytical Methods for the Determination of Biologically Derived Absorbed Species in Biomedical Elastomers

D. R. OWEN, R. ZONE, T. ARMER, and C. KILPATRICK

Tulane University, Polymer Laboratory, New Orleans, LA 70118

> *The calcification on textured neointimal-lined and smooth surface Biomer, a poly(urethane co-ether), during in vivo blood contact was studied with respect to the possible precursor role of a time-dependent sorption of lipids by the elastomer. Surface-deposited or imbibed biological species may act as precursor anchoring sites for the mineralization process. Recent studies have observed high levels of free, long-chain fatty acids (LCFA) in in vitro static Biomer samples after long-term pseudoplasma contact. Indications of free LCFA's and other lipids in textured tissue–lined Biomer samples were observed also. Rapid in vitro calcification occurred on these lipid-imbibed smooth Biomer surfaces when they were exposed to calcium-containing physiological solutions. Attempts made to reduce the lipophilicity of Biomer by the photoinitiation of a polyvinylpyrrolidone interpenetrating network polymer on the elastomer surface resulted in a decreased free LCFA sorption by the polymer.*

Advances in numerous areas have allowed marked increases in survival times of artificial heart device (AHD) and left ventricular assist device (LVAD) experiments. Successful clinical trials employing LVAD's for temporary post-operative assistance after coronary surgical procedures have been reported by several centers (1). As clinical use of circulatory assist devices progresses, longer term (i.e., ≥ 3–4 months) implantations will be needed; requiring not only initial surface hemocompatibility, but also long-term surface inertness or stability.

The increased longevities of animal implantations have caused unforeseen problems at the blood contacting surfaces. Increased mechanical and surface degradation of polymers employed as flexing components in assist devices have occurred. As is well known, the elastomeric polymers being used in AHD and LVAD applications (i.e., Biomer, Avcothane, and Hexsyn, etc.) were not specifically developed for this application. While short-term hemocompatibility appears to be satisfactory, long-term blood–polymer interactions are not understood. Anticipated future increases in long-term use of existing materials could result in AHD and LVAD material failures.

The search for elastomeric materials with good hemocompatibility and dynamic mechanical properties has resulted in, at present, only polyurethanes and poly(α-olefins) being used in prototype devices. One such material, Biomer, a poly(urethane co-ether) has found numerous applications in AHD and LVAD flexing components over the past ten years. The polyurethane has good flex strength and hydrolytic stability (2). In addition, the material has demonstrated short-term blood compatibility, with the rapid adsorbance of albumin rather than thrombus-forming proteins upon in vivo blood exposure (3). However, long-term exposure of Biomer has resulted in the formation of calcifications on the blood contact surface (4). Animal studies demonstrated that this type of calcification may cause stiffening and eventual failure of blood pump linings (5).

The exact cause of the observed mineralization process on blood-contacting synthetic materials has yet to be determined. Recent studies found mechanical strain to be a causative factor of surface calcification in textured neointimal lined LVAD bladders (6). Furthermore, calcification on smooth surface polyurethanes was observed in high stress areas (7). These findings do not give an indication of the nucleating species or the apparent anchoring sites. Recent work, however, has detected concentrations of the calcium-binding amino acid, γ-carboxyglutamic acid (GLA), in proteins isolated from calcified neointimal surfaces (8). The presence of GLA-containing proteins, also found to occur in human atherosclerotic plaque (9), on these LVAD surfaces in vivo would indicate a possible anchoring site for calcium.

Probably no single causal mechanism functions in the calcification process of neointima-lined or smooth surface polyurethanes. Rather, surface calcification is most likely a result of the combination and interaction of mechanical and surface chemical effects at the blood–surface interface. Mechanical damage to or physical imperfections on the polymeric substrate in smooth surface devices or the neointima lining of textured bladders may be capable of inducing a deposition and mineralization process. Calcification of tissue valve leaflets has been proposed to result from the diffusion of blood elements into mechanically disrupted tissue (10), thus providing a site for mineralization to occur. Likewise, deposits of calcium-chelating proteins or lipids in defects in neointimal tissue or the polymer substrate may act as precursor binding sites for the observed mineralization.

Recent evidence indicates that inorganic (11) and organic compounds (12) of blood are capable of penetrating into the type of amorphous elastomers used in AHD and LVAD flexing applications. Localized imbibement of biomolecules within Biomer may be facilitated by the rheological behavior of discrete phases in the polymer. These phases consist of either a hard (i.e., crystalline aromatic urethane) or soft (i.e., amorphous polyether) domain. The latter type domain will undergo conformational changes during flexation of the polymer. In particular, lipid diffusion in the amorphous domains may be enhanced during flexation due to increased mobility of the polyether segments.

The possibility that charged lipid species such as free long-chain fatty acids or amphipathic phospholipids may provide an anchoring site for surface calcium in vivo has led to an examination of the possible role of lipid sorptive processes at the elastomer surface.

Lipids have proven to be quite active in polymer environments (13–15). Investigations in the 1960's performed on silicone rubber heart valve poppets (16) demonstrated that polydimethylsiloxanes with low cross-link densities and low silica filler underwent significant lipid uptake in vivo.

Studies have demonstrated that the degree of lipid absorption depends on the lipophilicity of the polymer (17). Enhanced lipid absorption was observed in block copolymers in which the lipid polar and hydrocarbon segments associated simultaneously with hydrophilic and lipophilic polymer chain regions, respectively. These results are supported by studies that have demonstrated the sorption of lipids by acrylic hydrogels to be inversely proportional to the hydrophilicity of the polymer (18).

The occurrence of surface calcification on Biomer flexing components will require modification of the existing surface or replacement of the polymer with a more blood-compatible material. Alleviation of lipid sorption, assumed to have a significant role in calcium deposition, could be accomplished by altering overall lipophilicity of the surface. Alteration of the Biomer surface has thus been attempted by surface grafting a hydrophilic polymer, poly(N-vinylpyrrolidone) (PNVP), on the elastomer surface. This procedure, best described as developing an interpenetrating polymer network of PNVP, has shown decreased thrombogenicity in vivo by several investigators (19).

The experimental work described here relates to studies done to characterize the affinity of lipids for Biomer and to determine their role in observed calcification of AHD and LVAD elastomeric bladders in vivo.

Experimental

In Vitro Studies. A series of elastomers were soaked in a 37°C synthetic plasma solution (Table I), based on a formulation developed by Carmen and Kahn (20), containing biologically important low molecular weight molecules in blood. The elastomer test samples were exposed to the synthetic plasma for periods extending from 20 weeks to one year. Gravimetric analysis was performed biweekly for 20 weeks and again at 52 weeks.

Table I. Synthetic Lipid Solution Composition

Solution Component	Quantity of Test Solution S/1 g
NaCl	9.0
Glucose	1.0
Urea	0.25
Amino Acids	0.5
Cholic Acid	0.5
Sodium Palmitate	4.0
Palmitic Acid	1.5
Linoleic Acid	1.5
Cholestrol	1.0
Cholestrol Acetate	1.25
Cholesterol Palmitate	1.25
Lecithin	2.5
Tripalmitin	4.5

Materials evaluated in the 20-week in vitro study included Pellethane 2300 Series polyurethane (Upjohn, Inc.), polyphosphazenes PNF-200 and 200M (Firestone Co.), polyHexene-H (Goodrich, Inc.), and Biomer (Ethicon, Inc.). Biomer film was cast from a 10% solution in N,N'-dimethylacetamide (Aldrich) on a glass plate at 60°C. Samples were cut into ½ in. × 6 in. strips, with thicknesses measuring approximately 0.6 mm. Prior to exposure, samples were cleansed with a 1% Triton X-100 (Polysciences, Inc.) solution and rinsed with distilled water. They were then vacuum dried for 25 h, and weighed before exposure commenced.

Gravimetric analysis of elastomers in the study was performed biweekly. Sample strips were rinsed with Triton-X and distilled water, and then vacuum dried at 60°C, before weight gains were determined. Strips were subsequently re-exposed for an additional 2 weeks. Following the twentieth week, samples were exposed without intermittent weighings for 52 weeks.

An additional study was performed on Biomer strips to evaluate lipid sorption during the first 2 weeks of exposure. Samples, prepared from 0.3-mm-thick film, were cut into 5.5 mm × 50 mm strips. Before exposure samples were prepared, similar to the previously mentioned study, gravimetric analysis was performed on odd days for 2 weeks. Five samples were prepared per exposure period. Preweight sample preparations were performed as in the previous study.

An in vitro calcification study was performed on lipid-imbibed Biomer samples to study the effects of surface adsorbed/absorbed lipids on the formation of surface calcium salts in vitro. A high calcium-buffered physiological medium was developed, as described in Ref. 21, to study the effects of imbibed surface lipids on calcium deposition. To a standard dialysate solution (Diasol Low Calcium-120, Travenol Laboratories) was added 1.5mM calcium chloride and potassium phosphate. The solution pH was adjusted to 7 with dilute aqueous sodium hydroxide. Lipid-exposed polymer strips and polymer control strips were soaked in the solution for 1 week, and were subsequently dried and weighed.

In Vivo Studies. Segments of bovine-implanted Biomer LVAD bladders were obtained from researchers at the Thermo Electron Corporation. Segments that possessed observed calcifications were also obtained. In addition, a control bladder sample, steam sterilized at 121.1°C for 3 h, was obtained. Samples were vacuum dried at 50°C for 24 h, followed by a 24-h $CHCl_3$ solvent extraction. Extract solutions were reduced to 1 mL prior to gas chromatographic (GC) analysis.

Calcium deposits attached to bladder surfaces were acidified to retrieve entrapped calcium-complexed fatty acids. Deposits were removed from bladder surfaces by freeze-drying and subsequent mechanical abrasion. They were weighed, then placed in a 6N HCl solution for 10 min. Solid material was filtered off, and a $CHCl_3$ extraction of the aqueous medium was performed.

Solvent Extraction Studies. Techniques necessary to detect lipid species extracted from in vitro and in vivo exposed Biomer were developed. Extractions with a nonpolar swelling solvent (e.g., $CHCl_3$) employing a soxhlet apparatus were performed to extract preferentially lipophilic biological components from Biomer or previously isolated neointimal samples. Experimentation demonstrated the high solubility in chloroform of polymer-derived monomeric and oligomeric components. A separation of lipids from these components was therefore required.

Extractions were performed for 24 h. Extract solutions were reduced and charged with excess hexanes to precipitate polymer-derived oligomeric species. The hexane fraction, containing the soluble lipids, was collected following centrifugation. Solutions were reduced to 1-mL quantities.

The effectiveness of solvent extraction was evaluated by a lipid-doped polymer study. Selected lipids were dispersed in Biomer. Then, two sample films, one containing 1 mg, the other 10 mg of palmitic acid, cholesterol, and tripalmitin were cast from two consecutive castings each of 10% Biomer in dimethylacetamide (DMAC). Lipid concentrations of the 1-mg- and 10-mg-doped samples were calculated to be 0.1% and 1%, respectively. Following casting, a soxhlet extraction and quantitative analysis of extracted lipids were performed. The final extracted concentrations were compared with initial solution concentrations, resulting in an extraction efficiency ratio for each type of component.

Volatile GC Analysis. A Sigma 2 gas chromatograph (Perkin–Elmer) with flame ionization detection (FID) was used to determine quantitatively the amounts of lipids existing in extract solutions. Lipid separations as seen in Figure 1 were performed on a high-temperature column, 1% Dexsil 300 (Supelco, Inc.) without derivatization. Quantitative separations were produced by an 8°C/min, 100°–350°C temperature program. All components eluting from the column were reported as to their elution time (compared with standards for the in vitro study), and were quantitated using FID response.

Polyvinylpyrrolidone (PVNP) Grafting. PVNP was grafted onto Biomer by radiation copolymerization of N-vinylpyrollidone monomer (Polysciences, Inc.) onto the elastomer surface. Polymerization was ultraviolet radiation–initiated in a monomer solution containing 0.1% azobisisobutyronitrile (AIBN) (Polysciences, Inc.).

Prior to polymerization, the monomer solution was vacuum distilled, and purged with nitrogen. Square Biomer samples measuring 1.5 cm^2, with average thicknesses of 0.6 mm, were cut from film cast from a 10% solution in DMAC. Each sample was preswelled in a monomer solution containing AIBN initiator. Samples were then transferred to a dilute aqueous solution of monomer, and were irradiated on both surfaces for 20 min with a 400 W mercury vapor lamp. The reaction vessel was purged with nitrogen and cooled with air.

Results and Discussion

In Vitro Analytical Results. In vitro studies showed that Biomer and a series of other elastomers underwent sorption of lipid species from a synthetic plasma solution (Figure 1). The 20-week in vitro study on the elastomers showed that rapid sample weight gains occurred in the first 2 weeks

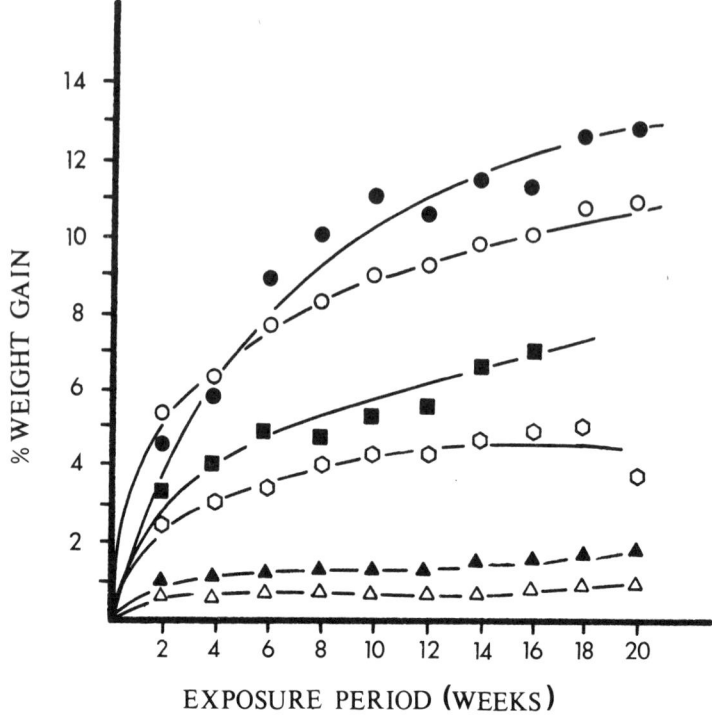

Figure 1. Elastomer weight gains due to in vitro lipid sorption. Key: ●, Pellethane Experimental; ○, Pellethane 2300 series; ■, PolyHexene-H; ⬡, Biomer; ▲, Polyphosphazene PNF 200; and △, Polyphosphazene PNF 200.

of exposure, followed by a slower rate of weight gain. Observed weight gains were the result of lipid sorption from the plasma solution. Water absorption by elastomers, observed in Biomer samples to approach 1% of the sample weight, did not contribute to calculated weight gains after an initial equilibrium period (See Table II.)

Table II. Lipid Weight Gain as a Function of PVP Grafting on Biomer

Exposure Period (days)	Extent PVP Grafting (% Weight Increase Biomer)	% Lipid Weight Gain
12	0	10.1
12	11	3.4
22	0	16.2
22	1.9	9.6
22	3.6	5.1
35	2.5	12.6
35	2.9	12.5
35	6.2	7.5
35	10.6	4.7

An additional in vitro study on Biomer further demonstrated a sorptive process occurring at the elastomer surface. A 2-week in vitro study exposing 0.3-mm-thick Biomer samples determined weight gains to approach 30 wt % of the elastomer after a 15-day exposure period (Figure 2). These significantly higher Biomer weight gains, as compared to those observed in samples exposed for 20 weeks, resulted from greater surface area-to-weight ratios of the 0.3-mm films. Identification of the types and amounts of lipids sorbed to sample surfaces was evaluated by GC analyses of soxhlet solvent extracts. Figure 3 shows the lipid separation obtained by the methods described.

Soxhlet extraction with a nonpolar solvent was effective in selectively removing adsorbed lipids (~50 μm within the polymer) in the elastomer. A solvent extraction study determined that chloroform soxhlet extraction for 24 h could extract entrapped lipid species in a lipid-doped polymer strip. An 800-mg film with an inner layer consisting of 1-mg quantities of palmitic acid, cholesterol, and tripalmitin was $CHCl_3$ extracted. Quantitative analysis by GC determined that the extraction removed 80% of palmitic acid and caused severe swelling of the elastomer, accounting for the high efficiency of removal of these substances. Chloroform also was found to extract considerable concentrations of polymer-derived species (i.e., oligomers, monomers). Figure 4 describes multiple volatile components contained within Biomer steam-sterilized LVAD bladders. Gravimetric analysis of samples soxhlet extracted

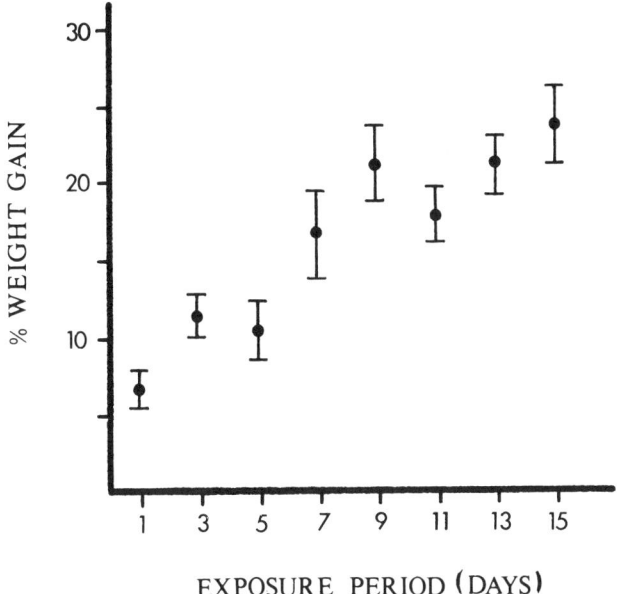

Figure 2. Biomer weight gains due to in vitro lipid sorption.

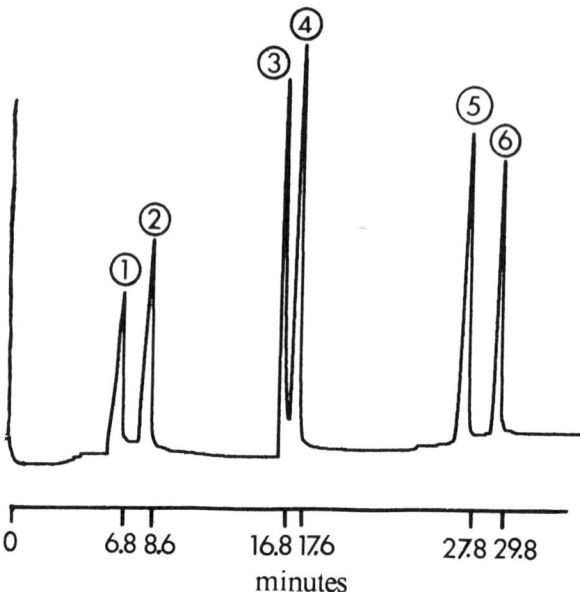

Figure 3. Chromatograph of a 1% solution of standard lipids in $CHCl_3$. Column conditions: 1% Dexsil 300; 100°–350°C at 8°C/min; and carrier—30 mL/min helium. Key: 1, palmitic acid; 2, linoleic acid; 3, cholesterol; 4, cholesterol acetate; 5, cholesterol palmitate; and 6, tripalmitin.

with $CHCl_3$ determined weight losses to be greater than 5% of the original elastomer weight. Recently, experimentation has determined that addition of excess hexanes to an extract solution effects a precipitation of the higher molecular weight oligomeric species, while solubilizing the lipids.

GC analyses on $CHCl_3$ extracts from in vitro studies detected high concentrations of palmitic and linoleic acids relative to other original solution concentrations (Figure 5). Selective sorption of free LCFA's from the plasma solution may occur by a rapid adsorptive process. Results of extractions on long-term (i.e., 1 year) in vitro samples indicated that higher molecular weight or bulky-shaped lipids occur at increased concentrations relative to the fatty acids. Comparing chromatographs from 3-day and 1-year sample extracts (Figure 6), cholesterol, and to a lesser extent the cholesterol esters and tripalmitin, are at increased concentrations relative to the fatty acids in 1-year exposed Biomer. These findings suggest that a size, as well as a solubility parameter–dependent absorptive process occurs over long durations. GC analyses also reveal the apparent absence of certain initially occurring monomeric or oligomeric species from 1-year in vitro samples. If slow in vitro or in vivo extraction of monomeric or oligomeric species occurs, subsequent formation of voids would permit increased absorption of size diffusion-limited species (e.g., high molecular weight lipids).

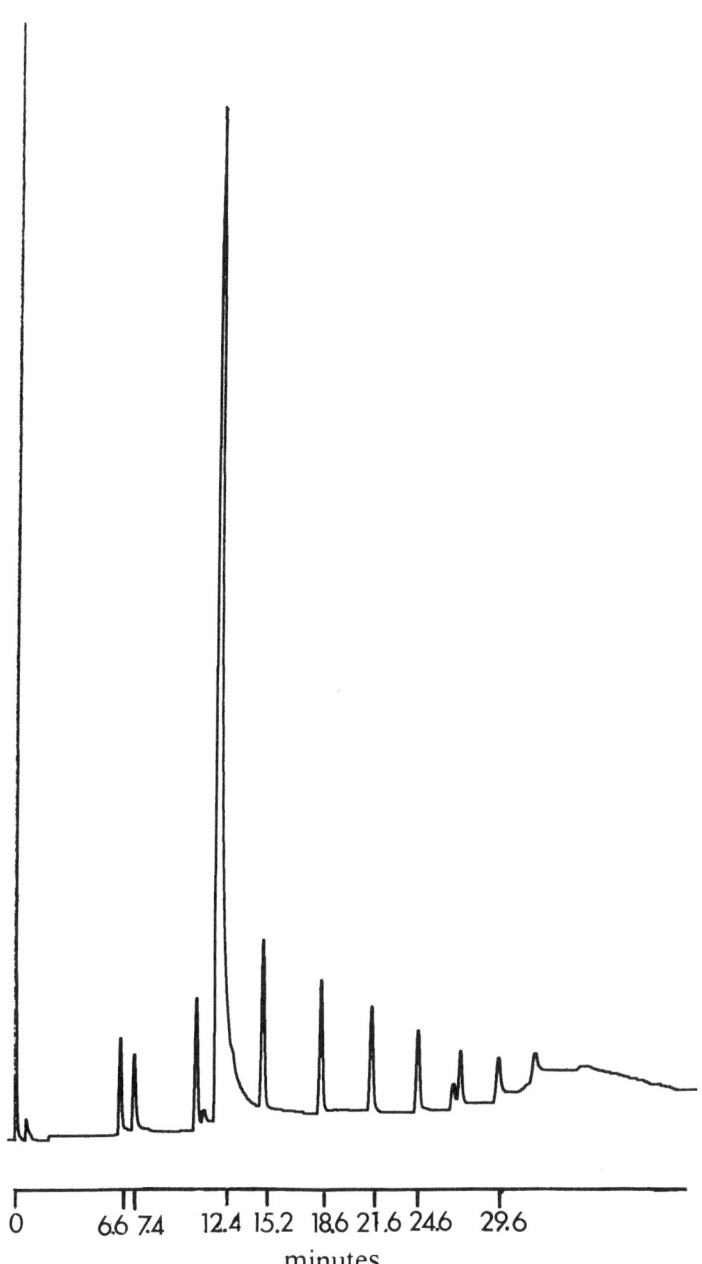

Figure 4. Chromatograph of $CHCl_3$ extract of steam-sterilized Biomer bladder. Column conditions: 1% Dexsil 300; 100°–350°C at 8°C/min; and carrier—30 mL/min helium.

A rapid calcification process on in vitro lipid-exposed Biomer samples occurred within a 1-week period. Strips exposed to the synthetic plasma for less than 2 weeks underwent a rapid surface calcium complexation following a 7-day exposure to a calcium-containing physiological medium (pH 7), whereas unexposed Biomer samples did not calcify. The development of calcium deposits as seen in in vivo bovine LVAD bladders probably would arise from this initial "nucleation" process.

PVP Grafting. The Biomer surface was modified to decrease its lipophilicity. The in situ polymerization of vinylpyrrolidone, after being allowed to swell the Biomer strips to a specific depth, was accomplished by photoinitiation. The resulting interpenetrating network polymer (i.e., PVNP) would be expected to increase surface hydrophilicity. Indeed, the aqueous contact angles on all grafted systems decreased from 10% to 25% of the original nongrafted value.

In Vivo Analytical Results. Indications of the presence of lipids at or within the polymer surface of bovine-implanted Biomer LVAD bladders and calcified neointimal areas were observed in GC solvent-extraction analyses. In addition, concentrations of polymer-derived species extracted from the Biomer bladder were detected. Although analytical techniques were effective in selectively separating lipids from extracted polymer components,

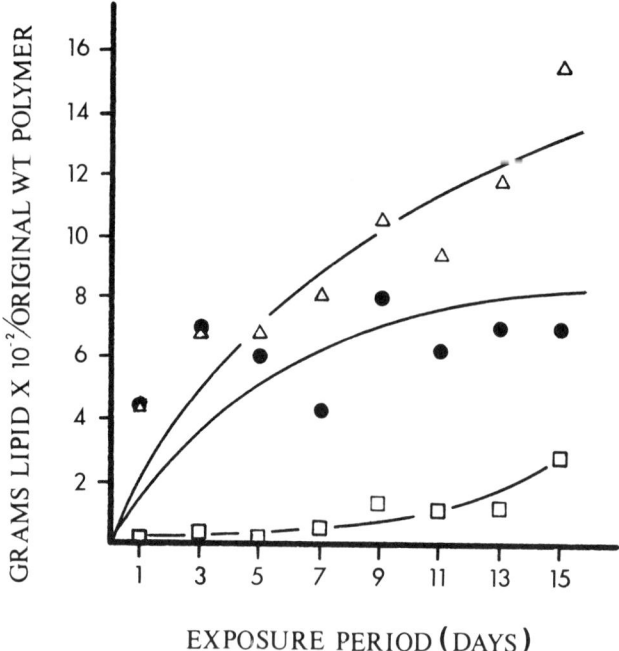

Figure 5. Weight of lipids $CHCl_3$ extracted from Biomer in vitro. Key: △, *palmitic acid;* ●, *linoleic acid; and* □, *cholesterol.*

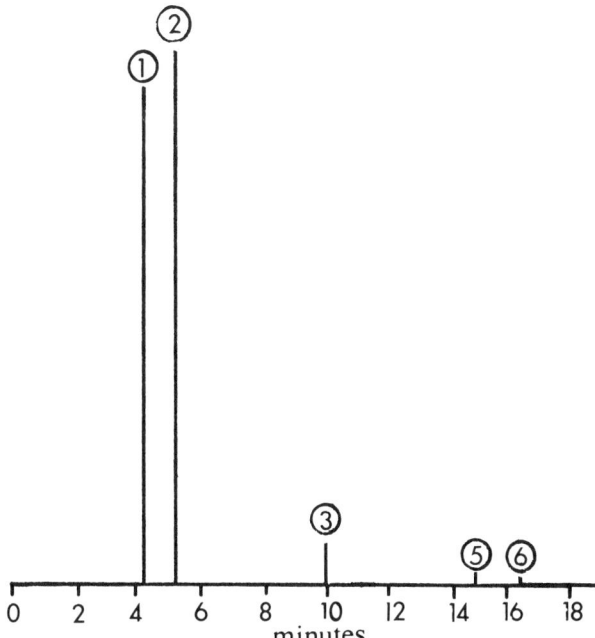
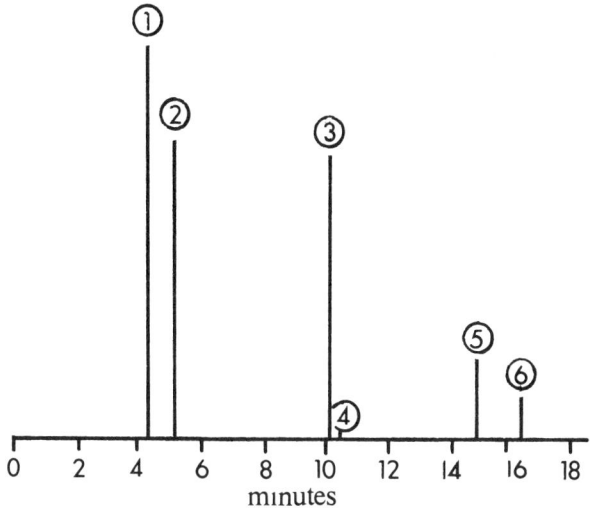

Figure 6. Reproduction of chromatographs from in vitro $CHCl_3$ extractions: (top) Biomer 3 days in vitro and (bottom) Biomer 1 year in vitro. Column conditions: 1% Dexsil 300; 100°–350°C at 15°C/min; and carrier—30 mL/min helium. Key: 1, palmitic acid; 2, linoleic acid; 3, cholesterol; 4, cholesterol acetate; 5, cholesterol palmitate; and 6, tripalmitin.

certain monomeric and oligomeric species remained in the extract solutions. As exhibited in Figure 6, a chromatograph of a steam-sterilized Biomer control sample, these components are well resolved and possess a wide range of retention times. Recent evidence indicates that these components are aromatic, presumably aromatic diisocyanate derivatives, and low molecular weight polyether molecules.

The first in vivo sample analyzed was retrieved from the noncalcified flex region of a 55-day implanted bladder. The sample chromatograph in Figure 7 shows that numerous species were extracted in addition to the labeled, previously detected polymer-derived components. Based on the lipid retention times determined previously (Figure 3), the peaks eluting between 7.2 and 12.2 min are assumed to be fatty acids. Those eluting between 12.2 and 18.4 min indicate cholesterol and cholesterol esters. While additional data are required to confirm these assumptions, the selectivity of the extraction and analysis suggests that these components are lipids. Although these peaks also may represent polymer-derived species, the long-term blood exposure would be expected to extract these components.

The second sample analyzed was retrieved from a lightly calcified flex region of a 106-day implanted bladder. The extract chromatograph of this sample in Figure 8 shows that several peaks appear at concentrations different than those seen previously in the control and shorter-term 55-day extract analyses. Several of the early eluting components, with retention times between 7.0 and 12.0 min, assumed previously to be fatty acids, were not detected. The absence of these peaks could be the result of calcium complexation of the fatty acids; the insolubility of fatty acid calcium salts in the extraction medium preventing their detection. The appearance of numerous peaks after 18.0 min could be explained in terms of long-term lipid sorption or diffusion into the bladder surface. The retention time of the peak eluting at 18.4 min indicates a cholesterol ester. Certain diglycerides and phospholipid fragments also have been determined to elute with similar retention times. Future efforts will center on determining if these species are indeed present. As indicated in the in vitro studies, the higher molecular weight lipid species (i.e., > 300 MW) may undergo a longer-term diffusion into the polymer, thus explaining their delayed appearance in the consecutive chromatographs. The appearance of these peaks must also be considered in terms of polymer-derived components. For instance, the previously undetected components eluting after 18 min may be polymer breakdown products. No indications of polymer breakdown exist, since numerous other peaks would be expected. A long-term diffusion of imbibed low molecular weight species to the surface during the implantation may also explain their presence in the chromatographs.

As previously mentioned, in vitro studies demonstrated a selectivity of Biomer for free LCFA's; extraction of in vivo samples would not be expected to extract identifiable concentrations of these species because of their susceptibility to calcium complexation.

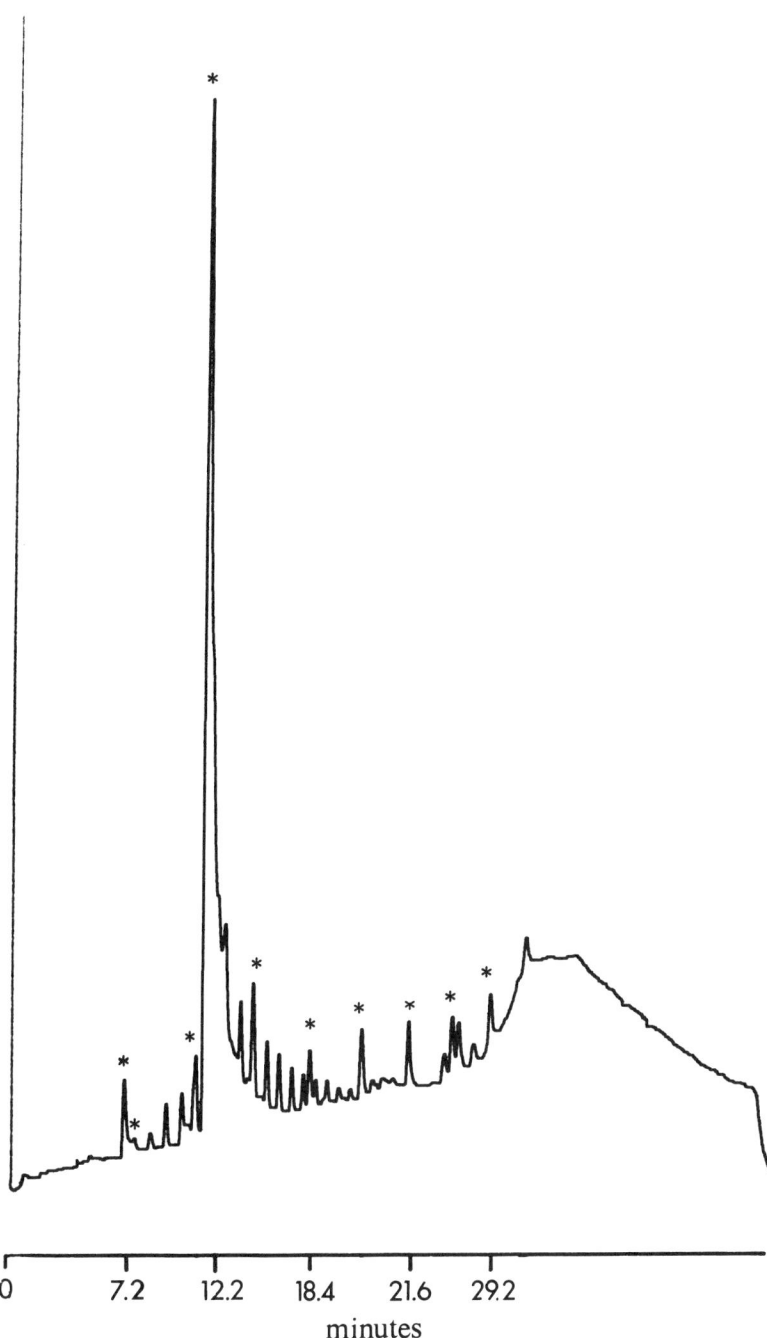

Figure 7. Chromatograph of $CHCl_3$ extraction on a 55-day in vitro LVAD bladder. Column conditions: 1% Dexsil 300; 100°–350°C at 8°C/min; and carrier–30 mL/min helium. Key: *, polymer derived.

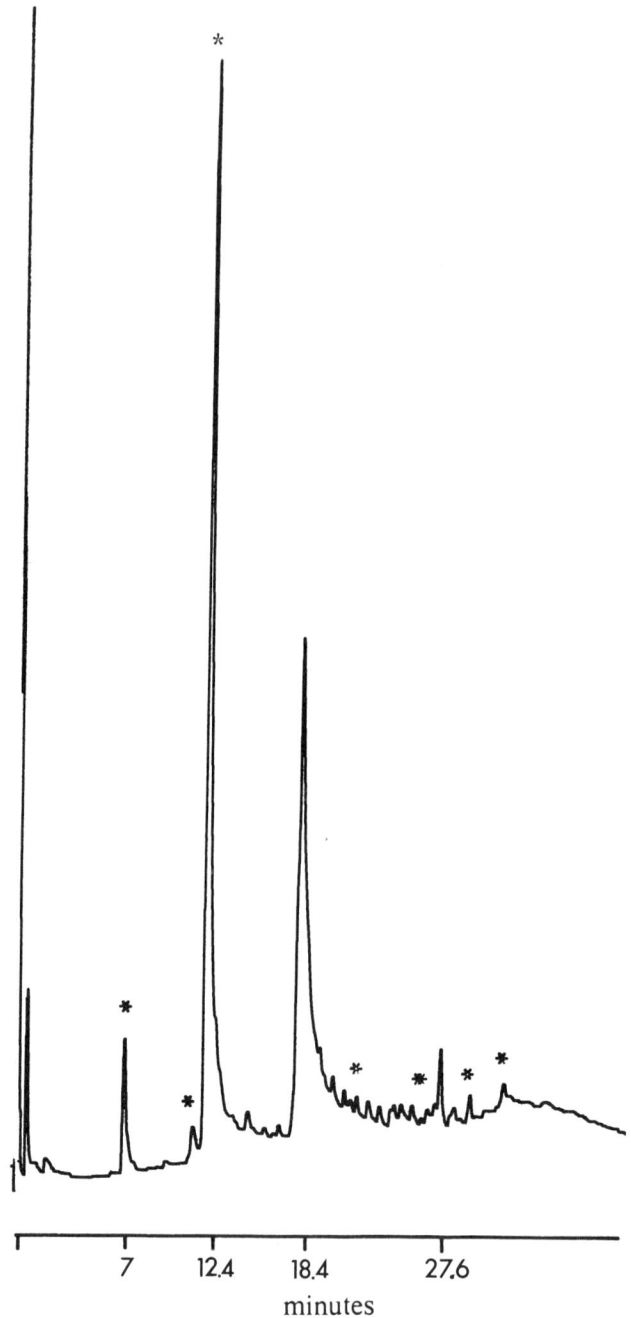

Figure 8. Chromatograph of a $CHCl_3$ extraction on a 106-day in vivo LVAD bladder. Column conditions: 1% Dexsil 300; 100°–350°C at 8°C/min; and carrier—30 mL/min helium. Key: *, polymer derived.

Extraction of a 30-mg calcium nodule detached from a 61-day bovine-implanted bladder segment immediately following acidification yielded a variety of fatty acids (Figure 9). This result was expected, since the initial complexation of free LCFA with calcium on the bladder surface would be assumed to initiate the mineralization. Entrapped LCFA could require acidification to convert them to $CHCl_3$-soluble species.

The mechanism for in vivo free LCFA deposition onto the polyurethane surface may result from a competitive desorption of albumin-bound LCFA's onto the lipophilic polymer soft segments. Albumin can carry upwards of 36 LCFA molecules (22), and Biomer has been shown to adsorb preferentially albumin during blood contact.

Conclusions

Polymer-derived monomeric and oligomeric species are readily extractable from Biomer LVAD bladders. Lipid sorption definitely occurs in vitro on/in various elastomers presently being used or considered for LVAD or AHD applications. Apparently, lipid sorption does occur in vivo, and may be involved in surface calcification observed on both smooth and textured

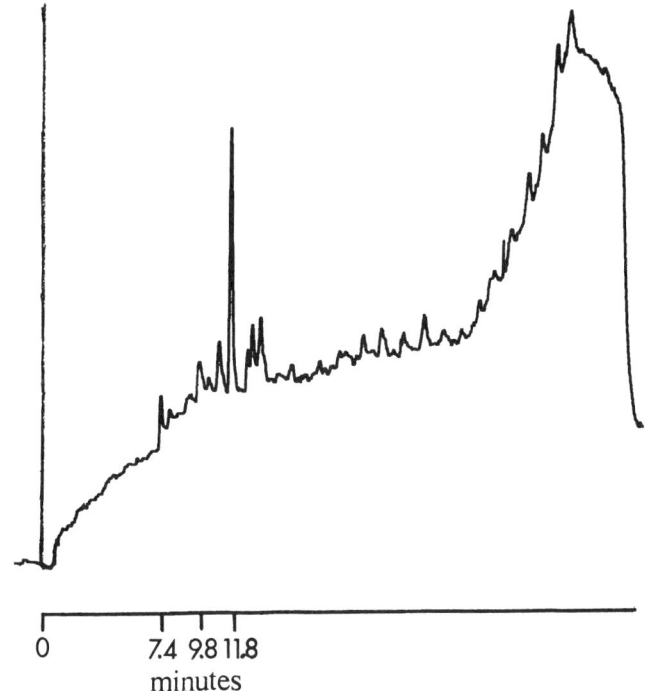

Figure 9. Chromatograph of a $CHCl_3$ extract from an acidified calcium nodule (LVAD #576). Column conditions: 1% Dexsil 300; 100°–350°C at 8°C/min; and carrier—30 mL/min helium.

neointimal-lined elastomer LVAD bladders. This effort has not shown that lipid sorption is necessarily the prime antecedent to the mineralization of smooth or neointimal-lined flexing polyurethane LVAD bladders. However, as in the natural atherosclerotic process, lipids are involved.

The difficulty in obtaining neointimal-lined or smooth surface LVAD or AHD polyurethane diaphragms with in vivo flexing times of six months precludes these obvious sources of information from being used extensively. The experimentalist in this area must therefore rely on in vitro experiments, for the short-term, and face the usual shortcomings of extrapolation to the in vivo situation.

Acknowledgments

The authors thank Dr. Michael Szycher at the Thermo Electron Corp. for providing in vivo LVAD samples. We would also like to acknowledge Dr. David Wasserman of the Ethicon Corp. for supplying the Biomer.

Literature Cited

1. Berger, R. L., McCormick, J. R.; Stetz, J. D.; Klein, M. D.; Ryan, T. J.; Carr, J.; Sweet, S.; Bernhard, W. F. *J. Am. Med. Assoc.* **1980**, *243* (1), 46.
2. Szycher, M.; Poirier, V.; Keiser, J. *Trans. Am. Soc. Artif. Intern. Organs* **1977**, *23*, 116.
3. Lyman, D. "Graft Materials in Vascular Surgery"; Dardik, H., Ed.; Symposia Specialists: Miami, 1978; p. 213.
4. Lawson, J. H.; Fukumasu, H.; Olsen, D. B.; Jarvik, R. K.; Kessler, T. R.; Coleman, D.; Pons, A. B.; Blaylock, R.; Kolff, W. J. *J. Thorac. Cardiovasc. Surg.* **1979**, *78*(1), 150.
5. Hennig, E.; Keilbach, H.; Böhme-Schmökel, D.; Bücherl, E. S. *Abstr. Amer. Soc. Artif. Intern. Organs* **1981**, *10*, 27.
6. Whalen, R. L.; Snow, J. L.; Harasaki, H.; Nose, Y. *Trans. Am. Soc. Artif. Intern. Organs* **1980**, *26*, 487.
7. Pierce, W. S.; Donacky, J. H.; Rosenberg, G.; Baier, R. E. *Science* **1980**, *208*, 601.
8. Lian, J.; Levy, R., personal communication.
9. Lian, J. B.; Skinner, M.; Glimcher, M. J.; Gallop, P. M. *Biochem. Biophys. Res. Commun.* **1976**, *71*, 349.
10. Harasaki, H.; Kiraly, R. J.; Jacobs, G. B.; Show, J. L.; Nose, Y. *J. Thorac. Cardiovasc. Surg.* **1980**, *79*, 125.
11. Coleman, D. L.; Lim, D.; Kessler, T.; Andrade, J. D. *Abstr. Am. Soc. Artif. Intern. Organs*, **1981**, *10*, 3.
12. McHenry, M. M.; Smeloff, E. A.; Fong, W. Y.; Miller, G. E., Jr.; Ryan, P. M. *J. Thorac. Cardiovasc. Surg.* **1970**, *59*(3), 413.
13. Meester, W. D.; Swanson, A. B. *J. Biomed. Mater. Res.* **1972**, *6*, 193.
14. Figge, K.; Kock, J. *Food Cosmet. Toxicol.* **1973**, *11*, p. 975
15. Weightman, B.; Simon, S.; Rose, R.; Paul, I.; Radin, E. *Biomed. Mater. Symp.* **1972**, *3*, 15.
16. Carmen, R.; Kahn, P. *J. Biomed. Mater. Res.* **1968**, *2*, 457.
17. Marsh, H. E., Jr.; Hsu, G. C.; Wallace, C. J.; Blackenhorn, D. H. *Am. Chem. Soc., Div. Org. Coat. Plast. Chem., Prepr.* (Chicago, Aug. 1973) *33*(2), p. 327.
18. Holly, F. J. *J. Polym. Sci., Polym. Symp.* **1979**, *66*, 409.

19. Boffa, G. A.; Lucien, N.; Favre, A.; Boffa, M. C. *J. Biomed. Mater. Res.* **1977**, *11*, 317.
20. Carmen, R.; Mutha, S. C. *J. Biomed. Mater. Res.* **1972**, *6*, 329.
21. Urry, D. W.; Long, M. M.; Hendrix, C. F.; Okamoto, K. *Biochemistry* **1976**, *15*(18), 4089.
22. Gurr, M. I.; James, A. T. "Lipid Biochemistry"; Cornell Univ. Press: New York, 1971; p. 182.

RECEIVED for review January 16, 1981. ACCEPTED November 11, 1981.

26
Effect of Electrical Signals on the Adsorption of Plasma Proteins to a High Copper Alloy

HERBERT J. MUELLER

Northwestern University, Department of Biological Materials, The McGaw Medical Center, Chicago, IL 60611 and American Dental Association, Council on Dental Materials, Instruments and Equipment, Division of Scientific Affairs, Chicago, IL 60611

> *Both potentiostatically controlled direct currents (−0.3, −0.5, and −0.7 V SCE) and pulsed sinusoidal signals (−0.27−−0.4 V) from 2 to 200 kHz produced copper surfaces (several % Zn) with increased resistance toward the adsorption of human albumin, γ-globulin, and fibrinogen. The ac procedures were, however, more effective. The 200-kHz surfaces almost consistently were free of all accumulated mass, whereas the lower frequencies produced surfaces with varying protein concentration. The scanning electron microscopic (SEM) analysis followed these events closely, showing, besides the adsorbed protein layer, the interaction of protein with the oxidized metal in the form of copper chloride phosphates. Potentiodynamic cyclic polarization indicated that addition of protein altered the charging and Faradaic currents. Decreased corrosion potentials ($i_a = i_c$) were observed with all proteins; increased current in the anodic traverse for albumin and globulin, and an inhibitory effect with fibrinogen.*

The normal surface charge on the endothelial lining of a vascular structure is negative and of the same sign as the cells in the flowing blood (1). Sialic acid, possessing a negative charge, is one of the main components in these linings. These natural surfaces are resistant to platelet aggregation and are considered the ideal nonthrombogenic surface (2). A thin polymeric film actually coats the endothelial cellular membranes, which in fact is the substance in direct contact with blood (3). Foreign materials in contact with blood demonstrate that within a few seconds, a thickening film of protein, mostly fibrinogen, is formed at the interface. After reaching a critical thickness of 100–200 Å, thrombogenic surfaces exhibit platelet adhesion leading to the general cascade for thrombus formation. Thrombogenic-resistant surfaces, however, exhibit platelet adhesion in a different form, which restricts further coagulation.

Relationship of Negative Surface Charge to Blood Compatibility

Comprehensive studies (1, 4–7) have been made regarding the compatibility of metals and alloys to flowing blood in ex vivo and in vivo applications. Thrombus formation will not occur if the electrode potential in blood is more negative than about +0.06 V [saturated calomel electrode (SCE)] for noble metals, or more negative than about −0.24 V for nonnoble metals. However, a dilemma is soon reached; that is, metals highly electronegative that are thrombus resistant are very corrosion prone, while metals highly electropositive that are corrosion resistant are thrombogenic. For example, the antithrombogenic characteristics of copper tubes implanted in dogs were improved greatly by the incorporation of either a direct polarized current (dc) or an alternating current (ac) at 200 kHz. Microscopic examination revealed that the ac surfaces exhibited deposits of fibrin and copper corrosion products without cellular material. Fibrous material with entrapped cellular matter was observed for the surfaces without cathodic currents. The dc surfaces exhibited intermediate behavior (5, 6).

The relationship of negative surface charge to increased blood compatibility is supported further by the fact that anionic polyelectrolyte hydrogels exhibit increased thrombogenic resistance (8), that surfaces coated with heparin (negatively charged) resist coagulation (9), that drugs increasing the surface charge negatively produce antithrombogenic behavior (7), and that proteins and their individual amino acids exhibit decreased surface coverage with increased negative electrode potential (10). However, an example is reported (8) showing decreased thrombogenicity for cationic hydrogels. Also, it is argued (3) that for very negative metals, adhesion and aggregation of proteins are overlooked because accumulated corrosion products are carried to other parts of the vascular system. This argument is likewise made for anionic polyelectrolytes that also degrade slowly. Several other examples are referenced (8). Furthermore, the high spontaneous potentials of carbon (+0.28 to +0.97 V) (11) really do not predict carbon's recognized good blood compatibility.

Interactions of Metals and Proteins

Besides the diversity in composition of metals and alloys employed with in vivo testing for blood compatibility, studies investigating the interaction between metals and proteins, either by immersion-induced effects or effects from polarization, mainly have been confined to platinum (7, 10, 12–15) and mercury (*10*, *16–19*). Platinum is useful because the +0.75–−0.80 V range will not exhibit any inherent oxidation and reduction peaks (*14*). Electrochemical reduction studies with mercury, as in polarography, are useful because of the high hydrogen overvoltage of this metal. Protein adsorption/desorption studies on gold (*20*), chromium and its oxide (*21*), and anodized tantalum (*22*) also have been made. Corrosion of metals by anodic polarization has been reported for 316LVM in calf's serum (*23*), for dental amalgam in human saliva and in albumin and mucin solutions (*24*, *25*), and for copper and nickel in amino acid solutions (*26*). Cystine, in contrast to bovine plasma albumin, had an inhibitory effect on the anodic polarization of copper. Corrosion rate measurements for in vivo applications are reported (*27–29*).

The interactions of proteins of albumin, γ-globulin, and fibrinogen with a metal surface are complex processes. The normal configuration and conformation of protein in solution are important to the nature of the ensuing binding mechanisms (*30*, *31*). Albumin (MW = 69,000, isoelectric point (IEP) = 5.4, and dimensions of 38 × 150 Å) forms a compact globule. Two structures have been proposed: The globule is either made of four compact subunits connected by short lengths of polypeptide chain, or the molecule is highly organized into a core covered by a less organized coating of polypeptide chain. γ-Globulin (MW = 150,000, IEP = 6.5, and a length of 270 Å) has a "Y"-shaped structure, whereas fibrinogen (MW = 340,000, IEP = 5.5, and dimensions of 90 × 450 Å) is chemically a dimer composed of a twin set of three polypeptide chains (globules). All three proteins contain an array of amino acid residues of aliphatic or aromatic nature, multifunctionality, and various amino acid side groups. Carboxyl, sulfhydryl, amino, as well as sulfide and disulfide groups are plentiful throughout the molecules. Because the isoelectric point of all three proteins is below the physiological pH of 7.4, a net negative charge exists.

Upon exposure to a protein solution, a metal exhibits a process of monolayer saturation formation (*20*). For gold in bovine serum albumin (BSA), this layer is about 7 Å; for chromium (*21*), about 12 Å; whereas chromium in fibrinogen is about 35 Å, and chromium oxide about 130 Å. At least two models are available to explain these adsorption processes related to electrochemical reduction. In the first case (*19*), portions of protein coming onto the free surface adsorb, unfold, and denature rapidly and irreversibly, and then flatten to form a monolayer tenaciously held onto the surface. The thickness is on the order of the polypeptide chain thickness, about 10 Å. Owing to the polypeptide chain rigidity, however, the monolayer cannot form tightly packed structures. It contains a great number of pores such that electron charge transfer to proteins in solution takes place via these surface discontinuities. In the second case (*32*), molecules of the first layer are deformed only in such a way that their biological activity and potential for electron exchange are both unaltered. The mechanism of charge transfer is thought to be a superimposition of electron transport by hopping through the adsorbed molecules and by exchange of already reduced molecules. Other models (*33*) include bimolecular adsorption layers and the jumping of electrons of over 10 Å from one layer into another. Selective desorption during reduction of the negatively charged hydrophilic surface regions of the flattened adsorbed protein with respect to the hydrophobic regions is, in addition, listed (34).

The interaction of protein with water is also an important consideration because the electrical conductivity of the adsorbed protein layer depends on the mechanism of charge transfer. The conduction in proteins with low water content is electronic, whereas at higher water contents it is protonic and/or due to small inorganic ions (35, 36). Water is considered (37) to exist in two structural forms: clusters (ordered) formed by hydrogen bonds, and free unbounded water (monomeric). Any factors, such as temperature, that favor monomeric water tend to increase the protein's catalytic activity, and factors favoring cluster formation tend to decrease catalytic activity. In addition, increased catalytic activity is probably related to increased binding properties to foreign surfaces.

Potentiostatic and cyclic voltammetry of protein solutions, particularly the fibrinogen, prothrombin, and thrombin/platinum interfaces, have been reported (12, 13), showing the modification in the current density–potential (j–U) behavior with protein additions. The voltammetry results show, besides the elimination of the reversible hydrogen peaks and the suppression of the platinum oxide reduction peak, the development of at least three new charge transfer and adsorption processes. Increasing concentration increases the peak currents. Electrolytic hydrogenation of fibrinogen occurs at the completion of cycling at about -0.7 V. Evidence is presented indicating the possible transformation of prothrombin into thrombin by electrolysis.

Referring the initial spontaneous potentials of metals to the j–U characteristics of the fibrinogen/platinum interface reveals (12) that the thrombogenic metals fall in the potential range where electropolymerization of fibrinogen into fibrin is apt to occur, whereas the thromboresistant metals fall where fibrinogen molecules are desorbed or undergo charge transfer.

This chapter further investigates the effect of surface charge on protein adsorption and charge transfer. Since most previous investigations concerning the electrochemistry of the adsorption/desorption processes of proteins have utilized metal electrodes of platinum or gold, inert to their surroundings, or a potential range where oxidation does not occur (reduction on mercury), electrochemical information is lacking pertaining to the systems involving the interactions of protein adsorption, charge transfer, and metal oxidation and reduction. Even though one of the requirements for a metallic prosthesis is to exhibit corrosion-free behavior, this study, nevertheless, can furnish electrochemical information about a corrodable metal and a protein system that can help to understand the processes occurring between dissolution of metal, and charge transfer and adsorption of protein. Behavior of protein in solution on electrodes inert to their environment, and behavior of a metal in solution void of protein additions, can not be used alone to predict the behavior of the combined oxidized metal/protein system.

As indicated, the blood compatibility of copper is greatly increased by the passage of cathodic electrical currents. Since the mechanism in decreasing the adsorption of blood components on metals by cathodic polarization is not fully understood, this study also was aimed at addressing more fully the desorption of some plasma proteins to a thrombogenic metal system, such as a high copper alloy, by the passage of either steady-state or cyclic-pulsating cathodic electrical signals. In addition, because the effects of variation in electronegativity and the effects of frequency variation in cathodic pulsation upon adsorption have not been reported thoroughly, this investigation relates these variables to the surface adsorption/desorption processes.

Experimental

Materials and Methods. High copper alloy commercial-grade rods (low zinc intensities, several percent, analyzed by energy dispersive x-ray analysis (EDAX)) machined to ⅜ in. diameter and 1 in. long were etched and finished through #600 grit metallographic paper. One end was subsequently finished to a 0.1-μm alumina polish. A threaded hole through the opposite face permitted the attachment of a stainless-steel rod which facilitated handling of the electrode and also placement into the protein solutions. Prior to immersion, all polished surfaces were held in an ultrasonic detergent and rinsed with ample quantities of deionized water. The samples were semi-immersed for periods on the order of hours, in the protein solutions at room temperature exposed to air, and with the polished surface about ¼ in. below the solution level. Aliquots of 15 mL of solution in a small glass beaker were used. Upon completion of immersion, all surfaces were rinsed with ample amounts (50–100 mL) of the phosphated saline supporting electrolyte under pressure from a wash bottle to remove all loosely clinging matter. Fixation was followed by immersion in a 10% formaldehyde phosphated saline solution for about 30 min. After drying with acetone, the surfaces were gold sputtered (Hummer II, Technics Inc.) with a film of about 300 Å.

For the electrochemical measurements, the copper–2% zinc alloy was mounted into epoxy (Buehler epoxide resin) by curing at room temperature for about 10 h. The finished metal surface had 1 cm² exposed. The reference electrode probe and both high-density graphite counter electrodes were also positioned into the beaker. The working electrodes were immersed in the solutions for up to 0.5 h prior to the cyclic voltammetry for monitoring the open circuit potential.

The blood components selected included the in vivo plasma protein concentrations (38) of human albumin at 46.2 g/L (Cohn Fraction V), human γ-globulin at 11.2 g/L (Cohn Fraction III), and human fibrinogen at 4 g/L (Cohn Fraction I). All proteins were obtained from ICN Pharmaceuticals. BSA (Sigma) was used for the polarization evaluations. The supporting electrolyte in all cases was a phosphated saline solution (38) composed of $0.114M$ NaCl, $0.0187M$ Na$_2$HPO$_4$, and $0.0046M$ NaH$_2$PO$_4 \cdot$ H$_2$O, with pH 7.4. The protein additions were added separately, and in combination, to yield four different protein solutions. The solutions used were then composed of (1) albumin at 46.2 g/L in supporting electrolyte; (2) γ-globulin at 11.6 g/L in supporting electrolyte; (3) fibrinogen at 4 g/L in supporting electrolyte; and (5) albumin at 46.2 g/L, globulin at 11.6 g/L, and fibrinogen at 4 g/L in supporting electrolyte. All solutions were prepared immediately before immersion of the copper–2% zinc electrodes.

Procedures. Cyclic voltammetry was obtained by using a potentiostat (model 6656 TR Wenking or model V 2LR Aardvark) in conjunction with the constant-sweep potential output from a polarography unit (model EUW-401, Heath Co.) or Aardvark model 3 scanning unit. For a sweep rate of 5 V/min, the polarography unit was used, whereas at 0.012 V/min, the scanning unit was used. These rates were chosen because rates on the order of 0.012 V/min represent Faradaic processes on the potential–current curves close to their equilibrium redox potentials. A higher rate of 5 V/min also was chosen, since rates of this magnitude are commonly used with polarography, and because these rates can generate the required profiles in only minutes. Hence, the longer-term experiment is avoided. Relationship of sweep rate to peak potentials and currents was not attempted. An oscilloscope (type 502A Tektronix) and a polaroid camera (model 606 EDAX International) were used to obtain the desired j–U profiles. An x–y Omnigraphic series 2000 (Houston Instruments) was used at the lower traverse rate.

The steady-state cathodic currents were obtained using the Wenking potentiostat by decreasing the electrode potential of the copper–2% zinc alloy from its rest state in protein solution of about -0.2 V to -0.3, -0.5, and -0.7 V. For all cases in this part of the investigation, the electrodes were always exposed to a cathodic signal throughout the entire length of immersion. The cathodic signals were actually impressed just momentarily prior to immersion. In no cases were the electrodes exposed to the open circuit potential (OCP) conditions. Current–time transients were monitored on a strip chart Omniscribe (Houston). The cathodic pulsating currents were obtained by superimposing a sinusoidal signal (0.15 V peak to peak) from a voltage oscillator (type 1310-A Genrad), at frequencies ranging from 2 to 200 kHz, to the control potential of -0.325 V (SCE). The oscilloscope was used to monitor the j–U characteristics.

Protein adsorption was assessed by observing surface characteristics using a scanning electron microscope (SEM) (Super Mini International Scientific Instruments). EDAX along with an EDAX peak identification computer (EPIC) were used to analyze the surface elemental distribution on the exposed copper–2% zinc electrodes. Photomicrographs are secondary electron images.

Results

Open Circuit Potentials. The open circuit 0.5 h potentials for the copper–2% zinc electrodes were more negative in the protein solutions (-0.20 to -0.25 V) than in supporting electrolyte (-0.12 to -0.15 V).

Cyclic Voltammetry—5 V/min. Figures 1a–e present the j–U behavior for the first cycle of copper–2% zinc in phosphated saline and in protein solutions. The corrosion potentials ($i_a = i_c$) during the forward scans were between -0.35 to -0.40 V in all cases. Two anodic peaks were observed for all protein solutions at -0.25 to -0.10 V and $+0.10$ to $+0.30$ V. The first peak in the supporting electrolyte was also observed, whereas j continued to increase, never reaching a peak up to the reversal potential of $+0.5$ V. Two main cathodic peaks were observed at -0.30 to -0.45 V and -0.65 to -0.75 V in all cases. A prepeak inflection also occurred at -0.2 to -0.3 V for both the albumin and globulin systems, and a small peak at -1.1 to -1.2 V for most systems. Cathodic currents increase sharply below about -1.5 V. Figures 2a–b represent the surface appearances after the first cycle of polar-

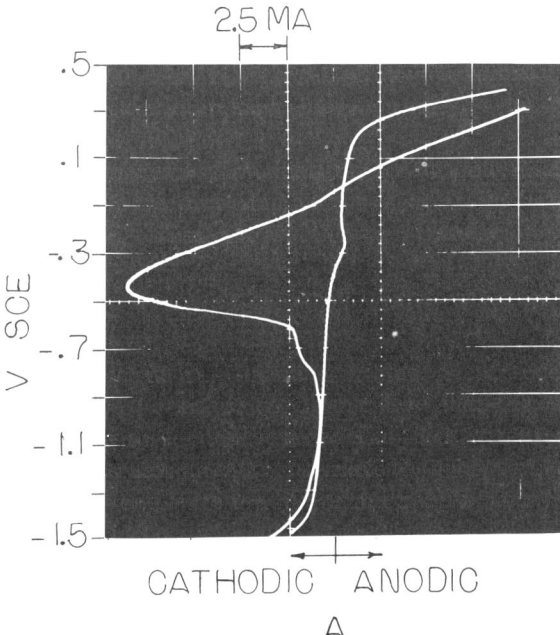

Figure 1a. Cyclic voltammetry of copper–2% zinc alloy at 5 V/min in phosphated saline composed of 0.11 M NaCl, 0.019 M Na_2HPO_4, and 0.005 M $NaH_2PO_4 \cdot H_2O$ at 25°C and at pH 7.4.

ization in phosphated saline and in the three protein combination solution. The surfaces from separate protein systems also exhibited similar behavior.

Cyclic Voltammetry—0.012 V/min. Figures 3a–f present the j–U behavior for the first cycle in protein-free and protein-containing solutions. The corrosion potential for copper–2% zinc in phosphated saline was −0.12 V, and between −0.22 and −0.26 V for protein solutions. The anodic behavior exhibited a peak at about 0 V, followed by passivation by almost two orders of magnitude for phosphated saline, and only about 0.5 orders of magnitude for systems containing albumin or globulin. Fibrinogen in supporting electrolyte exhibited a critical j for passivation, one order of magnitude less than for the other systems. Slight inflections also occurred in several regions of the profiles, possibly indicating the existence of additional peaks. The cathodic process for phosphated saline exhibited a peak at −0.075 V, with a small surge in j at $U = -0.025$ V. These potentials correspond to the two major peaks observed in albumin solution. Globulin and the combination protein systems exhibited a major peak at −0.13 V, which is at least one order of current magnitude larger than for the remaining systems. The reduction process for the fibrinogen solution was altered; that is, no similar reduction peak around −0.1 V occurred.

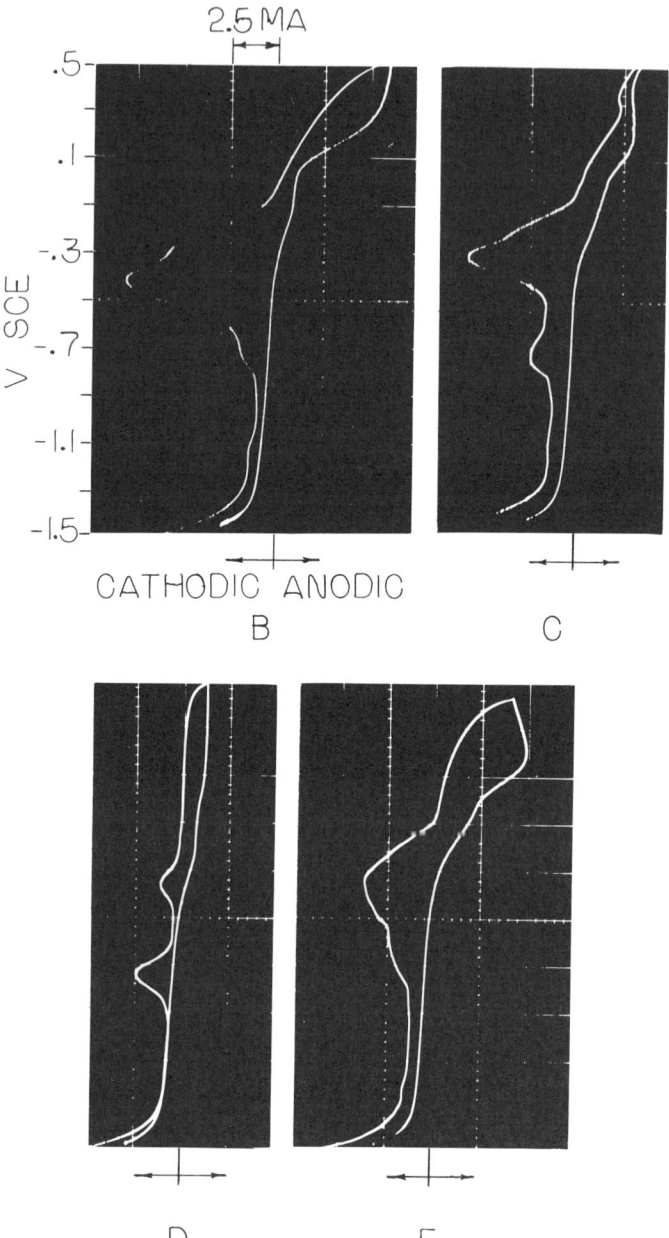

Figures 1b–e. Cyclic voltammetry of copper–2% zinc alloy at 5 V/min in phosphated saline supporting electrolyte as listed in Figure 1a, and with the additions of 46.2 g/L of BSA (b), 11.6 g/L of human γ-globulin (c), 4 g/L of human fibrinogen (d), and albumin–globulin–fibrinogen combination (e) at 25°C and at pH 7.4.

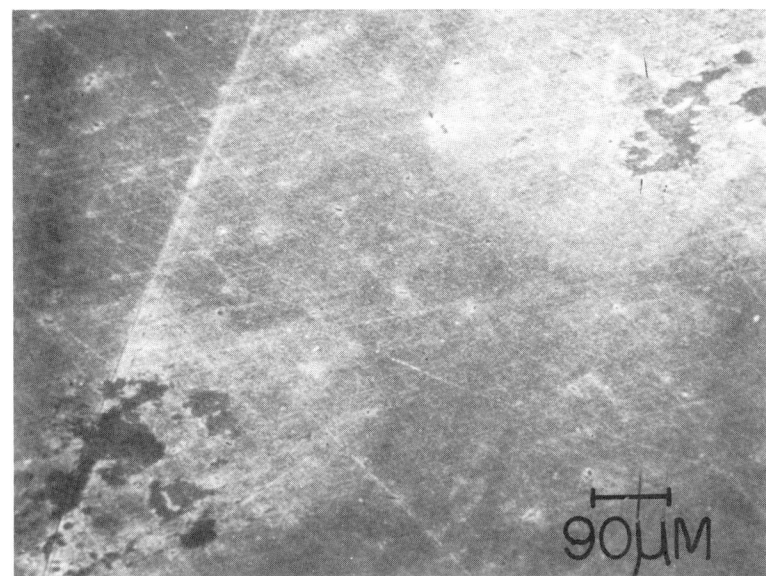

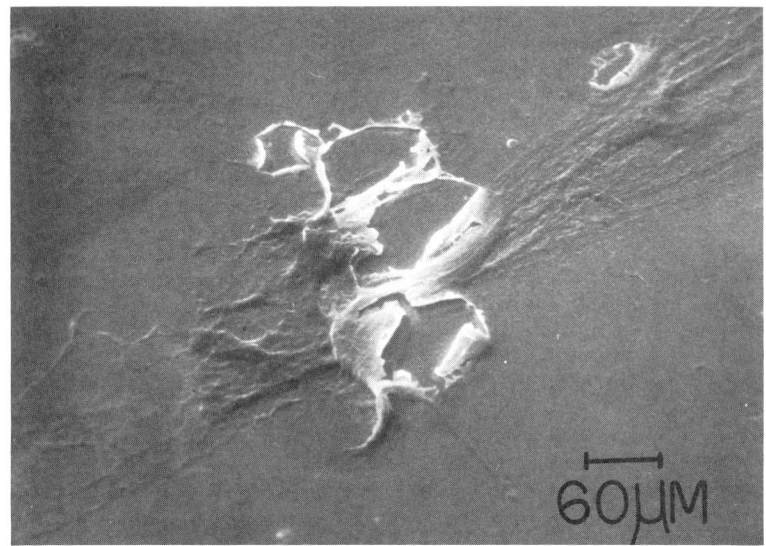

Figures 2a–b. SEM photomicrographs of copper–2% zinc alloy after first cycle of polarization at 5 V/min as shown in Figures 1a and 1e, respectively, for phosphated saline (a) and with a combination of BSA at 46.2 g/L, human γ-globulin at 11.6 g/L, and human fibrinogen at 4 g/L (b).

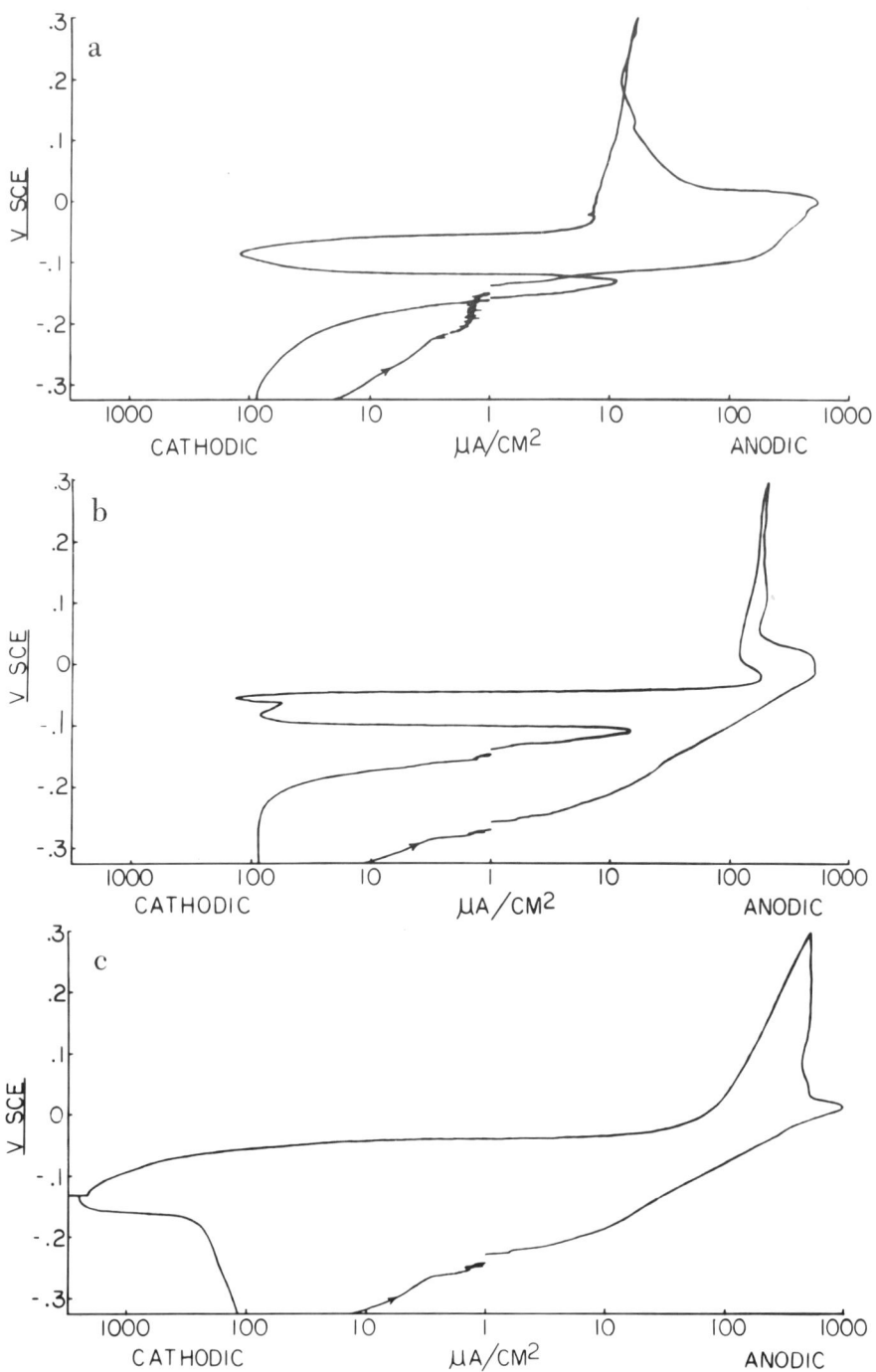

Figure 3a–c. Cyclic voltammetry of copper–2% zinc alloy at 0.012 V/min in phosphated saline supporting electrolyte as listed in Figure 1a (a), with addition of 46.2 g/L of BSA (b), and human γ-globulin (c).

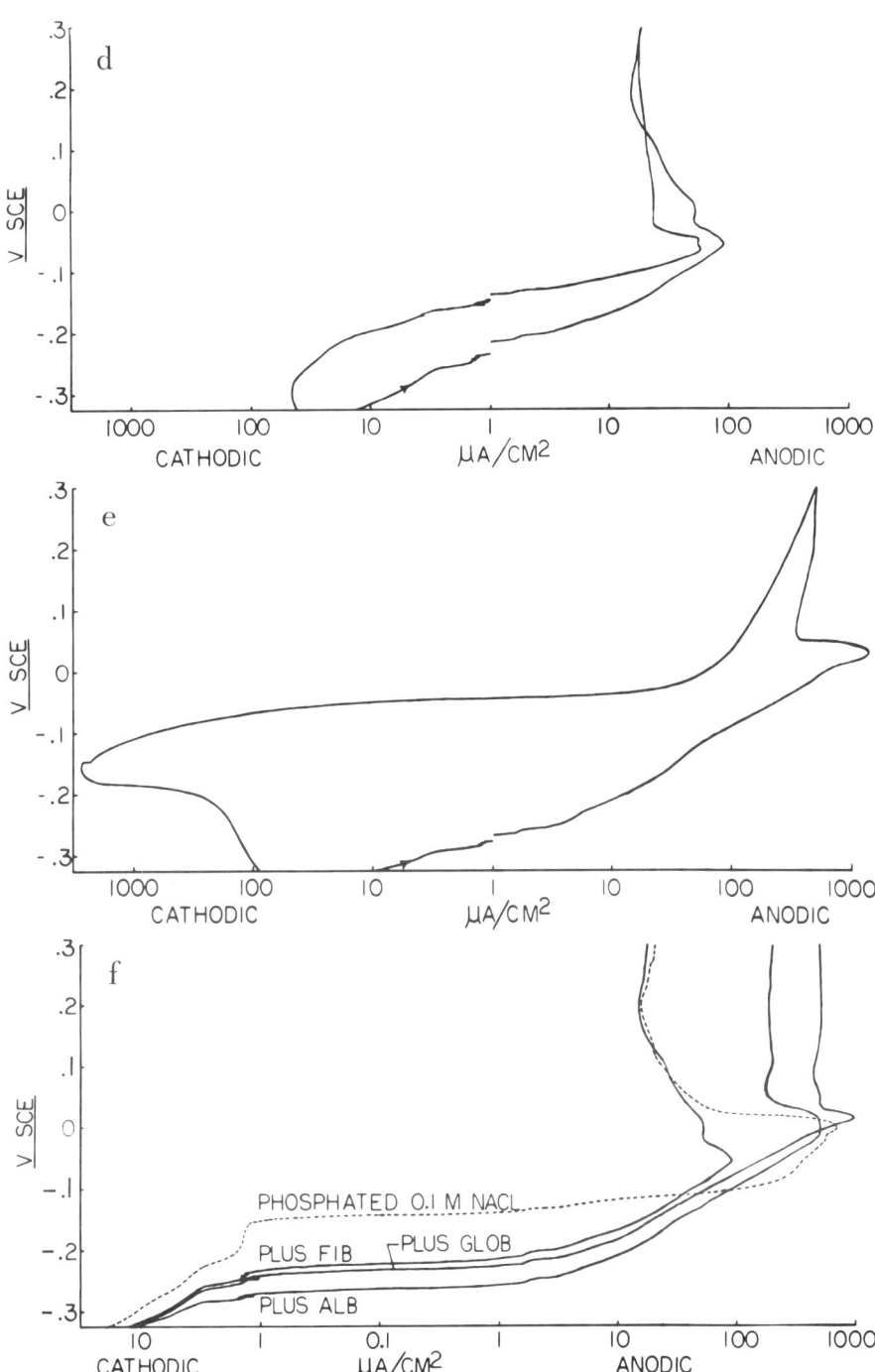

Figures 3d–f. Cyclic voltammetry of copper–2% zinc alloy at 0.012 V/min in phosphated saline supporting electrolyte with addition of 4 g/L of human fibrinogen (d), and albumin–globulin–fibrinogen combination (e), at 25° with at pH 7.4 (f).

Figure 4 presents the polarization results for the copper–2% zinc electrode in phosphated saline and in a fibrinogen solution due to repeated cycling (2nd for saline and 4th for fibrinogen) in only the cathodic regions. Because of cycling, the forward and return traces became reversible, except in the regions approaching the corrosion potential. Here the scan in the negative direction continued to exhibit a region of constant j at about 1 $\mu A/cm^2$. This region, however, has decreased from a range in potential of over 0.15 V for the first cycle in saline to about 0.1 V. The fibrinogen solution also exhibited a similar change. Tafel slopes for both systems in the potential range of -0.4 to -0.25 V were between 0.215 and 0.230 V/decade.

Current–Time Transients. The current–time potentiostatic behavior for the copper–2% zinc alloy in supporting electrolyte with and without fibrinogen is shown in Figure 5. The current initially decreased and then gradually increased, reaching a plateau and further decreasing at longer times. The current was less with the fibrinogen solution. Similar behavior was observed at -0.5 V. Differences in the j–t characteristics at -0.3 V were difficult to ascertain, even though current was slightly higher in the fibrinogen solution.

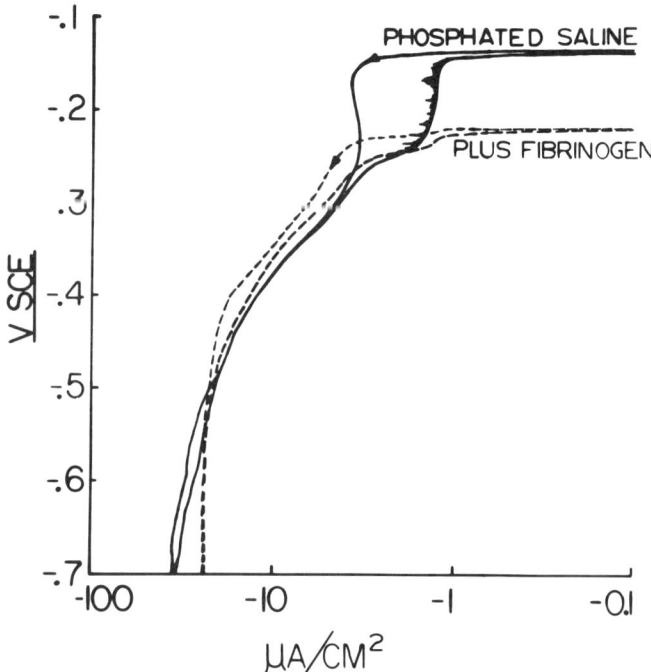

Figure 4. Cathodic cyclic traces for copper–2% zinc alloy in phosphated saline, as listed in Figure 1a, for the second cycle (a), and with the addition of 4 g/L of human fibrinogen for the fourth cycle (b) at 25° and at pH 7.4.

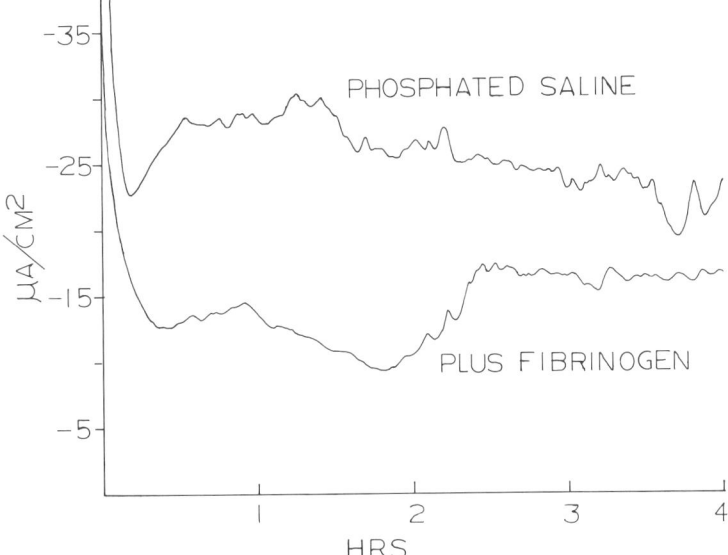

Figure 5. Cathodic current–time transients at −0.7 V SCE of copper–2% zinc alloy in phosphated saline, as listed in Figure 1a, and with the addition of 4 g/L of human fibrinogen at 25°C and at pH 7.4.

Steady-State Cathodic Polarization. Figures 6a–b present the photomicrographs for the etched and as-polished surfaces of the copper–2% zinc alloy. The circular dark regions could be inclusions or a second phase. The appearances after immersion in saline and in phosphated saline are presented in Figures 7a–b. For both solutions, corrosion product deposition was evident, being mainly oxides and chlorides of copper for saline-only solution, and with the addition of copper phosphates for the phosphated saline solution. Microstructural features, such as dendrites and coring effects, also were observed with the saline-only solution. The phosphated saline solution produced prismatic and orderly deposition of products covering the entire surface. Cathodic polarization at −0.3 V, shown in Figure 8, eliminated most of the copper phosphates from the surface.

For the albumin-containing phosphated saline solution, surface appearances corresponding to various stages of polarization are presented in Figures 9a–c. The as-immersed surface (Figure 9a) was mostly covered with a proteinaceous layer appearing thicker in specific regions. Some regions appeared void of protein, since polishing scratches, and pits can be observed. Polarization at −0.3 V (Figure 9b) did not change the surface appearance very significantly, since large areas that are covered with a protein layer can still be detected. Polarization at −0.5 V (Figure 9c) desorbed more of the protein mass; however, specific regions exhibiting protein accumulation can be detected.

426 BIOMATERIALS: INTERFACIAL PHENOMENA AND APPLICATIONS

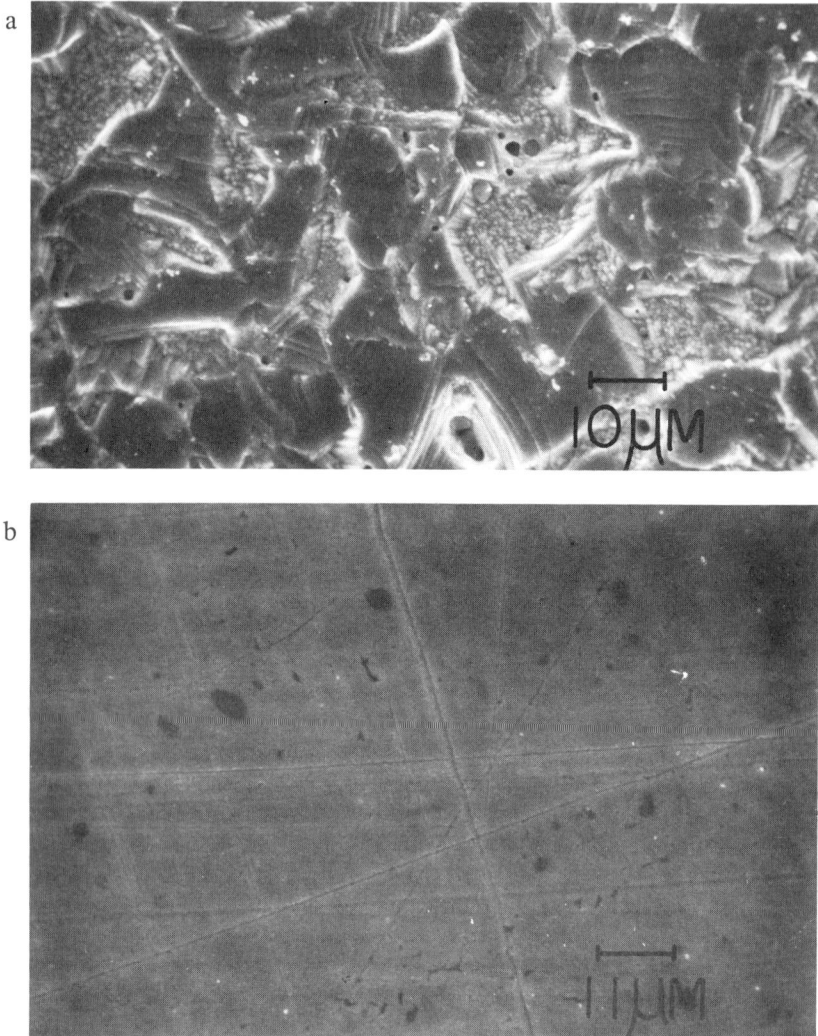

Figures 6a–b. SEM photomicrographs of copper–2% zinc alloy in the etched (a) and in the as-polished (b) conditions.

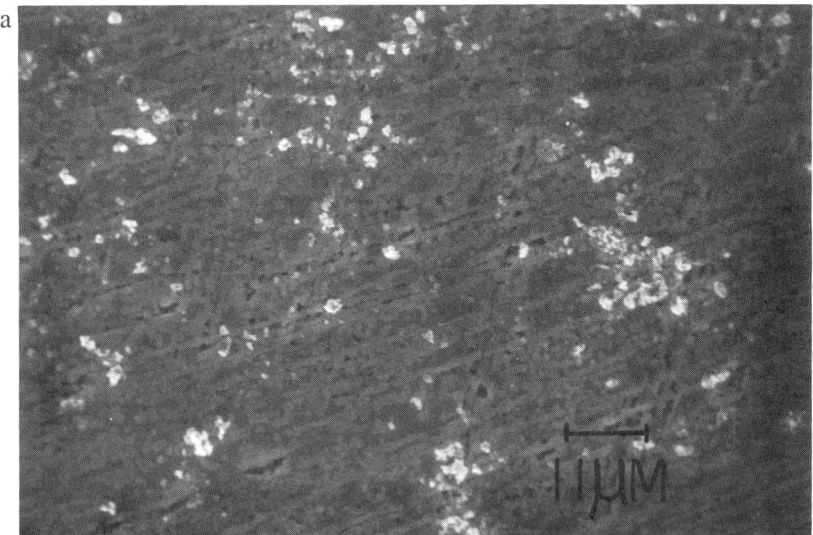

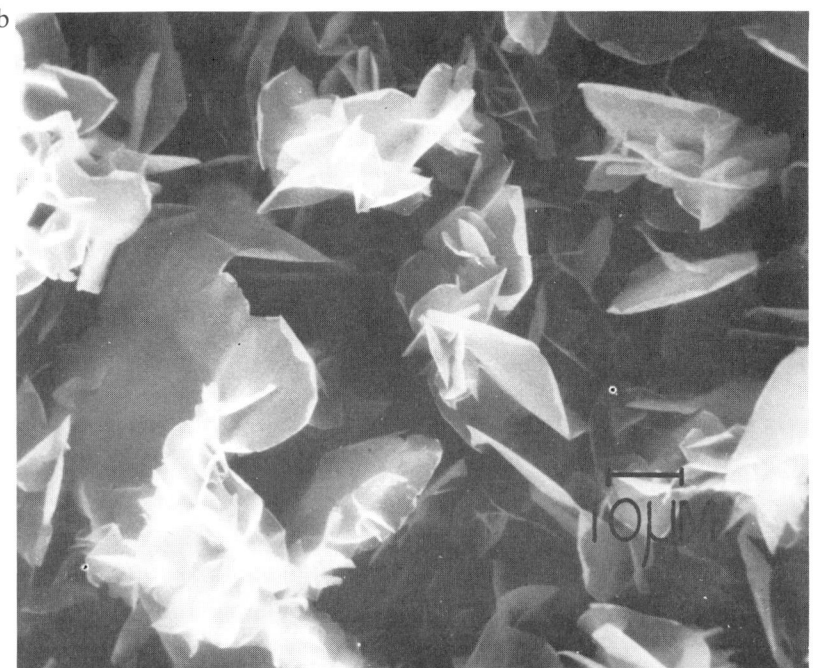

Figures 7a–b. SEM photomicrographs of copper–2% zinc alloy after immersion in 0.11 M NaCl only (a) and with additions of 0.019 M Na_2HPO_4 and 0.005 M $NaH_2PO_4 \cdot H_2O$ (b).

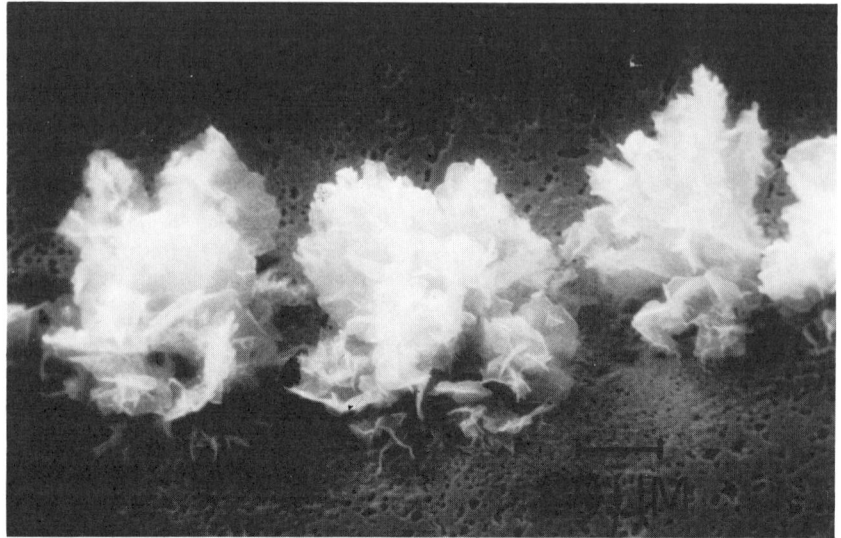

Figure 8. SEM photomicrograph of copper–2% zinc alloy after cathodic polarization at −0.7 V SCE in phosphated saline as listed in Figure 7.

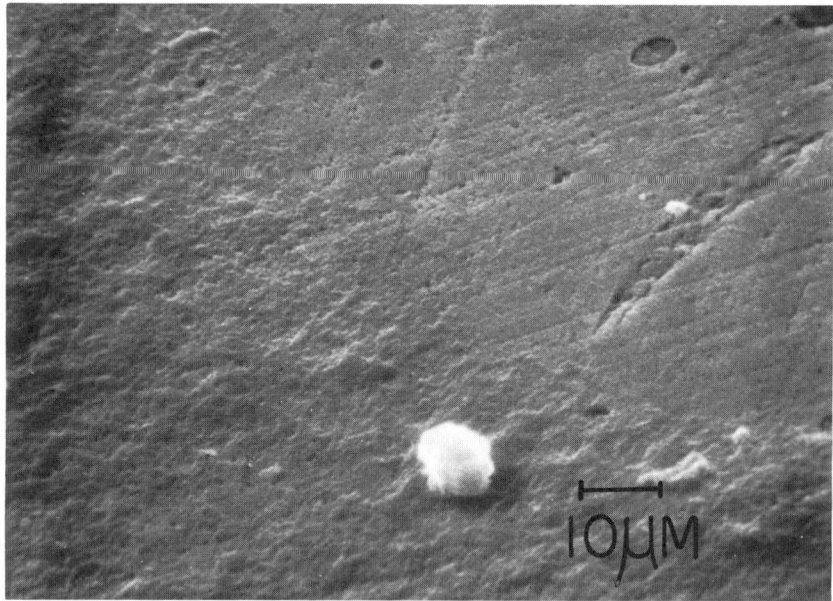

Figure 9a. SEM photomicrograph of copper–2% zinc alloy exposed for 4 h in 46.2 g/L of human albumin phosphated saline solution at 25°, pH 7.4, by immersion only.

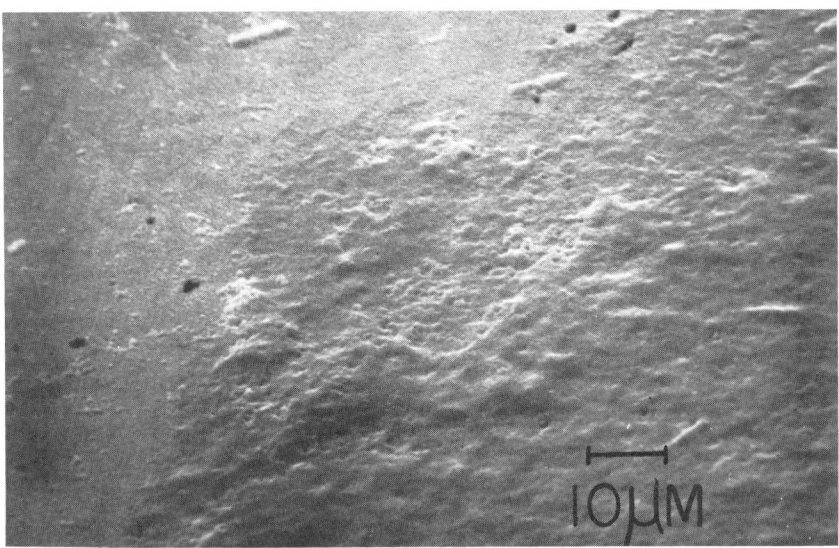

Figure 9b. SEM photomicrograph of copper–2% zinc alloy exposed for 4 h in 46.2 g/L of human albumin phosphated saline solution at 25°, pH 7.4, by cathodic polarization at −0.3 V SCE.

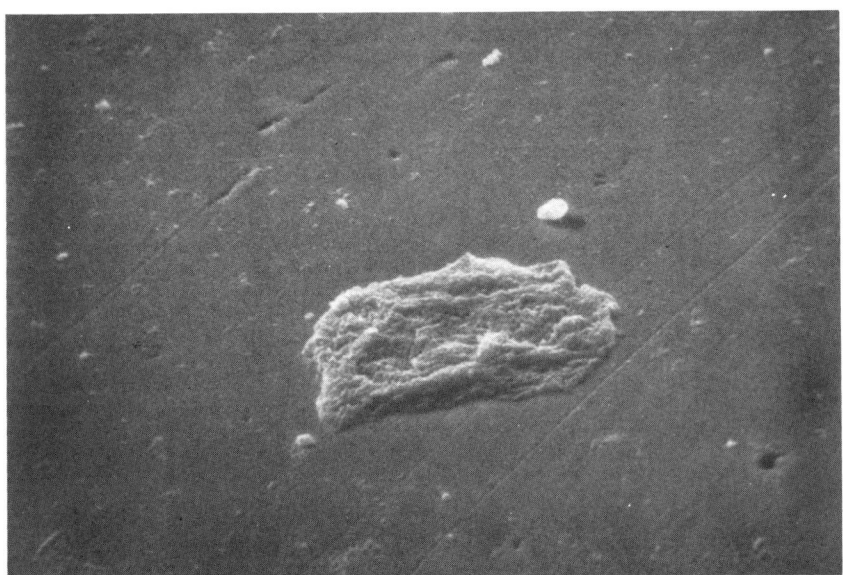

Figure 9c. SEM photomicrograph of copper–2% zinc alloy exposed for 4 h in 46.2 g/L of human albumin phosphated saline solution at 25°, pH 7.4, by cathodic polarization at −0.5 V SCE.

The phosphated saline γ-globulin system is presented in Figures 10a–e. The as-immersed surface (Figure 10a) exhibited protein accumulation and spherical-appearing corrosion products identified as copper chloride phosphates over an adsorbed protein layer. The underlying adsorbed protein layer as well as the accumulated protein masses were analyzed to contain copper and low chlorine concentrations. The complete EDAX spectra did not indicate zinc. Low silicon and calcium occasionally were identified. Specific regions of this layer broke away during the gold sputtering operation, leaving a discontinuous surface layer with bare copper–2% zinc areas exposed (Figure 10b). The −0.3 V polarized surface appeared entirely similar to the as-immersed surface (Figure 10c). The −0.5 V polarized surface (Figure 10d) still exhibited large protein masses distributed across the surface, but with some indications of specific regions being freed of protein. The −0.7 V surface (Figure 10e) was significantly desorbed of much of the protein mass; a few areas are exposing the metal surface. Some polishing scratches also can be observed.

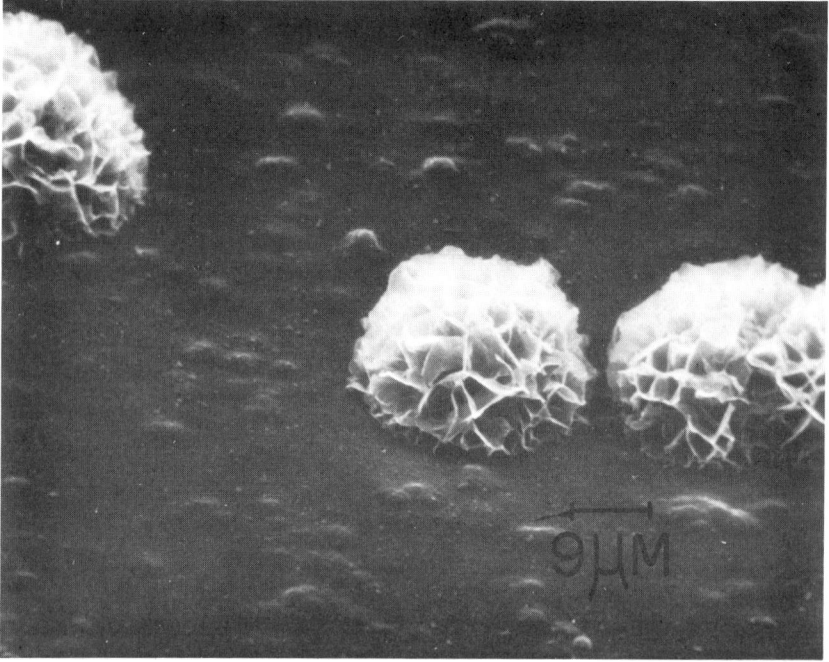

Figure 10a. SEM photomicrograph of copper–2% zinc alloy exposed for 4 h in 11.6 g/L γ-globulin phosphated saline solution at 25°, pH 7.4, by immersion only.

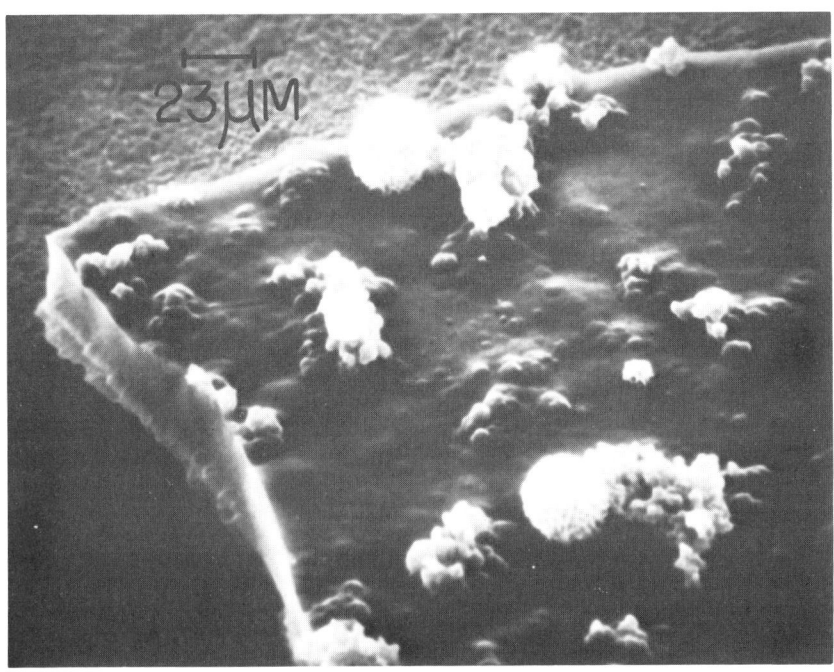

Figure 10b. SEM photomicrographs of copper–2% zinc alloy exposed for 4 h in 11.6 g/L of γ-globulin phosphated saline solution at 25°, pH 7.4, by immersion only.

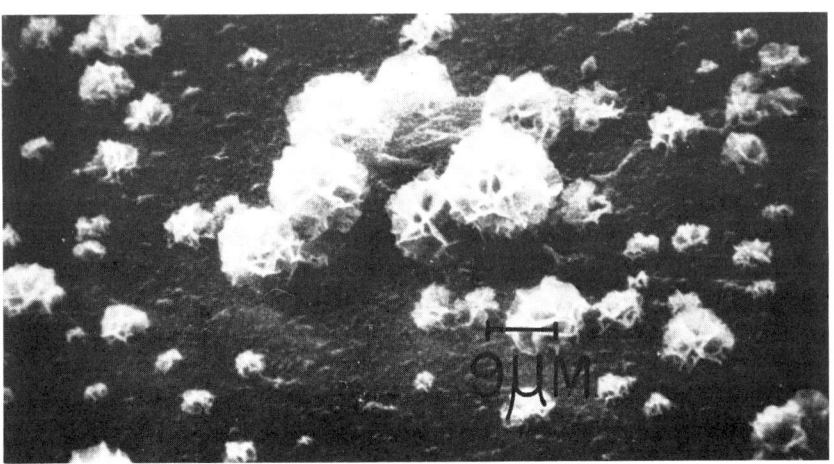

Figure 10c. SEM photomicrograph of copper–2% zinc alloy exposed for 4 h in 11.6 g/L γ-globulin phosphated saline solution at 25°, pH 7.4, by cathodic polarization at −0.3 V SCE.

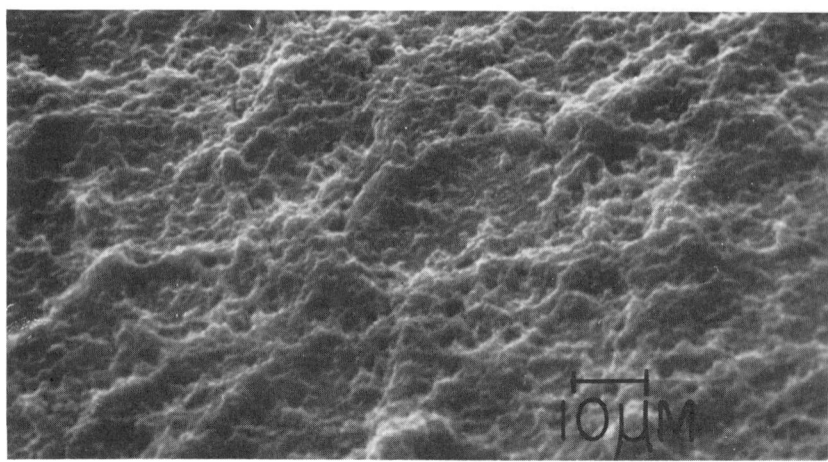

Figure 10d. SEM photomicrograph of copper–2% zinc alloy exposed for 4 h in 11.6 g/L of γ-globulin phosphated saline solution at 25°, pH 7.4, by cathodic polarization at −0.5 V SCE.

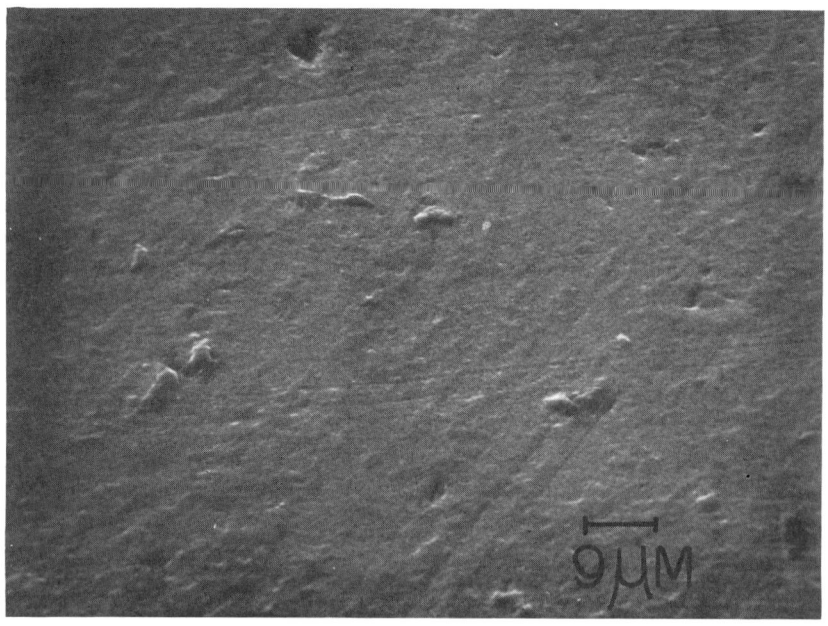

Figure 10e. SEM photomicrograph of copper–2% zinc alloy exposed for 4 h in 11.6 g/L of γ-globulin phosphated saline solution at 25°, pH 7.4, by cathodic polarization at −0.7 V SCE.

Analysis of the phosphated-saline fibrinogen system is shown in Figures 11a–f. Complete surface coverage occurred, with additional protein accumulation also taking place. Low chlorine concentrations were identified with the protein mass. However, no insoluble corrosion products were observed attached to the as-immersed surfaces (Figures 11a–b). Polarization at −0.3 V greatly diminished the protein accumulation over the underlying adsorbed protein layer. However, the basic underlying layer is still present, with occasional long fibers of protein (Figure 11c–d). Contrary to the as-immersed surface, copper chloride phosphates were observed here. The −0.5 V polarized surface (Figure 11e) appeared quite desorbed of protein mass, except for a few isolated long strands of fibrinogen fibers altered in appearance by the polarization process. The −0.7 V surface contained only a few isolated islands of remaining protein (Figure 11f).

Figures 12a–d present the surface appearances of copper–2% zinc alloy exposed to the phosphated-saline albumin–globulin–fibrinogen solution. The as-immersed surface (Figures 12a–b) exhibited a protein layer, protein accumulation, and copper chloride phosphates as corrosion products. Polarization at −0.3 V eliminated the outer surfaces of protein accumulation and of corrosion products. Only the underlying protein layer was observed (Figure 11c). Polarization at −0.5 V desorbed most of the protein (Figure 11d).

Pulsed Cathodic Polarization. Figure 13a presents two typical j–U profiles encountered as a function of frequency. At low frequencies (2 Hz), an elliptical pattern encompassing a range of current densities was observed,

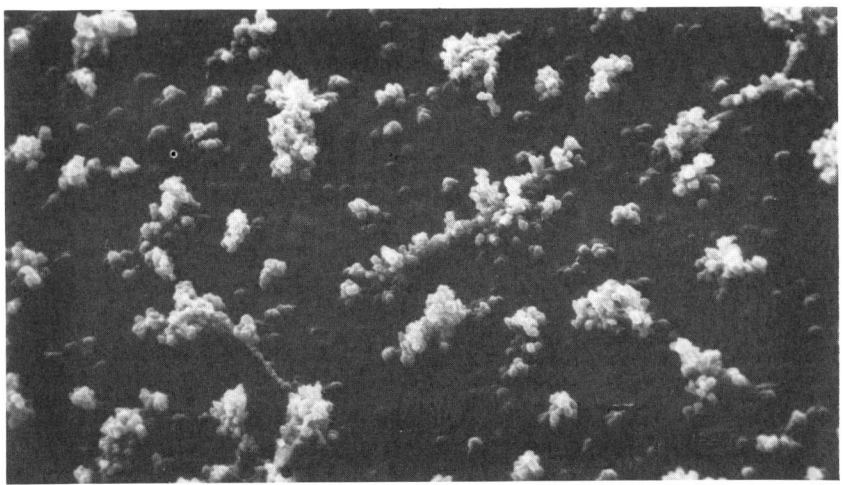

Figure 11a. SEM photomicrograph of copper–2% zinc alloy exposed for 4 h in 4 g/L of human fibrinogen phosphated saline solution at 25°, pH 7.4, by immersion only.

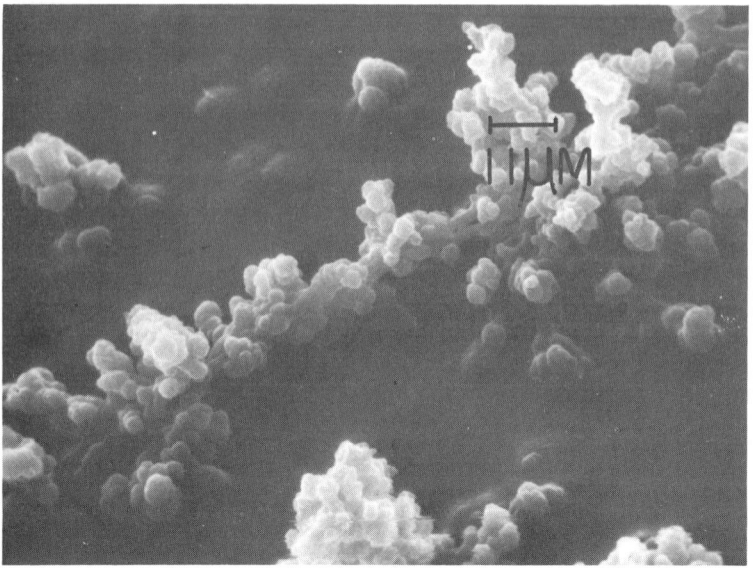

Figure 11b. SEM photomicrograph of copper–2% zinc alloy exposed for 4 h in 4 g/L of human fibrinogen phosphated saline solution at 25°, pH 7.4, by immersion only.

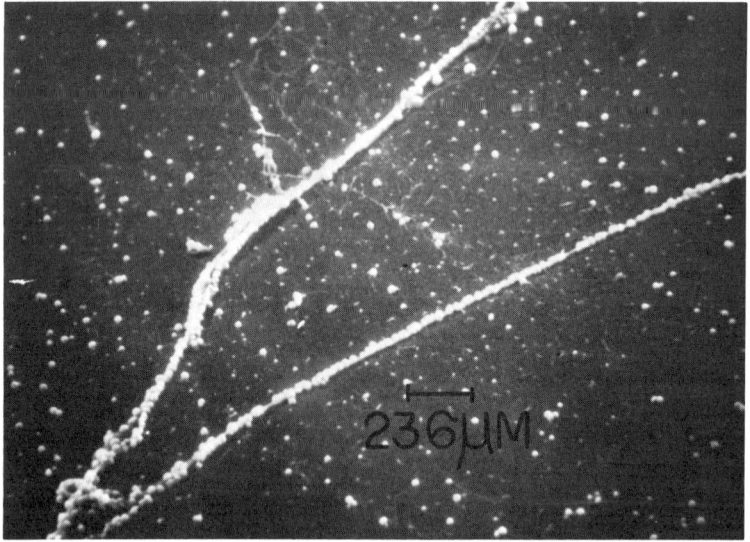

Figure 11c. SEM photomicrograph of copper–2% zinc alloy exposed for 4 h in 4 g/L of human fibrinogen phosphated saline solution at 25°, pH 7.4, by cathodic polarization at −0.3 V SCE.

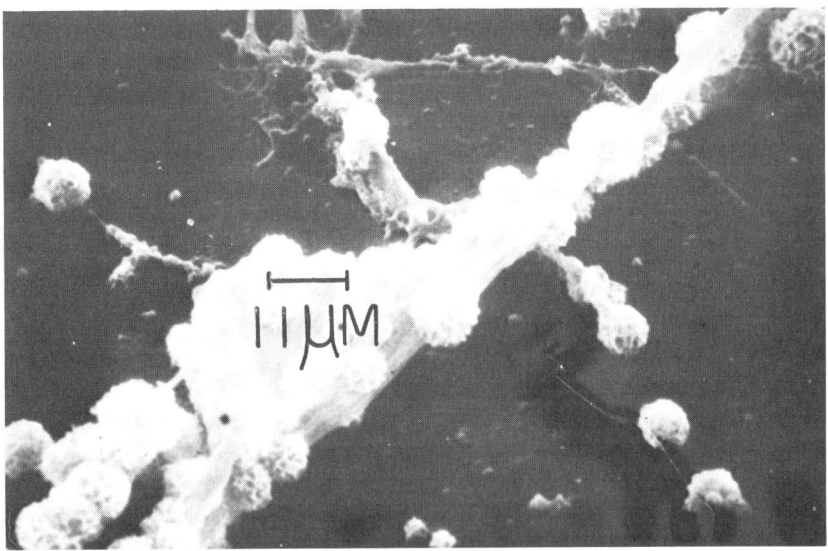

Figure 11d. SEM photomicrograph of copper–2% zinc alloy exposed for 4 h in 4 g/L of human fibrinogen phosphated saline solution at 25°, pH 7.4, by cathodic polarization at −0.3 V SCE.

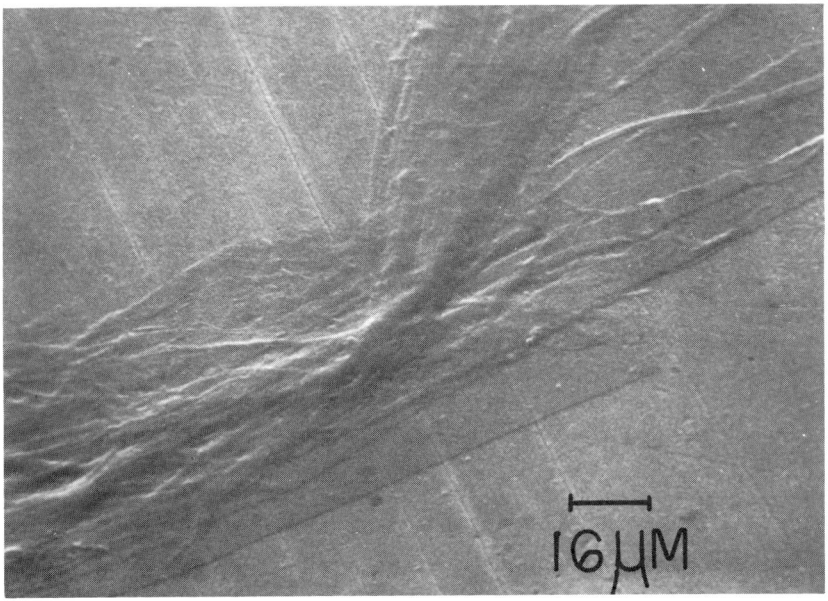

Figure 11e. SEM photomicrograph of copper–2% zinc alloy exposed for 4 h in 4 g/L of human fibrinogen phosphated saline solution at 25°, pH 7.4, by cathodic polarization at −0.5 V SCE.

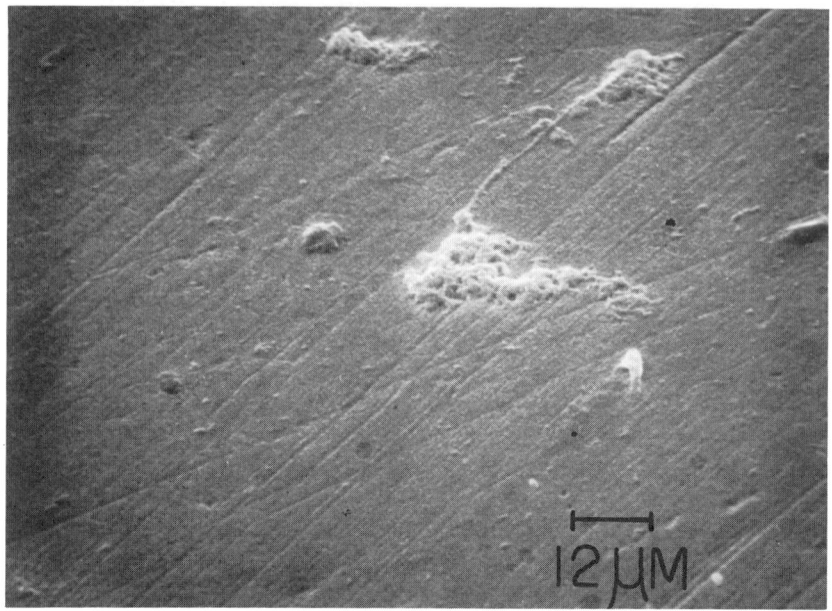

Figure 11f. SEM photomicrograph of copper–2% zinc alloy exposed for 4 h in 4 g/L of human fibrinogen phosphated saline solution at 25°, pH 7.4, by cathodic polarization at −0.7 V SCE.

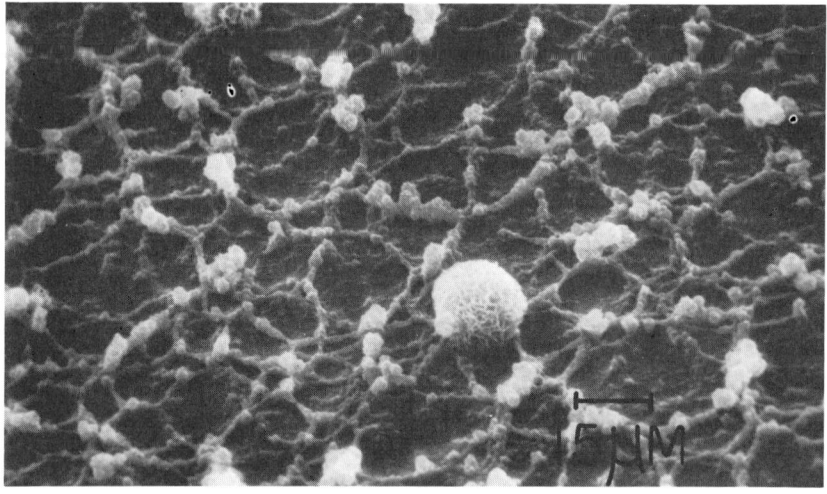

Figure 12a. SEM photomicrograph of copper–2% zinc alloy exposed for 4 h in 46.2 g/L of human albumin, 11.6 g/L of human γ-globulin, and 4 g/L of human fibrinogen combination phosphated saline solution at 25°, by immersion only.

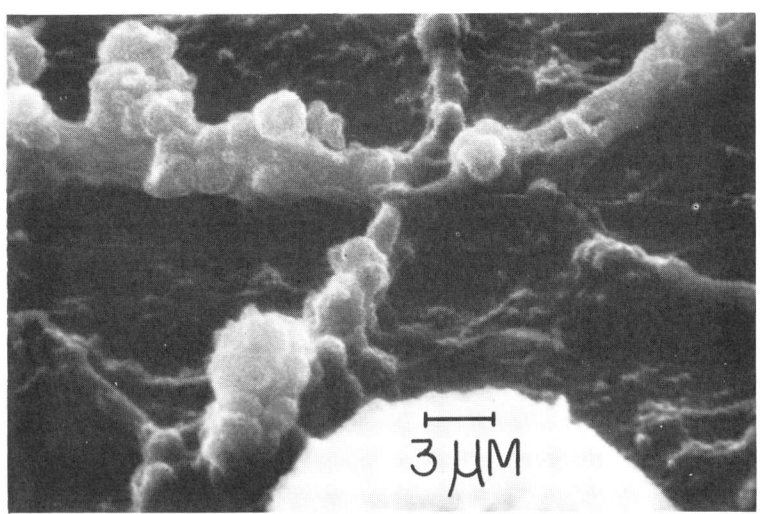

Figure 12b. SEM photomicrograph of copper–2% zinc alloy exposed for 4 h in 46.2 g/L of human albumin, 11.6 g/L of human γ-globulin, and 4 g/L of human fibrinogen combination phosphated saline solution at 25°, by immersion only.

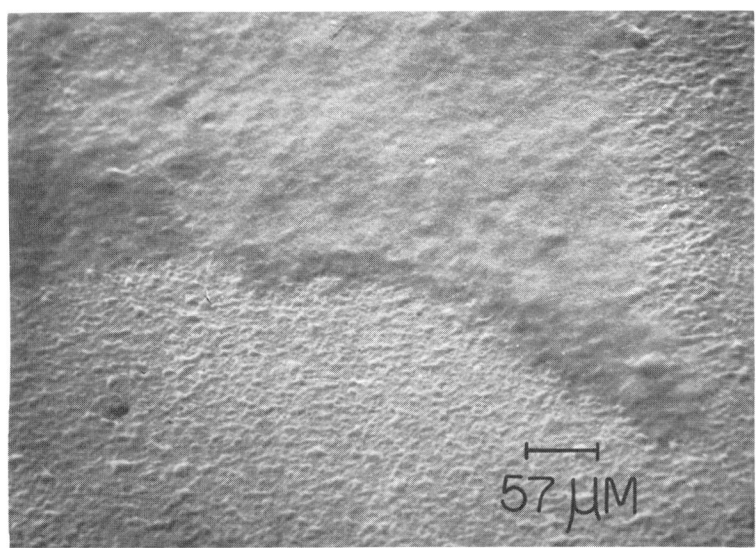

Figure 12c. SEM photomicrograph of copper–2% zinc alloy exposed for 4 h in 46.2 g/L of human albumin, 11.6 g/L of human γ-globulin, and 4 g/L of human fibrinogen combination phosphated saline solution at 25° by cathodic polarization at −0.3 V SCE.

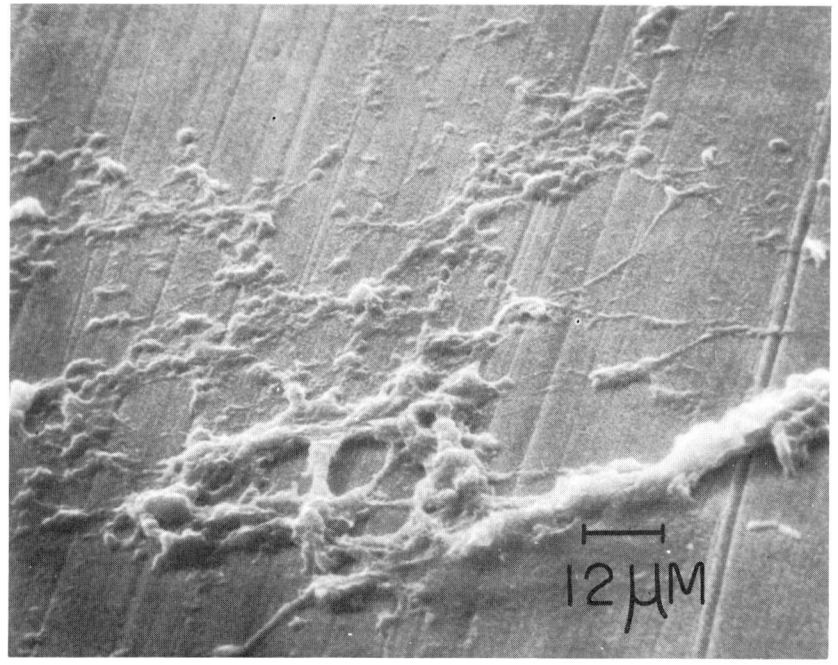

Figure 12d. SEM photomicrograph of copper–2% zinc alloy exposed for 4 h in 46.2 g/L of human albumin, 11.6 g/L of human γ-globulin, and 4 g/L of human fibrinogen combination phosphated saline solution at 25° by cathodic polarization at −0.5 V SCE.

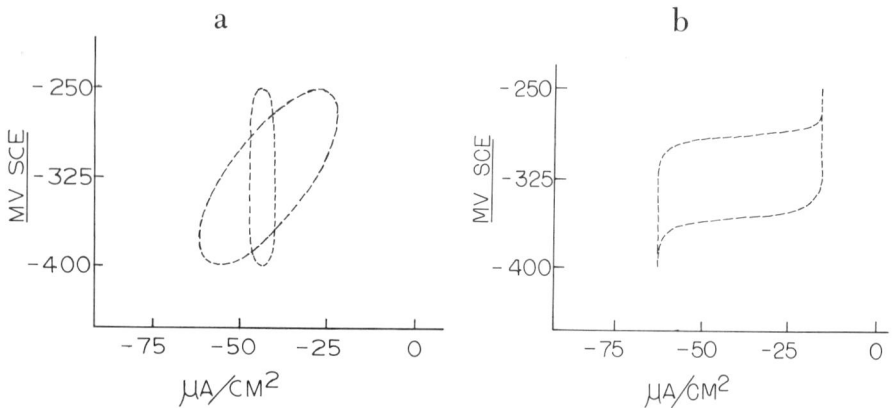

Figures 13a–b. Typical potential–current density patterns obtained for copper–2% zinc alloy in protein solutions cathodically polarized potentiodynamically at 2 Hz(broad), 200 kHz(flat) (a), and at 200 Hz (b).

whereas at high frequencies (200 kHz), the vertical pattern almost independent of current was seen. Intermediate frequencies (20–20 kHz) often exhibited patterns between these two extremes with, at times, the elliptical patterns replaced by the patterns of Figure 13b.

Figures 14a–c present the surface appearance of copper–2% zinc immersed in various protein solutions pulsed at 2 Hz. In albumin (Figure 14a), specific circular regions were beginning to be depleted of protein, with several of these regions exhibiting a swelling or a spalling of the underlying protein layer. With a globulin solution, the surface appeared desorbed of much of the protein (Figure 14b). Surface scratches were visible beneath the remaining attached protein mass. The copper/fibrinogen system again showed more protein accumulation (Figure 14c).

For copper–2% zinc exposed to globulin solutions, the surface appearances corresponding to 20 and 200 Hz and 2 and 20 kHz are presented in Figures 15a–d. At 20 Hz (Figure 15a), a desorbed surface with only a few isolated areas of protein was seen; however, more protein accumulation was

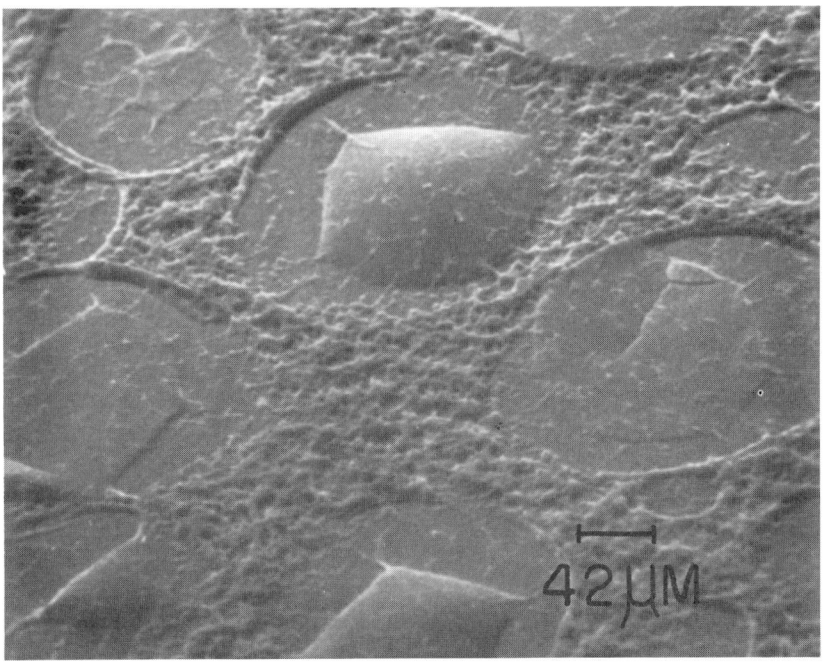

Figure 14a. SEM photomicrograph of copper–2% zinc alloy after employing a sinusoidal potential (−0.25 to −0.40 V SCE peak to peak) at a frequency of 2 Hz for 4 h with phosphated saline, as in Figure 1a, and incorporating human albumin at 46.2 g/L.

440 BIOMATERIALS: INTERFACIAL PHENOMENA AND APPLICATIONS

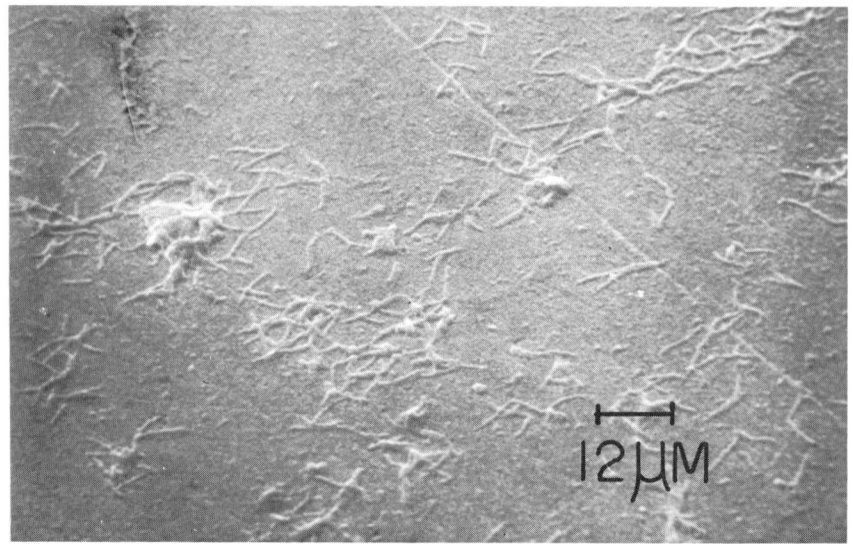

Figure 14b. SEM photomicrograph of copper–2% zinc alloy after employing a sinusoidal potential (−0.25 to −0.40 V SCE peak to peak) at a frequency of 2 Hz for 4 h with phosphated saline, as in Figure 1a, and incorporating human globulin at 11.6 g/L.

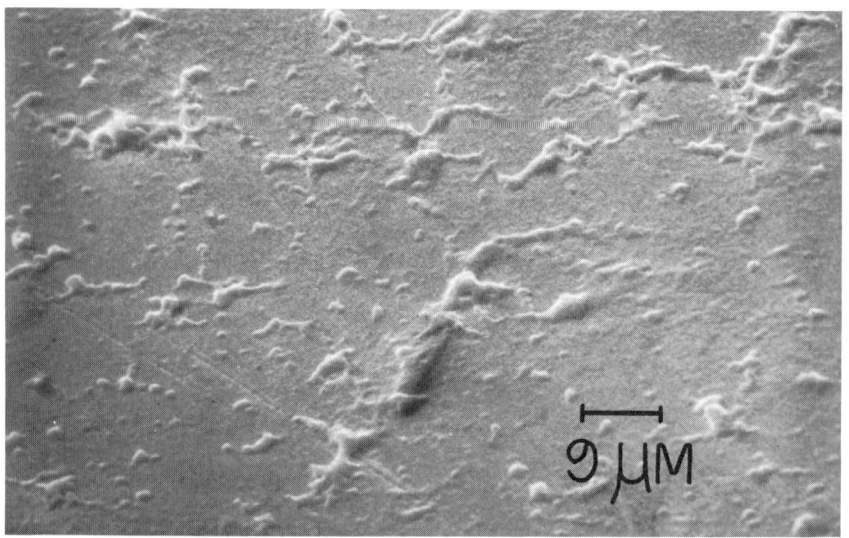

Figure 14c. SEM photomicrograph of copper–2% zinc alloy after employing a sinusoidal potential (−0.25 to −0.40 V SCE peak to peak) at a frequency of 2 Hz for 4 h with phosphated saline, as in Figure 1a, and incorporating human fibrinogen at 4 g/L.

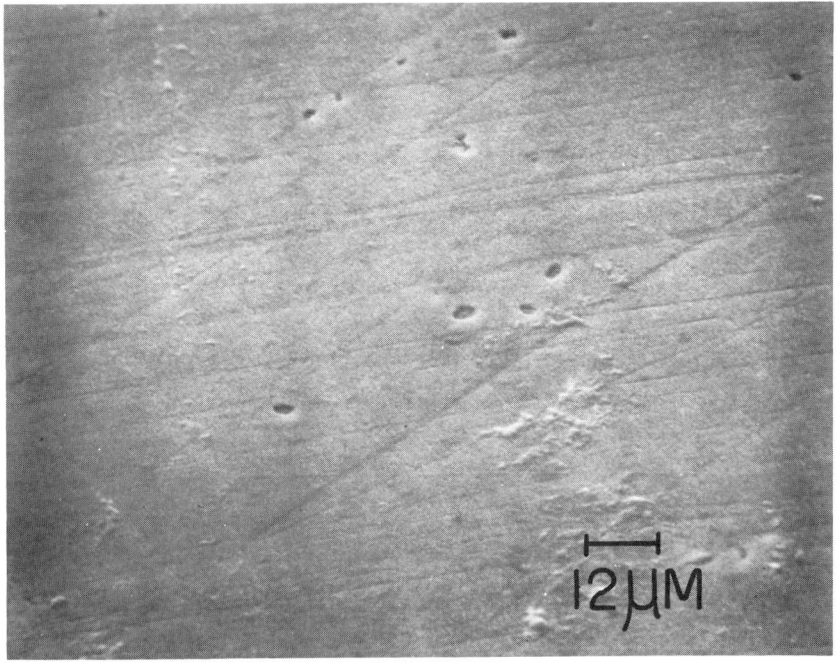

Figure 15a. SEM photomicrograph of copper–2% zinc alloy in phosphated saline solution, as in Figure 1a, for 4 h incorporating 11.6 g/L of human γ-globulin and with a sinusoidal potential (−0.25 to −0.40 V SCE peak to peak) at frequencies of 20 Hz.

observed at 200 Hz (Figure 15b). The 2 kHz (Figure 15c) and 20 kHz (Figure 15d) pulsed surfaces also exhibited surfaces with varying protein accumulations.

Figures 16a–d show the surface appearances of copper–2% zinc exposed to albumin, globulin, fibrinogen, and combination protein solutions, respectively, at 200 kHz. All surfaces represented desorbed protein states.

Discussion

The concentration of dissolved oxygen in water at 25°C in contact with air is 8 ppm (*39*). The concentration of dissolved oxygen in blood (*40*) compares favorably to this value, at 4.3 ppm. The major part of O_2, about 280 ppm in the blood, however, is bound with hemoglobulin, and is not considered available for reaction with the inner walls of a vascular prosthesis. Deaeration of the protein solutions for electrochemical measurements was not carried out for the same reason cited in the literature (*12, 13*); that is, denaturation of protein occurs with deaeration.

442   BIOMATERIALS: INTERFACIAL PHENOMENA AND APPLICATIONS

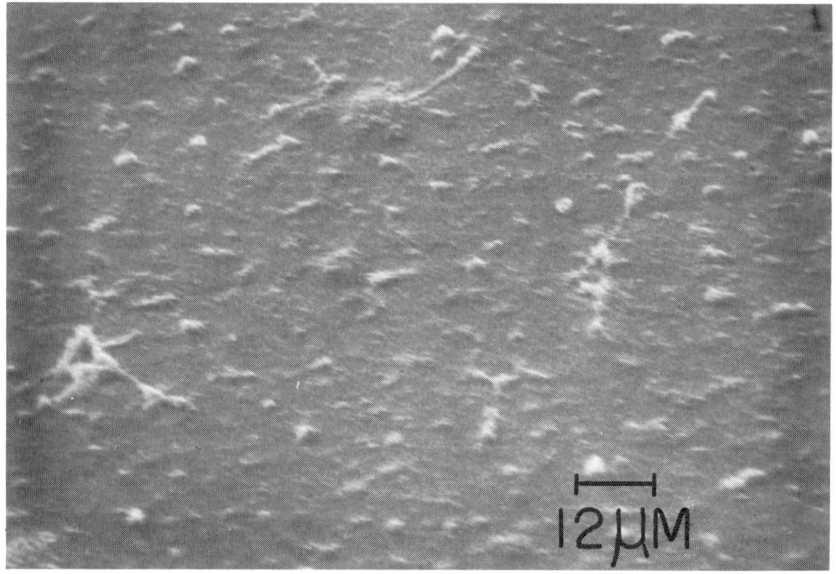

Figure 15b. SEM photomicrograph of copper–2% zinc alloy in phosphated saline solution, as in Figure 1a, for 4 h incorporating 11.6 g/L of human γ-globulin and with a sinusoidal potential (−0.25 to −0.40 V SCE peak to peak) at frequency of 200 Hz.

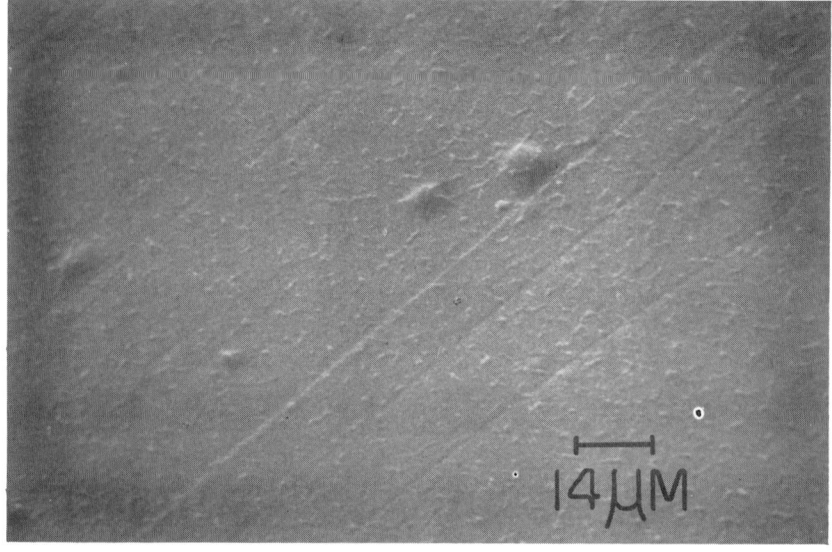

Figure 15c. SEM photomicrograph of copper–2% zinc alloy in phosphated saline solution, as in Figure 1a, for 4 h incorporating 11.6 g/L of human γ-globulin and with a sinusoidal potential (−0.25 to −0.40 V peak to peak) at 2 kHz.

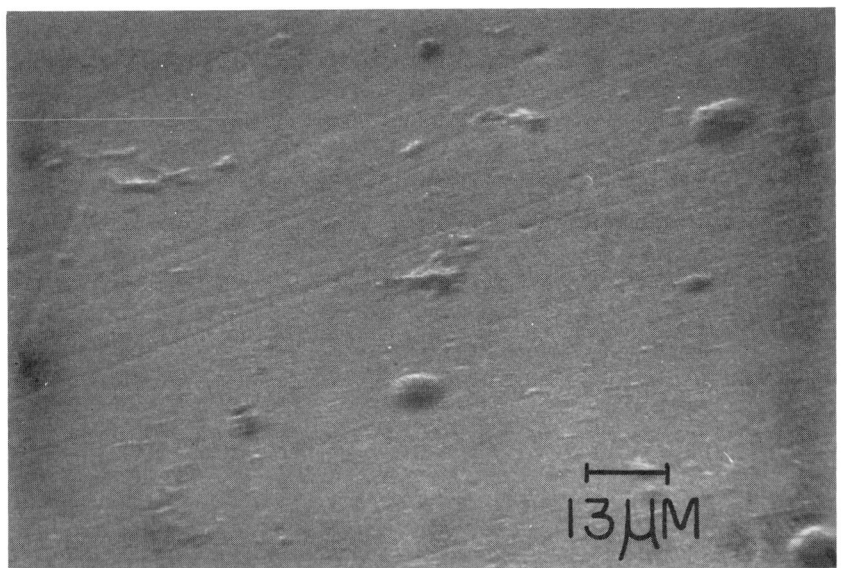

Figure 15d. SEM photomicrograph of copper–2% zinc alloy in phosphated saline solution, as in Figure 1a, for 4 h incorporating 11.6 g/L of human γ-globulin and with a sinusoidal potential (−0.25 to −0.40 V peak to peak at 20 kHz.

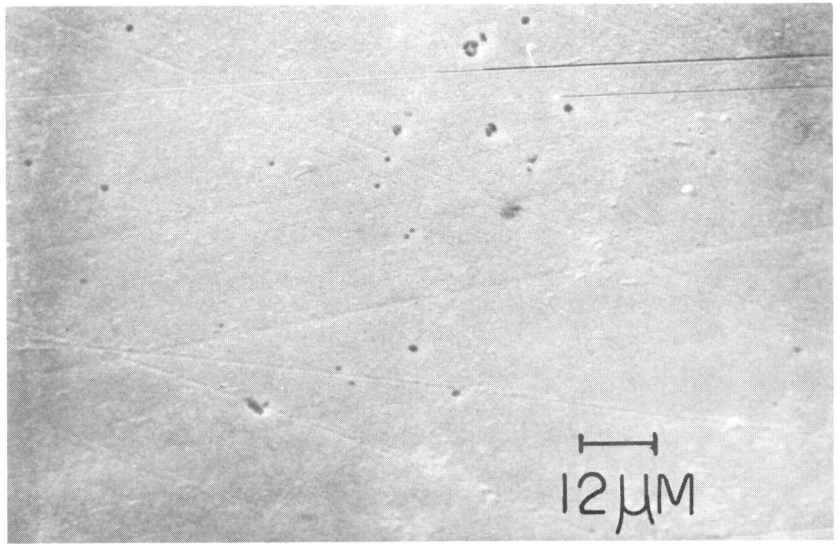

Figure 16a. SEM photomicrograph of copper–2% zinc alloy after employing a sinusoidal potential (−0.25 to −0.40 V SCE peak to peak) at a frequency of 200 kHz for 4 h with phosphated saline, as listed in Figure 1a, and incorporating human albumin at 46.2 g/L.

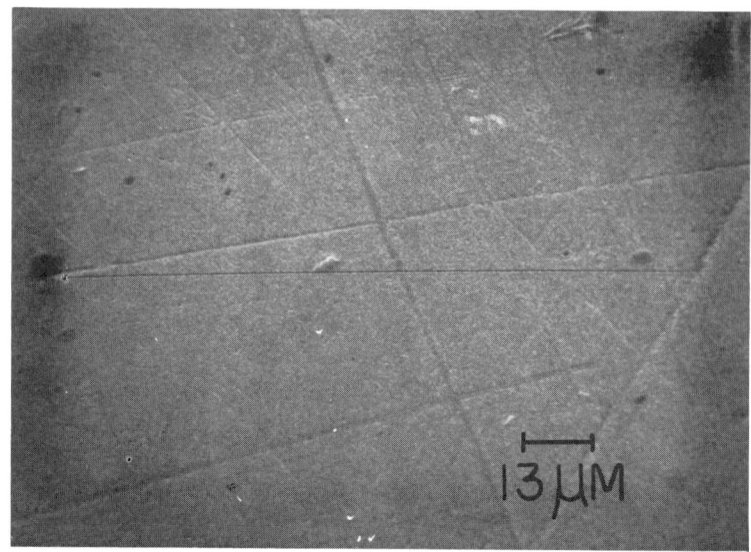

Figure 16b. SEM photomicrograph of copper–2% zinc alloy after employing a sinusoidal potential (−0.25 to −0.40 V SCE peak to peak) at a frequency of 200 kHz for 4 h with phosphated saline, as in Figure 1a, and incorporating human γ-globulin at 11.6 g/L.

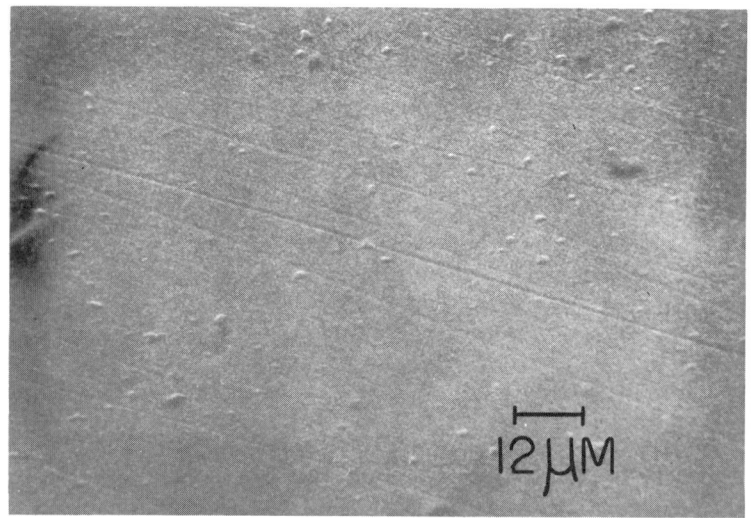

Figure 16c. SEM photomicrograph of copper–2% zinc alloy after employing a sinusoidal potential −0.25 to −0.40 V SCE peak to peak) at a frequency of 200 Hz for 4 h with phosphated saline, as in Figure 1a, and incorporating human fibrinogen at 4 g/L.

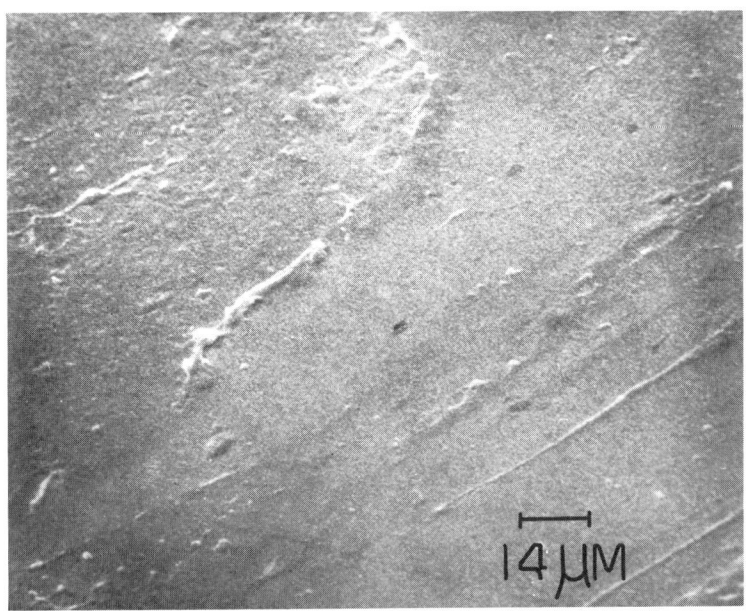

Figure 16d. SEM photomicrograph of copper–2% zinc alloy after employing a sinusoidal potential (−0.25 to −0.40 V SCE peak to peak) at a frequency of 200 Hz for 4 h with phosphated saline, as in Figure 1a, and incorporating combination albumin–globulin–fibrinogen.

Consideration also must be given to the possible changes in protein state with duration of the experiments. For the 5 V/min cyclic voltammetry experiments, results were completed within several minutes (for evaluations not including the 0.5-h OCP), whereas for the 0.012 V/min profiles, up to several hours were needed. Even longer times of 4 h were needed for the j–t transients and for the adsorption studies. Flocculation and coagulation as crude indications of protein denaturation (40) were not observed. Experiments at 37°C of up to 1 h with the plasma proteins (38) as well as electrochemical studies with fibrinogen solutions of up to 16 h (41) were reported with no adverse complications due to protein denaturation. Techniques of electrophoresis, isoelectric focusing, and optical rotation (30) certainly could have indicated possible changes in the protein solutions employed.

Even though zinc is at a low level of only 2% in the alloy, it cannot be overlooked in regard to its effect upon the alloy's interaction with protein. Admittedly, the presence of zinc in the material compounds the issues of protein adsorption that are under investigation. Zinc binds to proteins in various ways, and in some instances, an active competition for zinc exists between certain proteins and amino acids (42). In normal human sera, between 2 and 8% of zinc is ultrafilterable, implying that the remainder is bound to protein. Zinc in human saliva is likewise bound to various molecular weight fractions (43). However, zinc in the present investigation was undetectable with adsorbed protein or corrosion products. The zinc concentration levels could have been below the EDAX sensitivity limits. Background radiation also is always present with the analysis, so that low concentrations of an element can remain undetected or be difficult to evaluate. In addition, soluble zinc corrosion products were probably generated, and were concentrated into the bulk of the solution. Atomic absorption spectrophotometry could have been very useful here.

Because of zinc's high electronegativity, this element must have participated in some manner with the corrosion processes. About the only possible indications from the electrochemical and x-ray evaluations made, are the small reduction peaks observed at about -1.15 V for protein solutions on the 5 V/min cyclic voltamograms. These cathodic peaks for use as evidence in showing zinc corrosion may just as well be reduction of copper products, since cathodic peaks are shifted negatively with respect to their redox potentials at faster sweep rates.

Because of the complexity added to the present system by the incorporation of low zinc, comparisons of the data presented herein with available data based upon elemental copper must not be confused. Application of models based upon elemental copper to the present alloy system is hard to justify.

Polarization

The results presented here confirm the studies demonstrating changes in the polarization profiles of various materials with addition of protein to the electrolyte (12, 13, 23–25). The shifting of the polarization curve for protein solutions in the negative direction near the corrosion potential, and the increase in current relative to the background solution during the anodic traverse, agree with earlier potentiostatic results for the platinum/fibrinogen interface, the dental amalgam/human saliva and albumin and mucin interfaces, and the 316LVM/calf's serum interface. This study also shows that similar behavior is observed with the copper–2% zinc/albumin, γ-globulin, and fibrinogen interfaces.

At 5 V/min, a finely divided gas (H_2) was clinging very tenaciously to the surface of the electrode by traversing from -1.5 or -2.0 V to the reversal potential of $+0.5$ V, and occurred only for protein solutions. This observation indicates that diffusion of H_2 is greatly restricted in protein solutions. In supporting electrolyte, H_2 must be dissipated extremely fast into the bulk of the solution, because no accumulation of gas occurs. This formed gas interface can be considered a barrier to the flow of current, and hence can be responsible for the decrease in j relative to the background solution for U's greater than about $+0.3$ V, and also for the decrease in current during the cathodic cycle. This reasoning, however, does not explain the increased anodic behavior at U values less than about $+0.3$ V. An additional viewpoint taking into account the increase in local interfacial pH with H_2 formation can be used to explain changes in configuration, adsorption characteristics, and denaturation of the interfacial proteins, and hence changes in the observed electrochemical profiles.

The electrochemical reactions involving protein at the metal interface has been related to adsorption and charge transfer (12, 13, 41). When Faradaic currents (i_f) occur, the total current (i) is given by (44),

$$i = C_{dl}\,(dE/dt) + i_f$$

with the product of the capacitance of the electric double layer (C_{dl}) and sweep rate (dE/dt) equaling the double layer charging current. Three regions are associated with the double layer. The layer adjacent to the metal contains adsorbed ions, water dipoles, and a layer of nonadsorbed hydrated ions. The diffuse layer extends into the bulk of the solution and includes the opposing effects of the electric field and of thermal agitations.

In the present system with the copper–2% zinc electrodes, all three processes of protein adsorption, charge transfer, and Faradaic oxidations and reductions are possible. The peaks observed in the anodic and cathodic processes are related, respectively, to oxidations and reductions of the electrode. Copper oxides, chlorides, basic chlorides, phosphates, etc., as well as zinc products, are probable compounds for these electrochemical reactions. Increased Faradaic processes and charge transfer processes with protein solutions are factors for increasing the j–U profiles at U's less than $+0.3$ V. Since the sweep rate is a constant here, the capacitance of the double layer must increase for the protein solutions, if the increase in j is not all due to Faradaic processes. One analog of the electrical double layer capacitance incorporates three capacitors in series (44). Hence

$$\frac{1}{C_{dl}} = \frac{1}{C_1} + \frac{1}{C_2} + \frac{1}{C_3}$$

where C_1, C_2, and C_3 represent the capacitance of the adsorbed layer, nonadsorbed layer, and diffuse layer, respectively. Therefore, the smallest of the three capacitors mainly determines the resulting value.

Because of the higher initial potential of -0.3 V employed with the 0.012 V/min sweep rate, effects due to H_2 formation can be dismissed. Visual inspection of the electrode surfaces during cyclic polarization revealed that for all protein solutions employed, protein was grossly adsorbed upon the surface as the potential became progressively more positive. Regular and orderly alignment of individual protein segments occurred across the surface with some segments, especially for fibrinogen, exhibiting streamer-like strands extending into the bulk of the solution. With these observations, the inherent interactional properties of proteins themselves with the metal surface is of a prime importance in regard to electrochemistry, instead of the considerations based on an interfacial H_2 barrier or interfacial pH changes due to formed gas.

For the protein solutions, increased anodic behavior near the corrosion potential has increased either Faradaic or charge transfer processes. This reasoning is in line with the hypothesis (24) stating that the depolarization of O_2 on the cathodic sites for the protein solutions is hindered, thus shifting the corrosion potential and therefore the initial portion of the polarization curve in the negative direction. For fibrinogen solution, however, a decrease in the critical j needed for passivation, and a reduction process with small hysteresis effects, are observed. The anodic process, in this case, can be related to the adsorption of protein with decreased Faradaic processes. A theory put forth (26) for this inhibitory process observed with copper in cystine solutions is mentioned here, but caution must be exercised in applying it to the present system without reservation because of the added presence of zinc in the alloy. That is, the electrical conductivity of the Cu_2O film is increased due to the doping of the semiconductor by cystine (in the present case, by fibrinogen). A larger portion of the potential drop is transferred to the film/solution interface from the metal/film interface, consequently causing a decrease in the activity for copper dissolution. Passivation is observed. Another mechanism proposed here is the alteration in the electrical conductivity of the adsorbing film by a change in the water concentration and/or its structural form with polarization state. Kinetic factors, such as the inhibition caused by the largeness of the fibrinogen molecule in relationship to the formed pore diameters on the adsorbed protein layer, can account for the decreased cathodic reduction processes. This observation is, however, contrary to the globulin system which exhibits larger cathodic currents, possibly because of the larger pore diameters for electron transfer. The polarographic wave of globulin on a dropping mercury electrode (DME) exhibits a peak that is related to an adsorption/desorption process (45).

The consumption of electrons in the reduction processes observed with protein can be considered to be due to the saturation of unsaturated amino acids, splitting of disulfide bridges, hydrogenation of electroactive disulfide linkages, and in general, reaction with any electroactive R group from amino acid residues. One reduction reaction shown to occur with proteins is (46),

$$\text{Protein} + 2H^+ + e^- = \text{Protein}$$
$$\underset{S\text{——}S}{|\quad\quad|} \quad\quad\quad\quad \underset{SH\;\;SH}{|\quad\;\;|}$$

Concentration polarization as reflected by the limiting diffusion current is observed for protein-free solutions at U's slightly negative to the corrosion potential, and at potentials lower than about -0.5 V for both protein-free and protein-containing solutions. The activation polarization region with a Tafel slope of beta = 0.22 V is higher by almost a factor of 2 from the beta = 0.12

V given for copper in 0.15N NaOH and 0.1N HCl (47). Since Tafel slopes are usually between 0.06–0.12 V, and usually never above 0.18 V for H_2 overvoltage on engineering materials (48), concentration polarization appears to affect the entire measured cathodic polarization curves, as presented in Figure 4.

Pulsed Currents

Pulsed currents are more effective than steady-state currents for desorbing proteins. The changing electrical charge in the adsorbed proteins and in the other nonadsorbed proteins participating in the reduction processes produces an electrical oscillatory pattern effective in desorbing protein. A mechanical vibrational response in addition to the normal molecular vibrations, rotations, and translations occurs in the whole adsorbed protein molecule, as well as in the individual protein segments joined at specific sites to metal and other polymer molecules. The secondary and primary binding forces associated with intermolecular chain binding and metal-chain binding are, most importantly, also subjected to these additional electrical and mechanical vibrations. Hence, the polymer segments can be thought of as opening and closing with cycling until sufficient energy has been gained to separate them into desorbed molecules. The conversion of the applied electrical oscillations into a vibratory mechanical response can be thought to occur by considering the changing molecular electrical dipole moments with the state of the electrical input. If this acquired energy can overcome the binding energy, then desorption occurs. Furthermore, at the same time electrons are being consumed, that is, splitting of bridges, by the reduction process. Alteration in the conformation of the proteins to a less coiled structure is expected, so that the mechanical vibrational energy is more effective in surmounting the activation free-energy barrier.

Statistical models predicting the dielectric properties of polar and nonpolar molecules, regarded as interacting classical particles, with fluctuating dipole moment or polarizability have been made (49, 50). The internal motion of the molecules representing the displacement of positive charge relative to negative charge is represented by the application of the harmonic potential of the Drude oscillator. Expressions are given for the dielectric constant for various conditions and assumptions. Relating this calculable dielectric constant to the polarizability, and multiplying by an assumed field intensity, energies on the order of the binding energies for protein and cellular matter ($\Delta F^{adh} \sim -4$ erg/cm^2) (51) are obtainable.

Surface Measurements

Even though SEM is one technique to at least follow the surface appearance of materials by interactions with proteins, techniques with greater sensitivity in following the initial events of protein adsorption are needed. In addition to the measurement of adsorption isotherms and the use of ellipsometry, techniques such as Fourier transform infrared spectroscopy (FTIR) (52), electron spectroscopy for chemical analysis (ESCA) (53), and ultrasonic reflectivity (54) are available. The FTIR technique is extremely applicable, since adsorbance or reflection peaks can be identified by the method of subtraction, which is usually not included or is overlooked with the conventional analysis. ESCA is valuable because of its capability of evaluating both organic and metallic films. Even though the developments of ultrasonic reflectivity have not kept pace with the other listed methods, the technique warrants consideration for studies dealing with protein interaction because of the sensitivity in following surface changes.

Conclusions

The electrochemical characteristics of a high copper alloy (2% zinc) are altered by the additions of albumin, γ-globulin, and fibrinogen to a supporting phosphated-saline electrolyte. This study confirms previous reports indicating changes in polarization behavior with proteins. Contrary to studies indicating the electrochemistry of protein solutions with inert metal electrodes, the electrochemical profiles from this study can be related to Faradaic oxidation and reduction processes, in addition to adsorption and charge transfer. Hence, processes, such as diffusion of metallic ions through the adsorbed protein layer and the formation of complex organometallic compounds, are additional consequences with the system employed. Furthermore, the occurrence of reduction processes of electron transfer to acceptor groups in adsorbed protein layer, and to native protein molecules in solution, can be altered by the presence of the oxidized metallic ions.

All protein solutions shifted the corrosion potential $(i_a=i_c)$ in the negative direction due to the adsorption process. For albumin and globulin systems, an enhancement in the anodic current density was observed at potentials positive to the passivation potentials. However, fibrinogen solutions exhibited an inhibition in the polarization profiles.

Results presented here confirm earlier studies indicating the increased desorption of protein with direct and pulsed cathodic currents. For the steady-state currents, increased desorption occurred by increasing the surface electronegativity from the OCP to -0.3, -0.5, and -0.7 V (SCE). Pulsed currents generated by an input sinusoidal signal (200 kHz) between -0.25 to -0.40 V consistently desorbed the surface of more protein. Selective lower frequencies from 2 Hz also were effective or partially effective in producing desorbed surfaces. The relationship of frequency to the adsorption/desorption process is controlled by the changing molecular electrical dipole moment produced in protein segments oscillating between fixed sites bound to the metal surface or to the protein molecules. Hence, a conversion of electrical pulsations to mechanical oscillations is made.

Acknowledgments

The author's professional positions as a National Research Service Award recipient (Northwestern University) and as a Research Associate (American Dental Association) were possible through NIH DE 07042 and DE 05761, respectively.

Literature Cited

1. Nose, Y.; Levine, S. N., Eds. "Biomedical Engineering and Medical Physics"; Interscience: New York, 1970; 273.
2. Kim, S. W.; Wisniewski, S.; Lee, E. S.; Winn, M. L. *J. Biomed. Mater. Res. Sym.* **1977**, *8*, 23.
3. Vroman, L.; Leonard, E. F. *Ann. N.Y. Acad. Sci.* **1977**, *283*, 17.
4. Sawyer, P. N.; Srinivasen, S.; Chopra, P. S.; Martin, J. G.; Lucas, T.; Burrowes, C. B.; Sauvage, L. *J. Biomed. Mater. Res.* **1970**, *4*, 43.
5. Gileadi, E.; Stanczewski, B.; Parmeggiani, A.; Lucas, T.; Ranganathan, M.; Sawyer, P. N. *J. Biomed. Mater. Res.* **1972**, *6*, 489.
6. Lucas, T. R.; Stanczewski, B.; Ramasamy, N.; Srinivasan, S.; Kammlott, G. W.; Sawyer, P. N. *Biomater., Med. Devices, Artif. Organs* **1975**, *3*, 215.
7. Ramasamy, N.; Sawyer, P. N. *Bioelectrochem. Bioenerg.* **1977**, *4*, 137.
8. Vroman, L.; Leonard, E. F. *Ann. N.Y. Acad. Sci.* **1977**, *283*, 372.
9. Stoner, G. E.; Srinivasan, S. *J. Phys. Chem.* **1971**, *75*, 2107.
10. Stoner, G. E.; Srinivasan, S. *J. Phys. Chem.* **1970**, *74*, 1088.
11. Vroman, L.; Leonard, E. F. *Ann. N.Y. Acad. Sci.* **1977**, *283*, 536.
12. Ramasamy, N.; Ranganathan, M.; Duic, L.; Srinivasan, S.; Sawyer, P. N. *J. Electrochem. Soc.* **1973**, *120*, 354.
13. Duic, L.; Srinivasan, S.; Sawyer, P. N. *J. Electrochem. Soc.* **1973**, *120*, 348.
14. Morrissey, B. W.; Smith, L. E.; Stromberg, R. R.; Fenstermaker, C. A. *J. Colloid. Interface. Sci.* **1976**, *56*, 557.
15. Stoner, G.; Walker, L. *J. Biomed. Mater. Res.* **1969**, *3*, 645.
16. Matthews, D. B. *J. Biomed. Mater. Res.* **1969**, *3*, 475.
17. Stoner, G. E. *J. Biomed. Mater. Res.* **1969**, *3*, 655.
18. Kuznetsov, B. A.; Mestechkina, N. M.; Shumakovich, G. P. *Bioelectrochem. Bioenerg.* **1977**, *4*, 1.
19. Kuznetsov, B. A.; Shumakovich, G. P.; Mestechkina, N. M. *Bioelectrochem. Bioenerg.* **1977**, *4*, 512.
20. Azzam, R. M.; Rigby, P. G.; Krueger, J. A. *Phys. Med. Biol.* **1977**, *22*, 422.
21. Cuypers, P. A.; Hermens, W. T.; Hemker, H. C., *Anal. Biochem.* **1978**, *84*, 56.
22. Vroman, L.; Adams, A. L. *Surf. Sci.* **1969**, *16*, 438.
23. Brown, S. A.; Merritt, K. *J. Biomed. Mater. Res.* **1980**, *14*, 173.
24. Finkelstein, G. H.; Greener, E. H. *J. Oral Rehab.* **1977**, *4*, 355.
25. Finkelstein, G. H.; Greener, E. H. *J. Oral Rehab.* **1978**, *5*, 95.
26. Svare, C. W.; Belton, G.; Korostoff, E. *J. Biomed. Mater. Res.* **1970**, *4*, 457.
27. Jones, D. A.; Greene, N. D. *Corr.* **1966**, *22*, 198.
28. Greene, N. D.; Jones, D. A. *J. Mater.* **1966**, *1*, 345.
29. Colangelo, V. J.; Greene, N. D.; Kettelkamp, D. B.; Alexander, H.; Campbell, C. J. *J. Biomed. Mater. Res.* **1967**, *1*, 405.
30. Allison, A. C., Ed. "Structure and Function of Plasma Proteins"; Plenum: New York, Vol. I and Vol. II, 1974 and 1976.
31. Putnam, F. C., Ed. "The Plasma Proteins"; Academic: New York, 1975.
32. Scheller, F.; Prumke, H.-J. *J. Electroanal. Chem.* **1976**, *70*, 219.
33. Berg, H. *Bioelectrochem. Bioenerg.* **1976**, *3*, 359.
34. Kuznetsov, B. A.; Shumakovich, G. P. *Bioelectrochem. Bioenerg.* **1975**, *2*, 35.
35. Bruck, S. D. *J. Biomed. Mater. Res. Sym.* **1977**, *8*, 1.
36. Vroman, L.; Leonard, E. F. *Ann. N.Y. Acad. Sci.* **1977**, *283*, 332.

37. Nekrasova, V. K. *Bioelectrochem. Bioenerg.* **1975**, *2*, 43.
38. Bagnall, R. D. *J. Biomed. Mater. Res.* **1977**, *11*, 947.
39. Linke, W. F. "Solubilities of Inorganic and Metal–Organic Compounds"; American Chemical Society: Washington, D.C., 1965, Vol. II, 4th ed., 1228.
40. Oser, B. L., Ed. "Hawk's Physiological Chemistry"; McGraw–Hill: New York, 1965, 188 and 956.
41. Ramasamy, N.; Keates, J. S.; Srinivasan, S.; Sawyer, P. N. *Bioelectrochem. Bioenerg.* **1974**, *1*, 244.
42. Yunice, A. A.; King, R. W. Jr.; Kraikitpanitch, S.; Haygood, C. C.; Lindeman, R. D. *Am. J. Physiol.* **1978**, *235*(1), F40.
43. Baratieri, A.; Picarelli, A.; Piselli, D. *J. Dent. Res.* **1979**, *58*, 540.
44. Macdonald, D. D. "Transient Techniques in Electrochemistry"; Plenum: New York, 1977, 5 and 187.
45. Fontaine, M.; Rivat, C.; Ropartz, C.; Caullet, C. *Bull. Soc. Chim. Fr.* **1973**, 1873.
46. Fontaine, M.; Rivat, C.; Hamet, C.; Caullet, C. *Bioelectrochem. Bioenerg.* **1977**, *4*, 242.
47. Uhlig, H. H. "Corrosion and Corrosion Control"; John Wiley and Sons: New York, 1965, 48.
48. Stern, M.; Weisert, E. D. *Proc. Am. Soc. Test. Mater.* **1959**, *59*, 1280.
49. Hoye, J. S.; Stell, G. *J. Chem. Phys.* **1980**, *73*(1), 461.
50. Hoye, J. S.; Stell, G. *J. Chem. Phys.* **1980**, *72*(3), 1597.
51. Neumann, A. W.; Hope, C. J.; Ward, C. A.; Herbert, M. A.; Dunn, G. W.; Zingg, W. *J. Biomed. Mater. Res.* **1975**, *9*, 127.
52. Ferraro, J. R.; Basile, L. J. "Fourier Transform Infrared Spectroscopy"; Academic: New York, 1979, Vol. II, 165.
53. Carlson, T. A. "Photoelectron and Auger Spectroscopy"; Plenum: New York, 1975; Chap. 6.
54. Rollins, F. R. *Mater. Eval.* **1966**, *24*, 683.

RECEIVED for review January 16, 1981. ACCEPTED July 27, 1981.

27

Adsorption of Proteins from Artificial Tear Solutions to Poly(methyl methacrylate–2-hydroxyethyl methacrylate) Copolymers

FREDERICK H. ROYCE, JR., BUDDY D. RATNER, and THOMAS A. HORBETT

University of Washington, Department of Chemical Engineering and Center for Bioengineering, Seattle, WA 98195

> *Lens hazing and protein deposition are common problems for wearers of soft contact lenses. Previous experiments with hydrophobic–hydrophilic copolymers exposed to plasma showed protein adsorption to be minimal at intermediate copolymer compositions. Adsorption of proteins from artificial tear solutions to a series of polymers and copolymers ranging in composition from 100% poly(methyl methacrylate) (PMMA) to 100% poly(2-hydroxyethyl methacrylate) (PHEMA) was measured. The total protein adsorption due to the three major proteins in tear fluid (lysozyme, albumin, and immunoglobulins) was at a minimum value at copolymer compositions containing 50% or less PHEMA. The elution of the adsorbed proteins from these polymers and copolymers with various solutions also was investigated to assess the binding mechanism.*

Soft contact lenses, and to a lesser extent hard contact lenses, can accumulate foreign materials on their surfaces and possibly within their polymer matrices. The deposits are composed primarily of substances present in the tear fluid (1). The deposits cloud the lens, cause the wearer discomfort, and may be responsible for a variety of inflammatory conditions including giant papillary conjunctivitis. Manifestations of this syndrome consist of increased mucus, mild itching, decreased lens tolerance, and the development of giant papillae in the upper tarsal conjunctiva (2). Other complications possibly stemming from deposits on soft lenses include corneal vascularization, infiltrates, and infections (3).

Proteins are the major component of lens deposits. Other investigators have observed that on the Bausch and Lomb Soflens [cross-linked poly(hydroxyethyl methacrylate)], protein is present at significant levels, and that only a limited number of the various types of protein present in the tear fluid are deposited along with lipids and certain carbohydrates. The principle proteins present in the tear solution and found in these deposits are lysozyme, albumin, and γ-G-globulin (1, 7). Carbohydrates may be present in the form of glycoproteins such as γ-G-globulins. Little calcium is present at the surfaces of contact lenses (4) except when tear calcium concentration is elevated or there is a tear insufficiency (5). Ethylenediaminetetraacetonitrile (EDTA) therefore, does not aid in lens deposit removal (1). These considerations suggest that, in most cases, a material that would minimize protein adsorption may inhibit lens clouding and immunologic responses.

Recent experiments indicate that polymers that contain a balance of hydrophobic (nonpolar) and hydrophilic (polar) chemical groups show minimal protein adsorption and cell adhesion (6). With the intent of rationally designing a contact lens material that would minimize protein adsorption, the adsorption of lysozyme, albumin, and immunoglobulin G (IgG) to a series of hydrophobic and hydrophilic polymers and copolymers was measured. The polymers ranged from 100% poly(methyl methacrylate) (PMMA) to 100% poly(2-hydroxyethyl methacrylate) (PHEMA). Adsorption varied significantly for each protein, as did the elutability of the proteins from the surfaces.

Materials and Methods

Polymer Synthesis. Methyl methacrylate (MMA) was obtained from Polysciences, Inc. and was used after vacuum distillation; 2-hydroxyethyl methacrylate (HEMA) was received in highly purified form from Hydromed Sciences, Inc. Ethylene glycol dimethacrylate (EDMA) was obtained from Polysciences, Inc. and was used as received. Cross-linked polymer slabs 5 cm × 8 cm × 0.2 cm were formed by polymerization in a cell faced with Mylar film and separated by a gasket fashioned from Silastic tubing. Thirteen polymers and copolymers were synthesized ranging from 100% PMMA through 100% PHEMA. Aliquots of 1 mL of EDMA (cross-linking agent) and 0.15 g of azobisisobutyronitrile (AIBN, catalyst) were used per 20 mL of MMA/HEMA monomer, with composition expressed as volume percent of monomer less EDMA and AIBN. The cell assembly with the monomer mixture, cross-linking agent, and catalyst was cured in a constant temperature oven at 45°C. Disks of 1 cm diameter were cut on a specially adapted milling machine at high speed (~ 2500 rpm), with the polymer slabs affixed to a clean Plexiglas table with double-faced tape. Prior to each experiment, all polymer specimens, contained in mesh cases to prevent scoring, received the following ultrasonic cleaning regime: 30 min in reagent grade petroleum ether, 15 min in reagent grade methanol, another 30 min in reagent grade petroleum ether, and finally, 15 min in reagent grade methanol. The polymers were then blotted dry between filter paper and placed under vacuum over desiccant for 1 week. Prior to each experiment, all polymers were equilibrated for at least 1 week in a buffer solution (*see* below), and then transferred to fresh buffer. This ensured complete polymer hydration and elution of any remaining methanol.

Equilibrium Water Content. Samples were equilibrated in deionized water for 1 week, blotted and weighed, placed under vacuum for 2 days to remove the water, and reweighed. Water content was computed using the relationship:

$$(\text{g water})/(\text{g water} + \text{g polymer}) \times 100 = \% \text{ water content}$$

Measurement of Protein Adsorption. The artificial tear solution consisted of lysozyme (1.20 mg/mL), albumin (3.88 mg/mL), immunoglobulin G (IgG) (1.61 mg/mL), and buffer. Egg white lysozyme was purchased from Sigma Chemical Company (code L-6876). Bovine albumin, crystallized, (code 81-001-2) and immunoglobulin G ("electrophoretically pure"; code 64-140-1) were purchased from Miles Laboratories, Inc. A less purified immunoglobulin fraction was used in some experiments when it was not the protein to be radiolabeled. It was also purchased from Miles Laboratories (Pentex Bovine Gamma Globulins, Labile enzyme free, Fraction I, code 82-042-3). The buffer used throughout these experiments (CPBSz) was $0.01M$ citric acid, $0.01M$ phosphate, $0.12M$ NaCl, 0.02% sodium azide, pH 7.4. Except for the azide, all salts were reagent grade. The protein composition of this artificial tear solution is similar to human tear fluid (7).

Measurement of the adsorption of individual proteins to the polymer samples was determined with ^{125}I-labeled proteins prepared using the ICl method as described previously (8). The protein to be examined was added in small amounts at high specific activity to the tear solution to give a final specific activity of 100–2000 cpm/μg. The amount of protein absorbed in μg/cm^2 was calculated from the radioactivity of the films by using the specific activity of the tear solution and the planar surface area of the film. In these calculations, film surface area was determined to an accuracy of $\pm 2\%$ by averaging the diameters and thicknesses (measured with a cathetometer) of three samples and then calculating average surface area.

In the adsorption experiments, two samples from each of the 13 polymers were placed in separate test tubes containing CPBSz buffer. An equal volume of protein stock solution (at twice the concentration stated in the results), with the appropriate radiolabeled protein, was then added. Solutions were maintained at 37°C. After 2 h, the adsorption process was terminated by using a dilution-displacement rinse with ambient temperature CPBSz. In this rinsing technique, buffer is run through the test tube containing the polymer adsorbed with protein at about 800 mL/min for approximately 0.5 min, using a two-hole rubber stopper fitted with glass tubes for entrance and exit of buffer. Following the initial dilution-displacement rinse, the polymers were placed in fresh CPBSz and their radioactivity counted. On the next day, the polymers were again put in fresh CPBSz and recounted to obtain the "overnight soak rinse" adsorption figures. Radioactive counting was performed with a Searle 1025 γ-scintillation counter.

Elution Experiments. An experiment was performed to investigate qualitatively the nature of chemical binding at the polymer interface through the use of reagents thought to destabilize particular molecular interactions (9). The same polymers used in the albumin adsorption experiment retained enough protein (over 50%) to permit their reuse in the elution experiments. A 2% solution of SDS was used to break hydrophobic bonds. A $2M$ urea solution was used since it is thought to disrupt hydrogen bonds as well as interfere with hydrophobic bonds. Finally, $2M$ NaCl was employed to solvate ionic interactions. One sample from each pair of polymers was used for the SDS elution, while the other sample was used for the urea elution. After these experiments were complete, the polymers were subjected to the NaCl solution. The experiments consisted of an initial radioactive counting, followed by a 1 day soak in the reagent of interest, and transfer to fresh CPBSz for the final radioactive counting. The percent of eluted protein was then calculated.

Results

The water content of PHEMA was the highest of all the polymers studied (30%). The PHEMA/PMMA copolymers had reduced water contents depending on polymer composition, as illustrated in Figure 1.

Figure 2 summarizes the data for the three protein adsorption experiments performed. Each curve represents the amount of protein bound to the surface after the overnight soak rinse. The top curve indicates the total amount of protein adsorbed, and is simply a summation of the data for the three proteins studied. The curve was compiled using the data from three separate adsorption experiments, each of which examined one labeled protein at a time in the artificial tear solution.

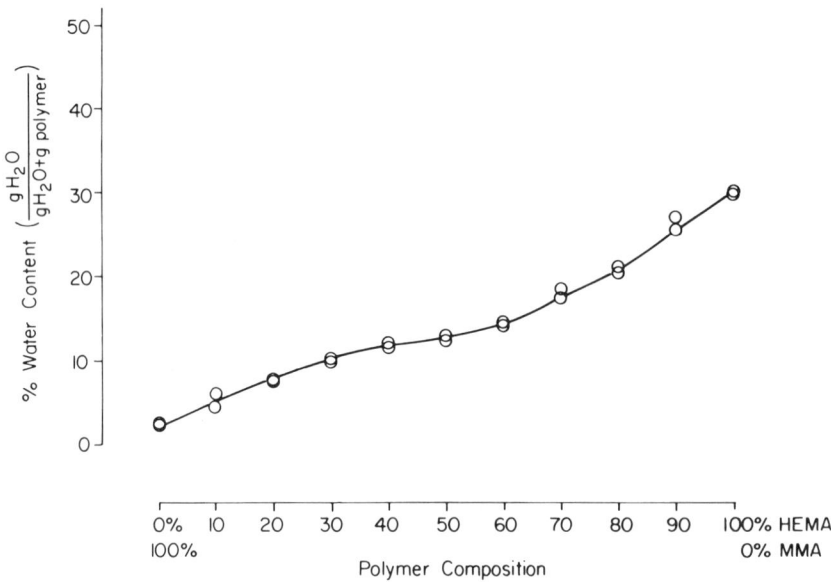

Figure 1. Effect of polymer composition on equilibrium water content for cross-linked PMMA/PHEMA copolymers.

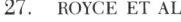

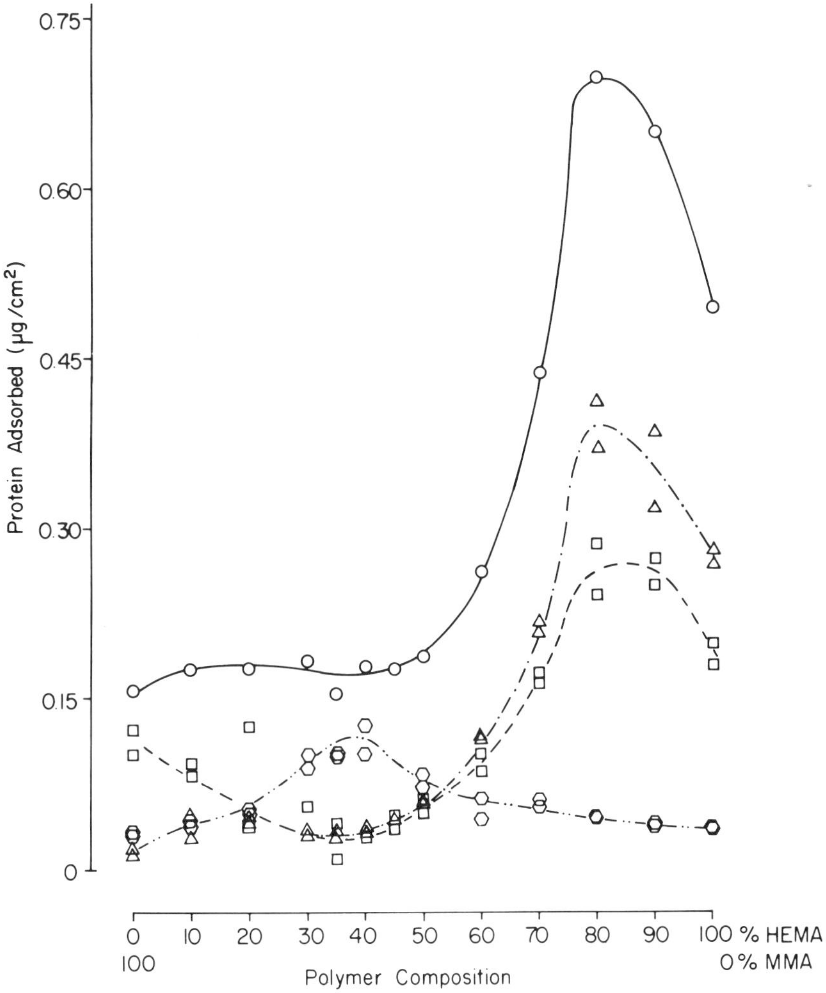

Figure 2. *Adsorption of lysozyme* (– – –, □), *albumin* (– · · – ·, △), *IgG* (– · · · – · ·, ○), *and total protein* (–, ○) *to PMMA/PHEMA copolymers from artificial tear solutions.*

Figure 3 presents a useful means of viewing the adsorption of the three proteins over the range of copolymers, namely, how surface enrichment (SE) varies with copolymer composition. Surface enrichment is defined as:

$$SE = \frac{\left(\dfrac{\mu g \text{ specific protein adsorbed}}{\mu g \text{ total protein adsorbed}}\right)}{\left(\dfrac{\mu g \text{ specific protein in bulk phase}}{\mu g \text{ total protein in bulk phase}}\right)}$$

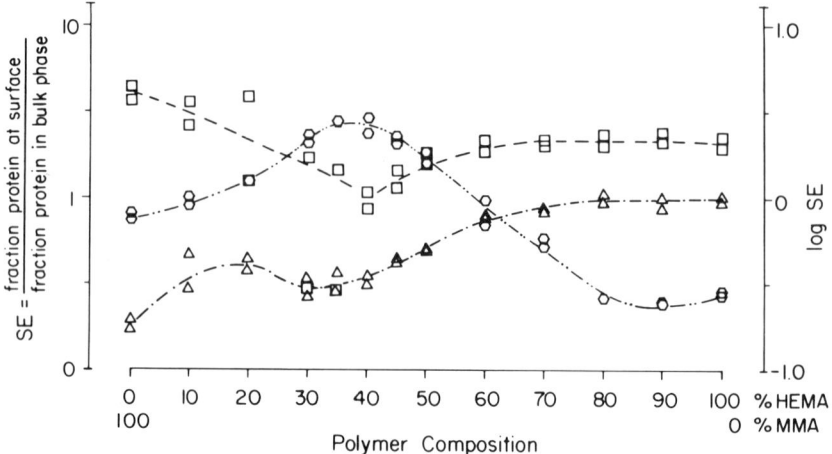

Figure 3. Surface enrichment for lysozyme (- - -, □), albumin (- · - · , △), and IgG (- · · - · · , ○) adsorbed onto PMMA/PHEMA copolymers from artificial tear solutions.

A surface enrichment greater than 1.0 means that the specific protein prefers the surface to the bulk phase and will be more readily adsorbed. Although albumin shows low surface enrichment, it is present in solutions at significantly higher concentration than lysozyme and the globulins.

To consider qualitatively chemical bonding of protein to the polymer surfaces and the ability of various solutions to elute this protein layer, three chemically distinct reagents were chosen. The three solutions used were SDS, a surfactant known to disrupt hydrophobic interactions; urea, a polar compound that disrupts hydrogen bonds and hydrophobic interactions; and NaCl, an ionic compound that should disrupt ionic bonds. The results of the SDS and urea elution of albumin from the polymer surface, expressed as percent albumin eluted, are shown in Figure 4. Within the limits of error of measurement, none of the remaining protein was elutable from the polymer surface with NaCl. The removal of over 50% of the albumin from PMMA by SDS, compared to less than 15% removal from PHEMA by this reagent, indicates a substantial difference in the mechanism by which albumin adsorbs to these two polymers (that is, hydrophobic bonding may be more important in albumin adsorption to PMMA than to PHEMA).

Discussion

The polymers and copolymers synthesized for these experiments had equilibrium water contents that varied with composition. The data in Figure 1 are in close agreement with published values (*10*). Since the 100% PHEMA specimen for this experiment is of the same material as the Bausch and Lomb

Soflens, the literature on this material might be used as a basis for comparison of experimental results.

Figure 2 shows that similar adsorption phenomena are exhibited by lysozyme and albumin. Related work seems to suggest that polymers that contain a certain balance of hydrophobic and hydrophilic chemical groups show minimized biological interaction (for example, low protein adsorption, low thrombus deposition, and low platelet consumption) (6). The adsorption of radiolabeled IgG, however, was maximal at intermediate copolymers. This result has a number of implications with respect to both the fundamental adsorption mechanism and the biocompatibility of these materials.

One might speculate on a number of chemical and physical factors that govern protein adsorption behavior. Previous experiments point to the importance of hydrophilicity as an influential factor (6), but this is certainly not the sole factor. In this polymer system, hydrophilicity (as governed by the surface concentration of HEMA) increases linearly with the bulk HEMA composition (11). The surface of a protein which is also soluble in aqueous media is probably of a polar nature. If protein adsorption could be characterized by polar interactions, then an adsorption trend that would parallel the

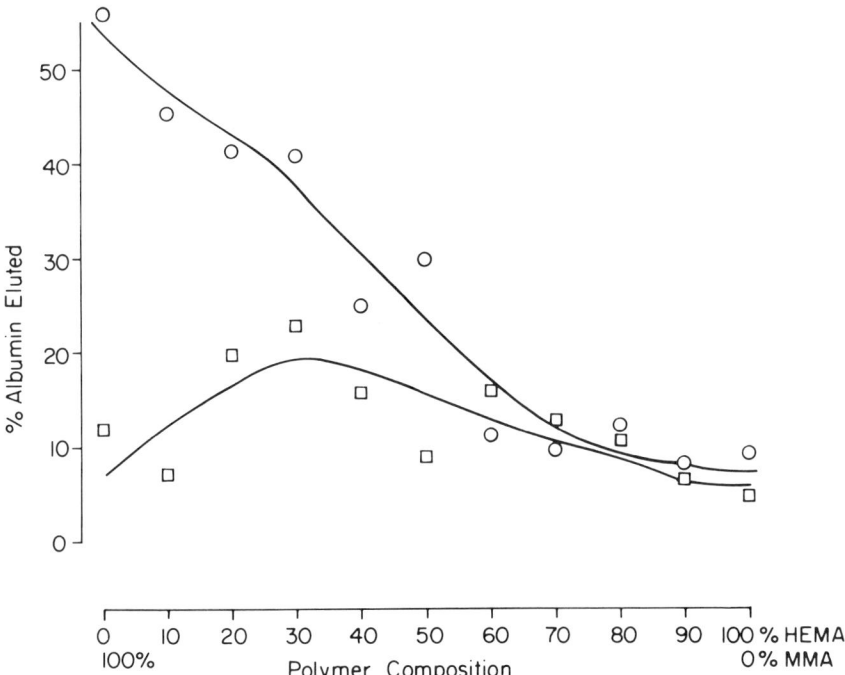

Figure 4. Elution of albumin adsorbed to PMMA/PHEMA copolymers with SDS (○) and urea (□).

surface concentration of hydrophilic groups in a linear manner should be evident. The data in Figure 2 and Figure 3 do not support this idea. Chain flexibility for the hydrophilic copolymers (and possibly for the protein itself) may be sufficiently great to allow molecular rearrangements to occur, leading to minimized interaction. Models considering such molecular rearrangements can be used to rationalize either maxima or minima in adsorption levels as a function of composition.

Another possible explanation for the protein adsorption behavior is the effect of surface texture or roughness. Although all the polymers were cast against an identical, relatively smooth Mylar film (in these experiments), any slight surface texture in the Mylar impressed in the polymer should be expanded in proportion to the degree of swelling (Figure 1). Therefore, surface texture, and consequently, surface area available for adsorption, may vary among the polymers.

Swelling degree also will influence the pore size in polymeric gels thereby potentially affecting protein adsorption values. Investigators have shown the effective pore size of cross-linked PHEMA gels formed in solution to be on the order of 5 Å (12, 13). The PHEMA gels cross-linked without solvent present which are similar to the type prepared here have been shown to have pore radii up to 30 Å (14). In addition, lysozyme (but not albumin) penetration into cross-linked PHEMA gels recently has been observed (15). The discussion for Figures 2 and 3 considered primarily monolayer protein adsorption. In fact, the data in Figure 2 indicate that for polymers above 70% PHEMA, the amounts of protein adsorbed correspond to multiple layers based upon calculations using the Stokes radii of the proteins. This could be an indication of protein penetration or free radioactive iodide dissociated from the protein. These penetration processes will be strongly influenced by the pore size of the gels. Alternately, multilayer film formation may be occurring, implying a change in the mechanism of interaction at high PHEMA levels. These possibilities are being investigated.

Of the solutions used in the elution experiments, SDS removed the most bound protein, suggesting that hydrophobic bonding may be an important factor in the protein surface interaction. Figure 4 shows that elution of albumin by SDS decreases linearly with hydrophilicity. Some elution of albumin by the urea also was observed, but it was considerably less than with SDS, and possibly indicates the ability of urea to disrupt weakly both hydrogen bonds and hydrophobic interactions. NaCl was ineffective in removing albumin, which suggests that ionic interactions are not nearly as significant as hydrophobic/hydrophilic interactions in protein binding to these electrostatically neutral polymeric materials.

Giant papillary conjuctivitis may be caused by an immunologic response to the lens deposits (2). Lens cleaning procedures, especially heat disinfection, may denature proteins, while shear forces created by the eyelids moving over the lens may also contribute to further denaturation and subsequent desorption of the adsorbed proteins. In addition, drying of the outer surface of the lens may result in further protein denaturation. These adsorbed, denatured proteins might then serve as antigens.

The onset of contact lens rejection, which may be immunologic in nature, occurs more rapidly for soft (PHEMA) lenses than for hard (PMMA) lenses [2]. This reaction may be a direct consequence of the total level of protein that accumulates on the lenses. Alternately, it may be a consequence of specific adsorbed proteins within the protein film.

The data presented here indicate that contact lenses formed of certain copolymers of PMMA and PHEMA may exhibit the desirable low adsorption levels seen for the pure PMMA polymers. The results also show some of the other benefits associated with soft lenses (for example, increased oxygen transport, comfort). However, the surface enrichment of the IgG protein on the intermediate copolymer lenses may have undesirable effects with respect to biological interaction.

Conclusions

The accumulation of proteins on contact lenses has long been viewed as an undesirable event. In this study, the effect of polymer composition on both the total amount of protein on the materials, and on the specific proteins on each polymer composition was documented. The importance of these factors for biological response is not known, so this situation remains a fertile area for investigation. This study also demonstrated that a linear variation in material composition will not necessarily result in a linear variation in absorbed layer protein composition. The minima and maxima noted at intermediate copolymer compositions have strong implications for both understanding the mechanism of protein adsorption and for biological response. Investigation is underway to explore further protein interaction with hydrophobic–hydrophilic copolymer materials.

Acknowledgments

This work was supported by a grant from the University of Washington Graduate Research Fund and, in part, under N.H.L.B.I. Grants 19419 and 22163. The assistance received from Medicornea Intraocular, Inc., Seattle, Washington, in machining the polymers used in these experiments is appreciated. We would also like to thank Barbara Pederson for her expert technical assistance.

Literature Cited

1. Wedler, F. C. *J. Biomed. Mater. Res.* **1977**, *11*, 523–35.
2. Allansmith, M. R.; Korb, D. R.; Greiner, J. V.; Henriquez, A. S.; Simon, M. A.; Finnemore, V. M. *Am. J. Ophthalmol.* **1977**, *83* (5), 697.

3. Dohlman, C. H.; Boruchoff, S. A.; Mobilia, E. F. *Arch. Opthalmol.* **1973**, *90*, 367.
4. Dohlman, C. H.; Mobilia, E.; Drago, D.; Havenor, V.; Gavin, M. *Ann. Ophthalmol.* **1975**, *7*, 345.
5. Klintworth, G. K.; Reed, J. W.; Hawkins, H. K.; Ingram, P. *Invest. Ophthalmol. Visual Sci.* **1977**, *16* (2), 158–61.
6. Ratner, B. D.; Hoffman, A. S.; Hanson, S. R.; Harker, L. A.; Whiffen, J. D. *J. Polym. Sci. Polym. Symp.* **1979**, *66*, Part C, 363–375.
7. Iwata, S. *Int. Ophthalmology Clinics*, **1973**, *13* (1), 34.
8. Weathersby, P. K.; Horbett, T. A.; Hoffman, A. S. *Trans. Am. Soc. Artif. Intern. Organs* **1976**, *22*, 242.
9. Pigott, G. H.; Gilding, D. K.; Askill, I. M.,; Ives, C. L. *Trans 11th Int. Biomater. Symp. Soc. Biomat.* **1979**, *3*, 142.
10. Fatt, I. In "Soft Contact Lenses: Clinical and Applied Technology"; Ruben, M., Ed.; John Wiley and Sons: New York, 1978, p. 107.
11. Ratner, B. D.; Hoffman, A. S. In "Adhesion and Adsorption of Polymersm," Part B; Lee, L., Ed.; Plenum: New York, 1980; pp. 691–706.
12. Refojo, M. F. *J. Appl. Polym. Sci.* **1965**, *9*, 3417.
13. Ratner, B. D.; Miller, I. F. *J. Biomed. Mater. Res.* **1973**, *7*, 353–367.
14. Haldon, R. A.; Lee, B. E. *Br. Polym. J.* **1972**, *4*, 491.
15. Refojo, M. F.; Leong, F. L. *J. Polym. Sci. Polym. Symp.* **1979**, *66*, 227–237.

RECEIVED for review January 16, 1981. ACCEPTED April 27, 1981.

NEW BIOMATERIALS SYSTEMS AND APPLICATIONS

28

Structure, Testing, and Applications of Biomaterials

NICHOLAS A. PEPPAS

Purdue University, School of Chemical Engineering, West Lafayette, IN 47907

The term *biomaterials* encompasses all materials used for medical applications that are interfaced with living systems. Although this definition addresses specifically materials used in contact with living systems (intracorporeal uses), other systems developed for extracorporeal uses (*1–4*) are also commonly classified as biomaterials.

Biomedical materials include metals, ceramics, natural polymers (biopolymers), and synthetic polymers of simple or complex chemical and/or physical structure. This volume addresses, to a large measure, fundamental research on phenomena related to the use of synthetic polymers as *blood-compatible* biomaterials. Relevant research stems from major efforts to investigate clotting phenomena related to the response of blood in contact with polymeric surfaces, and to develop systems with nonthrombogenic behavior in short- and long-term applications. These systems can be used as implants or replacements, and they include artificial hearts, lung oxygenators, hemodialysis systems, artificial blood vessels, artificial pancreas, catheters, etc. (*5*).

Other biomedical applications of polymers include sustained and controlled drug delivery formulations for implantation, transdermal and transcorneal uses, intrauterine devices, etc. (*6, 7*). Major developments have been reported recently on the use of biomaterials for skin replacement (*8*), reconstruction of vocal cords (*9*), ophthalmic applications such as therapeutic contact lenses, artificial corneas, intraocular lenses, and vitreous implants (*10*), craniofacial, maxillofacial, and related replacements in reconstructive surgery (*1*), and neurostimulating and other electrical-stimulating electrodes (*1*). Orthopedic applications include artificial tendons (*11*), prostheses, long bone repair, and articular cartilage replacement (*1*). Finally, dental materials and implants (*12, 13*) are also often considered as biomaterials.

This chapter presents a brief analysis of important physical, chemical, and biological properties of biomaterials, which can serve as the basis for development of new candidate polymers.

Criteria

Candidate polymers for biomedical applications must comply with a variety of requirements characteristic of most biomaterials. These requirements arise either from the specific chemical or physical structure of the polymers (chemical, physical, and mechanical criteria) or from the physiological environment where they will be used (biological criteria). Table I summarizes major criteria for the design and selection of polymers as biomaterials.

Biomaterials must be free from elutable impurities, such as additives and residual substances. Additives include stabilizers, antioxidants, plasticizers, and fillers which are added to commercial polymers to impart specific physical or mechanical properties. Since long- and short-term migration of these components to the adjacent tissues and biological fluids is highly undesirable, additives must be eliminated before use. In addition, favorable polymer properties can be achieved without using additives via block or random copolymerization of the candidate homopolymer with other monomers. Graft copolymerization is also used to obtain polymer surfaces with

Table I. Criteria for Development of Biomaterials

Chemical and Physical Structure
- Chemically inert materials
- Materials free from leachable impurities, additives, and compounds remaining after polymerization and cross-linking
- Materials with desirable physical structure (crystallinity, entanglements, equilibrium swelling)
- Materials with minimal mechanical degradation and environmental aging
- Other desirable properties (permeability, friction, electrical properties, etc.)

Mechanical Behavior and Materials Processing
- Materials with satisfactory mechanical properties in tension, compression, and shear
- Readily processable systems by conventional processing methods

Biological Interactions
- Nontoxic materials
- Noncarcinogenic materials
- Materials that do not cause teratological effects
- Sterilizable materials
- Nonbiodegradable systems (unless biodegradation is desired)
- Materials that do not induce inflammatory reactions
- Materials that do not cause thrombosis
- Materials that do not alter the stability of biological fluids

uniform properties (*14*). Initiator residues can be avoided by employing polymerization reactions induced by ultraviolet radiation, electron beams, or γ-rays, which usually produce polymer grades of high purity. Solvent residues and emulsifiers are usually the result of solution, suspension, or emulsion polymerization methods. They can be eliminated by proper devolatilization or avoided by switching to bulk polymerization techniques (*15*). Ultrapure grades of biomaterials have been prepared recently by plasma polymerization. Some residual monomers of the polymerization reactions are toxic even at levels of a few ppm. Although removal by devolatilization and related techniques is used to minimize this residue, it is not always possible to eliminate long-term diffusion of small amounts of monomers to the tissue.

Candidate biomaterials must fulfill certain requirements related to the physical and mechanical properties of the polymer. Parameters of interest include the geometry of the device, implant or component, degree of swelling at equilibrium, degree of cross-linking, volume degree of crystallinity, size of crystallites, sequence and size of "blocks" and "hard/soft segments" (for certain types of polymers), elastic properties, response to tensile, shear, or compressive stresses under stress–relaxation, creep, quasi-equilibrium or oscillatory loading, tear propagation, fatigue resistance, and time–temperature viscoelastic behavior.

Proper design of biomaterials, especially for long-term applications, should consider mechanical degradation and environmental aging problems. Thermal degradation is of lesser importance in biomaterials, due to the relatively small fluctuations of the temperature in most biomedical applications.

Biomaterials should be cast readily or molded in films, rods, tubings, or more complex geometrical shapes. Injection and rotational molding, reaction injection molding, and casting are desirable polymer processing techniques.

Finally, chemically inert systems are required in most biomedical applications. Chemical (e.g., hydrolytic) cleavage should be avoided. Exceptions include biodegradable or bioerodible controlled-release systems, which biodegrade by enzymatic or chemical mechanisms at prescribed rates.

Biological and physiological criteria are related to the specific applications of biomaterials in the body. Fundamentals of blood compatibility are analyzed expertly in the overview by Hoffman (*16*) included in this volume. Blood-compatible biomaterials should not cause cancer or teratological effects, and they should not be toxic. Toxicity may be related to functional groups of the polymer surface structure, or to migration of residual monomers under quiescent or flow conditions.

Biomaterials should be sterilizable, without any alterations in form or properties, and without permanent adsorption of sterilizing agents. They should not induce inflammatory reactions when in contact with natural tissue, and they should not degrade in the presence of naturally circulating enzymes in biological fluids.

Depending on the specific application, additional properties may be necessary. For example, adequate drug permeation through polymer matrices is important for controlled-release systems. Low friction properties are desirable in articular cartilage materials. Hematological criteria call for materials that do not cause thrombosis, do not alter the stability of soluble or cellular materials in the blood, and do not allow allergic, toxic, aging, or cell fragility reactions.

Testing of Physical Properties

Determination of the physical properties of polymeric systems is necessary before they can be used as biomaterials. Depending on the application

Table II. Major Tests of Physical Behavior of Biomaterials

Macromolecular Structure
- Molecular weights and molecular weight distributions by dilute solution viscometry, light scattering, membrane osmometry, and gel permeation chromatography
- Degree of cross-linking and degree of swelling by swelling experiments, dilatometry, laser light scattering, and rubber elasticity
- Ordered (crystalline) structure by differential scanning calorimetry, x-ray diffraction, electron microscopy, infrared spectroscopy, sonic modulus, mechanical testing, etc.

Other Properties and Macroscopic Structure
- Thermal characterization by differential scanning calorimetry, thermogravimetric analysis, and thermomechanical analysis
- Friction properties
- Electrical properties
- Porosity by porosimetry
- Permeation analysis by solute diffusion studies

Mechanical Behavior
- Tensile, compressive, and shear experiments
- Stress–relaxation experiments
- Creep experiments
- Testing under oscillatory loading
- Accelerated aging tests

Surface Characterization
- Roughness analysis
- Contact-angle measurements
- X-ray photoelectron spectroscopy
- Total reflectance infrared spectroscopy
- Auger electron spectroscopy
- Secondary ion mass spectrometry

considered, a range of physical analyses will have to be carried out. Table II summarizes some of the important experiments for a preliminary evaluation of candidate materials. Extensive analysis of physical and physicochemical techniques for the investigation of the structure of homopolymers, copolymers, blends, and composites can be found in standard references (17–19).

The macromolecular structure can be investigated in terms of the size, branching, and distribution of the macromolecular chains, the ordered structure and orientation of the polymer, and the thermodynamic compatibility of the system with biological fluids. The first type of analysis calls for evaluation of the molecular weight distribution of the bulk polymer before, during, and after implantation. Analysis of the ordered structure refers to investigation of the crystalline structure of the macromolecular chains and its possible alteration due to application of stresses or to the possible swelling by biological fluids. Thermodynamic compatibility testing refers to the dynamic and equilibrium swelling behavior of biomaterials.

Other properties related to the structure of the candidate biomaterials include thermal, electrical, and tribological properties. Analysis of solute diffusion can be obtained by porosimetry (for microscopic pores) and by diffusion/permeation experiments (for molecular-size structures of entangled or cross-linked chains).

Mechanical properties can be determined by a variety of standard tests, under both static and dynamic loading. Accelerated aging tests are necessary for long-term implantation applications.

Surface characterization is very important in the development of blood-compatible biomaterials, since the surface characteristics of the polymer have been linked to polymer–tissue and polymer–blood interactions. Further information on surface characterization of biomaterials can be found elsewhere (20, 21).

Evaluation of Toxicity of Polymers as Biomaterials

Among various experimental investigations, toxicity studies of potential biomaterials are required to evaluate the ability of these systems to remain biologically inert during implantation or while in contact with biological fluids.

Table III summarizes a series of recommended toxicity tests that are reported in recent guidelines of NIH (20). Toxicity experiments must be performed at logical points during the biomaterial development. Level I includes tests that are necessary for evaluating commonly used biomaterials, that is, polymers that were biocompatible in previous investigations. Level II tests are recommended for the assessment of new, modified, and previously untested polymers.

Table III. Toxicity Evaluation of Polymers for Biomedical Applications

Level I: Initial Screening and Quality Control of Polymers
- Agar overlay response of materials
- Agar overlay response of materials extracts
- Inhibition of cell growth by water extracts of materials
- Intradermal irritation test for materials extracts and leachable components

Level II: Initial Evaluation of Novel Biomaterials
- Tissue culture test on materials
- Tissue culture test on materials extracts
- Cell growth in contact with test materials
- Hemolytic activity test
- Intramascular implantation of materials
- Test of osmotic fragility of erythrocytes
- In vitro mutagenicity test
- Test of material extracts by perfusion of isolated rabbit heart

Source: Adapted from Ref. 20.

Tests assessing the carcinogenicity, teratogenicity, and mutagenicity of biomaterials are described in recent reviews (3, 20, 22). Due to the complexity of these tests, a wide range of experimental protocols can be followed, although none of these protocols is well enough established to be recommended as a standard test. However, polymeric materials designed intelligently and fabricated for medical applications should have little trouble passing these toxicity tests, since the techniques that can be used for reducing leachable components have been well established.

Finally, manufacture of conventional or novel biomaterials is not complete without proper sterilization. Sterilization methods include heat, steam, irradiation, and gaseous treatment (23, 24). Heat and steam sterilization can be recommended for polymers that are relatively stable and do not exhibit dimensional changes in the range 30°–150°C. Radiation sterilization at low dose levels (usually 0.5–2 Mrads) may be used for many hydrophilic biomaterials. However, radiation can cause major structural changes of the biomaterial, such as cross-linking or degradation. Gaseous sterilization employs ethylene oxide, formaldehyde, and other sterilants. Residues of some of these sterilizing agents on biomaterials have caused mononuclear cell leukemia and malignant neoplasms in laboratory animals. Therefore, the proper choice of sterilization method for a candidate polymer for biomedical applications depends on careful optimization of a variety of effects of the method on the chemical, mechanical, and surface properties of biomaterials. Various tests for evaluating sterility of biomaterials are summarized in an NIH report (20).

Conclusions

Important considerations in the development of new or modified polymers for biomedical applications include macromolecular structure, physical, chemical, and biological properties, and behavior of the biomaterials in the physiological environment. Although systematic investigation of polymer properties is highly recommended before a particular use, the suggested tests may be minimized in the case of previously tested and well-documented biomaterials. In general, the process of selection, design, and evaluation of new biomaterials is long and painstaking. Just one example, indicative of the synthetic thinking and optimization of properties required in the design of new biomaterials, is the recently reported work on the development of collagen-based materials for skin replacement (8, 25). Similar experience can be obtained by studying the case histories of development of cellulose acetate dialysis membranes, porous polytetrafluoroethylene vascular grafts, ethylene–vinyl acetate copolymers for controlled-release of drugs, poly(2-hydroxyethyl methacrylate) (PHEMA) for soft therapeutic contact lenses, etc.

A wide range of polymeric materials has been proposed, tested, or actually used for biomedical applications. Table IV attempts to summarize

Table IV. Commercially Available and Potentially Useful Blood-Compatible Polymers

Polymer Group	References
Hydrogels (Water-swollen networks)	26, 27
PHEMA	28–30
Other nonionic hydrogels	27, 31
Polyelectrolyte networks	32, 33
Interpenetrating networks	3
Polyurethanes	
Segmented polyurethanes	34–37
Segmented polyether–polyurethanes	38
Polyurethane-based block copolymers and blends	39–40
Heparinized polymers	
Polyolefin-based systems	41, 42
Hydrogels	43, 44
Other polymers	45
Fibrinolytic enzyme-immobilized polymers	46, 47
Modified collagen	48
Silicone elastomers	3
Pyrolitic carbons	49
Other polymeric systems	
Polyesters causing pseudoneointima formation	50
Polyphosphazenes (inorganic polymers)	51

major categories of polymeric materials, which are either moderately successful or promising for blood-compatible applications. Major references reviewing the structure and biocompatibility of these polymers are included also. This list only indicates the complexity of the problem of development of biomaterials and of the great potential of polymers in biomedical applications.

Acknowledgment

The author thanks B. D. Ratner for helpful suggestions.

Literature Cited

1. Park, J. B. "Biomaterials," Plenum: New York, 1979.
2. Szycher, M.; Robinson, W. J. "Synthetic Biomedical Polymers," Technomic: Westport, Connecticut, 1980.
3. Bruck, S. D. "Properties of Biomaterials in the Physiological Environment," CRC: Boca Raton, Florida, 1980.
4. Bruck, S. D. "Blood Compatible Synthetic Polymers," Thomas: Springfield, Illinois, 1974.
5. Bruck, S. D. *Ann. N.Y. Acad. Sci.* **1977**, *283*, 332.
6. Langer, R. *Chem. Eng. Commun.* **1980** *6*, 1.
7. Langer, R.; Peppas, N. A. *Biomaterials (Gildford, Engl.)*, **1981**, *2*, 195.
8. Yannas, I. V.; Burke, J. F. *J. Biomed. Mater. Res.* **1980**, *14*, 65.
9. Peppas, N. A.; Benner, R. E., Jr. *Biomaterials (Gildford, Engl.)* **1980**, *1*, 158.
10. Refojo, M. F. In "Synthetic Biomedical Polymers," Szycher, M.; Robinson, W. J., Jr., Eds.; Technomic: Westport, Connecticut, 1980; p. 171.
11. Hodge, J. W., Jr.; Wade, C. W. R. In "Synthetic Biomedical Polymers," Szycher, M.; Robinson, W. J., Jr., Eds.; Technomic: Westport, Connecticut, 1980; p. 201.
12. Brauer, G. M. *Polym. Plast. Technol. Eng.* **1977**, *9*, 87.
13. Grant, A. *Br. Polym. J.* **1978**, *10*, 241.
14. Ratner, B. D.; Hoffman, A. S. In "Synthetic Biomedical Polymers," Szycher, M.; Robinson, W. J., Jr., Eds.; Technomic: Westport, Connecticut, 1980; p. 133.
15. Odian, G. "Principles of Polymerization," McGraw Hill: New York, 1981.
16. Hoffman, A. S. et al. Chapter 6 in this book.
17. Rabek, J. F. "Experimental Methods in Polymer Chemistry," Wiley: New York, 1980.
18. Fava, R. A., Ed. "Methods in Experimental Physics: Polymers," Academic: New York, 1980; Vol. 16A, 16B, 16C.
19. Ferry, J. D. "Viscoelastic Properties of Polymers," Wiley: New York, 1981.
20. Keller, K. H.; Andrade, J. D.; Baier, R. E.; Dillingham, E. O.; Ely, J.; Altieri, F. D.; Morrisey, B. W.; Klein, E. "Guidelines for Physicochemical Characterization of Biomaterials," National Heart, Lung, Blood Institute, N.I.H. pub. No. 80–2186, 1980.
21. Ratner, B. D. Chapter 2 in this book.
22. Autian, J. *Artif. Organs*, **1977**, *1*, 53.
23. Bruck, S. D. *J. Biomed. Mater. Res.* **1971**, *5*, 139.
24. Block, B.; Hastings, G. W. "Plastics in Surgery"; Thomas: Springfield, Illinois, 1967.
25. Yannas, I. V. et al. Chapter 29 this book.
26. Ratner, B. D.; Hoffman, A. S. In "Hydrogels for Medical and Related Applications," Andrade, J. D., Ed.; ACS Symposium Series, No. 31, American Chemical Society: Washington, DC, 1976; p. 1.

27. Ratner, B. D. In "Biocompatibility of Clinical Implant Materials," Williams, D. F., Ed.; CRC: Boca Raton, Florida, 1981.
28. Gregonis, D. E.; Chen, C. M.; Andrade, J. D. In "Hydrogels for Medical and Related Applications," Andrade, J. D., Ed.; ACS Symposium Series, No. 31, American Chemical Society: Washington, DC, 1976; p. 88.
29. Hoffman, A. S. *Radiat. Phys. Chem.*, **1977**, *9*, 207.
30. Pedley, D. G.; Skelby, P. J.; Tighe, B. J. *Br. Polym. J.* **1980**, *12*, 99.
31. Peppas, N. A.; Merrill, E. W. *J. Biomed. Mater. Res.* **1977**, *11*, 423.
32. Bruck, S. D. *J. Biomed. Mater. Res.* **1973**, *7*, 387.
33. Bruck, S. D. *Ann. N.Y. Acad. Sci.* **1977**, *283*, 332.
34. Ulrich, H.; Bonk, H. W.; Colovos, G. C. In "Synthetic Biomedical Polymers," Szycher, M.; Robinson, W. J., Eds.; Technomic: Westport, Connecticut, 1980; p. 29 and literature cited therein.
35. Phillips, W. M.; Pierce, W. S.; Rosenberg, G.; Donachy, J. H. In "Synthetic Biomedical Polymers," Szycher, M.; Robinson, W. J., Eds.; Technomic: Westport, Connecticut, 1980; p. 39.
36. Szycher, M.; Poirier, V.; Keiser, J. *Trans. Am. Soc. Artif. Intern. Organs* **1977**, *23*, 116.
37. Lyman, D. J.; Seare, W. J., Jr.; Albo, D., Jr.; Bergman, S.; Lamb, J.; Metcalf, L. C.; Richards, K. *Int. J. Polym. Mater.* **1977**, *5*, 211.
38. Brash, J. L.; Fritzinger, B. K.; Bruck, S. D. *J. Biomed. Mater. Res.* **1973**, *7*, 313.
39. Nyilas, E. *J. Biomed. Mater. Res.* **1972**, *6*, 97.
40. Nyilas, E.; Ward, R. S., Jr. *J. Biomed. Mater. Res.* **1977**, *11*, 69.
41. Leininger, R. I.; Epstein, M. M.; Falb, R. D.; Grode, G. A. *Trans. Am. Soc. Artif. Intern. Organs* **1966**, *12*, 151.
42. Grode, G. A.; Falb, R. D.; Crowley, J. P. *J. Biomed. Mater. Res.* **1972**, *6*, 77.
43. Merrill, E. W.; Salzman, E. W.; Wong, P. S. L.; Ashford, T. P.; Brown, A. H.; Austen, W. G. *J. Appl. Physiol.* **1970**, *29*, 723.
44. Peppas, N. A.; Gehr, T. W. B. *Trans. Am. Soc. Artif. Intern. Organs* **1978**, *24*, 404.
45. Holland, F. F.; Gidden, H. E.; Mason, R. G.; Klein, E. *Am. Soc. Artif. Intern. Organs* **1978**, *1*, 24.
46. Ohshiro, T.; Kosaki, G. *Artif. Organs* **1980**, *4*, 58.
47. Sugitachi, A.; Tanaka, M.; Kawahara, T.; Takagi, K. *Trans. Am. Soc. Artif. Intern. Organs* **1980**, *26*, 274.
48. Silver, F. H.; Yannas, I. V.; Salzman, E. W. *Thromb. Res.* **1978**, *13*, 267.
49. Sharp, W. V.; Teague, P. C.; Scott, D. L. *Trans. Am. Soc. Artif. Intern. Organs* **1978**, *24*, 223.
50. Bruck, S. D. *Int. J. Artif. Organs* **1979**, *2*, 31.
51. Allcock, H. R. *Acc. Chem. Res.* **1979**, *12*, 351.

RECEIVED for review June 15, 1981. ACCEPTED June 29, 1981.

29

Design Principles and Preliminary Clinical Performance of an Artificial Skin

I. V. YANNAS—Massachusetts Institute of Technology, Fibers and Polymers Laboratories, Department of Mechanical Engineering and Harvard–MIT Division of Health Sciences and Technology, Cambridge, MA 02139

J. F. BURKE—Massachusetts General Hospital and Harvard Medical School, Boston, MA 02114

M. WARPEHOSKI, P. STASIKELIS, E. M. SKRABUT, D. P. ORGILL and D. GIARD—Massachusetts Institute of Technology, Cambridge, MA 02139

We designed and successfully tested a novel family of polymeric membranes for treating patients with extensive skin loss. Stage 1 membranes consisted of a highly porous bottom layer of a covalently cross-linked collagen–glycosaminoglycan network and a top layer of a conventional silicone elastomer. Stage 2 membranes, studied so far only with guinea pigs, were prepared by seeding the bottom layer of Stage 1 membranes with autologous epidermal (basal) cells, prepared 4 h or less before grafting. Prompt and long-term closure of full-thickness skin wounds in guinea pigs and in humans occurred. Infection, exudation, and host–graft rejection were absent while synthesis of neoepidermal and neodermal tissue took place in the presence of the polymeric template.

Loss of skin exposes an organism directly to the environment. Such exposure reveals two vital functions of skin, namely, control of bacterial infection and of fluid loss. Unless treated, extensive skin loss can lead to death due to either of these causes. In the United States approximately 10,000 individuals die every year due to extensive skin loss sustained in a fire, while at least 130,000 others are treated in hospitals for extensive burns. Skin loss can, of course, also result from a large number of causes not related to fire injury.

0065-2393/82/0199-0475$06.00/0
© 1982 American Chemical Society

Being a highly differentiated organ with a multiplicity of functions, skin should not be looked at simply as a membrane that passively controls the traffic of bacteria and moisture at the interface between the individual and the environment. Skin is an actively metabolizing organ, and our work shows that attempts to design its replacement become successful if they incorporate this important fact. For convenience we have termed this replacement an artificial skin.

A 10-year effort to design an artificial skin (1) has yielded a bilayer polymeric membrane comprising a top silicone elastomeric layer and a bottom layer consisting of a novel, highly porous cross-linked collagen–glycosaminoglycan (GAG) network. The polymeric bilayer is termed a Stage 1 membrane, indicative of its ability to treat the needs of the patient immediately after and up to about 45 days following injury. A Stage 2 membrane prepared by seeding Stage 1 membranes with epidermal (basal) cells prior to grafting addresses the long-term needs of the patient, particularly the control of disfiguring scars and crippling contractures that normally result when a deep wound is not closed with an autograft.

We report the highlights of our effort to design and study Stage 1 membranes with animals and humans. A preliminary account of the performance of Stage 2 membranes is presented also.

Summary of Design Principles

Design Stages. A staged design corresponding to patient survival and patient rehabilitation, respectively, was used. Stage 1 is a wound closure that prevents, in a single application, bacterial infection and fluid loss even with the largest, full thickness injuries over a period of not less than 30 days. Stage 2 membranes are advanced versions of Stage 1 membranes capable, in addition, of controlling scar formation.

The Physical Chemistry of Wound Closure. The efficient wetting of the wound bed by the graft is essential. Without such wetting, microscopic air pockets lodge themselves at the graft–wound bed interface and form sites of bacterial proliferation (1). Wetting of a freshly excised wound bed can be achieved by reducing the bending rigidity of the membrane to a level that is sufficiently low to ensure draping over the rough wound bed as well as over surfaces of negative curvature (e.g., clavicle, popliteal region). In addition, the surface energy of the graft–air surface must be no higher than that of the wound–air surface.

Once achieved, this air-free graft–wound interface must be maintained. Two major events can destroy the intimate interfacial contact. The first is a history of mechanical loads, primarily shear forces and peel forces, to which a graft is accidentally exposed during clinical manipulations of the patient. The second is a force arising from shrinkage of the graft due to dehydration or, conversely, an internal peel force arising from swelling (edema) at the graft–wound bed interface caused by the inability of tissue moisture to escape.

These physicochemical properties were incorporated into a bilayer polymeric membrane. The top (silicone) layer renders the graft suturable and the grafted site aseptic, while the thickness of the layer is adjusted to provide the required optimal moisture flux rate (about 1 mg/cm^2/h). The bottom (collagen–GAG) layer is susceptible to degradation by enzymes, for example, collagenases, released by the wound and surrounding dermal tissue. Because this layer is highly porous, it is populated rapidly by mesenchymal cells that synthesize new connective tissue. Matching (2, 3) of the time constants for biodegradation and new tissue synthesis appears to be responsible for the observed development of substantial peel strengths, amounting to about 45 N/m (45 g/cm) 10 days after grafting. The controlled biochemical interaction between the collagen–GAG layer and the wound bed appears to be indispensable in maintaining the integrity of the graft–wound bed bond, thereby protecting the wound from infection and fluid loss.

Limiting Dimensions of the Graft. Migration of cells from the wound bed in a direction roughly normal to the plane of the membrane must be considered in light of two major parameters: mean pore size and thickness. If the characteristic pore size is lower than about 5 μm, the advance of migrating cells is limited by the biodegradation rate of the collagen–GAG matrix. On the other hand, if the thickness of a sufficiently porous nonvascularized layer exceeds a certain limit, the motility of migrating fibroblasts is limited by the diffusivity of critical nutrients originating at the wound bed (1).

In the event of adequate vascularization of the collagen–GAG layer, following migration of endothelial cells in it, nutrient transport can proceed via blood capillaries. A simple mathematical model based on the analysis of Thiele (4), and modified by Wagner (5) and Weisz (6), relating the reactivity and diffusive flow in porous catalyst particles can be used (1) to gain insight into this process.

The limiting dimension of the graft in the plane is determined primarily by the migration velocity of epithelial cell sheets advancing from the wound edge. At approximate speeds of about 0.25 mm/day, epithelial cell sheets advancing from opposite wound edges are observed to cover the surface of a wound with a length of 3 cm within about 60 days, a period that is barely acceptable clinically. This mechanism would be inadequate as a means of epithelializing massive wounds of about 30 cm resulting from extensive burns. One successful approach that we used involves seeding of the collagen–GAG layer, before grafting, with autologous epidermal cells. Following grafting, these cells proliferate in the sterile interior of the graft and form sheets of mature, keratinized epidermis. This approach appears to overcome the limitation with respect to length of wound that can be grafted effectively by a single application. The role of contraction as a process that accelerates wound closure was neglected in this qualitative discussion.

Constraints on the Selection of Chemical Components. The physicochemical, mechanical, and biochemical attributes of an effective lower layer appear to be met by a cross-linked collagen–chondroitin 6-sulfate network (7). A detailed rationale for use of these macromolecular components is presented elsewhere (1).

Experimental

The materials used and the detailed procedures employed in preparation of Stage 1 membranes are described elsewhere in detail (7–10). Stage 2 membranes were prepared by seeding the collagen–GAG layer of Stage 1 membranes with autologous epidermal (basal) cells. Epidermal cells were harvested from the animal, and basal cells were separated by the method of Prunieras et al. (11, 12). A suspension of cells was seeded into the porous collagen–GAG layer by a variety of methods, including inoculation using a hypodermic syringe and a centrifugal force field to drive the cells into the porous membrane. The entire procedure starting with cell harvest from the animal and ending with grafting of the seeded membrane on the animal lasted 4 h. Promptness of wound closure following skin injury was thereby maintained.

The animal model used was a 3 × 1.5–cm, full-thickness excised skin wound on the guinea pig, described elsewhere (1).

Human subjects, all victims of extensive burns, were grafted with segments of the bilayer membrane following primary excision of burned eschar. Techniques previously used with autografting (13) were generally used. Grafts were applied on the excised surface, free from devitalized tissue, on which meticulous hemostasis had been obtained. Following placement on the wound bed, grafts were carefully sutured under slight tension, avoiding wrinkling of the thin membrane.

Results

Grafting of Full-Thickness Wounds in Guinea Pigs. Results obtained by grafting more than 120 animals with Stage 1 membranes showed clear differences between the performance of the bilayer membrane described here and that of the allograft. By Day 14, the allograft was generally well on its way to being rejected as the wound was undergoing strong contraction. By contrast, 3 × 1.5–cm wounds covered with the bilayer membrane showed little contraction on that day, and the gross appearance of the graft gave no evidence of rejection. Histological study of the region grafted with the bilayer membrane showed no evidence of rejection over the entire period of observation of grafted animals (up to 400 days). No immunosuppression was used.

Significant delay in onset of wound contraction occurred with wounds grafted with Stage 1 membranes compared to the ungrafted controls. We observed a delay in "half-life" of the 3 × 1.5–cm wound (the time necessary for the wound area to contract to 50% of the original area) from about 13 days with the ungrafted controls to about 28 days with grafted wounds.

The histological evidence shows that epidermal migration consistently occurred over, rather than under, the bottom (collagen–GAG) layer of Stage 1 membranes. Coverage of the bottom layer of the 3 × 1.5–cm graft by the advancing epidermis was complete by Days 30 to 40. The top (silicone) layer of the graft was ejected spontaneously at about the same time, revealing a scar, while the histological evidence clearly indicated completion of epithelialization over the entire area.

Recently, Stage 2 membranes were used successfully in animal studies to seed the wound bed with autologous epidermal (basal) cells (see Experimental section). When transferred to the wound bed, which was maintained sterile by the grafted membrane, inoculated basal cells migrated extensively and formed confluent sheets of mature, keratinized epidermis at the interface between the silicone layer and the collagen–GAG layer. Most of the epidermal sheet formation occurred in locations that were clearly removed from the wound edge. Formation of mature, keratinized epidermis occured in less than 2 weeks following grafting of the full-thickness wound by the cell-inoculated polymeric membrane. This finding suggests that the additional manipulation of inoculating Stage 1 membranes with autologous epidermal cells extends almost indefinitely the area of skin loss that can be closed by a single application of this bilayer membrane.

Grafting of Human Subjects. Seven extensively burned (50 to 95% body area) human subjects, 5- to 60-year-old males and females, were grafted with rectangular pieces of cell-free Stage 1 membrane, ranging from 5 × 10 to 15 × 25 cm. The grafts remained in place from 25 to 46 days. During this period no infection or inflammation was noted, and no immunosuppression was used. Occasional lifting of the edge of the graft was treated as with an autograft (13), by debriding the edge. Whenever the graft was next to intact epidermis, the epidermal edge migrated between the two layers of the membranes over a distance of a few millimeters. Between 25 and 46 days following grafting the silicone layer was removed, and thin layers of autoepidermal grafts were harvested and placed on top of the neodermal tissue that had replaced the original collagen–GAG layer. This procedure left minimal scarring both at the donor site and at the graft site. A detailed discussion of the human studies appears elsewhere (14).

Discussion

Experiments with animals have shown that closure of 3 × 1.5–cm, full-thickness skin wounds with Stage 1 membranes provides prompt, reliable protection against infection and fluid loss by a single application. Subsequent removal is not necessary. These findings are the first successful effort to promptly close large, full-thickness wounds, not requiring replacement or the use of an autograft.

Promptness of closure of full-thickness skin wounds is essential. Failure to close large wounds satisfactorily within 3–7 days following injury increases mortality significantly (15). Recently, cultured autologous epidermal cells (16) and a reconstituted collagen lattice populated with cultured autologous fibroblasts and epidermal cells (17) were grafted onto full-thickness skin wounds in humans 5 weeks following cell harvesting (16), or were grafted on rats at least 2 weeks following cell harvesting (17). Because they require culturing of cells prior to grafting, these interesting procedures (16, 17) do not appear to meet the criterion of promptness of wound closure following injury.

In contrast, Stage 1 membranes are available in sterile containers and are ready for use in a matter of minutes. Stage 2 membranes (see Experimental section) require no more than a 4-h interval between harvesting of cells and grafting, because cells seeded into the membranes before grafting are cultured inside the graft, which is maintained sterile by the silicone membrane, rather than outside of it. This seeding procedure yields, therefore, a graft that induces the wound tissue itself to generate new tissue in vivo. There is no dependence on an ex vivo tissue culture medium to generate such tissue during a lengthy procedure before grafting. Promptness of treatment is thereby assured by using these bilayer polymer membranes.

Long-term function is also an important characteristic of a skin graft. Currently, cadaver skin, maintained in a frozen skin bank (18), is used successfully as an adequate but temporary wound closure. Cadaver skin is normally used with immunosuppression, in order to delay host–graft rejection, but such treatement greatly increases the risk of infection. In contrast with cadaver grafts, porcine skin grafts are commercially available, but they are normally removed between the third and ninth days. Several membranes based on synthetic and natural polymers have been used, but failure to control infection has been a consistent problem. Autografting remains a standard treatment because it provides for functional replacement of skin over an indefinite period of time. Nevertheless, harvesting of a split-thickness autograft is a serious operation and, in cases where the injury is massive, sufficient autograft is unavailable. Lastly, harvesting of a split-thickness autograft normally leaves a scarred donor site.

Stage 1 membranes are not rejected and therefore appear to be superior to cadaver and porcine skin grafts. In studies of Stage 1 membranes with extensively burned humans, the silicone (top) layer was electively removed between 25 and 46 days after grafting and replaced by autoepidermal grafts. This procedure eventually yielded a relatively scar-free donor site and a largely scar-free treatment site that appeared to require no further manipulation.

Stage 2 membranes, studied so far only with animals, do not appear to require eventual replacement of the silicone layer by autoepidermal grafts. Instead, these advanced membranes induce wound tissue to construct both neoepidermal and neodermal tissue, thereby leading to an apparently functional reconstruction of skin (19). Therefore, Stage 2 membranes appear to compare favorable in performance with the autograft itself. Development of these membranes is in progress.

Acknowledgment

This work was supported in part by NIH grants HL 14322, GM 23946, and GM 21700. We thank V. M. Ingram, F. O. Schmitt, and R. L. Trelstad for useful discussions.

Literature Cited

1. Yannas, I. V.; Burke, J. F. *J. Biomed. Mater. Res.* **1980**, *14*, 65–81.
2. Yannas, I. V.; Burke, J. F.; Umbreit, M.; Stasikelis, P. *Fed. Proc.*, **1979**, *38*, 988.
3. Yannas, I.V.; Burke, J. F.; Huang, C.; Gordon, P. L. *J. Biomed. Mater. Res.* **1975**, *9*, 623–628.
4. Thiele, E. W. *Ind. Eng. Chem., Ind. Ed.* **1939**, *31*, 916–920.
5. Wagner, C. Z. *Phys. Chem. (Leipzig)* **1943**, *193*, 1–5.
6. Weisz, P. B.; Prater, C. D. In "Advances in Catalysis and Related Subjects;" Frankenburg, W. G.; Komerewsky, V. I.; Rideal, E., Ed. Academic: New York, 1954. Vol. 6, pp. 143–196.
7. Yannas, I. V.; Burke, J. F.; Gordon, P. L.; Huang, C.; Rubenstein, R. H. *J. Biomed, Mater. Res.* **1980**, *14*, 511–528.
8. Dagalakis, N.; Fink, J.; Stasikelis, P.; Burke, J. F.; Yannas, I. V. *J. Biomed. Mater. Res.* **1980**, *14*, 511–528.
9. Yannas, I. V.; Burke, J. F.; Huang, C.; Gordon, P. L. *Am. Chem. Soc., Polymer Prepr.* (Chicago, Aug., 1975), *16*(2), 209–214.
10. Yannas, I. V.; Burke, J. F.; Gordon, P. L.; Huang, C. US Patent 4060081, 1977; Yannis, I. V.; Gordon, P. L.; Huang, C.; Silver, F. H.; Burke, J. F., U.S. Patent 42 80954, 1981.
11. Prunieras, M.; Delescluse, C.; Regnier, M. *J. Invest. Dermatol.* **1976**, *67*, 58–65.
12. Regnier, M.; Delescluse, C.; Prunieras, M. *Acta Dermatovener (Stockholm)* **1973**, *53*, 241–247.
13. Burke, J. F.; Bondoc, C. C.; Quinby, W. C. *J. Trauma* **1974**, *14*, 389–394.
14. Burke, J. F.; Yannis, I. V.; Quinby, W. C.; Bondoc, C. C.; Jung, W. K. *Ann. Surg.* **1981**, *194*, 413–428.
15. Shires, G. T.; Black, E. A. *J. Trauma* **1979**, *19*, 855–936
16. O'Connor, N. E.; Mulliken, J. B.; Banks-Schlegel, S.; Kehinde, O.; Green, H. *Lancet* **1981**–I, 75–78.
17. Bell, E.; Ehrlich, H. P.; Buttle, D. J.; Nakatsumi, T. *Science* **1981**, *211*, 1052–1054.
18. Bondoc, C. C.; Burke, J. F. *Ann. Surg.* **1971**, *158*, 371.
19. Yannis, I. V.; Burke, J. F.; Orgill, D. P.; Skrabut, E. M. *Science* **1982**, *215*, 174–176.

Received for review January 16, 1981. Accepted July 11, 1981.

30

Collagenase Immobilized on Cellulose Acetate Membranes

Y. CHEN, N. S. MASON, and R. E. SPARKS

Washington University, Department of Chemical Engineering, St. Louis, MO 63130

D. W. SCHARP and W. F. BALLINGER

Washington University, Department of Surgery, St. Louis, MO 63130

> *Collagenase covalently attached to cellulose acetate membranes, following periodate activation of the membrane, maintained its enzymatic activity and permanence of attachment for more than 6 weeks. The length of spacer between the enzyme and the membrane was studied with enzymes attached directly, through ethylenediamine and through ethylenediamine plus succinnic anhydride. Enzyme activity was measured by determining the degradation rate of a pigskin gelatin solution, and stability of the bond was measured by observing continued degradation after the enzyme–membrane was removed from the solution. The longest spacer resulted in the highest enzyme activity.*

Interest is growing rapidly in supplying blood glucose control in diabetics through the use of chambers in which Islets of Langerhans are interfaced with the blood supply through a permeable membrane. The object is to provide adequate insulin release in response to blood glucose, while isolating the cells from immune response. Consideration is being given to both intravascular and extravascular islet-transplantation chambers.

A problem that arises in the consideration of an extravascular device is that synthetic materials placed in the body tissues rapidly become covered with cells (polymorphonuclear leukocytes and macrophages) and surrounded with relatively impervious fibrous tissue. This could decrease the diffusion rates of glucose and insulin, eventually rendering a chamber useless. One possible solution to this problem is the attachment of proteolytic enzymes to the surface of the chamber to prevent formation and attachment of fibrous tissue at the interface.

It was reported by Jolley (1) that a cellulosic chamber (Millipore Corporation) coated with covalently bound collagenase and implanted in the rat peritoneal cavity had stayed sufficiently permeable to maintain some of the enclosed dog islet cells viable in the chamber for 6 months. The major problem was the growth of fibroblasts, which were contaminants in the transplanted islet suspension, inside the chamber. Visual evidence indicated a striking difference in the appearance of the chambers with and without the bound enzymes. The control chambers were covered with white, dense tissue, whereas the chambers having the surface-bound enzymes were surrounded with relatively transparent gelatinous material. Apparently, the bound collagenase did not permit the initiation of tissue organization.

Islet isolation methods that yield islets free of contaminating fibroblasts now have been developed. Successful prevention of the growth of dense fibrous tissue on extravascular chambers containing these purified islets would raise new possibilities in the design of islet-transplantation chambers. This chapter contains the initial results of binding enzymes to Millipore AA cellulose ester membranes for application in such chambers. The enzyme chosen for study was collagenase from *Clostridium histolyticum* (Worthington Biochemicals, Inc.).

Enzyme Attachment

The methods of attaching enzymes covalently to insoluble functionalized polymers have been reviewed by Zaborsky (2). The most frequently used methods for cellulosic substrates involve activation in base with cyanogen bromide, resulting in a reactive imidocarbonate $\begin{array}{c}-O \\ -O\end{array}\!\!\!>\!C=NH$, activation with sodium nitrite, resulting in an activated azide $OC(=O)N_3$, or activation with cyanuric chloride leading to the s-triazinyl derivative of cellulose:

$$-O-\underset{\underset{Cl}{N}}{\overset{N}{\underset{\|}{\bigcirc}}}-Cl$$

A recent method reported by Royer et al. (3), involves peridoate oxidation in cold borate buffer at pH 4 to obtain adjacent aldehyde groups on some of the anhydroglucose units. Attachment of the enzyme is then through the formation of a Schiff base with a primary amine group on the enzyme, followed by reduction with sodium borohydride. This binding method was chosen because it avoids the possible degradation of the cellulose ester in basic conditions such as those employed in cyanogen bromide activation. One set of test membranes was produced by binding the enzyme directly to the activated substrate. These membranes are referred to as "direct-coupled membranes."

Cuatrecasas et at. (4) and Schmer (5) found that an increase in the extent of binding and in biological activity sometimes resulted if there was a spacer or "arm" between the substrate and the biologically active molecule. In a second test membrane, formed to test for this effect, a spacer was introduced between the substrate and the enzyme by first binding ethylenediamine to the activated cellulosic substrate and then coupling the amine to the enzyme through a carboxyl group on the enzyme using a water-soluble carbodiimide, 1-(3-dimethylaminopropyl)-3-ethylcarbodiimide hydrochloride, as described by Cuatrescasas (6). The reactions are

$$R'-N=C=N-R'' + HO\overset{O}{\underset{\|}{C}}-ENZ \rightarrow \begin{array}{c} R' \\ | \\ HN \\ \diagdown \\ C-O\overset{O}{\underset{\|}{C}}-ENZ \\ \diagup \\ HN \\ | \\ R'' \end{array}$$

$$>\!\!CH-NH-(CH_2)_2-NH_2 \;+\; \begin{array}{c} R' \\ | \\ HN \\ \diagdown \\ C-O\overset{O}{\underset{\|}{C}}-ENZ \rightarrow \\ \diagup \\ HN \\ | \\ R'' \end{array}$$

$$>\!\!CH-NH-(CH_2)_2-NH-\overset{O}{\underset{\|}{C}}-ENZ \;+\; \begin{array}{c} R' \\ | \\ HN \\ \diagdown \\ C=O + H^+ \\ \diagup \\ HN \\ | \\ R'' \end{array}$$

The enzyme–membrane products formed by these reactions are called "aminoethyl-coupled membranes."

To provide a test of the effect of spacer length on enzyme activity, a third membrane–enzyme system was formed by reacting the product of the reaction between ethylenediamine and the cellulose ester membrane with succinyl anhydride, then coupling this product to an amine on the enzyme using the carbodiimide route. The product may be represented as:

$$\diagdown\!\!\!\!\text{CH}\!-\!\text{NH}\!-\!(\text{CH}_2)_2\!-\!\text{NH}\!-\!\overset{\overset{\text{O}}{\|}}{\text{C}}\!-\!(\text{CH}_2)_2\!-\!\overset{\overset{\text{O}}{\|}}{\text{C}}\!-\!\text{NH}\!-\!\text{ENZ}$$

These membranes were referred to as "succinyl aminoethyl–coupled membranes."

Enzyme–Membrane Testing

Activity and Stability of the Enzyme–Membrane Bond. The activity of soluble collagenase is generally determined with solid bovine achilles tendon collagen as the substrate by measuring the amount of L-leucine liberated. This is a specific test that distinguishes collagenase from other proteases, as shown by Decker (7). Due to the difficulty of contacting a bound enzyme with a solid substrate, a solution of gelatin, a degraded form of collagen, was used as the substrate to test the activity and stability of the bound enzymes.

The enzyme–membranes were placed in a well-agitated 1–2 wt % pigskin gelatin (pI ~ 8.5 where pI is the pH of the isoelectric point of the gelatin) solution at 25°C and also at 37°C. After varying periods of time the reduced viscosity of the solution was measured with a Cannon–Ubbelohde No. 1 capillary viscometer. The decrease in viscosity of the gelatin solutions containing enzyme–membranes was compared to the viscosity decrease of control solutions and solutions to which a known amount of soluble enzyme was added.

To test for the stability of enzyme attachment, the membrane was removed from the gelatin solution, and the solution viscosity measurements continued as a function of time. Any subsequent decrease in solution viscosity measured how much unbound or poorly bound enzyme was present on the membrane.

Figure 1 contains the data from four consecutive tests of the enzymatic activity of control membranes (no bound enzyme) and the aminoethyl-coupled and succinyl aminoethyl–coupled membrane systems. Between each section of the test, the membrane was removed from the gelatin solution, rinsed with deionized water, and then placed in a fresh gelatin solution. This is indicated in Figure 1 by the vertical arrows at the bottom of the figure. The viscosity of the remaining solution is indicated by the dashed lines. The first three tests were carried out with a 1 wt % gelatin solution, and the fourth test with a 1.5 wt % gelatin solution.

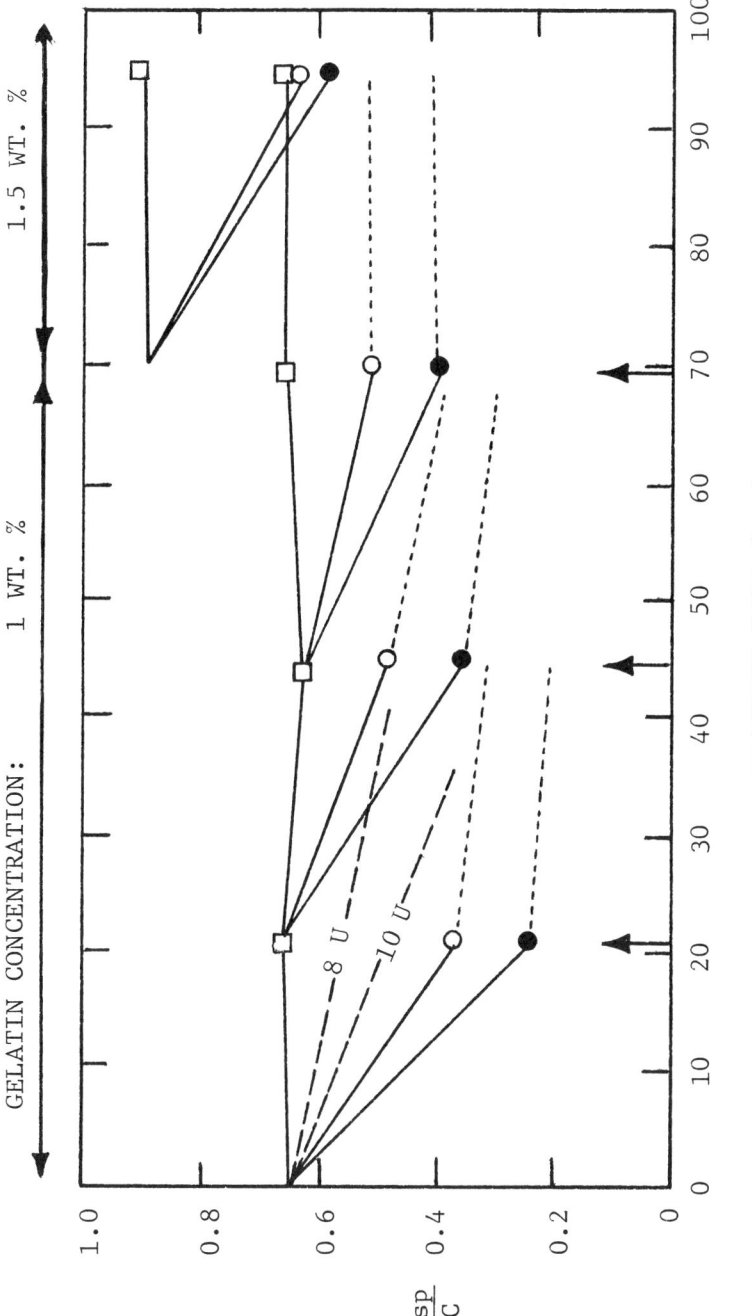

Figure 1. Binding stability of collagenase to Millipore membrane at 37° C. Key: □, control; ○, aminoethyl-coupled membrane; ●, succinyl aminoethyl-coupled membrane; ———, enzyme solution (calibration); and - - -, supernatant, after removing membrane.

The solution viscosity decreased substantially only when the membrane was immersed in the solution, indicating that most of the enzymatic activity is associated with bound enzymes. The high activity of the membrane remaining at 96 h and the lack of residual enzyme in solution at that time indicate that the membrane–enzyme bond is stable. The membrane contains approximately 1 U of active enzyme per cm^2, estimated from a comparison of the reactivities of the bound enzyme and the free enzyme. The enzyme attached to the membrane by the longest spacer, in the succinyl aminoethyl-coupled membrane system, exhibited the highest activity.

Long-Term Enzyme Stability. The activity of the bound enzyme for over 900 h is shown in Figure 2. The data indicate that only a small decrease in activity occurs during this time; hence, long-term stability appears to be obtainable. [The differences in initial viscosity of the gelatin solutions are due to slight differences in solution preparation at 25°C where gelatin is known to form intermolecular networks, mainly through hydrogen bonds, as shown by Pouradier and Venet (8).]

Enzyme Kinetics. The change in the number-average molecular weight of gelatin with time was determined as follows. Measurements of viscosity at known concentrations were extrapolated to infinite dilution to obtain the intrinsic viscosity $\{\eta\}$ from Huggins and Kramer's equations,

$$\frac{\eta_{sp}}{C} = \{\eta\} + K'\{\eta\}^2 C \tag{1}$$

$$\frac{\ln \eta_r}{C} = \{\eta\} - K''\{\eta\}^2 C \tag{2}$$

where K' and K'' were determined by calibration with five different samples of partially degraded gelatin (0.354 and −0.146, respectively).

The number-average molecular weight was obtained from the intrinsic viscosity, through the Mark–Howink equation, with constants determined by Pouradier and Venet (9) on a similar photographic-grade gelatin. Thus,

$$\{\eta\} = 1.66 \times 10^{-5} \{M_n\}^{0.885} \tag{3}$$

The data for change in molecular weight with time do not follow Michaelis–Menten kinetics, but appear to follow pseudo first-order kinetics, expressed as

$$\frac{dM_n}{dt} = -k\, M_n \tag{4}$$

where k is a function of the enzyme activity per unit area of the membrane. When k was examined as a function of time (Figure 3), an initial rapid change in enzyme activity was observed. However, the rate stabilized after about 100 h. The few data points for the direct-coupled membrane indicated that it was only slightly less active than the aminoethyl-coupled membrane, whereas the succinyl aminoethyl–coupled membrane maintained a rate constant 50% higher than that of the aminoethyl-coupled membrane. Hence, the longest spacer had a definite and persistent effect in permitting a faster reaction rate.

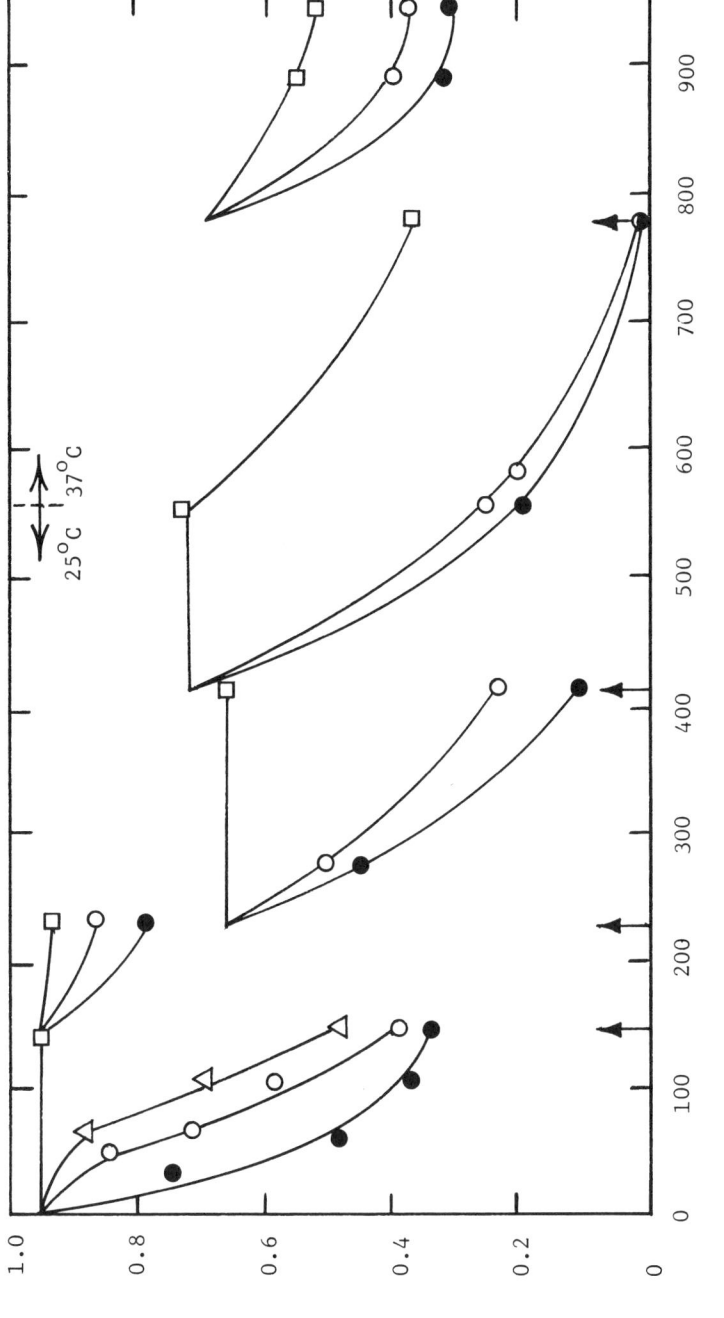

Figure 2. Long-term tests of bound enzyme activity. Key: □, control; ○, aminoethyl-coupled membrane; ●, succinyl aminoethyl-coupled membrane; and △, direct-coupled membrane.

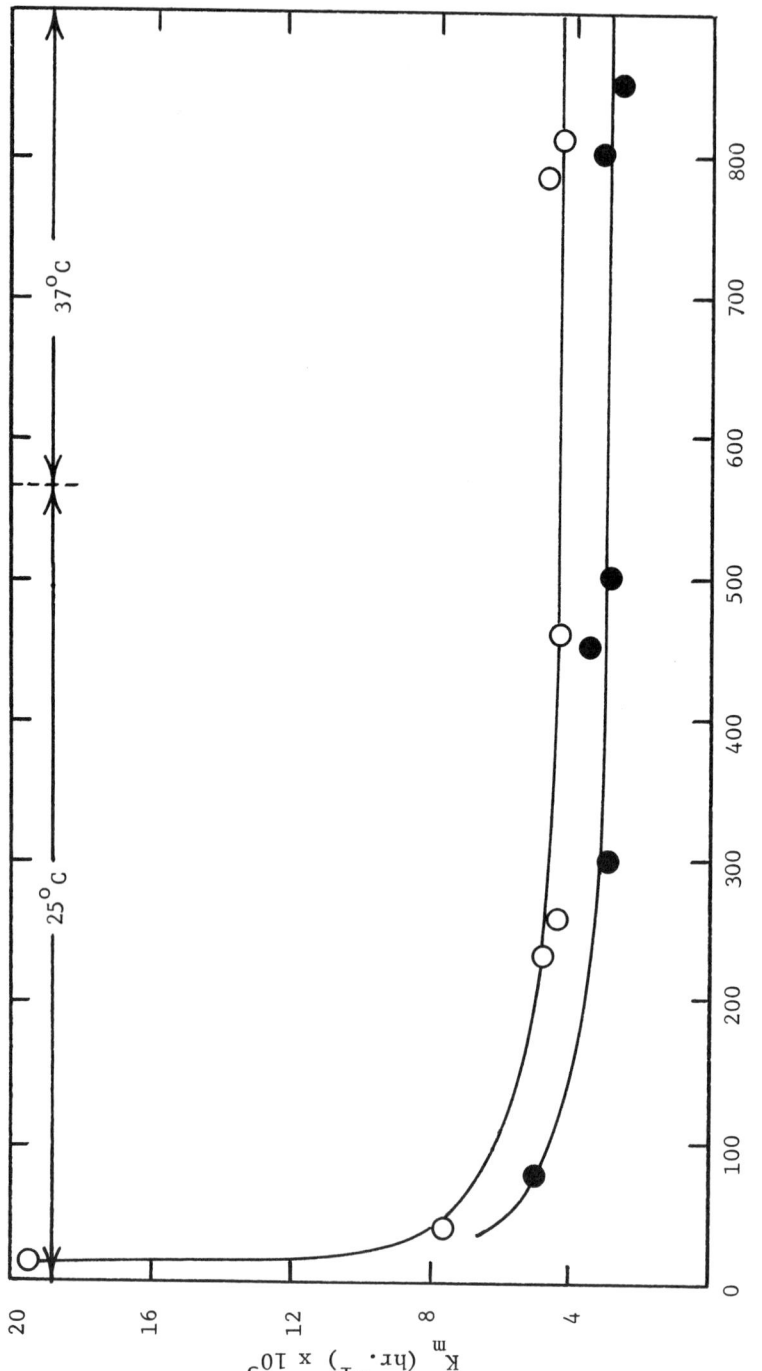

Figure 3. Change in first-order constant with time. Key: ○, *succinyl aminoethyl-coupled membrane and* ●, *aminoethyl-coupled membrane.*

Conclusions

- Gentle periodate oxidation is effective for activation of cellulose ester polymers in preparation for reaction with enzymes.
- Enzymes can be readily bound to these activated polymers using carbodiimides.
- Gelatin degradation is attactive as an indicator of proteolytic enzyme activity.
- Bonds between enzymes and cellulose ester membranes are stable for many weeks, and enzyme activity is retained for many weeks.
- The longest spacer permits the highest enzymatic activity in these enzyme–membrane systems.

Literature Cited

1. Jolley W. B.; Hinshaw, D. B.; Cole, T. W.; Alvoid, L. F. *Transplant Proc.* **1977**, *9*, 363.
2. Zaborsky, O. R. "Immobilized Enzymes": CRC: Cleveland, 1973.
3. Royer, G. P.; Liberatore, F. M.; Green, G. M. *Biochem. Biophys. Res. Comun.* **1975**, *64*, 478.
4. Cuatrecasas, P.; Wilcheck, M.; Anfisen, C. B. *Proc. Natl. Acad. Sci. U.S.A.* **1968**, *61*, 636.
5. Schmer, G. *Trans. Am. Soc. Artif. Intern. Organs* **1972**, *18*, 321.
6. Cuatrecasas, P. *J. Biol. Chem.* **1970**, *245*, 3059.
7. Decker, L. A. "Worthington Enzyme Manual," Worthington Biochemicals, Inc.: Freehold, N.J., 1977.
8. Pouradier, J.; Venet, A. M. *J. Chim. Phys.* **1950**, *47*, 13.
9. Pouradier, J.; Venet, A. M. *J. Chim. Phys.* **1952**, *49*, 87.

RECEIVED for review February 24, 1981. ACCEPTED May 14, 1981.

31

A System for Heparin Removal

R. LANGER

Massachusetts Institute of Technology, Department of Nutrition and Food Science, Cambridge, MA 02139 and Children's Hospital Medical Center, Department of Surgery, Boston, MA 02115

R. J. LINHARDT, P. M. GALLIHER, M. M. FLANAGAN, and C. L. COONEY

Massachusetts Institute of Technology, Department of Nutrition and Food Science, Cambridge, MA 02139

M. D. KLEIN

University of Michigan, Section of Pediatric Surgery, Ann Arbor, MI 48109

> *Extracorporeal medical machines rely on systemic heparinization to improve blood compatibility. However, heparin can lead to serious complications such as hemorrhaging. We propose a new approach to control heparin levels by employing a blood filter containing immobilized heparinase. Such a filter could potentially enable heparinization of an extracorporeal circuit without simultaneous heparinization of the patient. The principal findings of our work thus far include (1) increasing volumetric enzyme production over 1000-fold from previously published procedures; (2) purifying heparinase by over 1000-fold from the crude cell extracts; (3) characterizing the biochemical properties of heparinase; (4) isolating the first heparinase inhibitors; (5) immobilizing heparinase with 91% activity recovery and excellent stability; and (6) demonstrating that columns as small as 1.5 mL can remove clinically used quantities of heparin in aqueous medium and in blood.*

Extracorporeal medical machines (e.g., artificial kidney, pump-oxygenator) perfused with blood have been an effective part of the therapeutic armamentarium for many years. These devices all rely on systemic heparinization to provide blood compatibility. Despite continuous efforts to improve anticoagulation techniques, many patients still develop coagulation abnormalities with the use of these devices (1–3). Even longer perfusion times may occur with machines such as the membrane oxygenator. In such cases, the drawbacks of systemic heparinization are multiplied (4). A number of approaches have been attempted to solve this problem. These include: (1) administration of compounds to neutralize heparin (5); (2) development of heparin substitutes (6); (3) bonding of heparin (7–12) or other substances (13) to the extracorporeal device; and (4) development of new blood–compatible materials for construction of the extracorporeal device (14). In spite of these efforts, heparinization continues to be used extensively in all extracorporeal treatments, and control of blood heparin levels remains a serious problem.

We propose a new approach that would allow the full heparinization of the extracorporeal device, yet could enable, on-demand, elimination of heparin in the patient's bloodstream. This approach consists of a blood filter containing immobilized heparinase, which could be placed at the effluent of any extracorporeal device (Figure 1). Such a filter could theoretically be used to eliminate heparin after it had served its purpose in the extracorporeal device and before it returned to the patient. In this chapter we discuss our efforts to develop such a filter. Our work has focused on several areas: (1) enzyme production; (2) enzyme purification; (3) characterization of heparinase; (4) immobilization of heparinase; and (5) in vitro testing of immobilized heparinase.

Experimental

Materials. Heparin, as the sodium salt, from porcine intestinal mucosa, was purchased from Sigma Chemical Co. (Grade II, 153 USP k units). Azure A dye was purchased from Fisher Scientific Co. (A-970, certified biological stain, total dye content 70%).

The following polymer supports used in the immobilization were obtained preactivated: (1) Sepharose-CNBr 4B from Pharmacia; (2) polyacrylamide polyacetyl and enzacryl AH from Aldrich Chemical Co.; and (3) polyacrylamide NHS active ester (PAN 1000) as a gift from George M. Whitesides, MIT, Department of Chemistry.

The unactivated polymer supports were obtained from the following sources: (1) poly(2-hydroxyethyl methacrylate) (PHEMA) from Polysciences Inc. and PHEMA (Spheron) from Hydron Inc.; (2) Dacron (poly(ethyleneterephthalate)) from Aldrich Chemical Company; (3) poly(methyl (methacrylate) (PMA) 7% divinyl benzene cross-linked) from Rohm and Haas Company; and (4) silicone (Masterflex silicone tubing) from Cole-Parmer. The activating agents used were: (1) cyanogen bromide (CNBr), hexamethylene diisocyanate, and Woodwards K reagent from Aldrich Chemical Company; (2) 1-ethyl-3-(3-dimethylaminopropyl)carbodiimide (EDC) from Calbiochem–Behring Corporation; (3) glutaraldehyde (EM grade 25%) from Polysciences, Inc.; and (4) organosilane ester (A-1100) from Union Carbide Corporation, Silicones division.

The heparinase inhibitors were purchased from the following sources: (1) poly(vinyl sulfate) from Sigma Chemical Company; (2) polyanethole sulfonate from Calbiochem Corporation; and (3) polystyrene sulfonate (aqueous solution MW 70,000) from Polysciences Inc.

The purification used hydroxylapatite (HTP) from Biorad Inc., protamine sulfate, bovine serum albumin (BSA), and polylysine (Type VI) from Sigma Chemical Company, and epoxy-activated Sepharose from Pharmacia Inc. Sodium dodecyl sulfate (SDS) gel electrophoresis and isoelectric focusing (IEF) were performed using chemicals and equipment from Biorad Inc.

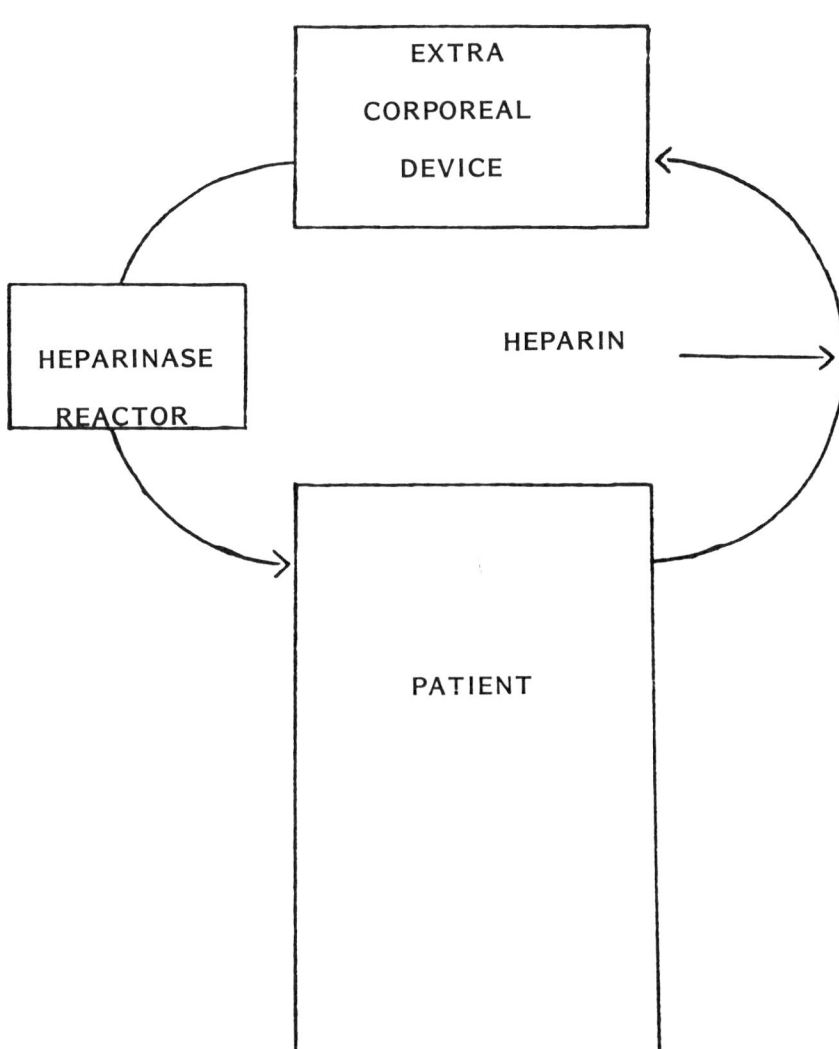

Figure 1. Proposed heparin circuit. The extracorporeal device could be a renal dialysis unit or a pump-oxygenator. The heparinase reactor could be part of a blood filter to be used either continuously (in which case heparin would be added continuously at the start of the circuit) or at the end of an operation. Heparin could thus be confined to the extracorporeal circuit.

Chondroitinase ABC from *Proteus vulgaris* was purchased from Sigma Chemical Company. All inorganic chemicals were reagent grade.

All chemicals used in heparinase production are as described previously (15).

Analytical Determinations. PROTEIN CONTENT. Protein was measured by the method of Lowry (16).

HEPARINASE ACTIVITY. Several assays were used to follow heparinase activity. These assays followed (1) the disappearance of heparin, (2) the appearance of heparin degradation products, or (3) the loss of the physiological function of heparin in anticoagulation. The basis of these assays and explanations as to when they are routinely used are listed below.

1. *Metachromasia in Azure A.* This assay measures heparinase activity by following the disappearance of heparin. Jacques (17) proposed that Azure A dye molecules dimerize in the presence of heparin, resulting in a decrease in the π-delocalization. This effect is observed as a shift in the absorption maximum from λ max = 620 nm to λ max = 520 nm. Since heparinase cleaves the α-linkage of heparin, its action causes chain shortening, resulting in less metachromasia. The presence of heparin or heparin-derived polysaccharide chains of hexasaccharide or larger (18) can be measured easily and reproducibly at levels of 1–10 μg/mL in crude (i.e., fermentation broths and cell sonicates) and purified preparations. Experimental details for utilizing this assay were reported in a previous publication (15).

2. a. *Reducing Sugar Assay.* With each cleavage of the heparin chain by heparinase (which is an α-eliminase), one reducing end group is formed and one α-β-unsaturated end group. The increase in reducing capacity, therefore, gives a measure of enzyme activity and product formation. This assay has been used routinely in assaying crude preparations of heparinase. The reducing capacity of the products produced from heparin at different stages in the purification of heparinase is variable. For example, the reducing capacity of products produced by the action of purified heparinase is lower than that obtained by the action of crude heparinase preparations. This result is apparently due to enzymes in crude preparations that cause further degradation of the products formed by heparinase. The Park and Johnson method (19) of measuring reducing sugars was used throughout these studies.

b. *Ultraviolet Assay.* The α-β-unsaturated acid end group resulting from heparin cleavage is a chromophore with a λ max at approximately 232 nm and a molar absorptivity of about $5 \times 10^5 \, M^{-1}$ (20). The action of heparinase can be measured by sampling the reaction mixture, quenching it in 0.03N hydrochloric acid, and measuring the absorbance. This assay can only be used to measure activity in relatively pure preparations due to two factors: (1) high concentration of protein interferes with the measurement of product, and (2) contaminating enzymes are capable of acting on the heparinase-derived product, resulting in the loss of the chromophore being measured. Because of its accuracy and ease of performing, this assay was the method of choice for measuring heparinase activity in the more purified heparinase preparations.

3. *Assays Measuring the Loss of Heparin's Biological Activity.* The loss of heparin's biological activity through the action of heparinase can be tested by a number of available assays. Three assays were chosen for their ease of use and the range of activity they measure. Whole blood recalcification time (21) involves the measurement of heparin in citrated whole blood by recalcifying the blood and measuring the clotting time. Factor X_a Assay (22) involves measuring the heparin in citrated plasma which has been enriched in Factor X_a by recalcifying and measuring the clotting time. Thrombin–antithrombin time (23) determines the action of heparin on the thrombin–antithrombin interaction by measuring the appearance of the chromophore released by thrombin from a synthetic polypeptide substrate. In each of these assays a standard curve was constructed with each determination.

Results

Heparinase Production. The objective of these studies was to develop an understanding of what factors influence heparinase production by *Flavobacterium heparinum* (15). This was done by studying the kinetics of microbial growth and heparinase production, and by developing a simple, defined medium to support this growth and production. A 1000-fold increase in volumetric heparinase production over previously reported results was obtained by implementing improved techniques of microbial cultivation and environmental and genetic manipulations. These improvements and our findings are summarized below.

The wild type strain of *Flavobacterium heparinum* produces a nonextracellular heparinase in the growth stage only when heparin is supplied to the growth medium as an inducer (15). Enzyme production occurs during growth, so factors affecting growth can directly affect enzyme production. A reliable heparinase production scheme was first worked out by growing the bacteria in a complex protein digest medium. Inducer was provided at the time of inoculation of the sterile medium. Growth was initially exponential, and heparin was rapidly taken up by the cell at a rate of 1.1 g/g cell-h (Figure 2). Enzyme specific activity began to increase just as heparin uptake was finishing, and increased at a volumetric rate of 375 units/L-h. At the onset of the stationary cell growth phase, enzyme production stopped, and a deactivation was observed, resulting in an 86% loss of total activity within 4 h. To avoid this deactivation, the kinetics of enzyme production had to be understood. Timely harvest was thus important to obtain highly active heparinase. Fifteen fermentations were performed, all yielding a total enzyme level on the average of 9600 units of heparinase/L of fermentor broth, demonstrating the reliability of this method.

To understand better the environmental factors governing enzyme production, a defined growth medium was developed. This medium was the result of nutritional requirement experiments performed to elucidate the growth factors required by this bacterium. The bacterium was a histidine auxotroph with an additional (though not obligate) requirement for methionine. No vitamin requirement was observed. This result permitted the use of the following defined growth medium: glucose (main carbon source), heparin (inducer), $(NH_4)_2SO_4$ (nitrogen source), K_2HPO_4, Na_2HPO_4, L-histidine, L-methionine, trace salts, and $MgSO_4 \cdot 7H_2O$. A 30% increase in growth rate was observed using this medium. Volumetric heparinase production was increased fourfold over the complex medium production to 1480 units/L-h. Additionally, higher cell densities were obtained routinely in this defined medium. A typical production run using 20 g/L of glucose results in a tenfold increase in total enzyme obtained to 96,000 units/L fermentor broth. This fermentation has been repeated eight times to date, demonstrating the reliability of this method. In addition, the product heparinase is

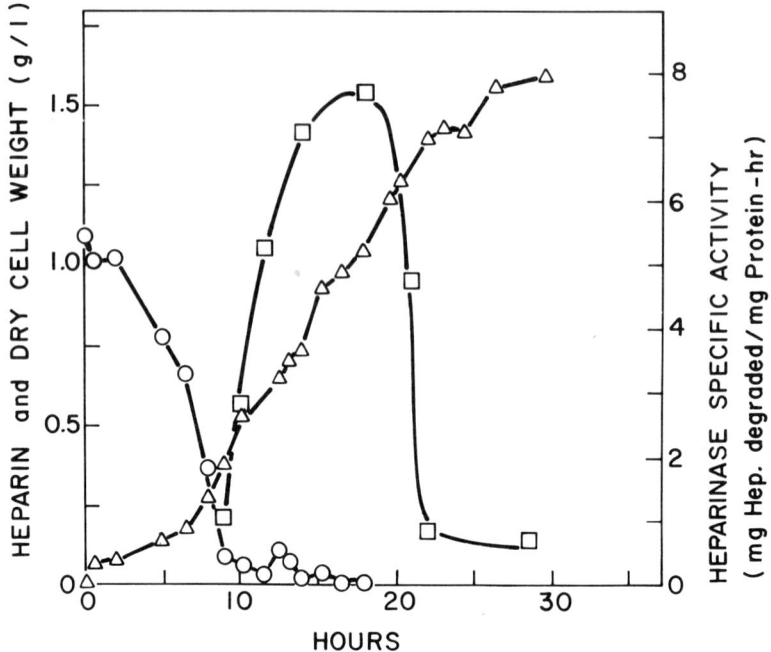

Figure 2. Results of a typical fermentation on complex medium showing heparin (○), heparinase specific activity (□), and dry cell weight (△) as a function of time as determined in a 2-L fermentor (15).

more stable, since no rapid loss of the enzyme occurs in this medium (Figure 3), and allows more flexibility and reliability for product recovery. The use of this defined medium also permitted tests concerning the effect of medium components and environmental factors on enzyme production. Optimum initial glucose and $(NH_4)_2SO_4$ concentrations were 8 g/L and 0.5 g/L, respectively. The effect of temperature on growth rate and enzyme production was studied. Optimum growth temperature was 29°C, whereas optimum temperature for enzyme production was 24°C. The maximum phosphate concentration not deleterious to growth was 20mM.

Other methods of increasing the specific heparinase production of *Flavobacteria* currently are under study. A strain improvement program of mutation and selection has been implemented using ultraviolet and γ-irradiation, followed by growth selection methods. Many mutant cultures have been obtained using these methods. Of those currently under investigation, one particular mutant has provided a twofold increase in specific productivity of heparinase over the wild type in defined medium. Genetic manipulation studies will be the main focus of continuing work, with the ultimate objective of obtaining a constitutive mutant capable of producing heparinase at high levels.

Purification of Heparinase. The objectives of our work on the purification of heparinase were twofold: (1) to adapt previous purification schemes of Hovingh and Linker (24) to large-scale production of heparinase; and (2) to purify heparinase to homogeneity. The first goal has been met largely by moving from a column to a batch purification. The cell pellet produced from centrifugation of the fermentation broth at 10,000 × g was resuspended at 100 mg/mL protein in 0.01M phosphate buffer at pH 7.0, and disrupted sonically; the nucleic acids were precipitated with 12.5 mg/mL of protamine sulfate; and the protein solution was added to 4 g of hydroxylapatite per g of protein. The hydroxylapatite-bound protein was then washed stepwise with increasing concentrations of NaCl and sodium phosphate (from 0.0M and 0.01M to 0.50M and 0.25M, respectively). The resulting enzyme preparation (HA), obtained in a 0.125M NaCl and 0.07M sodium phosphate wash, was of sufficient purity to have its activity determined by any of the available assays.

As a further purification technique, affinity chromatography was explored. In preliminary experiments, a heparin–Sepharose column failed to bind heparinase. We therefore searched for a competitive and reversible heparinase inhibitor to act as a ligand. Three synthetic heparin substitutes—poly(vinyl sulfate), polyanethole sulfonate, and polystyrene sulfonate—met these requirements. The inhibitory effect of poly(vinyl sulfate) ($K_i = 3.0 \times 10^{-8} M$; MW ~ 10,000) appeared to be linked to the presence of sulfate groups because inhibition was lost when poly(vinyl sulfate) was hydrolyzed.

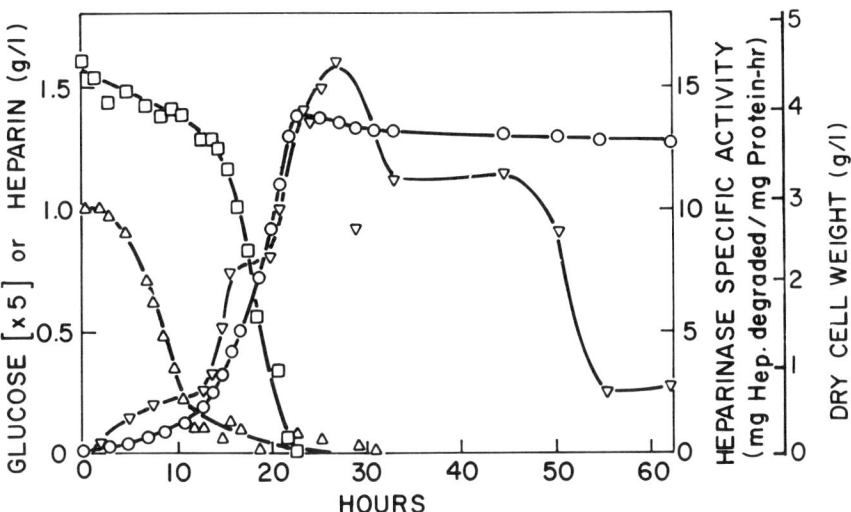

Figure 3. Results of a typical fermentation on defined medium showing dry cell weight (○), glucose (□), heparin (△), and heparinase specific activity (▽) as a function of time in a 2-L fermentor (15).

An affinity column was prepared by immobilizing partially hydrolyzed poly(vinyl sulfate) on epoxy-activated Sepharose (25). Heparinase (HA purified) was bound to this column, and was released at either high or low pH (11 or 4) with 5–10% total activity recovery and up to 500% enrichment (21).

IEF also was applied towards the HA-purified enzyme to obtain highly pure heparinase. The enzyme was loaded onto a prefocused acrylamide gel at pH 7.0. After IEF, the enzymatic activity was recovered at pH 8.5 ± 0.5. The resulting enzyme had a specific activity of about 5000 units/mg protein, having undergone an enrichment of 50-fold (21).

The purification of heparinase has been followed by SDS gel electrophoresis. The crude sonicate gave more than 20 major bands; the HA purified enzyme, 3 major bands; and the IEF purified enzyme, 2 major bands. A summary of the specific activities, protein recoveries, and enzyme purity obtained using our purification procedures is listed in Table I.

Properties of Heparinase. Our studies of the structure of heparinase show it to have a molecular weight of $51,000 \pm 6,000$ by Sephadex G-200 gel exclusion chromatography, and $45,700 \pm 1,600$ without subunits by SDS gel electrophoresis.

The enzyme is very specific, acting only on heparin ($Km = 4.2 \times 10^{-5}M$) and heparin monosulfate. Heparinase acts endolytically as an α-1, 4-eliminase cleaving heparin ($MW \cong 10,000$) at 7 to 8 sites (42).

Detailed studies have been performed on the activity and stability of heparinase. Hydroxylapatite-purified heparinase (HA) is stable to freeze–thawing and freeze-drying, with 90 and 87% recovered activity, respectively. Highly purified heparinase requires the addition of BSA or polylysine (0.05%) and glycerol (7.5%) to permit 100% activity recovery on freeze–thawing.

The effect of salts on heparinase activity was examined. An activity maximum was obtained in $0.162M$ sodium chloride; however, the maximum enzyme stability occurred at a somewhat higher concentration. The effect of the cations Ca^{2+}, Fe^{2+}, Fe^{3+}, Zn^{2+}, Cu^{2+}, Mo^{2+}, Co^{2+}, Mn^{2+}, Sn^{2+}, Cd^{2+}, Pb^{2+}, Li^{+}, K^{+}, Hg^{2+}, Mg^{2+}, NH_4^{+}, Al^{3+}, Ba^{2+}, was tested using the HA-purified heparinase. Slight inhibition was shown by Ba^{2+}, NH_4^{+}, and Pb^{+}, but total loss of activity occurred for Hg^{2+} at $10^{-5}M$.

Table I. Heparinase Purification

Procedure	Specific Activity[a]	Protein (mg)	Major SDS Bands
Whole cells	4.3	1000	—
Sonicate	7.9	730	20
Protamine precipitate	12.5	480	—
Hydroxylapatite purified	88	45	3
Affinity chromatography	2,000	—	—
Isoelectric focusing	5,000	—	2

[a]Milligrams of heparin degraded per milligram of protein per hour (15).

Studies of the effect of pH on HA heparinase activity and stability determined that the activity maximum occurs at pH 5.8, while the stability maximum occurs at pH 7.0.

HA heparinase has an activity maximum at 30°C (Figure 4), but greater stability at lower temperature; $t_{1/2}$ denaturation at 4°C was 125 h and $t_{1/2}$ denaturation at 30°C was 25 h (Figure 5).

Heparinase Immobilization. Heparinase has been immobilized on a variety of supports, with a widely differing degree of success. The best results have been obtained on Sepharose and polyacrylamide. Low levels of activity recovery occurred on PHEMA. The other supports tested gave either no activity recovery or only barely detectable levels of activity (Table II).

To check several of the immobilization methods, chondroitinase ABC (from *Proteus vulgaris*) was used as a control. A summary of the activity recoveries of immobilized heparinase and chondroitinase is listed in Table II.

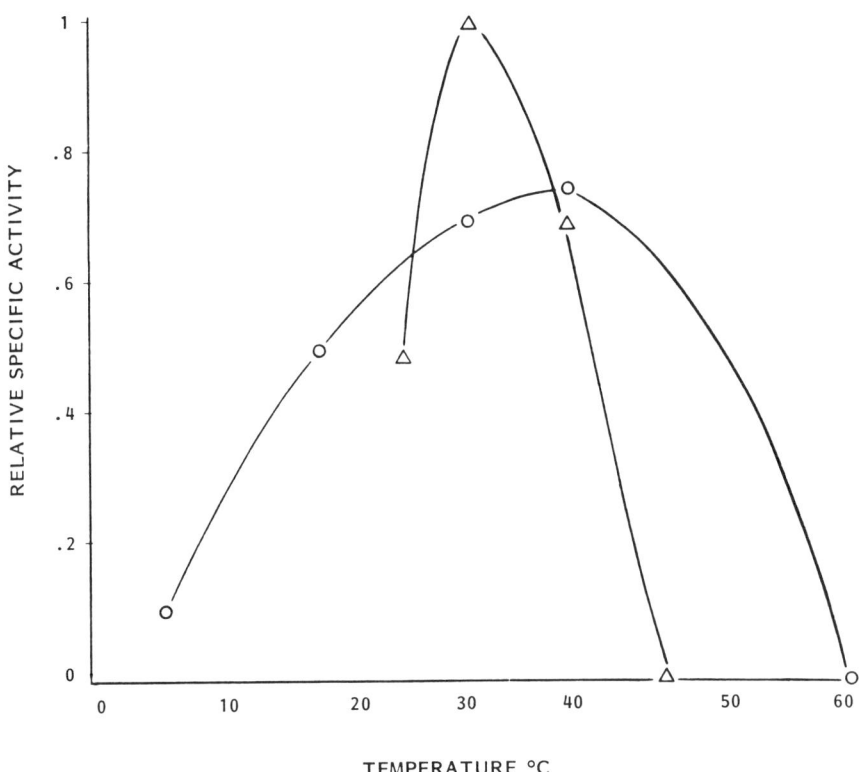

Figure 4. Activity profile of heparinase. Key: △, *specific activity of native enzyme, and* ○, *specific activity of the Sepharose-immobilized enzyme.*

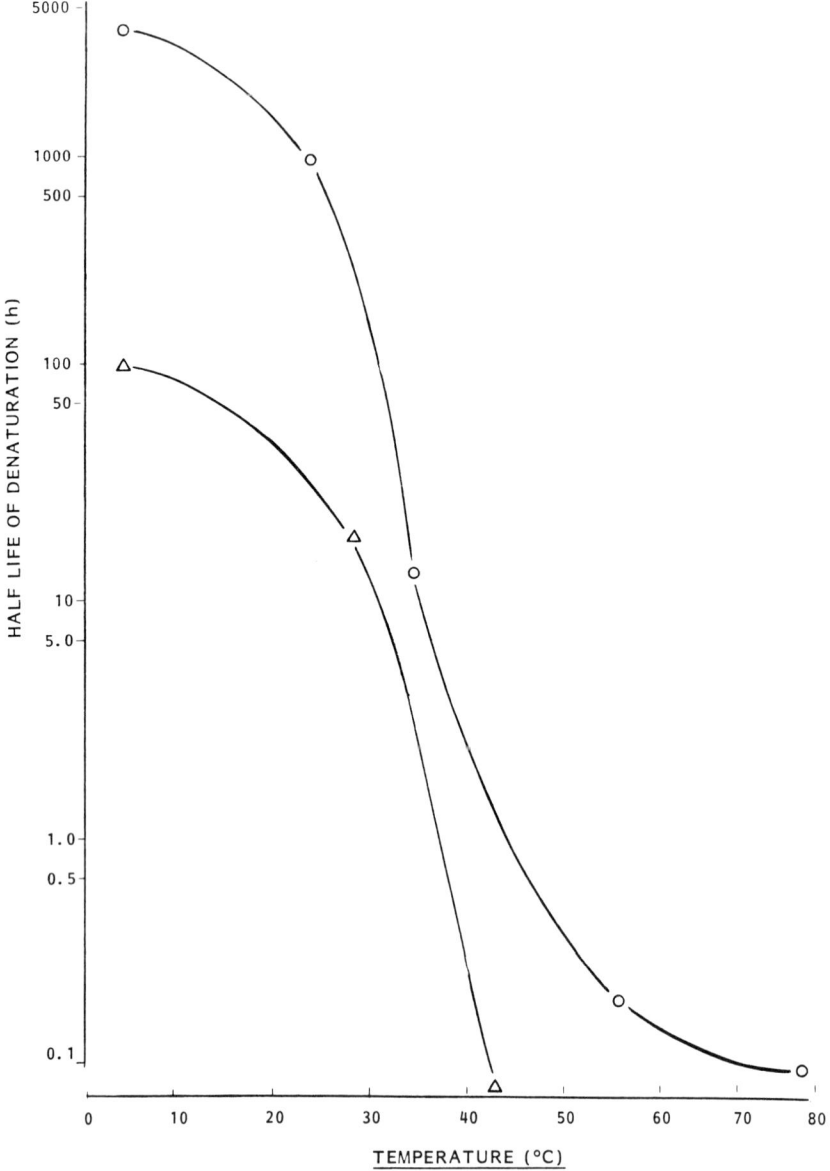

Figure 5. Stability of heparinase. Key: △, *half life of denaturation of native enzyme, and* ○, *half life of denaturation of Sepharose-immobilized enzyme.*

Table II. Enzyme Immobilization on Various Polymer Supports

Carrier	Coupled By	Ref.	% Activity Heparinase	Immobilized Chondroitinase
Sepharose	CNBr	(26)	91	0.8
Polyacrylamide	NHS active ester	(27)	56	—
	Polyacetal(aldehyde)	(28)	1.2	—
	Acyl hydrazide	(28)	0.7	—
PHEMA	CNBr	(26, 29)	1.6	—
PHEMA(Spheron)	CNBr	(26, 29)	0.03	2.2
PMA–CO_2H	EDC	(30)	0.01	0.4
PMA–$CONH(CH_2)_2OH$	CNBr	(26, 30)	0.0	—
PMA–BSA	$(CH_2)_6(CHO)_2$	(30)	0.0	—
PMA–$(CH_2)_2NH_2$	$(CH_2)_6(CHO)_2$	(30)	0.0	—
PMA–$(CH_2)_6NH_2$	$(CH_2)_6(CHO)_2$	(30)	0.0	—
Dacron	$(EtO)_3Si(CH_2)_3N=CH(CH_2)_3CHO$	(31)	0.2	10.0
Dacron–NH_2	$(CH_2)_6(CNO)_2$	(32)	0.0	—
	$(CH_2)_6(CHO)_2$	(33)	1.0	—
Dacron–CO_2H	Woodwards K reagent	(34)	0.2	—
Silicone–NH_2	$(CH_2)_6(CHO)_2$	(35)	0.0	0.4

The CNBr-activated Sepharose 4B support (1 g dry weight) was swelled in 25 mL of hydrochloric acid (0.001M), and then washed with 100 mL of 0.5M NaCl, 0.1M NaHCO$_3$ buffer at pH 8.3. To this support 5.5 mL of hydroxylapatite-purified heparinase (0.2 mg/mL protein with an activity of 88 units/mg protein in 0.2M phosphate buffer at pH 7.0) and 60 mg of heparin were added. The mixture was shaken overnight at 4°C, after which the beads were washed and blocked overnight at 4°C with a solution of lysine at pH 8.2 in 0.5M NaCl, 0.1M NaHCO$_3$ buffer solution. This support showed an uptake of 87% of the protein and an immobilization of 91% of the heparinase activity.

At present, we are continuing our efforts to immobilize heparinase to support materials in order to achieve higher yields. While this work is in progress, we have begun to explore the properties of immobilized heparinase using heparinase–Sepharose as a model.

Heparinase, immobilized on Sepharose, has enhanced thermal stability. This effect is especially noticeable in the low-temperature storage of this enzyme. At 4°C the immobilized enzyme has a half life of denaturation of > 3600 h, compared with a 125-h half life of the native enzyme at the same temperature (Figure 5). The greater stability of the immobilized enzyme is also seen at higher temperatures: 25°C, $t_{1/2}$ = 1,000 h; 37°C, $t_{1/2}$ = 15 h; and 60°C, $t_{1/2}$ = 0.2 h.

Along with enhanced stability, the activity profile of the enzyme is broadened over a larger temperature range as a result of the immobilization. The activity maximum is shifted to a slightly higher temperature, from T = 30°C for the free enzyme to T = 37°C for the Sepharose-immobilized enzyme (Figure 4). This result may reflect the temperature dependence on the rate of substrate diffusion into the support. The pH maximum of both the native and immobilized (on Sepharose) enzyme are identical (data not shown).

The apparent K_m of the immobilized enzyme is $1.2 \times 10^{-3}M$ (this can be determined by replotting the data in Figure 6 on a Lineweaver–Burk plot). This K_m is considerably higher than the K_m determined for the free enzyme ($K_m = 4.2 \times 10^{-5}M$).

In Vitro Studies on Immobilized Heparinase. Initial experiments have been conducted to test the effectiveness of immobilized heparinase in removing heparin in vitro. Controls consisted of Sepharose–heparinase that was denatured by heating at 100°C for 30 min. In one set of experiments, both active and denatured immobilized heparinase were loaded into two columns, both with a 1.5-mL bed volume. Solutions of heparin, BSA (60

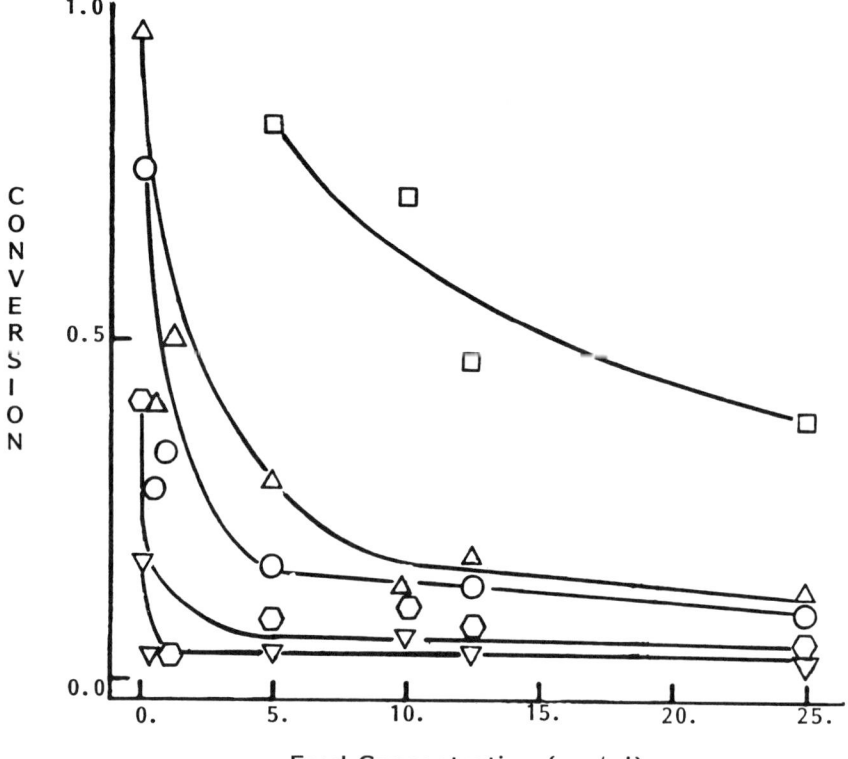

Figure 6. The conversion of heparin to products as the result of passing a sodium acetate buffer (pH 7.0, 0.25M) containing heparin through a 1.5-mL Sepharose–heparinase column. The conversion was measured as both a function of feed concentration (x-axis) and flow rate (mL/min). Key: □, 0.1; △, 0.2; ○, 0.3; ◇, 0.4; ▽, 0.5.

mg/mL), and salts were passed through each column at a flow rate of 0.5 mL/min. The concentrations of the nonheparin species were chosen to mimic physiological concentrations. The heparin levels in the solution increased in stepwise fashion from 15 µg/mL to 75 µg/mL, as shown in Figure 7. As the heparin level in the input solutions increased, the difference in the heparin recovered at the outlet of the control and active columns also increased (Figure 7). Even at 66 µg/mL the heparin was largely removed by the active

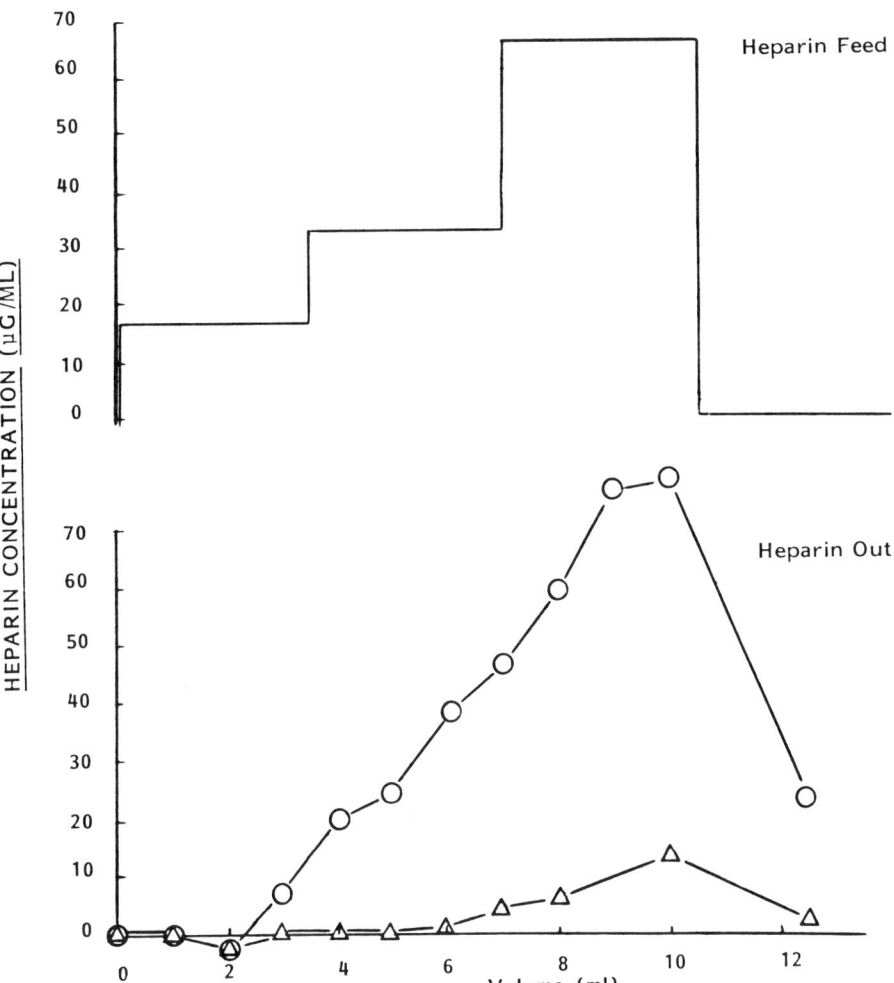

Figure 7. Heparin removal from a protein/salt solution by a 1.5-mL column packed with Sepharose-immobilized heparinase. The upper portion represents the stepped increase of heparin input; the bottom portion measures heparin output from both the Sepharose-immobilized enzyme (△) and the heat-denatured Sepharose-immobilized enzyme (○).

heparinase column, while the denatured heparinase column had no effect. Clinically used levels of heparin are on the order of 5–10 μg/mL.

In a second experiment, the effect of both heparin concentration and flow rate on heparin degradation was examined. The same size column as was used in the previous experiment was employed. As shown in Figure 6, at low flow rates this small column was fully capable of degrading very large quantities of heparin (more than 100-fold in excess of clinically used amounts) in a single pass.

We have just begun a series of experiments in which citrated rabbit blood, heparinized at a level of 10 units/mL (153 units/mg), was passed through a Sepharose–heparinase column (0.5mL) at a flow rate of 0.5 mL/min (Figure 8). After 5 min the blood leaving the bottom of the column was sampled and assayed for heparin by whole blood clotting time and Factor X_a heparin assays. In the active column, 50% of the heparin was removed. However, when the same heparinized blood was treated with a control column, less than a 5% decrease in anticoagulant activity was observed.

Discussion

These studies provide initial data for developing a system to remove heparin in extracorporeal therapy. Because the amount of data on heparinase has been limited, until now, and the methods of producing it inadequate for large scale use (24), the focus of our research thus far has been on developing the necessary technology for enzyme production and purification. The principal contributions of our studies have been (1) increasing production levels of heparinase by over 1000-fold (15) from previously published procedures (24), (2) purifying heparinase by over 1000-fold from the crude cell extracts, (3) characterizing the properties of heparinase and isolating the first heparinase inhibitors, (4) immobilizing the enzyme with 91% activity recovery and excellent stability, and (5) demonstrating that columns as small as 1.5 mL can remove clinically used quantities of heparin in aqueous medium and in blood.

The development of the heparin removal system is still at an early stage. Work currently is being directed toward (1) completing the purification of heparinase, (2) immobilizing heparinase to additional supports, and (3) testing the blood compatibility and effectiveness of heparinase reactors in vitro and in vivo.

One of the critical factors in our research has been the adaptation and use of multiple assays to follow heparinase activity. Particularly important were assays (e.g., Azure A) used in monitoring the fermentation and early stages of purification. By utilizing three different approaches for assaying heparin (disappearance of heparin, appearance of reaction products, and disappearance of heparin's biological activity), the occurrence of any artifacts in the production and purification procedures, and activity tests, was avoided.

While our studies on heparinase production and purification have been encouraging, less success has been achieved in the immobilization procedures (Table II). Studies are in progress to understand better the important parameters in immobilization procedures and in establishing new supports. Initial results indicate that a noncharged support with a high surface area is best (Table II). Additionally, our preliminary evidence is that high levels of heparinase (> 1 mg/mL) and the presence of substrate in the immobilization reaction enhance the recovery of immobilized enzyme activity.

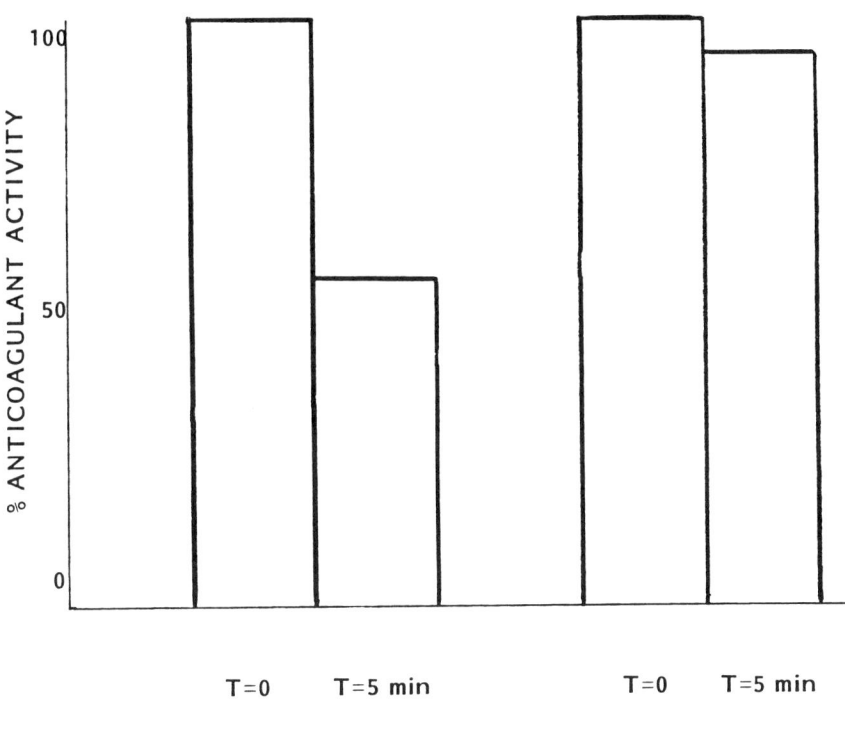

Figure 8. In vitro heparin removal from citrated rabbit blood by passing heparin through a 500-µL Sepharose–heparinase column at a flow rate of 0.5 mL/min. The anticoagulant activity as measured by both Factor X_a and whole blood clotting time is shown for the untreated blood and for the blood cycled through either the natured or denatured Sepharose–heparinase column for 5 min.

Heparinase immobilized on a negatively charged support probably will result in substrate repulsion, and thus reduced activity due to the strong negative charge of heparin. This result may, in fact, explain the apparent poor activities of some of the immobilized heparinase preparations listed in Table II.

The initial tests of immobilized heparinase on heparinized blood were limited to short time periods (<5 min). At later times, apparent decreases in heparin levels were observed in the control columns, although at a slower rate than with the active column. This effect may be due to blood damage occurring on the column. Such damage by Sepharose is not unexpected (37), and research is in progress to use either a different support with better blood compatibility or a Sepharose column with a lower bed-to-blood volume ratio.

At present, synthetic blood filters are routinely placed at the effluent of extracorporeal devices such as the pump-oxygenator or artificial kidney to remove clots or aggregates formed during the perfusion. The filters used in oxygenators can be as large as 2 L, whereas those used in renal dialysis are only several milliliters. With further development, heparinase could be immobilized to polymers in these filters. In this case, the filter could remove both clots and heparin.

The use of such a filter is anticipated to be general. Ideally it could be used during the entire operation to prevent high levels of heparin from ever entering the patient. Such an approach would require that heparin be added continuously to the extracorporeal unit either by infusion (2) or controlled release (38). The filter could be used at the very end of the perfusion to neutralize heparin, similar to the way protamine is currently used. However, the specificity of heparinase and the fact that it is immobilized could eliminate the toxic effects caused in some cases by protamine (39). The toxicity of heparinase reaction products and immunological effects remain to be tested. Nevertheless, the results obtained to date indicate that small volumes of immobilized heparinase can remove clinically used levels of heparin. Although work is still at an early stage, many of the feasibility questions (e.g., stability, activity) of the heparinase reactor have been addressed, and work is in progress to develop further the heparin removal system. Finally, we hope that the studies conducted will not only act as a first step towards developing a heparinase reactor, but that they will also aid and encourage other studies using this enzyme to examine the structure of heparin (40), to develop new assays for heparin (41), and to understand better the action of eliminase enzymes (42).

Acknowledgments

This work was supported by the National Institutes of Health Grant No. GM25810. The authors thank G. Fitzgerald and S. Hoffberg for their technical assistance.

Literature Cited

1. Gervin, A. S. *Surg. Gynecol. Obstet.* **1975**, *140*, 789.
2. Swartz, R. D.; Port, F. K. *Kidney Int.* **1979**, *16*, 513.
3. Basu, D.; Gallus, M.; Hirsh, J.; Cade, J. *N. Engl. J. Med.* **1972**, *287*, 324.
4. Fletcher, J. R.; McKee, A. E.; Mills, M.; Snyder, K. C.; Herman, C. M. *Surgery* **1976**, *80*, 214.
5. Jastrzebski, J.; Hilgard, P.; Sykes, M. K. *Cardiovas. Res.* **1975**, *9*, 691.
6. Berglin, E.; Hansson, H. A.; Teger–Nilsson, A. C.; William-Olsson, G. *Thromb. Res.* **1976**, *9*, 81.
7. Schmer, G. *Trans. Am. Soc. Artif. Intern. Organs* **1972**, *18*, 321.
8. Lagergren, H. R.; Eriksson, J. C. *Trans. Am. Soc. Artif. Intern. Organs* **1971**, *17*, 10.
9. Leininger, R. D.; Falb, R. D.; Grode, G. A. *Ann. N.Y. Acad. Sci.* **1968**, *146*, 11.
10. Yen, S. P. S.; Rembaum, A. *J. Biomed. Mater. Res. Symp.* **1971**, *1*, 83.
11. Hersh, L. S.; Gott, V. L.; Najjar, F. *J. Biomed. Mater. Res. Symp.* **1972**, *3*, 85.
12. Rea, W. J.; Whitley, D.; Eberle, J. W. *Trans. Am. Soc. Artif. Intern. Organs* **1972**, *18*, 316.
13. Kusserow, B. K.; Larrow, R.; Nichols, J. *Trans. Am. Soc. Artif. Intern. Organs* **1971**, *17*, 1.
14. Kolff, W. J.; Stellwag, F. *Ann. N.Y. Acad. Sci.* **1977**, *283*, 443.
15. Galliher, P. M.; Cooney, C. L.; Langer, R.; Linhardt, R. J. *Appl. Environ. Micro.* **1981**, *41*, 360.
16. Lowry, O. H.; Rosebrough, N. J.; Farr, A. L.; Randall, R. J. *J. Biol. Chem.* **1951**, *193*, 265.
17. Jacques, L. B. *Science* **1979**, *206*, 528.
18. Dietrich, C. P. *Biochem. J.* **1968**, *108*, 647.
19. Park, J. T.; Johnson, M. J. *J. Biol. Chem.* **1949**, *181*, 149.
20. Linker, A.; Hovingh, P.; *Bioch.* **1972**, *11*, 563.
21. Linhardt, R. J.; Langer, R.; Cooney, C. L.; Galliher, P. M.; Flanagan, M. M.; Hoffberg, S. M., unpublished data.
22. Yin, E. T.; Wessler, S.; Butler, J. *J. Lab. Clin. Med.* **1973**, *81*, 298.
23. Lam, L. H.; Silbert, J. E.; Rosenberg, R. D. *Biochem. Biophys. Res. Commun.* **1976**, *69*, 570.
24. Linker, A.; Hovingh, P. *Methods Enzymol.* **1972**, *28*, 902.
25. Vretblad, P. *Biochem. Biophys. Acta* **1976**, *434*, 169.
26. March, S. C.; Parikh, I.; Cuatrecasas, P. *Anal. Biochem.* **1974**, *60*, 149.
27. Pollak, A.; Blumenfeld, H.; Wax, M.; Baughn, R. L.; Whitesides, G. M. *J. Am. Chem. Soc.* **1980**, *102*, 6324.
28. Epton, R.; Hibbert, B. L.; Thomas, T. H. *Methods Enzymol.* **1976**, *44*, 84.
29. Turkova, J. *Methods Enzymol.* **1976**, *44*, 66.
30. Dincer, A. K. Ph.D. Dissertation, Massachusetts Institute of Technology, 1977.
31. Hersh, L. S. *J. Polymer Sci.* **1974**, *47*, 55.
32. Ozawa, H. *J. Biochem.* **1967**, *62*, 419.
33. Allison, J. P.; Davidson, L.; Hartman, A.; Kitto, B. *Biochem. Biophys. Res. Commun.* **1972**, *47*, 66.
34. Wagner, T.; Hsu, C. J.; Kelleher, G. *Biochem. J.* **1968**, *108*, 892.
35. Garnett, J. L.; Kenyon, R. S.; Liddy, M. J. *J. Chem. Soc. Chem. Commun.* **1974**, 735.
36. Chibata, I. "Immobilized Enzymes", Halsted: New York, 1978.
37. Berk, P. D.; Plotz, P. H.; Scharschmidt, B. F. "Biomedical Applications of Immobilized Enzymes and Proteins", Chang, T. M. S., Ed.; Plenum: New York, 1977, Vol. I, p. 297.
38. Langer, R. *Chem. Eng. Commun.* **1980**, *6*, 1.
39. Jastrzebski, J.; Sykes, M. K.; Woods, D. G. *Thorax* **1974**, *29*, 534.
40. Lindahl, U.; Backstrom, G.; Hook, M.; Thurnberg, L.; Fransson, L.; Linker, A. *Proc. Nat. Acad. Sci.* **1979**, *76*, 3198.
41. Hutt, E. D.; Kingdom, H. S. *J. Lab. Clin. Med.* **1972**, *79*, 1027.
42. Linhardt, R. J.; Fitzgerald, G. L.; Cooney, C. L.; Langer, R. *Biochem. Biophys. Acta*, in press.

RECEIVED for review January 16, 1981. ACCEPTED September 8, 1981.

32
Implantable Micropump for Insulin Delivery
Effect of a Rate-Controlling Membrane

MICHAEL V. SEFTON

University of Toronto, Department of Chemical Engineering and Applied Chemistry, Toronto, Ontario M5S 1A4, Canada

Using a controlled-release micropump with a 1.2-µm cellulose acetate membrane inserted between the insulin reservoir and the micropump solenoid, and a concentration-difference driving force (100 U/mL), the basal insulin delivery rate was 0.3 U/day and the degree of augmentation was 83 × at maximum power input. This delivery rate remained constant during the 8-h experiment, in contrast with the performance of 1-µm Nucleopore membranes upon which occlusive precipitates quickly formed to lower the basal rate. The suggested inherent reliability of the device, the small reservoir, and the apparent absence of a problem with insulin precipitation may prove to be significant advantages of the controlled-release micropump. With this device, diabetologists will be able to assess the potential benefits to be derived from open-loop insulin delivery systems.

An estimated five million people in North America and 30 million in the world are diabetic. Almost half of these people require repeated, often daily, injections of insulin to maintain approximately normal glucose levels. While gross metabolic control is achieved, diabetics are still subject to unavoidable complications. Conventional insulin therapy is inadequate for the restoration of normoglycemia sufficient to prevent these degenerative sequelae of diabetes (1). Hence, artificial pancreata have been designed and developed to deliver insulin continuously in direct response to the physiological need to provide the finer control of glycemia necessary for homeostasis in insulin-dependent diabetes.

The connection between glycemia and the degenerative vascular complications of diabetes which, in turn, cause premature death, is based on a limited amount of indirect evidence (2). Proof of a direct causal relationship between normoglycemia and the degenerative sequelae of diabetes must await the results of clinical trials of the various artificial pancreata currently under development around the world.

The Artificial Pancreas

Whether open-loop or closed-loop control is envisaged, the artificial pancreas consists of an insulin delivery mechanism or pump attached to an appropriate reservoir and to a power supply/control package (Figure 1). The inadequacies of current glucose sensors (3, 4) make open-loop control the only practical operating mode envisaged at this time for the long-term treatment of a large number of insulin-dependent diabetics.

Open-loop control systems are characterized by operation at two levels: basal delivery up to and following the absorption of meals, and augmented delivery for short periods associated with the absorption of meals adjusted to the insulin requirement of the respective meal. Augmented flow rates have ranged from 4× basal (5) to 15× basal (6, 7), and augmented periods have varied from a single bolus injection/meal in humans (8) to 7 h/day in dogs (9).

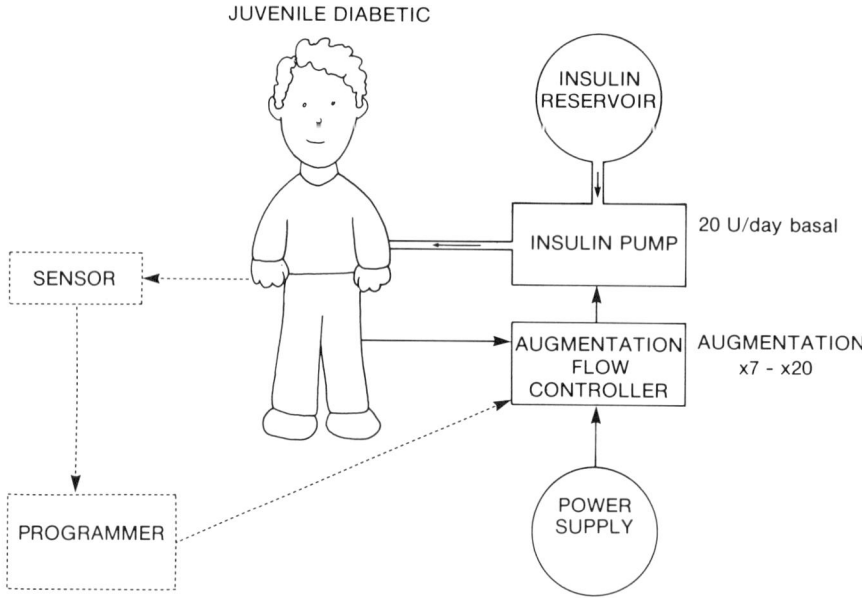

Figure 1. Artificial pancreas block diagram. Closed-loop control (---) uses the sensor and programmers to direct flow controller. In open-loop control (—), augmentation is initiated by the diabetic, without the sensor. Typical design criteria are indicated on the right-hand side of the drawing.

The characteristics and limitations of these devices recently were reviewed (4), and were the subject of a recent symposium (10). Subsequent to this review, other researchers have reported their success using open-loop insulin delivery systems to maintain normoglycemia in dogs (7, 9) and in humans (8, 11–14). The effects of this restoration of normoglycemia on diabetic metabolism and blood chemistry are beginning to be reported (15–19), but no clear evidence of long-term beneficial effects of normoglycemia have yet been obtained.

Insulin Pumps

Unlike the bedside or portable insulin delivery systems for which commercially available peristaltic or syringe pumps may be used, the key component of an implantable (open-loop) artificial pancreas is the specially developed miniature insulin pump.

Although numerous devices have been developed (20) for the controlled delivery of pharmaceuticals, only three have been used for insulin delivery and can be characterized as implantable (7, 11, 21). Other devices for insulin delivery are or have been under development, but little is known of their performance characteristics (22, 23).

The primary limitation currently facing the development and use of these implantable micropumps is the precipitation of insulin on the pump components (7, 11, 14, 31), although bicarbonate (33), certain serum components (25), or amino acides (32) may minimize or prevent insulin aggregation. These precipitates, if they accumulate, tend to occlude the flow channels in the pump and particularly the fine bore tubing or valves that are integral parts of these devices. Additional concern is related to the reliability and inherent safety of these devices and to their ability to use small, concentrated insulin reservoirs.

Controlled-Release Micropump

The controlled-release micropump (Figure 2) is a recently invented device that uses the principles of membrane transport and controlled release of drugs to deliver insulin at variable rates (20, 26). With a suitable supply of insulin connected to the pump, the concentration and/or pressure difference across the membrane results in diffusion or bulk transport through the membrane(s). This process is the basal delivery and requires no external power source. Augmented delivery is achieved by repeated compression of the foam membrane by the coated mild-steel piston. The piston is the core of the solenoid, and compression is effected when current is applied to the solenoid coil. Interruption of the current causes the membrane to relax, drawing more drug into the membrane in preparation for the next compression cycle.

Energy consumption is low since power is consumed only during the postprandial delivery phase, and even then only during the compression

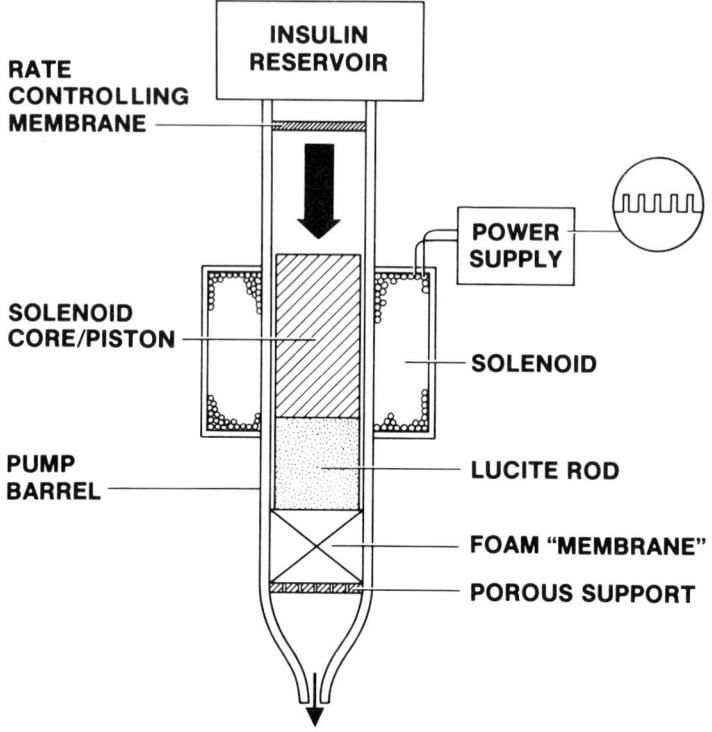

Figure 2. Schematic of the controlled-release micropump. Rate-controlling membrane is not present in early prototypes (26).

portion of the cycle (power for typical therapeutic use: 60 W peak × 5 ms "on" time = 0.3 J/compression stroke, with a frequency of 30 strokes/min).

This chapter reports on the continued development of this pump with particular emphasis on the use of a rate-controlling membrane to lower the basal rate and raise the degree of augmentation to clinically acceptable levels.

Experimental

Micropump Fabrication. Lucite prototypes were prepared as described earlier (26). Glass prototypes with 2000 turns of 36-gauge wire ($R = 80\ \Omega$) were prepared as described before (20) except that the sintered glass disk was glued to the end of the 11.3-cm long glass tube (7-mm o.d.), and a 7-cm length of tapered tubing (a portion of pasteur pipette) was glued to the disk and used as the pump outlet. The lucite spacer was 5 mm long, making the nominal magnetic field gap 1.7 cm. The power supply (26) provided an interrupted dc current for the solenoid with an "on" time of of 5 ms at a frequency of 30 strokes/min for these experiments.

Membranes. A 1-cm thick, approximately 5-mm-diameter disk of HYPOL nonwicking hydrophilic polyurethane foam was used in all experiments. Only disks with an air permeability of $5 \pm 1 \times 10^{-7}$ cm^2 at an air flow rate of 850 cm^3/min were used. No specific conditioning of the foam was done nor was any attempt made to remove extractables from the cured foam.

To improve the delivery, 13-mm-diameter rate-controlling membranes held in a Swinnex filter chamber (Millipore Corp.) were inserted in the delivery line between the insulin reservoir and the micropump. The effective membrane area was 0.7 cm^2. Membranes investigated were 1-μm and 8-μm pore size polycarbonate filters (Nuclepore Corp.), 0.45-μm cellulosic microporous filters (Amicon Corp.), Cuprophane PT-150 (from Ultra-Flow 145 Dialyser, Travenol Laboratories), and 0.2-μm and 1.2-μm pore size cellulose acetate filters (Schleicher and Schuell OE 66 and ST 69).

Pressure-Difference Driving Force. The falling head permeameter (26) was used to measure the volumetric flow rate through the controlled-release micropump with a pressure difference driving force. The pressure difference in this permeameter is the difference in height of insulin solution in an open vertical graduated pipette or tube, acting as the upstream reservoir, and the constant height of liquid in a downstream reservoir in which the pump outlet is immersed. The rate of decrease of insulin solution in the upstream reservoir was measured and converted to overall flow resistance, or basal and augmented flow rates as required. Different pipettes or tubes were used to cover a range of flow rates: 2-mL pipette (3.36-mm i.d.), 0.5-mL pipette (1.96-mm i.d.), or a length of PE20 Intramedic tubing (0.38-mm i.d., Clay Adams). The resistances of the permeameter itself and the filter chamber were estimated by measuring the flow resistance without a membrane and without the controlled-release micropump. Unfortunately, the resistance of the PE20 tubing, unlike the others, was very dependent on the height in the permeameter (i.e., length of tubing), complicating the correction for the resistance. The feed reservoir consisted of 0.4 U/mL mixed bovine/porcine insulin (Toronto Insulin, Connaught Laboratories Ltd.) in 0.05M phosphate-buffered saline (pH 7.4) containing 1% formaldehyde.

Concentration-Difference Driving Force. A shorter glass prototype in which the membrane held in the Swinnex chamber was attached directly to the pump barrel was used for these experiments. The pump barrel (7-mm o.d. glass tube) was 4 cm long with the membrane held approximately 5 cm from the sintered glass disk. The tapered glass tube was replaced with the male end (1 cm long) of a 1-mL syringe (Plastipak, B-D). All other components were the same as the previously described glass prototype. The pump including filter chamber weighed 40 g.

Insulin delivery rate was determined by following the increase in ^{125}I-insulin concentration in a 2-mL downstream reservoir. The reservoir was connected via a siphon to a test tube that fit into the sampling well of a NaI scintillation detector. A 1-mL sample of the downstream solution was taken by appropriate manipulation of the siphon arm heights. The detector was connected to an Eberline MS-2 Scaler (Datamex Ltd.). The insulin reservoir solution contained 100 U/mL Toronto insulin and approximately 0.5 μCi/mL of ^{125}I-insulin (Amersham-Searle).

Care had to be taken to fill the micropump with liquid since the presence of air bubbles in any of the lines would reduce the delivery rate. The portion of the pump below the membrane was filled with insulin-free phosphate buffered saline containing 0.5% (w/v) m-cresol (a preservative) via a tube connected to the pump outlet. When this portion was full, the membrane was laid onto the membrane support portion of the chamber, and the upper half of the chamber was reconnected to the controlled-release micropump. The upper half of the chamber constituted the 1-cm^3 upstream reservoir for these experiments and was filled with radioactive feed solution through a needle inserted horizontally into the side of the membrane chamber. The top of the chamber was connected to a plastic three-way valve using the appropriate Luer-lok connections to permit filling. The valve was turned to seal the chamber and eliminate the pressure difference before the experiment. One of the ports of the valve was used to collect a sample of feed solution to measure its concentration and to avoid the problem of correcting for adsorption. Neither upstream nor downstream reservoirs were stirred. Care was taken to avoid dilution of the upstream solution with insulin-free saline.

Results

The effects of operating parameters (voltage, frequency of compression, and pressure difference) and some design parameters were demonstrated in earlier publications (20, 26). The results presented here focus on the effect of a rate-controlling membrane between the solenoid and the insulin reservoir.

Pressure-Difference Driving Force. The effect of a 1-μm polycarbonate microporous filter on basal and augmented delivery in the controlled-release micropump due to a pressure difference is shown in Figure 3. As the pressure difference was lowered (i.e., as the liquid level dropped in the falling head permeameter) the basal flow rate was reduced to less than 0.2 mL/day (pressure difference, approximately 0.8 cm H_2O). At this basal rate, operation with a 100-U/mL reservoir becomes practical. More importantly, the degree of augmentation was increased to more than 10× from the

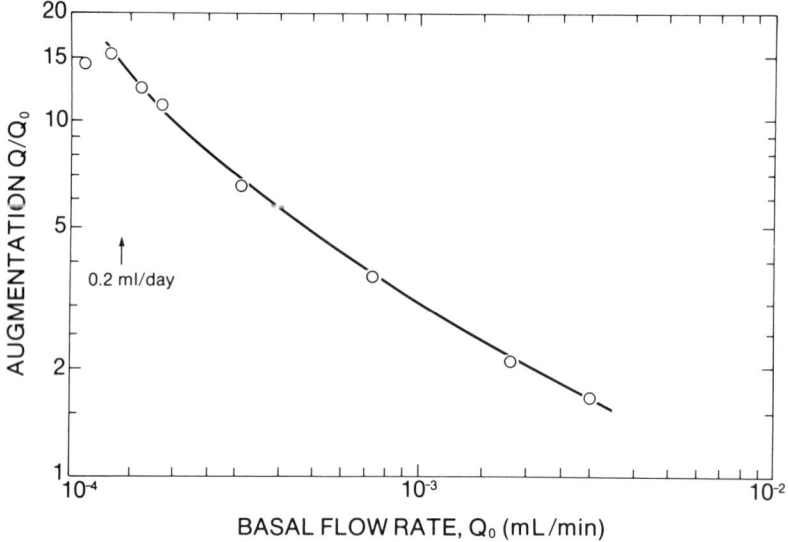

Figure 3. Degree of augmentation with a 1-μm polycarbonate filter as the rate-controlling membrane as a function of initial basal flow. (26).

Basal flow was varied by lowering the pressure difference from 3000 dyn/cm^2 to 800 dyn/cm^2 in the falling head permeameter. The PE20 tubing used in the permeameter to give an overall initial basal pump resistance varying from 1×10^6 to 7.6×10^6 $dyn \cdot min/cm^5$. Augmentations were measured at a time-averaged power input of 250 mW (90 V, 80 Ω).

1.5–2 × that was obtained without this membrane. Under these conditions the controlled-release micropump meets the minimum design criteria for an insulin delivery system. Since these data were obtained with the PE20 tubing in the permeameter, and the PE20 tubing offered an additional significant resistance to flow (ranging from 7×10^5–3×10^6 dynes·min/cm^5), the basal flow rates were lower, at any pressure difference, than would have been obtained without the permeameter. Other membranes similarly lowered the basal rate in accordance with their resistance relative to that of the rest of the pump and the permeameter. The resistance of the membrane was determined by difference between the total resistance and the resistance without a membrane for the various permeameters.

While the 1-μm polycarbonate membrane provided the appropriate resistance to give the desired basal rate, this resistance was very time dependent (Table I). Unlike the 8-μm polycarbonate or 0.45-μm cellulosic membrane, the flow resistance through the 1-μm membrane increased sixfold over a 5-h period. This was attributed to the formation of an insulin precipitate on the membrane which blocked the pores of the membrane. Figure 4 shows these precipitates for a membrane that had been placed between the Hypol foam and the porous disk in an earlier prototype (26). Presumably, the larger pores in the 8-μm polycarbonate membrane were not significantly affected by the precipitates, and fewer precipitates had formed on the more hydrophilic 0.45-μm membrane during the time of the experiments. In other experiments (27) the permeability of Cuprophane and other hydrophilic membranes was measured over a 7-day period without any noticeable decrease in rate. The apparent difference in behavior of hydrophilic and hydrophobic membranes is not currently known, although this difference probably reflects differences in the adsorption pattern of insulin on the different membranes (34).

Table I. Effect of Membrane on Basal Flowrate Decay

Membrane	$R_m^{\circ\ a}$	$R_m^t/R_m^{\circ\ b}$ Time (h)				
		0	1	2	3	5
8-μm Polycarbonate (Nuclepore)	630	1	1.01	1.03	—	—
1-μm Polycarbonate (Nuclepore)[c]	3.4×10^3	1	1.4	2	2.7	5.9
0.45-μm Cellulosic (Amicon)	2.6×10^5	1	1.01	1.025	1.045	1.084

Note: Data determined by interpolation.
[a] R_m^t = membrane resistance at time t; R_m° = initial membrane resistance (dyn min/cm^5).
[b] R_m° = total resistance − resistance without membrane
[c] R° determined from 2-mL pipette, all others using 0.5-mL pipette.

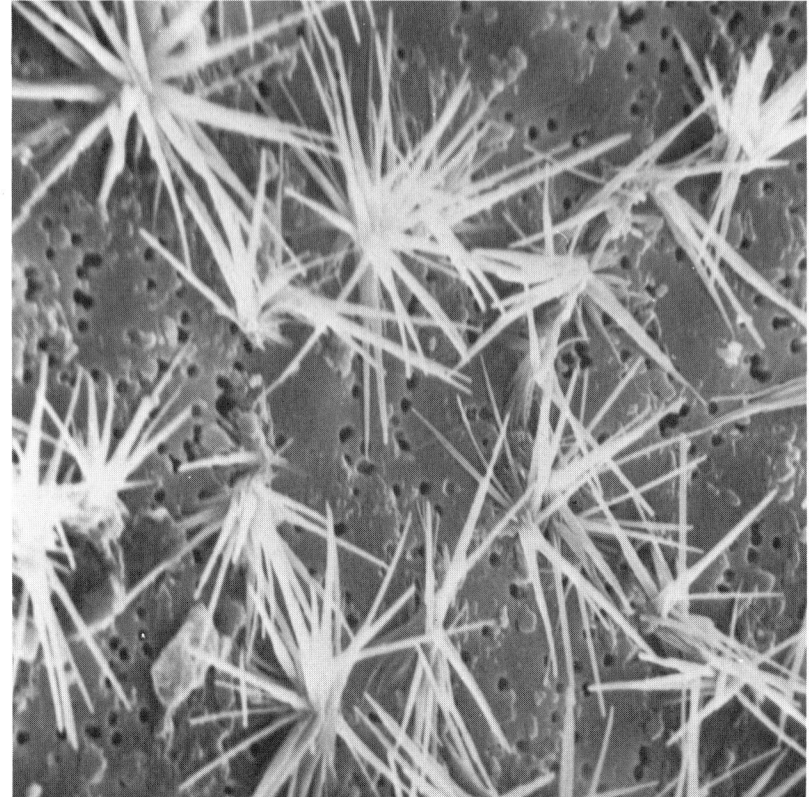

Figure 4. *Scanning electron micrograph of precipitates on 1-µm polycarbonate filter after 2 h of use. This membrane was placed between the foam membrane and the porous support (26).*

Concentration-Difference Driving Force. The realization that high augmentations were best obtained at low pressure differences led to the design of a prototype that used a concentration-difference driving force. The basal and augmented flows through this device are shown in Figure 5 for various hydrophilic membranes. From the 100-U/mL reservoir, basal rates ranged from less than 0.3 to 1.1 U/day, while degrees of augmentation for the 1.2-µm cellulose acetate membrane were as high as 83 × the basal rate at 100 V (time-averaged power = 310 mW). Because of the less-than-detectable basal rate for the other membranes, these augmentations were also very high, although the augmented flow rates were lower than for the 1.2-µm cellulose acetate membrane. The significant diffusion resistance of the controlled-release micropump itself is also apparent from Figure 5. Comparing basal rates, the pump barrel, outlet, and membrane chamber offer approximately 27% of the total resistance of the micropump with the 1.2-µm cellulose acetate membrane. During the 8-h maximum duration of these experiments, no noticeable decrease in insulin delivery rate was noted, that is, after a short initial unsteady-state period, the rate of increase of insulin concentration in the downstream reservoir was constant. The duration of these unsteady-state periods is obviously important to the design of the augmented delivery programs. To minimize these time lags, the current prototype has been shortened further to give a device with a total diffusion path of approximately 2 cm.

Discussion

Although the initial prototypes were designed for use with an insulin reservoir supplying drug to the pump inlet at constant pressure (20, 26), these more recent experiments indicate that the device performs better (higher augmentation/power ratio) and at the required insulin basal rate (~20 U/day) with a constant-concentration upstream reservoir. Further-

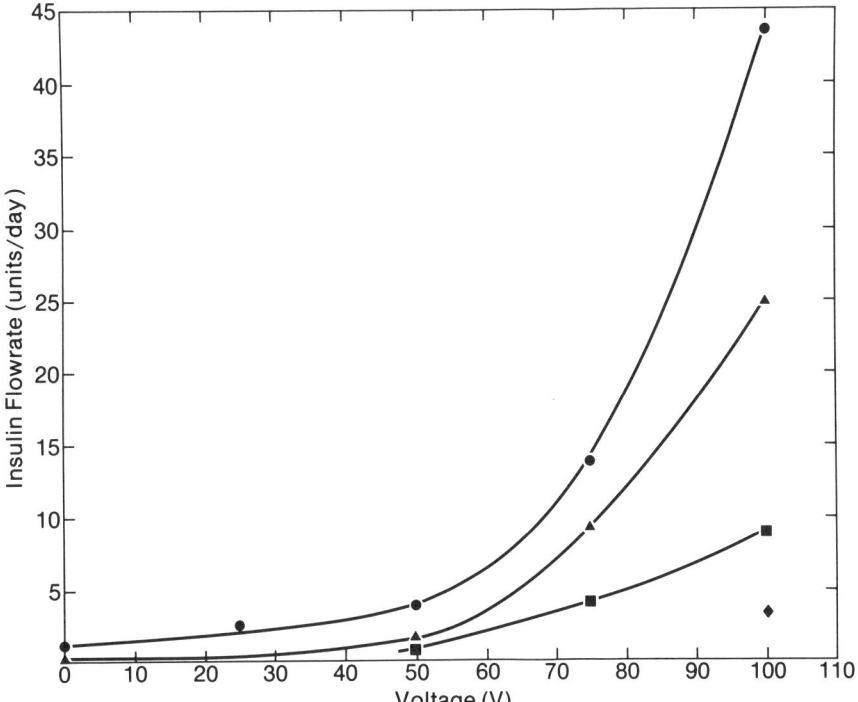

Figure 5. Basal and augmented insulin delivery rates with various membranes as rate-controlling membranes, using a concentration-difference (100 U/mL) driving force. Peak voltage used as abscissa (R = 80 Ω, 30 strokes/min, 5 ms "on time"); voltage = 0 corresponds to basal rate.
Key: ●, no membrane; ▲, 1.2-μm cellulose acetate;
■, 0.2-μm cellulose acetate; and ◆, Cuprophane.

more, the maintenance of a constant-pressure difference, particularly at these low levels, in vivo is not a simple matter. The constant-concentration reservoir, on the other hand, would simply be a chamber containing insulin at unit activity (solid insulin dispersed in a nontoxic medium) separated from the pump itself by the hydrophilic rate-controlling membrane. These reservoirs would contain 10,000–20,000 U/cm^3; consequently, at a consumption rate of 50 U/day, a 2-cm^3 reservoir could contain enough insulin for 1–2 years without a refill. Therefore, the total mass of the device (without power pack) could be kept to less than 50 g and yet be useful for more than 1 year. A similar solid insulin reservoir has been used for constant rate-controlled release of insulin (28), and the insulin activity has been retained for more than 8 months at 37°C in this form (29).

Augmented delivery is achieved without valves in the controlled-release micropump, and hence the mechanical unreliability associated with the inadvertent opening and sticking of valves, with complex motors, or with the peristaltic action of a rotating metal component on a soft plastic tube is avoided. Furthermore, in the controlled-release micropump, basal delivery is not achieved by regulating a large flow rate as it is done in valve-operated systems. The reliability associated with the repeated compression of the foam is, however, of great concern. Results acquired to date indicate that for a pump fabricated with only limited care, a life of 1100 h (for continuous augmented delivery) can be expected (30); this result corresponds to a life of 1 year of normal use.

Insulin deposition in the controlled-release micropump is not expected to be important. While it was significant in one of the prototypes (Figure 4), changing the rate controlling membrane from a hydrophobic polycarbonate filter to a hydrophilic Cuprophane or cellulose acetate membrane has apparently eliminated the problem. Although the situation may be different as longer-term experiments are performed, presumably the problems that may arise may relate more to the biological stability of the insulin reservoir than to insulin deposition.

The mechanism of action of the controlled-release micropump is unclear. With a pressure difference, the rapid oscillatory movement of the piston during augmented delivery may be responsible for the increased delivery rate by lowering the overall resistance of the micropump to bulk flow (35). When only a concentration difference exists, on the other hand, augmentation can be attributed to a pressure difference superimposed during piston movement on the basal concentration difference, or to a mixing effect associated with piston movement. The physical relationship between piston movement and augmentation remains to be defined.

A number of concerns regarding open-loop delivery of insulin in general, and delivery of insulin by the controlled-release micropump, in particular, remain to be resolved. The optimum site of insulin delivery (intravenous or subcutaneous), the tissue reaction to the pump outlet, the optimum method of adjusting the basal rate for patient-to-patient variability, pump reliability, and the time lags between steady-state basal and augmented delivery rates must be determined or assessed. Furthermore, whether the restoration of nomoglycemia leads to reduction of or prevention of the degenerative complications of diabetes must be determined. In addition, proof that open-loop control of glycemia results in a better degree of control than multiple injection therapy or, alternatively, that there is a subgroup of diabetics for whom open-loop insulin delivery would be the preferred mode of treatment remains to be shown. These questions must be addressed before open-loop delivery of insulin with the controlled-release micropump becomes a clinically acceptable mode of therapy.

Conclusions

The controlled-release micropump is a simple means of delivering insulin at variable rates to control the glucose level of insulin-dependent diabetics at physiological levels. Operating with a concentration-difference driving force, the controlled-release micropump delivers insulin at a low constant rate which can be augmented more than 80 × in one prototype by repeated compression of a foam membrane. The suggested inherent reliability of the device, the small reservoir, and the apparent absence of a problem with insulin precipitation may prove to be significant advantages of the controlled-released micropump compared to other proposed insulin delivery systems.

With this device, diabetologists and biomedical researchers will be able to examine the relationship between safe and reliable metabolic control and the incidence of degenerative complications, and to assess the potential benefits to be derived from open-loop insulin delivery systems.

Acknowledgments

The support of the J. P. Bickell Foundation and the technical assistance of K. J. Burns, P. J. Cahill, and R. Sirisko are gratefully acknowledged.

Literature Cited

1. Cahill, G. F.; Etzwiler, D. D.; Freinkel, N. *Diabetes* **1976,** *25,* 237–239.
2. Tchobroutsky, G., *Diabetologia* **1978,** *15,* 143–152.
3. Albisser, A. M.; Leibel, B. S. *Clinics in Endocrin and Metab.* **1977,** *6*(2), 457.
4. Santiago, J. V.; Clemens, A. H.; Clarke, W. L.; Kipnis, D. M. *Diabetes* **1979,** *28,* 71–84.
5. Hepp, K. D.; Renner, R.; von Funcke, H. J.; Mehnert, H.; Haerten, R.; Kresse, H. *Horm. Metab. Res. Suppl.* **1977,** *7,* 72–76.
6. Slama, G.; Hautecouverture, M.; Assan, R.; Tchobroutsky, G. *Diabetes* **1974,** *23,* 732.
7. Blackshear, P. J.; Rohde, T. D.; Grotteng, J. C.; Dorman, F. D.; Perkins, P. R.; Varco, R. L.; Buchwald, H. *Diabetes* **1979,** *28,* 634–639.

8. Tamborlane, W. V.; Sherwin, R. S.; Genel, M.; Felig, P. *N. Engl. J. Med.* **1979**, *300*(11), 573–578.
9. Goriya, Y.; Bahoric, A.; Marliss, E. B.; Zimman, B.; Albisser, A. M.; *Diabetes* **1979**, *28*, 558–564.
10. "Feedback-controlled and preprogrammed insulin infusion in diabetes mellitus." Workshop Schloss Reisenberg. *Horm. Metab. Res. Suppl.* **1979**, *8*, 1–211.
11. Irsigler, K.; Kritz, H. *Diabetes* **1979**, *28*, 196–203.
12. Pickup, J. C.; White, M. C.; Keen, H.; Parsons, J. A.; Alberti, K. G. M. M. *Lancet*, **1979**, October 27, 870–873.
13. Kolendorf, K.; Bojesen, J.; Lorup, B. *Diabetologia* **1980**, *18*, 141–145.
14. Champion, M.; Shepherd, G.; Rodger, N. W.; Dupre, J. *Diabetes Astr.* **1979**, *28*(156), 383.
15. Pickup, J. C.; Keen, H.; Parson, J. A.; Alberti, K. G. M. M.; Rowe, A. S. *Lancet* **1979**, June 16, 1255–1257.
16. Tamborlane, W. V.; Sherwin, R. S.; Genel, M.; Felig, P. *Lancet* **1979**, June 16, 1258–1261.
17. Bolli, G.; Cartechinni, M. G.; Compagnucci, P.; Santeusanio, F.; Massi-Bendeti, M.; Calabrese, G.; Puxeddu, A.; Brunetti, P. *Diabetologia* **1980**, *18*, 125–130.
18. Gertner, J. M.; Tamborlane, W. V.; Horst, R. L.; Sherwin, R. S.; Felig, P.; Genel, M. *J. Clin. Endocrinol. Metab.* **1980**, *50*, 862–866.
19. Hanna, A. K.; Zinman, B.; Nakhooda, A. F.; Minuk, H. L.; Stokes, E. F.; Albisser, A. M.; Leibell, B. S.; Marliss, E. B. *Metabolism* **1980**, *29*(4), 321–332.
20. Sefton, M. V.; Lusher, H. M.; Firth, S. R.; Waher, M. U. *Ann. Biomed. Eng.* **1979**, *7*, 329–343.
21. Albisser, A. M.; Jackman, W. J.; Ferguson, R.; Bahoric, A.; Goriya, Y. *Med. Prog. Technol.* **1978**, *5*, 187–193.
22. Thomas, L. J.; Bessman, S. P. *Trans. Am. Soc. Artif. Intern. Organs* **1975**, *21*, 516–520.
23. Nalecz, M.; Lewandowski, J.; Werynski, A.; Zawicki, I. *Artif. Organs* **1978**, 305–309.
24. Lougheed, W.; Albisser, A. M. *Int. J. Artif. Organs* **1980**, *3*, 50–56.
25. Albisser, A. M.; Lougheed, W.; Perlman, K.; Bahoric, A. *Diabetes* **1980**, *29*(3), 241–243.
26. Sefton, M. V.; Burns, K. J. *Ind. Eng. Chem. Prod. Res. Dev.* **1981**, *20*, 1–5.
27. Sefton, M. V.; Nishimura, E. *J. Pharm. Sci.* **1980**, *69*, 208–209.
28. Creque, H. M.; Langer, R.; Folkman, J. *Diabetes* **1980**, *29*, 37–40.
29. Langer, R. S., personal communication.
30. Burns, K. J. M.A.Sc. Thesis, University of Toronto, 1980.
31. Lougheed, W. D., Woulfe-Flanagan, H.; Clement, J. R.; Albisser, A. M. *Diabetologia* **1980**, *19*, 1–9.
32. Bringer, J.; Heldt, A.; Grodsky, G. M. *Diabetes* **1981**, *30*, 83–85.
33. Lougheed, W. D.; Fischer, U.; Perlman, K.; Albisser, A. M. *Diabetologia* **1981**, *20*, 51–53.
34. Antonacci, G.; Sefton, M. V. unpublished data.
35. Treen, M. E. B.A.Sc. Thesis, University of Toronto, 1979.

RECEIVED for review January 16, 1981. ACCEPTED September 30, 1981.

INDEX

A

N-Acetylated diaminoalkane agarose
  gels 167f
N-Acetylated heparin, proton NMR
  spectrum...................... 172f
Acidified calcium nodule,
  chromatogram 409f
Acrylamide-grafted Silastic 4, 63f, 69t
Acrylic hydrogels, lipid sorption........ 397
Adhesion of platelets onto artificial
  surfaces......................... 82
Adhesion of sheared and unsheared
  leukocytes...................... 213
Adsorbed lipids in elastomer, Soxhlet
  extraction 401
Adsorbed protein(s)
  circular dichroism 240, 248
  denaturation..................... 239
  fibrin deposition 325f
  general properties................. 235
  interfaces 233
  layer, organization................. 236
  microcalorimetric studies............ 240
  platelet deposition................. 325f
  SDS-polyacrylamide gel electorphoretic,
    analysis........................ 72f
  structure......................... 239
  substrates, fibrin deposition ...323f, 327f,
                                      328f
  substrates, platelet deposition..323f, 328f,
                                      329f
Adsorbed species, biologically derived,
  experimental design 397
Adsorption
  albumin................. 259f, 309f, 317
  dynamics for albumin and γ-globulin. 366f
  fibrinogen.... 237, 282f, 285f, 286f, 288f,
                                        317
  fibronectin 317
  γ-globulin........................ 317
  hemoglobin 283
  interfacial 351
  intensity, circular dichroism spectra .. 253
  proteins........................245, 277
    from artificial tear solutions........ 453
    on biomaterials 233
    chromatographic examination 254
    from complex mixtures............ 234
    at interfaces 235
    on polymers..................... 293
  plasma protein(s)................... 192
  whole plasma..................... 237
Adsorption–desorption dynamics for albumin
  and γ-globulin................... 365f
Adsorption isotherm................... 357
  albumin..................257f, 364, 365f
  bovine γ-globulin 362, 363f
  proteins......................256, 450
AES (Auger electron spectroscopy) 17

Affinity chromatography, heparinase
  purification..................... 499
Affluent profiles, proteins 256
Agarose gels, heparin immobilization .. 174t
Albumin........................270, 294
  adsorption....76, 238, 293, 313, 317, 364,
                                        453
  contact lens polymers.. 457f, 458f, 459f
  copper.....................413, 417
  critical-point dry technique........ 305f
  defatted........................ 309f
                                365f, 366f
  enhancement.................... 294
  isotherm.................... 364, 365f
  methyl-coated surface............ 259f
  polymers....................... 308f
  PVC............................. 338
  quartz.......................... 253
  Silastic......................... 338
  sintered Teflon.............. 304f, 307f
  affinity........................... 293
  attenuated total reflection spectrum.. 384f
  band intensity ratios............... 376f
  binding, enhancement 308f
  circular dichroism 253f
  coated on PVC.................... 341f
  conformation of fibrinogen adsorbate.. 312
  deposit 271
  desorption 257f, 260, 262f
  desorption dynamics........... 366, 367f
  effect on adsorption of Cohn I
    fraction 294
  effects on cellular interactions with
    foreign materials 235t
  emergent front on treated glass
    beads......................... 255f
  emission spectrum 367
  exchange, by fibronectin on amine-coated
    surface........................ 261f
  fluorescence emission spectra 368f
  FTIR spectroscopy 373
  and intact plasma 272f
  interaction with metal surface........ 415
  lens deposits 454
  morphology 304
  photochemical effects............... 362
  polarization in solution.............. 425
  red cell effect 290
  represent 250f
  transmission spectra 374f, 375t, 377f,
                                      378f
  tyrosine fluorescence 368
Albumin–fibrinogen adsorption.... 312, 313,
                                      317
Albumin–fibrinogen mixture
  attenuated total reflection
    spectrum...................... 385f
  band frequency changes and Raman
    assignments 390t
  kinetics plot intensities............. 386f

523

Albumin-fibrinogen mixture (continued)
  spectrum.................... 391f, 292f
Albumin-globulins mixture, transmission
  spectra 379f, 380f, 381f
Aliphatic urethane model compounds ... 119
Alkyl halides and polyurethanes, reaction
  scheme 297f
Alkyl isocyanates and polyurethanes,
  reaction scheme................. 298f
Aminoethyl-coupled membranes 485
Anchoring site on polymers............ 397
Animal model for thromboresistance of
  polymers........................ 25
Anodized tantalum-sputtered glass...... 266
Anticoagulant activity(ies) assay 168
  derivatized end group 171
  heparins
    derivatized and immobilized....... 161
    effect of derivatization 164
    carboxylic derivatives............ 170t
    hydroxyl derivatives 171t
Anticoagulation techniques 493
Antifibrinogen 238, 273
  binding........................... 237
Antigenic protein 237
Antiplatelet agents 210, 218
Antithrombin III........... 150, 151t, 154f
Artificial pancreas 512
Artificial skin
  clinical advantages.................. 480
  collagen–glycosaminoglycan network .. 475
  design and performance......... 475–476
  evaluation........................ 478
  silicone elastomer 475
Artificial tear solutions................. 453
Aspirin, effect on thrombogenesis 57t
Atomic organization and surface
  crystallinity..................... 13t
Attenuated total reflectance IR
  spectroscopy..................... 19
Attenuated total reflection
  polymer surface and protein
    adsorption...................... 384
  protein layer 385
  protein solutions 382
  protein studies..................... 372
Auger electron spectroscopy (AES) 17
Augmented delivery, controlled-release
  micropump..................... 520
Autologous vein segments.............. 54

B

Band intensity ratios for albumin 376f
Binding mechanism, tearfilm proteins... 453
Binding stability of collagenase........ 487f
Block copolymer 133
  hydrophobic polyurethane............ 82
  lipid adsorption 397
  plasma interaction................... 81
Block copolyurethanes 109, 110, 128
Blood coagulation 91, 234t
Blood compatibility
  heparinization 493
  polyacrylamide surfaces 60
  with polymers 293

Blood compatibility (continued)
  properties....................... 109
  relationship to negative surface charge 414
  Stellite alloy heart valves............. 20
Blood filter, heparinase 493, 494
Blood flow rates...................... 225
Blood glucose control in diabetics 483
Blood heparin levels.................. 494
Blood interaction(s)
  with filters 228
  at foreign interfaces 4t, 5t
  with grafts 59
  mathematical model 33
  with polymers 76, 181, 294, 317, 347, 396,
                                           469
  with surface 36, 371, 265
Blood microemboli 221, 225
Blood microparticle flow resistance 222
Blood-compatible
  biomaterials 465
  materials......................... 147
  polymers......................... 471t
Blood-handling devices 221
Biocompatibility
  environment..................... 233
  process, cellular events 233
  synthetic polymers, effects on adsorbed
    proteins....................... 234t
Biological criteria of biomaterials 467
Biological environment, role in blood
  interactions at foreign interfaces..... 4t
Biological interactions, criteria for
  biomaterials 466t
Biological processes influenced by proteins
  at interfaces 234t
Biomaterials
  biological and physiological criteria ... 467
  and blood microemboli production.... 221
  blood-compatible................. 465
  constant-pressure filtration 227t
  development criteria............... 466t
  -induction of microemboli 224
  interactions with blood......... 3, 4t, 291
  mechanical degradation and
    environmental aging problems 467
  molecular orientation 10
  parallel-disc apparatus 224f
  physical behavior................. 468t
  platelet and fibrin deposition 317
  properties....................465, 467
  protein adsorption.................. 233
  surface characterization 20
  sterilization....................... 470
  structure......................... 465
  thrombus formation on coated rod.... 46f
  thrombus formation evaluation 44f
  toxicity.......................... 469
Biomedical elastomers 395
Biomer 396
  affinity of lipids 397
  bladder(s)
    chromatogram 403f, 408f
    lipids 404, 409
  calcification........................ 395
  flexing components................. 397
  free long-chain fatty acid adsorption .. 406

INDEX 525

Biomer (*continued*)
  lipid(s)
    adsorbed........................ 405f
    extracted....................... 404f
    sorption.....................398, 399
    weight gain..................... 400t
  lipophilicity 395
  polymerization of vinylpyrrolidone.... 404
  sorption of lipids................398, 399
  weight gains due to lipid sorption ... 401f
Bound heparin, in vitro activity 152
Bound thrombin–antithrombin
  III 150, 151t, 154
Bound water associated with
  polyphosphazene, DSC 188
Bovine γ-globulin(s) 357
  adsorption isotherm 362, 363f
  adsorption on sintered Teflon 302f
  fluorescence emission spectra....... 368f
Bovine serum albumin................ 357

C

Calcium deposition................... 397
Calcification......................... 294
  Biomer 395
  elastomeric bladders................ 397
  in blood–foreign material interactions .. 7t
Cannula composition 73t
Cannula platelet consumption........... 78
Carboxyl group determinations of
  heparin........................ 167
Carboxylic derivatization of
  heparin....................164, 170
Catheter studies, paired................ 31t
Carotid artery catheter region-of-interest
  scintillation counting............. 28f
Cell adhesion............... 293, 294, 312
  effects on adsorbed proteins 234t
  and protein adsorption.............. 454
Cell contents, effect on fibrinogen
  adsorption....................... 286
Cellular events, biocompatibility process 233
Cellular interactions with foreign
  materials...................... 235t
Cellular interactions sensitivity......... 233
Cellular reactions to proteins 241
Cellulose acetate membranes
  collagenase immobilization 483
  enzyme activity long-term tests 489f
  enzyme attachment............484, 486
  enzyme kinetics................... 488
  enzyme stability 488
Cellulose ester membranes............. 484
Chemical structure of block
  copolyurethanes.................. 110
Chemical structure, criteria for
  biomaterials 466t
Chemiluminescence levels............. 214
Cholesterol and cholesterol esters 406
Chromatogram
  acidified calcium nodule............ 409f
  Biomer bladder 403f, 408f
  examination of protein adsorption 254
  lipids........................... 402f
    adsorbed on Biomer............. 405f

Chromatogram (*continued*)
  lipids (*continued*)
    Biomer bladder 407f
Circular dichroism
  adsorbed proteins 240, 246, 248
  adsorption intensity 253
  albumin......................... 253f
  protein structure determination 246
Closure of full-thickness skin wounds ... 479
Clotting factors, surface-activated....... 273
Clotting tests, in vitro 149
Clot
  dissolution 348
  formation 348
  weight distribution 52f
Clot-promoting surfaces................ 267
Cohn I fibrinogen 293, 299, 304
  adsorption..................303f, 307
Collagen–glycosaminoglycan network,
  artificial skin.................... 475
Collagenase, binding stability......... 487f
Collagenase immobilized on cellulose
  acetate membranes............. 483
Complement C3 effects on cellular
  interactions with foreign materials . 235t
Complexation of LiBr with
  copolyether-urethane–ureas........ 133
Composition
  adsorbed protein...............236, 237
  thrombus formed on coated rods 49f
Concentration–difference driving force,
  insulin micropump 515, 518
Concentration of proteins at interfaces .. 236
Conductimetric titration curve for heparin
  derivative 168f
Conjunctivitis, giant papillary......453, 460
Constant-pressure filtration
  blood–filter interaction.............. 228
  flow rate curves.................... 227
  test
    blood microemboli 221
    filter pore size and filtration
      pressure 228
    for microemboli.................. 223
    results......................... 226f
    results for three biomaterials....... 227t
Controlled-release micropump
  augmented delivery 520
  insulin delivery 511, 513
  insulin deposition 520
  mechanism of action................ 520
  schematic 514f
Contact-activated coagulation 293
Contact angle, analysis of copolymers ... 86t
Contact angle measurements.......19, 184
Contact lenses, soft............453, 458–459
  accumulation of proteins 461
  copolymers, elution of adsorbed
    albumin...................... 459f
  polymers, adsorption of lysozyme,
    albumin, and IgG 457f, 458f
  polymers, water content 456
  rejection......................... 461
Contamination
  fluoropolymer 9, 10
  polymer 10

Contamination (continued)
silicone 10
surface 9, 10
Teflon 10
Copolyether-urethane–ureas
bulk morphology 115
complexation of LiBr 133
DSC 134
FTIR 129
internal reflectance 130f
LiBr effect on water absorption
 properties 135
and model polymer films 113
phase separation 115
polyether segment molecular weight .. 109
ratios of carbon 1s bands 128t
salt complex 133
synthesis 110
transmission spectra 116f, 117f
block–See Block copolymers
contact angle analysis 86t
critical surface tensions 90
hydrophilic, protein adsorption ... 460
hydrophobic polyurethane 82
platelet adhesion 90t
surface energy analysis 86t
synthetic structure 115
Copolyurethane(s) 133
FTIR analysis 137
hydrogels
 loss modulus and storage modulus vs.
  temperature 143f
 spectra 134
 tensile strengths 136
interaction with LiBr 136
IR analysis 137
morphology 135, 141
water absorption at saturation point .. 136t
Copper
adsorption of serum proteins 417
surfaces, resistant to serum proteins .. 413
Copper–zinc alloy
and albumin–globulin–fibrinogen
 solution 433
cyclic voltammetry 419f
electrodes 447
steady-state cathodic polarization 425
Copper cation concentration 63f
Corrosion potential, protein solutions .. 448, 450
Couette test system 43
Covalently heparinized materials 148
Critical-point dry technique 305f
Critical surface tensions for copolymers .. 90
Critical surface tension of
polyphosphazenes 188t
Cyclic voltammetry, proteins 416–420, 422f, 423f

D

Deconvolution spectrum, proteins 382
Defatted albumin adsorption 309f
Denaturation
adsorbed proteins 239
fibrinogen 247

Deposition
fibrinogen 48, 273
platelets 48, 54
red blood cells 48
Derivatization, effect on heparin
anticoagulant activity 164
Derivatization, heparin 170
Derivatized and immobilized heparins .. 161
Design principles, artificial skin 476
Desorption
albumin 260, 262f, 366
denatured protein 262
γ-globulin 366, 367f
protein, kinetics 387f
Dielectric mechanical measurements of
triblock copolymer 199
Dielectric spectra polyphosphazene 186f
Dielectric spectra unirradiated
polyphosphazene 185f
Difference dielectric measurements 179
Difference dielectric spectra of
polyphosphazenes 187f
Differential scanning calorimetry
(DSC) 103
bound water associated with
polyphosphazene 188
copolyether-urethane–ureas 134
LiBr–copolyurethane complexes 138t
Diol polyethers 101
Dipolar interaction, LiBr and urethane
groups 141
Dipyridamole 209, 210
Divinylsulfone-mediated N-acetylated
heparin hydroxyl group
derivatization 166f
Divinylsulfone-mediated 2-aminoethyl
hydrogen sulfate heparin
derivative 173f
Domain-like aggregates 127
Domain-matrix morphology 109
Drugs, effects on thrombus formation 54
Drugs in blood–foreign material
interactions 7t
DSC—See Differential scanning calorimetry
Dynamic mechanical measurements of
triblock copolymer 199
Dynamic mechanical spectra of triblock
copolymer 201f

E

Effluent profile, proteins 256
Elastomers
adsorption of long-chain fatty acids ... 402
biomedical, determination 395
bladders, calcification 397
lipid sorption 395, 399, 409
Elastomer weight gains due to lipid
sorption 400f
Electrical signals, effect on plasma protein
adsorption 413
Electrochemical reactions, protein at metal
interface 447
Electrochemistry of adsorption–desorption
processes of proteins 416
Electrolytic hydrogenation of fibrinogen .. 416

INDEX

Electron microscopy, gold decoration
  transmission 294
Electron spectroscopy for chemical analysis
  (ESCA)
  experiment, information derived
    from 16t
  instrument using a hemispherical electron
    analyzer 17f
  polyacrylamide–Silastic .. 66f, 67f, 68f, 70f
  pure polyacrylamide film cast on glass. 71f
  reasons for use 14
  Silastic tubing 66f
Electronic particle counting, leukocytes . 211
Electrophoresis, proteins 287, 289f
Elemental ratios for Silastic and
  acrylamide-grafted Silastic 69t
Emboli 327
Embolization and thrombosis,
  components 3
Embolication and thrombogenesis on
  polyacrylamide hydrogel surfaces 78
Energetics of protein binding 262
Energetics, surface 9
Energy dispersive analysis of x-rays,
  extracted hydrogel 134
Enzymes
  activity 486, 489f
  attachment, cellulose acetate
    membrane 484, 486
  immobilization, heparinase–
    Sepharose 503
  production, heparinase 497
  stability and kinetics 486, 488
Epichlorohydrin in heparin hydroxyl group
  derivatization 166f
Epidermal migration, skin graft 478
Erthrocytes, in blood–foreign material
  interactions 7t
Erthrocyte-poor blood 275
ESCA—*See* Electron spectroscopy for
  chemical analysis
Extracorporeal
  blood studies 178
  medical machines, heparinzation 493
  shafts 179
Extrinisic fluorescence, protein
  adsorption 354

F

Factor XII 265
Fatty acid 406
Fermentation, heparinase 498f, 499f
Filter–blood interaction, constant-pressure
  filtration 228
Filter pore size and filtration pressure .. 228
Filtration curve for microemboli-laden
  blood 225
Flow rates
  blood 225
  curves, constant-pressure filtration 227
Flow resistance
  blood microparticle 22
  microemboli 221–222
Flow time behavior of protein adsorption 393

Flowing attenuated total reflection
  spectrum, albumin 384f
Flowing attenuated total reflection
  spectrum, albumin–fibrinogen
  mixture 385f
Flowing protein solution, kinetics of
  desorption 387
Flowing systems, protein adsorption 382
Fluid shear
  dependence of protein adsorption ... 306f
  effects on adsorbed protein 306
  stress, protein adsorption 294
Fluorescence data for γ-globulin on
  quartz 359f
Fluorescence emission polarization
  studies 364
Fluorescence emission spectra 368f
Fluorescence, protein adsorption 351
Fourier transform infrared spectroscopy
  (FTIR) 114
  albumin 373
  albumin–γ-globulins mixture 383f
  copolyether-urethane–ureas 115, 129
  copolyurethanes 137
  fibrinogen 373
  γ-globulin 373
  instruments 19
  protein adsorption analysis 450
  proteins mixture 375
  protein–surface studies 371
  protein structure at surfaces 239, 240
  segmented polyurethanes 103
Fibrin 304
  deposition 342
  on adsorbed protein 325f
  on adsorbed protein substrates 323f,
                                   327f, 328f
  and platelet deposition
    biomaterials, role of plasma
      proteins 317
    curves 322
    experimental design 318
    on α₂-macroglobulin-coated PVC 335f
    α₂-macroglobulin-coated Silastic 336f
    polymers 191
    profiles 317
  formation 157, 348
  polymerization 341
Fibrinogen 265, 267, 275, 277, 294,
                                414, 447
  adsorption 91, 92, 237, 238, 266, 283,
                        293, 308f, 313, 317, 331
  to Cu 413, 417
  effect of red cells 280
  on glass 282f, 285f, 286f, 288f
  kinetics 239
  on PVC 327, 340
  on Silastic 327, 340
  SBS block copolymer 92
  conversion reaction, kininogen 240
  deposited in narrow spaces 267
  deposition 48, 271, 273
  effects on cellular interactions with
    foreign materials 235t
  electrolytic hydrogenation 416
  FTIR spectroscopy 373

Fibrinogen (continued)
   interaction with metal surface........ 415
   interaction, model................... 92
   kinetics of adsorption 283
   left by normal plasma between lens and
      glass slide...................... 274f
   left between convex lens and glass
      slide........................... 268f
   left by intact plasma between convex lens
      and anodized tantalum-sputtered glass
      slide........................... 269f
   radii............................. 271t
   representation 250f
   ring left by plasma 270f
   surface denaturation 247
Fibrinogen-coated PVC 343f, 344f
Fibronigen–albumin mixture
   adsorption........................ 371
   spectral changes 388
Fibrinogen–platinum interface 416
Fibrinolytic enzyme-immobilized
   polymers........................ 471t
Fibronectin.......... 260, 310, 317, 318
   adsorption on PVC and Silastic....... 334
   on amine-coated surface............ 261f
   plasma........................... 256
Fibronectin-coated PVC......... 337f, 339f
Fibronectin-coated Silastic............ 340f
Foreign body reaction around soft tissue
   implants 233
Foreign material–blood interactions...... 5t
Free long-chain fatty acid adsorption,
   Biomer 406
FTIR—See Fourier transform infrared
   spectroscopy
Functional group derivatization of
   heparin 164

G

Gel permeation chromatography 101
Genetic manipulation studies, heparinase
   production 498
Glass
   fibrinogen adsorption 92
   surface for studying biological
      interactions..................... 10
   transition of polyphosphazene........ 181
Glass–fibrinogen system........... 277, 278
Glycoproteins....................... 312
Glycoprotein–polymer interaction 293
Ghost cells
   preparation...................... 281f
   SEM 279f
γ-Globulin 294
   adsorption....................... 317
   to Cu........................413, 417
   –desorption dynamics....... 365f, 366f
   on PVC......................... 331
   on Silastic....................... 331
   on sintered Teflon.......... 301f, 302f
   confomational changes 363
   desorption 366, 367f
   FTIR spectroscopy................ 373
   interaction with metal surface........ 415
   photochemical effects 362

γ-Globulin (continued)
   photochemical susceptibility 362
   platelet release reaction 318
   protein emission spectrum........... 367
   on quartz, fluorescence data 359f
   representation 251f
   transmission spectra 378f
γ-Globulin-coated PVC 332f
γ-G-Globulin, lens deposits............ 454
Gold decoration transmission electron
   microscopy................... 293, 294
   protein adsorption on polymers 310
Gold nucleus (i)
   density, γ-globulin adsorbate 299
   distributions, Teflon 299
   on Teflon 300f
Graft level as a function of length for
   polyacrylamide-Silastic shunts...... 64f
Graft–wound bed interface, artificial
   skin............................ 476
Growth medium, heparinase
   production 497

H

Hematological profile during typical ex vivo
   test procedure.................... 45f
Hemispherical electron analyzer, ESCA
   instrument use................... 17f
Hemocompatibility effect of molecular
   motions of the polymer interface ... 177
Hemodialysis, shear stress levels 217
Hemodynamic parameters............. 48
Hemodynamics, role in blood–foreign
   material interactions............... 5t
Hemoglobin
   adsorption................... 283, 290
   blood–surface phenomena 290
   in supernatant as a function of time.. 284f
Heparin
   activity, assay curve 169f
   activity, activated partial thromboplastin
      time assays..................... 169
   anticoagulant activity(ies)........... 161
   N-acetylated and derivatized....... 168
   effect of derivatization 164
   bound, in vitro activity.............. 152
   carboxyl and sulfate group
      determinations................. 167
   carboxylic derivatives, anticoagulant
      activities..................... 170t
   carboxylic derivatization............ 164
   circuit for removal................ 495f
   complex 148
   conversion 504f
   on cyanogen bromide-activated
      surfaces..................... 163
   degradation 506
   derivatives, activated partial
      thromboplastin time 170
   derivatization 170
   derivatized and immobilized,
      anticoagulant activity 161
   effects of concentration on thrombus
      formation 56f
   fate of surface bound 147, 149t

Heparin (continued)
  functional group derivatization 164
  hydroxyl derivatives, anticoagulant
    activities 171t
  hydroxyl group derivatization 165
  immobilization 166, 171
    N-acetylated diaminoalkane agarose
      gels 167f
    to agarose gels 174t
    to polymer surface 163
    spacer groups 164
    stability 150
    thromboresistant surfaces 164
  long-term use 148
  and platelets, interaction 157
  removal
    from citrated rabbit blood 507f
    experimental design 494
    extracorporeal therapy 506
    protein–salt solutions 505f
    side effects 162
    system 493, 506
  surfaces, prolonged clotting times 171
Heparin–PNA beads, prolongation of
  thrombin time 152
Heparin–poly(vinyl alcohol) 148
  beads
    recalcification time of plasma 153f
    thrombin affinity 150
    thrombin binding 152
    thrombin time of plasma 152f
  displacement of bound radiolabeled
    protein 155f
  linkage 156
  preparation 149
  thrombin binding 156
Heparinase
  activity 506
  enzyme production 497
  fermentation 498f, 499f
  immobilization on polymer supports . 503t
  immobilized, in vitro studies 504
  improved production, purification,
    characterization of properties 493
  inhibitors, isolation 493
  kinetics of enzyme production 497
  production 497
    environmental factors and growth
      medium 497
    genetic manipulation studies 498
  purification 499
    affinity chromatography 499
  reactor 508
  stability 502f
  thermal stability 503
Heparinase–Sepharose, enzyme
  immobilization 503
Heparinization 157
  blood compatibility 493
  extracorporeal medical machines 493
Heparinized
  beads 154f
  gels 171, 174
  glutaraldehyde-stabilized surfaces 163
  materials, long-term use 157
  polymers, blood-compatible 471t

Heparinized (continued)
  surfaces, coagulation factors 174
  surfaces in blood–foreign material
    interactions 7t
High pressure liquid chromatography
  (HPLC), proteins 255
Histopathology of recovered thrombus .. 32f
Host–graft rejection 480
  artificial skin 475
Hydrated (frozen) samples and ESCA
  technique 16
Hydrodynamics and thrombus formation 46,
                                        48
Hydrogel(s)
  blood-compatible 471t
  bulk morphology 135
  copolyurethene, tensile strengths 136
  formation 133
  internal reflectance spectra 144f
  materials 59
  morphology 142
  preparation 134
  tensile strength vs. concentration of
    LiBr 137f
  water absorption vs. concentration of
    LiBr 135f
  water absorption curves 133, 135
Hydrophilic copolymers, protein
  adsorption 460
Hydrophobic
  bonding, protein surface interaction .. 460
  interaction 290
  polyurethane block copolymer 82
Hydrophobic–hydrophilic
  copolymers 453
  interactions, protein binding 460
Hydroxyl-derivatized heparin 170
Hydroxyl group derivatization of
  heparin 165
Hysteresis effects, protein adsorption ... 363

I

IgG–See Immunoglobulin G
Ion scattering spectroscopy 18
Ionic model to correlate and interrelate
  properties of copolymer to
  thrombogenesis 195
Inactivation of thrombin by antithrombin
  III 154f
Inhibition of thrombus formation 48
Immobilized heparins
  anticoagulant activity 161
  directly to polymer surface 163
  stability 150
Immunoglobulin, protein adsorption 453
Immunoglobulin G (IgG)
  adsorption to contact lens polymers .. 457f,
                                      458f
  effects on cellular interactions with
    foreign materials 235t
  red cell effect 290
Implant polymers 294
Implantable micropump for insulin
  delivery 511
Implants, major reactions 233

Infection exudation, artificial skin....... 475
Influence of interfacial protein layer 235
Insulin
  delivery
    controlled-release micropump...... 513
    implantable micropump, effect of
      rate-controlling membrane 511
    mechanism..................... 512
    open-loop.................520, 521
    rate micropump.............511, 515
    rates with various membranes..... 519f
    systems, open-loop............... 511
  deposition in controlled-release
    micropump..................... 520
  micropump
    concentration-difference driving... 515, 518
    design factors.................... 520
    effect of membranes............. 517t
    effect of polycarbonate filter....... 516
    pressure-difference driving force .. 515, 516
    rate controlling membrane 516
    precipitates, SEM micrograph 518f
    precipitation...................... 511
    pumps........................... 513
Interaction(s)
  blood–biomaterial.................3, 291
  blood, at foreign interfaces 4t
  blood–foreign material 5t
  blood–polymer............ 294, 347, 396
  blood–surface...................... 371
  experimental design of specific test .. 36
  cellular, sensitivity 233
  dipolar, LiBr and urethane groups.... 141
  grafted polyacrylamide–Silastic surfaces
    with blood 59
  heparin–platelets.................... 157
  hydrophobic....................... 290
  hydrophobic–hydrophilic, protein
    binding......................... 460
  LiBr
    and urethane group 137
    and segmented
      copolyether-urethane–ureas...... 134
    and copolyurethanes............... 136
  metal–protein...................... 414
  model of fibrinogen.................. 92
  plasma, on block copolymers.......... 81
  platelet–protein..................... 318
  polymer–blood..................... 469
  polymer–tissue..................... 469
  protein adsorption................... 416
  protein–surface 245, 318, 346
  protein–thrombus................... 318
  protein–water...................... 416
  receptor–protein 233
  red cell–surface..................... 291
  tissue–material..................... 233
  urethane interface and polyether
    matrix......................... 123
  urethane NH groups and polyether... 125
  urethane NH groups and polyether or
    urethane alkoxy oxygens 123
Interfaces
  absorbed proteins 233, 235
  behavior of proteins 234

Interfaces (continued)
  biological processes influenced by
    proteins...................... 234t
  blood–polymer.................... 317
  concentration and localization of
    proteins......................... 236
  structure of proteins................ 240
Interfacial
  adsorption......................... 351
  behavior of proteins 260
  fluorescence signals, adsorbed
    protein 359
  photochemistry 361
  protein fluorescence................. 364
  protein adsorption.................. 352
  protein layer 235
Intermolecular interactions in polyether
  matrix 124
Intermolecular interactions,
  polyether-urethane–ureas 126
Internal reflection evanescent wave
  excitation, protein adsorption 352
Internal reflectance fluorescense
  exponential decay curves 355f
  protein adsorption, experimental
    design......................... 354
  quantitation assumptions, protein
    adsorption...................... 360
  principles 352
  rectangular coordinate system....... 353f
  schematic 356f
  spectra, copolyether-urethane–ureas . 130f
  spectra of hydrogels 144f
Intrinsic fluorescence, protein
  adsorption..................352, 359
IR, Fourier transform—See Fourier
  transform infrared spectroscopy
IR spectra
  albumin and γ-globulin mixture...... 382
  aliphatic urethane III and urethane IV
    model compounds................ 121
  copolyurethanes.................... 137
  copolyurethanes with LiBr 134
  polyether-urethane–ureas 118, 119
  polyphosphazenes 184
  transmission studies of proteins 372
Islet suspension, transplanted.......... 484
Islet-transplantation chambers......... 483
  cellulose ester membranes.......... 484

K

Kinetics
  adsorption of proteins.............. 238
  desorption, flowing protein solution... 387
  enzyme production, heparinase 497
  fibrinogen adsorption 239
  of interaction with surfaces of proteins 245
  plot of intensity for albumin–fibrinogen
    mixture...................... 386f
  of protein desorption 387f
  of thrombus accumulation 54
Kininogen.................. 265, 273, 290
  fibrinogen conversion reaction 240
  left by normal plasma between lens and
    glass slide..................... 274f

INDEX

L

Laser scattering technique............. 77
Lens deposits....................... 460
   lysozyme, albumin, and γ-globulin ... 454
Lens hazing........................ 453
Leukocyte
   adhesion
      antiplatelet drugs, effect 213
      measurement................... 212
      sheared and unsheared........... 213f
   in blood–foreign material interactions .. 7t
   in electronic particle counting........ 211
   in protein adsorption 346
   suspensions, changes in electronic particle count........................ 212f
   in thrombogenesis on artificial surfaces. 77
Leukocyte β-blucuronidase activity 215f
Leukocyte integrity of dipyridamole RA-233 and prostaglandin E_1 210
Leukocyte response, analysis of shear stress....................... 209–212
Leukocyte peak chemiluminescence ... 214f
Leukocyte phagocytosis 218
Lipid adsorption
   on Biomer 404, 405f, 407f
   block copolymers................... 397
Lipids
   chromatogram 402f
   extracted from Biomer............. 404f
   sorption
      Biomer bladders 409
      Biomer weight gains........ 400t, 401f
      elastomer weight gains........... 400f
      polymers, various 398
Lipophilicity of Biomer 395
Liquid-scintillation counting, tritium-labeled free heparin levels 169
Lithium bromide
   effect on water absorption properties of copolyether-urethane-ureas........ 135
   interaction with copolyurethanes 136
   interaction with segmented, copolyether-urethane–ureas........ 134
   and urethane groups, dipolar interaction 141
Lithium bromide complexation with copolyether-urethane–ureas........ 133
   DSC dissociation temperatures...... 138t
   loss tangent vs. temperature........ 138f
   transmission spectra 139f, 140f
Localization of proteins at interfaces 236
Long-chain fatty acids
   adsorption on elastomers............ 402
   deposition onto polyurethane 409
Long-term function, skin graft 480
Long-term tests of enzyme activity, cellulose acetate membrane....... 489f
Loss of cytochemically assayed LAP ... 217f
Loss modulus and storage modulus vs. temperature for copolyurethane hydrogels 143f
Lysozyme
   adsorption to contact lens polymers.. 457f, 458f
   lens deposits 454
   protein adsorption................. 453

M

$α_2$-Macroglobulin................... 346
   adsorption on PVC and Silastic....... 334
$α_2$-Macroglobulin-coated PVC, platelets and fibrin......................... 335f
$α_2$-Macroglobulin-coated Silastic, platelets and fibrin..................... 336f
Macromolecular adsorption on thin polymer films 354
Macroscopic structure, tests of physical behavior of biomaterials.......... 468t
Mass spectroscopy of polyphosphazenes . 184
Mathematical modeling, blood–materials interactions..................... 33
Mechanical behavior
   and materials processing, criteria for biomaterials 466t
   tests of physical behavior of biomaterials 468t
Mechanical spectra, dynamic, of triblock copolymer..................... 201f
Mechanism of adsorption inhibition..... 278
Mechanism for inhibition of thrombus formation 48
Membranes
   cellulose acetate, binding of collagenase 483, 487f
   for use with insulin micropump 514
Membrane–enzyme testing............ 486
Metal–protein interaction 414
Methemoglobin...................286, 290
Microcalorimetric studies of adsorbed proteins....................... 240
Microemboli
   biomaterial-induced 224
   concentrations 227
   constant-pressure filtration 221, 223
   flow-resistant
      criteria 222
      method to count 221
      screen filtration pressure test 222
   production, three types of materials .. 228
Microemboli-laden blood, filtration curve........................... 225
Microparticle, blood, flow resistance.... 222
Micropump
   controlled-release, for insulin delivery................ 511, 513, 514
   fabrication........................ 514
   for insulin delivery, implantable, rate controlling membrane 511
Migration velocity of epithelial cell sheets, skin graft...................... 477
Mineralization process 395
Mobility of groups attached to polymer segments....................... 39
Model
   fibrinogen interaction................ 92
   ionic, to correlate and interrelate properties of copolymer to thrombogenesis 195
   for in vivo platelet and thrombus kinetics 25
   to predict thrombogenic responses of polymeric substrates............. 195
   structure determination 33

Model (continued)
  thrombogenesis 203
Modified collagen, blood-compatible ... 471t
Molecular motions
  effect on thrombogenesis 203
  polyphosphazene 181, 192
  polymer interface 177, 178
Molecular template to orient polymer
  chains 11
Molecular weight of polyether
  segment 109, 115
Morphological changes,
  copolyurethanes 134, 135
Morphological structures of bulk and surface
  of block copolyurethanes 110
Morphology
  copolyether-urethane–ureas 115
  copolyurethane 141
  effects of LiBr 133
  hydrogels 135, 142
  phase-separated 115
  polyether-urethane–urea 118
  polyphosphazene 180
  surface, of copolyether-urethane-
    ureas 115
  triblock copolymer 197

N

NMR analysis of derivatized heparins ... 165
Nomarski microscopy 83

O

Open-loop glucose control systems 512
Open-loop insulin delivery ... 511, 520, 521
Optical scattering cuvette 62f
Organization of adsorbed protein layer .. 236
Orientation, polymer chain surface 11
Outer radii of rings of platelets left by
  heparinized blood 272t
Oxidation, common surface reaction 12
Oxyhemoglobin 286, 290

P

Pancreas, artificial—See also Artificial
  pancreas 512, 513
Pannus formation 294
Parallel-disc apparatus for exposing blood to
  biomaterials 224f
Partial coverage gold nuclei 299
Partial gold decoration 308, 311
Pellethane 2363–80A 309f
Periodate oxidation 491
Perpendicular polarization-mode electric
  field amplitide equation 352
Phagocytosis 214
Phase separation
  copolyether-urethane–ureas 115
  polyether-urethanes 118
Phosphodiesterase inhibitors 218
Phosphorus x-ray dispersion map of
  polyphosphazene 181f, 182f, 183f
Photochemical effects, γ-globulin and
  albumin 362

Photochemistry, interfacial 361
Photoeffects, conventional
  spectrofluorometric conditions 361
Physical behavior of biomaterials 468t
Physical chemistry of wound closure 476
Physical properties, polymeric systems
  tests 468
Physiochemical behavior of a surface 91
Plasma
  fibronectin 256
  interaction on block copolymers 81
  recalcification time 149, 152
  in narrow spaces of clot-promoting
    surfaces 265
Plasma protein(s)
  adsorption 238
    to Cu 413, 417
    to polyphosphazene surface 192
  affecting cellular interactions with foreign
    materials 235
  role in initiating platelet and fibrin
    deposition on biomaterials 317
  structural changes 245
Platelet
  accumulation 33
  activation, polyurethane 96
  adhesion 91, 265, 275, 291, 293, 318,
              331, 335, 341–343, 348, 414
    for copolymers 90t
  heparinized glutaraldehyde-stabilized
    surfaces 163
  plasma interaction on block
    copolymer 81
  in blood–foreign material interactions .. 6t
  in clot on polyphosphazene-coated
    shafts 191t
  consumption 73–74
  content in thrombus 32
  deposition 157
    on adsorbed protein 325f
    on adsorbed protein substrates ... 323f,
                                    328f, 329f
  phosphazene polymers 191
    on PVC 324
    on rod 54
    on Silastic 326
  interaction with heparin 157
  microaggregate 216, 217
  kinetics 33
  retention 27, 105, 275
  index 38, 40, 95, 96, 105f
  in vitro test 37f
  polyethylene catheters 30f
  on polymer surfaces, in vitro
    experiments 35, 38
  and thrombus dissolution 28f
  and thrombus kinetics 25
  triblock polymer 199
Platelet and fibrin deposition
  curves 322
  on biomaterials 317
  experimental design 318
  on α$_2$-macroglobulin-coated PVC 335f
  on α$_2$-macroglobulin-coated Silastic .. 336f
  measurements 320
  profiles 317

Platelet and fibrin deposition (continued)
  phosphazene polymers 191
  rates 48
Platelet–protein interactions 318
Plexiglass, effects on blood flow rates ... 225
Polarization
  curve for protein solutions 446
  electronic transitions, proteins 252f
  protein accumulation 433
Polyacrylamide
  hydrogel(s)
    surfaces, thrombogenesis and
      embolization 78
  surfaces
    blood compatibility 60
    thrombogenicity 74
Polyacrylamide-grafted substrates, platelet
  consumption 74t
Polyacrylamide-silastic
  cannulae, thromboemboli generated
    grafts 74
  eluates 76
  ESCA C1s spectra 70f
  hydrogel surfaces 78
  shunts
    graft level as a function of length ... 64f
    thromboembolic propensity 72
  surfaces
    with blood, interaction of grafted 59
    grafted, thrombotic events 59
  thromboemboli volume and platelet
    consumption 75f
  tubing
    dehydrated, ESCA C1s
      spectra 67f, 68f
    SEM 65f
Polycarbonate discs 225
Polycarbonate membrane 517
Polydimethylsiloxane 294
  platelet retention index 38
Polyelectrolyte hydrogels 414
Polyelectrolyte adsorption 203
Polyethers
  platelet retention index values 96
  segment, molecular weight 109, 110, 115
  soft segments segmented
    polyurethanes 95
Polyether-urethane, phase separation ... 118
Polyether-urethane–urea
  films
    spectra 114
    surfaces 128
    IR spectrum 118, 119
    morphologies 118
Polyethylene 290
  catheters, platelet retention
    behavior 30, 30f
  complex surface structure due to
    oxidation 12
Poly(ethylene oxide)
  chemical shifts 97t
  platelet retention index 38
PolyHexene-H, lipid sorption 398
Poly(hexyl acrylate) 38
Poly(2-hydroxyethyl methacrylate) 453

Polymers
  albumin preadsorption 308f
  animal model assessing
    thromboresistance 25
  biomedical application, criteria 466
  chain surface orientation 11
  composition, effect on equilibrium water
    content 456
  interface 177, 178
  platelet retention index $\bar{\rho}$ 38f
  protein adsorption 293
  and cell adhesion 454
  supports, heparinase immobilization . 503t
  segments, mobility of groups attached .. 39
  surface, immobilization of heparin 163
  surface, protein adsorption 384
  surfaces, platelet retention 35
  toxicity 469, 470t
Polymer-based implants 293
Polymer–blood interactions ... 347, 396, 469
Polymer–blood interface 317
Polymer-coated rods 54t
Polymer–tissue interactions 469
Polymer–salt complexes, morphological
  changes resulting from 134
Polymeric gels, protein adsorption values 460
Polymeric material
  at blood–polymer interface, molecular
    elements 35
  to thrombogenesis, surface
    properties 177
Polymeric membranes for patients with
  skin loss 475
Polymeric substrates, model to predict
  thrombogenic responses 195
Polymeric systems, testing of physical
  properties 468
Poly(methyl acrylate), platelet retention
  index 38
Poly(methyl methacrylate) 453
  casting solvent 11
  platelet retention index 30
Poly(methyl methacrylate-2-hydroxyethyl
  methacrylate) copolymers 453
Polypropylene glycol 125
Poly(propylene oxide) 38, 97t
Polypropylene surface after exposure to
  flowing blood 51f
Polystyrene–beads 41
  effects on blood flow rates 225
  platelet retention index 38
Polystyrene–poly(ethylene oxide) 84
  Nomarski micrograph of surface
    texture 88f, 89f
  TEM 85f, 87f
Poly(tetramethylene oxide), platelet
  retention index 38, 97t
Poly[(trifluoroethoxy)
  (fluoroalkoxy)phosphazene] 177, 178
  adsorption of plasma protein onto
    surface 192
  blood interfacing surface 181
  contact angle measurements 184
  dielectric spectra 185f, 186f, 187f
  exposed to canine blood,
    SEM 190f, 191f

Poly[(trifluoroethoxy)(fluoroalkoxy)
phosphazene] *(continued)*
  effect of primary and secondary molecular
    motions on thrombogenesis........ 181
  fibrin deposition 191
  function of irradiation dose 189f
  function of UV irradiation 188t
  glass transition..................... 181
  IR spectra......................... 184
  lipid sorption 398
  mass spectra....................... 184
  molecular motions.............. 181, 192
  morphology 180
  phosphorus x-ray dispersion map 181f,
    182f-183f
  platelet deposition.................. 191
  polymers, thrombogenic response 188
  TEM 180f, 182f-183f
  tensile stress–strain measurements.... 188
  thrombogenic response 192
  x-ray dispersion spectra 184f
Polyurea, platelet retention index 38
Polyurethane 82, 294
  analyzed by ESCA 21
  and alkyl halides, reaction scheme ... 297f
  and alkyl isocyanates, reaction
    scheme 298f
  block copolymer, hydrophobic 82
  blood-compatible................... 471t
  hard-segment phase, platelet
    activation 96
  lipid sorption 398
  partial coverage gold nuclei.......... 299
  platelet attachment.................. 91
  protein adsorbates.................. 293
  segmented 95, 103
    bulk and surface composition 104t
    characteristics 102t
    critical study 95
    FTIR............................ 103
    vs. platelet retention index 105f
    polyether 96
    surface and bulk composition 104t
    synthesis........................ 97
    type I 98, 99f, 107
    type II or III 98, 100f
    x-ray photoelectron spectroscopy ... 103
  surface energy data.................. 89
  thrombin adsorption................. 96
Polyurethane–silicone rubber
  copolymer......................... 294
Poly(vinyl alcohol) (PVA)
  beads
    recalcification time of plasma incubated
      with......................... 153f
    thrombin affinity 150
    thrombin time of plasma 152f
  platelet retention index 38
Polyvinyl chloride (PVC)
  absorption fibrinogen and von Willebrand
    factor.......................... 340
  albumin adsorption................. 338
  albumin-coated 341f
  arteriovenous shunts................ 317
  fibrinogen-coated............. 343f, 344f
  fibronectin adsorption..........327, 334
  fibronectin-coated 337f, 339f

Polyvinyl chloride (PVC) *(continued)*
  γ-globulin adsorption 331
  γ-globulin-coated................... 332f
  α_2-macroglobulin absorption 334
  protein adsorption............. 324f, 327
  test data 330t
  protein and thrombus response 322
  von Willebrand factor-coated 345f
Potentiostatic voltammetry of protein
  solutions 416
PNF—*See* Poly[(trifluoroethoxy)
  (fluoroalkoxy)phosphazene]
Pressure–difference driving force, insulin
  micropump 514, 515, 516
Proliferation of fibrin fibrils............. 52
Prolonged partial thromboplastin
  times 152, 156
Propst diagram 14f
Prostaglandin therapy................. 218
Prostaglandin E$_1$ 209, 210
Protein(s)
  accumulation 425, 433
  adsorption..................... 266, 291
    albumin....................... 453
    from artificial tear solutions.... 453, 454
    attenuated total reflection, polymer
      surface...................... 384
    on biomaterials 233
    blood–foreign material interactions .. 6t
    from blood plasma............... 76
    and cell adhesion, polymers 454
    and charge transfer..........416, 447
    chemical and physical factors 459
    chromatographic examination 254
    from complex mixtures........... 234
    Cu 445
    and desorption...............245, 294
    dog model 347
    dynamics...................... 357
    effects on biocompatibility of synthetic
      polymers..................... 234t
    effects on cell adhesion 234t
    effects on immunology........... 234t
    electrochemical reactions.......... 447
    electrochemical reduction 415
    extrinsic fluorescence 354
    flow time behavior 393
    flowing systems 382
    fluid shear stress................. 294
    on Fluorofilm, fluid shear
      dependence 306f
    FTIR analysis................... 450
    gold decoration, TEM 310
    hydrophilic copolymers 460
    hydrophobic–hydrophilic
      copolymers.................. 453
    hysteresis effects 363
    immunoglobulins................ 453
    at interfaces 233, 234
    interfacial protein fluorescence..... 352
    internal reflectance fluorescence.... 354
    internal reflection evanescent wave
      excitation 352
    intrinsic fluorescence 354
    isotherm(s) 236, 450
    leukocytes...................... 346
    lysozyme....................... 453

Protein(s) (continued)
  adsorption (continued)
    partial gold decoration
      methodology 311, 313
    polymeric gels 460
    on polymers 293–294
    on polyurethane 293
    proterties 235
    pulsed cathodic polarization 433
    on PVC 317, 324f, 327, 330t
    red cells, influence 277, 278
    signal intensity 360
    on Silastic 326f
    on silicone rubber 293
    structure 239
    surface texture or roughness 460
    onto surfaces 245
    solid–aqueous buffer solution
      interfaces 351
    on Teflon 293
    in thrombotic response of blood to
      polymers 69
    total internal reflection intrinsic
      fluorescence 351
  adsorption–desorption
    dynamics 364
    information, interpretation 260
    kinetics 246
    rates 388
  affinity for surfaces 236
  antigenic 237
  attenuated total reflection studies 372
  bacterial nuclease, representation ... 248f, 249f
  behavior at interfaces 234
  binding
    energetics 262
    hydrophobic–hydrophilic
      interactions 460
  cellular reaction 241
  circular dichroism 246
  composition, site density, and
    reactivity 236
  conformational changes 388
  on contact lenses, accumulation 461
  deposition 320, 453
  desorbing, pulsed currents 449
  effluent profile 256
  electrophoresis 289f
  emission spectrum, albumin, tryptophan,
    and γ-globulin 367
  high pressure liquid chromatography .. 255
  hydrogen bond structure 373
  induced desorption 262
  interfacial 233, 260
    adsorption 235
    biological processes influenced 234t
    concentration and localization 236
    structure 240
  IR transmission studies 372
  mixture, FTIR spectroscopy 375
  in narrow spaces of clot-promoting
    surfaces 265
  plasma
    adsorption to high Cu alloy 413
    and cellular interactions with foreign
      materials 235t

Protein(s) (continued)
  plasma (continued)
    role in initiating platelet and fibrin
      deposition on biomaterials 317
    proportion of activating and
      passivating 242
    polarization of electronic transitions .. 252f
    and polyelectrolyte adsorption of
      thrombogenesis model 203
    reduction reaction 448
  solutions
    attenuated total reflection 382
    corrosion potential 448, 450
    cyclic voltammetry 418, 419
    polarization curve 446
    potentiostatic and cyclic
      voltammetry 416
    spectral identification in mixtures 381
    structural changes 246, 373
    instrumental technique 239, 240
    interpretation 246
    and kinetics of interaction with
      surfaces 245
  at surfaces
    FTIR 239, 240
    total internal reflectance
      fluorescence 239, 240
    on tetradecane–trimethylsilane-coated
      glass 251t
    and thrombus response to PVC and
      Silastic 322
Protein-coated surfaces, thrombotic
  response 327
Protein–metal interaction 414, 415
Protein–platelet interactions 318
Protein–polymer binding 310
Protein–polymer sorption studies 294
Protein–protein binding 304, 310
Protein–protein exchange processes 258
Protein–receptor interaction 233
Protein–surface interactions ... 318, 346, 371, 460
Protein–thrombus interaction 318
Protein–water interactions 416
Prothrombin zymogen form 174
Proton NMR spectrum of N-acetylated
  heparin 172f
Proton NMR spectrum of
  divinylsulfone-mediated 2-aminoethyl
  hydrogen sulfate heparin
  derivative 173f
Pulsed cathodic polarization, protein
  adsorption 433
Pulsed currents, desorbing proteins 449
Purification of heparinase 499
Pure polyacrylamide film cast on glass,
  ESCA spectra 71f
PVA—See Poly(vinyl alcohol)
PVC—See Polyvinyl chloride
Pyrolitic carbons, blood-compatible
  polymers 471t

R

Rate-controlling membrane, insulin
  micropump 516
Reaction scheme, polyurethanes and alkyl
  halides 297f

Reaction scheme, polyurethanes and alkyl
   isocyanates 298f
Reactivity of proteins 236
Recalcification time of plasma incubated
   with PVA and heparin-PVA
   beads......................... 153f
Receptor–protein interaction........... 233
Recovered thrombus, histopathology.... 32f
Rectangular coordinate system, internal
   reflection fluorescence 353f
Reduction reaction, proteins........... 448
Red blood cells
   and components, influence on protein
      adsorption..................... 277
   deposition rates.................... 48
   effect on adsorption of albumin and
      fibrinogen to polyethylene surfaces . 277
   interactions........................ 291
Red cell effect 277, 283, 290
   quantity of fibrinogen adsorbed to glass
      surface......................... 280
   membrane-related.................. 277
   preparation, distribution of cell
      volume 281f
   albumin and IgG................... 290
Red cell–surface interactions........... 291
Red thrombus formation 147
Resistance, flow, blood microparticle.... 222
Routes to the formation of blood thrombi.. 3

S

SBS—See Styrene–butadiene–styrene
Scanning Auger microprobe (SAM) 18
Scanning electron microscopy (SEM)
   of copper–zinc alloy 426f, 427f
   after cathodic polarization 428f
   with albumin 429f, 436f–439f, 443f,
                                        445f
   with albumin–globulin fibrinogen . 115f
   with fibrinogen .. 433f-438f, 440f, 444f,
                                        445f
   with γ-globulin .. 430f–432f, 436f–438f,
                                 440f–443f, 445f
   in saline and proteins............. 420f
   ghost cell 279f
   insulin precipitates 518f
   phosphazene 190f, 191f
   polyacrylamide–Silastic.............. 65f
   polypropylene surface after exposure to
      flowing blood................... 51f
Schematic
   controlled-release micropump....... 514f
   internal reflectance fluorescence..... 356f
   optical scattering cuvette............ 62f
   total internal reflectance fluorescence
      data..................... 358f, 361f
Screen filtration pressure test, flow-resistant
   microemboli..................... 222
Secondary bonding occurring within a pure
   urea domain.................... 123
Secondary ion mass spectrometry........ 18
Segmental surface experiments to test
   sensitization of blood 53f
Segmented copolyether-urethane–ureas,
   interaction with LiBr 134
Segmented polyether polyurethanes 95

Segmented polyurethanes 95, 103
   characteristics 102t
   critical study 95
   FTIR............................ 103
   vs. platelet retention index 105f
   surface and bulk composition 104t
   type I 98, 99f, 107
   type II or III 98, 100f
   synthesis........................ 97
   x-ray photoelectron spectroscopy 103
SEM—See Scanning electron microscopy
Sensitization of clotting factors 52
Sepharose–heparinase enzyme
   immobilization................... 503
Sequence and mechanistic aspects of
   thrombotic events................. 60
Shear, effects on thrombus formation 48, 50f
Shear stress
   leukocyte response 209, 212
   levels during hemodialysis........... 217
   release of LAP.................... 215f
Side chain motion and chemistry,
   thrombogenesis model 203
Silastic.............................4, 61
   albumin adsorption................ 338
   arteriovenous shunts, proteins
      adsorbed..................... 317
   clot weight distribution 52f
   elemental ratios.................... 69t
   eluates........................... 76
   fibrinogen adsorption 340
   fibronectin adsorption..........327, 334
   fibronectin-coated................. 340f
   γ-globulin adsorption 331
   grafted, thrombotic events........... 59
   α$_2$-macroglobulin adsorption 334
   platelet consumption 75f, 78
   platelet deposition................. 326
   protein adsorption.............326f, 330t
   shunts, thromboembolic propensity.... 72
   surfaces interaction with blood........ 59
   thromboemboli volume 75f
   tubing
      ESCA spectra 66f, 67f
      SEM 65f
   von Willebrand factor adsorption 340
Silicone
   contamination 10
   elastomer
      artificial skin.................... 475
      blood-compatible............... 471t
   rubber
      partial coverage gold nuclei........ 299
      protein adsorbates............... 293
SIMS (Secondary ion mass
   spectrometry).................... 18
Site density of proteins 236
Skin, artificial, design and
   performance.................... 475
   See also Artificial skin
Skin graft
   epidermal migration................ 478
   full-thickness wounds in guinea pigs ... 478
   human subjects 479
   limiting dimensions................ 477
   long-term function 480

Skin graft (continued)
  migration velocity of epithelial cell
    sheets 477
  wound contraction 478
Skin wounds, closure of full-thickness ... 479
Soflens 458–459
Soft tissue implants, foreign body
    reaction 233
Solid–aqueous buffer solution interfaces,
    protein adsorption 351
Sorption of lipids
  acrylic hydrogels 397
  elastomer 395
Soxhlet extraction, adsorbed lipids in
    elastomer 401
Spacer group distance, heparinized
    gels 174
Spacer length, effect on enzyme
    activity 486
Spacer between substrate and biologically
    active molecule 485
Spatial relations in thrombus formation ... 50
Spatially resolved surface chemistry
    analysis 13t
Spectral analysis, copolyether-
    urethane–ureas 115
Spectral changes
  fibrinogen–albumin mixture 388
  protein structural changes 373
Spectroscopies used to study surfaces ... 14f
Stability
  enzyme attachment, cellulose acetate
    membrane 486
  heparinase 502f
  immobilized heparin 150
Steady-state cathodic polarization Cu–zinc
    alloy 425
Stellite alloy heart valves, blood
    compatibility 20
Sterility, biomaterials 470
Structural changes, plasma proteins 245
Structure of protein(s)
  adsorbed 239
  determination by circular dichroism
    spectroscopy 246
  at interfaces 240
  serum 247
  surfaces, interaction kinetics 245
Styrene–butadiene–styrene 83
  block copolymer 82
  fibrinogen adsorption 92
  platelets attached 91
  Nomarski micrograph of surface
    texture 85f
TEM
  irregular styrene domains 83f
  spherical styrene domains 84f
Succinyl aminoethyl-coupled
    membranes 486
Sulfate determinations of heparin 167
Surface
  analysis methods 13t
  analytical methods, comparison 15f
  bound heparin, fate 147, 149t
  and bulk composition of segmented
    polyurethanes 104t

Surface (continued)
  calcification on Biomer flexing
    components 397
  characterization
    biomaterials science 20
    materials for blood contact
      applications 9
    techniques 12
    tests of physical behavior,
      biomaterials 468t
  chemical reactions 11
  contaminations 9–10
  crystallinity and atomic organization .. 13t
  denaturation
    adsorbed albumin 254
    fibrinogen 247
  electrical properties 13t
  energetics 9
  energy, analysis of copolymers 86t
  energy data, polyurethane 89
  free energy distribution 294
  hydrophobicity/hydrophilicity 177
  interactions with blood 36, 371
  interaction with proteins 245, 318
  interactions with red cells 291
  microcrystallinity 177
  morphologies of block
    copolyurethanes 128
  morphology of
    copolyether-urethane–ureas 115
  orientation, polymer chain surface 11
  properties 9, 177
  texture
    acrylamide-grafted silastic and
      ungrafted silastic 63
    protein adsorption behavior 460
    protein adsorption and desorption .. 294
  thrombosis 241
  topography 13t
Surface-induced thrombogenesis 161
Surface chemistry
  analysis 13t
  and molecular motions on
    thrombogenesis 203
  related to complex blood interactions
    responses 21
Surface–protein studies, FTIR 371
Synoptic flow chart of thrombogenesis . 207f
Synthesis
  copolyether-urethane–ureas 110
  segmented polyurethanes 97, 98, 99f

T

Tearfilm proteins, binding mechanism ... 453
Teflon
  Cohn I fibrinogen adsorbed 303f
  gold nuclei 300f
    distributions 299
  protein adsorbates 293
Teflon, sintered,
  albumin adsorbed 304f
  albumin preadsorbed 307f
  bovine γ-globulin 302f
  γ-globulin adsorbed 301f, 302f
TEM—See Transmission electron
  microscopy

Tensile stress–strain measurements of
  polyphosphazenes 188
  as a function of irradiation dose 189f
Tensile strength vs. concentration of LiBr
  for hydrogel 137f
Tensile strengths of copolyurethane
  hydrogels 136
Tetradecane–trimethylsilane-coated glass,
  protein structure 251t
Thermal stability, heparinase 503
Thermodynamic analysis 13t
Thrombin
  adsorption 174
    on polyurethanes 96
    and heparin-PVA beads 150, 152, 156
  inactivation by antithrombin III on
    heparinized beads 154f
  time of plasma in presence of PVA and
    heparin-PVA beads 152f
Thromboemboli generated grafts of
  polyacrylamide–silastic and silastic
  cannulae 7
Thromboembolic potential,
  polyacrylamide–Silastic surfaces 77
Thromboembolic propensity,
  polyacrylamide–Silastic and Silastic
  shunts 72
Thrombogenesis 148, 195, 293, 294
  See also Thrombosis, Thrombus formation
  effect of aspirin 57t
  effect of drugs 54
  model 203, 207f
  protein and polyelectrolyte
    adsorption 203
  schematic 204f, 205f, 206f
  synoptic flow chart 207f
  molecular motions 177
  on phosphazene polymers 188, 192
  on polyacrylamide hydrogel surfaces ... 78
  on polymeric substrates 195
  surface chemistry and molecular
    motions 203
  surface-induced 161
  surface properties of polymeric
    materials 177
Thrombogenicity 76, 322, 346
  adsorbed fibrinogen 318
  vein segments placed on polymer-coated
    rods 54t
Thromboplastin time
  activated partial 168–170, 175f
  prolonged partial 156
Thromboresistence 148, 307, 311
  ionically heparinized catheters 152
  polymers 25
Thromboresistant surfaces, immobilized
  heparin 162, 164
Thrombosis 317
  and embolization, components 3
  on grafted polyacrylamide–Silastic
    surfaces 59
  protein-coated surfaces 327
  surface 233, 241
Thrombus
  deposition 317, 329
  patterns 322

Thrombus (continued)
  dissolution 317
  and platelet retention 28f
  distributed over length of shaft in
    biomaterial test chamber 47f
  formation 161, 317, 318, 414
  characterization 45
  effects of drugs 54
  effects of heparin concentration 56f
  effects of shear 43, 48, 50f
  and hydrodynamics 48
  mechanism for inhibition 48
  on rods coated with different
    materials 49f
  spatial relations 50
  statistics 49
  on surface
    biomaterial coated rod 46f
    in contact with blood 43
    ex vivo test system 43
  growth and dissolution 29f
  histopathology 32f
  platelet concentration and thrombus
    weight, correlation 31f
  platelet content 32
  prevention 161
  propagation in vascular prostheses 54
  and protein response to PVC and
    Silastic 322
  red 3
  white 3
Tissue–material interactions 233
Tissue–polymer interactions 469
Transmission circular dichroism,
  conformational changes 364
Transmission electron microscopy
  polyphosphazene 182f–183f
  triblock copolymer 197f, 198f, 199f,
                                       202f
Transmission spectra
  albumin 374f, 377f, 378f
  aqueous solutions 375t
  albumin, γ-globulin, and
    albumin–γ-globulin mixture 378f
  albumin–globulins mixture 379f, 380f,
                                       381f
  copolyether-urethane–ureas 116f
  LiBr–copolyurethane complexes 139f, 140f
  mixtures of model proteins 375
  polypropylene glycol–urethane I
    mixture 122f
  polypropylene glycol–urethane I–urea I
    mixture 126f
  urea I and urea II 124f
  urethane I and urethane III 120f
Transient thrombus deposition
  measurements, experimental
  arrangement 321f
Transplanted islet suspension 484
Triblock copolymer
  dielectric and dynamic mechanical
  measurements 199
  dynamic mechanical spectra 201f
  morphology 197
  properties and synthesis 196
  schematic 204, 205f, 206f

INDEX

Triblock copolymer (*continued*)
TEM 197f, 198f, 199f, 202f
x-ray dispersion analysis............. 197
x-ray spectra..................... 200f
Triblock polymer, platelets 199
Tryptophan, protein emission
spectrum........................ 367
L-Tryptophan, fluorescence emission
spectra 368f
Total fluorescence signal, adsorbed
protein 359
Total internal reflectance fluorescence data,
schematic 358f, 361f
Total internal reflectance fluorescence,
protein structure at surfaces ...239, 240
Total internal reflection intrinsic
fluorescence.................... 351
Toxicity of polymers 469, 470
Two-step adsorption experiment,
proteins....................... 258f

U

Urea model compounds, spectra 124
Urethane interface, mixing with polyether
matrix 129
Urethane I and III, transmission
spectra 120f
Urethane III and IV model compounds
IR spectra...................... 121

V

Visible spectra of hemolysate preparation
and hemoglobin................. 287f
von Willebrand factor..............318, 345
absorption......................... 340
von Willebrand factor-coated PVC..... 345f

W

Water adsorption of hydrogens 135
vs. concentration of LiBr for
hydrogels 135f
of copolyurethanes at saturation
point 136t
properties of copolyether-urethane–ureas,
effect of LiBr.................... 135
Water content
polyphosphazene as a function of UV
irradiation..................... 188t
soft contact lens polymers 456
Water–protein interactions 416
White thrombi........................ 3
Wound closure, physical chemistry 476
Wound contraction, skin graft.......... 478

X

X-ray dispersion spectra of
polyphosphazene................ 184f
X-ray dispersion spectra of triblock
copolymer.................. 197, 200f
X-ray photoelectron spectroscopy segmented
polyurethanes 103
X-ray, phosphorus, dispersion map of
polyphosphazene................ 181f

Z

Zinc electronegativity.................. 446

Copy Editor: Susan Moses
Production Editor: Cynthia Hale
Indexer: L. Luan Corrigan
Managing Editor: Janet D. Shoff

Typesetting: Circle Graphics, Inc. Washington, DC
Printing: Maple Press Company, York, Pa